AF327974

1997
YEAR BOOK OF
NEUROLOGY AND
NEUROSURGERY®

Statement of Purpose

The YEAR BOOK Service

The YEAR BOOK series was devised in 1901 by practicing health professionals who observed that the literature of medicine and related disciplines had become so voluminous that no one individual could read and place in perspective every potential advance in a major specialty. In the final decade of the 20th century, this recognition is more acutely true than it was in 1901.

More than merely a series of books, YEAR BOOK volumes are the tangible results of a unique service designed to accomplish the following:

- to *survey* a wide range of journals of proven value
- to *select* from those journals papers representing significant advances and statements of important clinical principles
- to provide *abstracts* of those articles that are readable, convenient summaries of their key points
- to provide *commentary* about those articles to place them in perspective.

These publications grow out of a unique process that calls on the talents of outstanding authorities in clinical and fundamental disciplines, trained literature specialists, and professional writers, all supported by the resources of Mosby, the world's preeminent publisher for the health professions.

The Literature Base

Mosby and its Editors survey more than 1,000 journals published worldwide, covering the full range of the health professions. On an annual basis, the publisher examines usage patterns and polls its expert authorities to add new journals to the literature base and to delete journals that are no longer useful as potential YEAR BOOK sources.

The Literature Survey

The publisher's team of literature specialists, all of whom are trained and experienced health professionals, examines every original, peer-reviewed article in each journal issue. More than 250,000 articles per year are scanned systematically, including title, text, illustrations, tables, and references. Each scan is compared, article by article, to the search strategies that the publisher has developed in consultation with the 270 outside experts who form the pool of YEAR BOOK editors. A given article may be reviewed by any number of editors, from one to a dozen or more, regardless of the discipline for which the paper was originally published. In turn, each editor who receives the article reviews it to determine whether or not the article should be included in the YEAR BOOK. This decision is based on the article's inherent quality, its probable usefulness to readers of that YEAR BOOK, and the editor's goal to represent a balanced picture of a given field in each volume of the YEAR BOOK. In addition, the editor indicates when to include figures and tables from the article to help the YEAR BOOK reader better understand the information.

Of the quarter million articles scanned each year, only 5% are selected for detailed analysis within the YEAR BOOK series, thereby assuring readers of the high value of every selection.

The Abstract

The publisher's abstracting staff is headed by a seasoned health care professional and includes individuals with training in the life sciences, medicine, and other areas, plus extensive experience in writing for the health professions and related industries. Each selected article is assigned to a specific writer on this abstracting staff. The abstracter, guided in many cases by notations supplied by the expert editor, writes a structured, condensed summary designed so that the reader can rapidly acquire the essential information contained in the article.

The Commentary

The YEAR BOOK editorial boards, sometimes assisted by guest commentators, write comments that place each article in perspective for the reader. This provides the reader with the equivalent of a personal consultation with a leading international authority—an opportunity to better understand the value of the article and to benefit from the authority's thought processes in assessing the article.

Additional Editorial Features

The editorial boards of each YEAR BOOK organize the abstracts and comments to provide a logical and satisfying sequence of information. To enhance the organization, editors also provide introductions to sections or individual chapters, comments linking a number of abstracts, citations to additional literature, and other features.

The published YEAR BOOK contains enhanced bibliographic citations for each selected article, including extended listings of multiple authors and identification of author affiliations. Each YEAR BOOK contains a Table of Contents specific to that year's volume. From year to year, the Table of Contents for a given YEAR BOOK will vary depending on developments within the field.

Every YEAR BOOK contains a list of the journals from which papers have been selected. This list represents a subset of the more than 1,000 journals surveyed by the publisher and occasionally reflects a particularly pertinent article from a journal that is not surveyed on a routine basis.

Finally, each volume contains a comprehensive subject index and an index to authors of each selected paper.

The 1997 Year Book Series

Year Book of Allergy, Asthma, and Clinical Immunology: Drs. Rosenwasser, Borish, Gelfand, Leung, Nelson, and Szefler

Year Book of Anesthesiology and Pain Management®: Drs. Tinker, Abram, Chestnut, Roizen, Rothenberg, and Wood

Year Book of Cardiology®: Drs. Schlant, Collins, Gersh, Graham, Kaplan, and Waldo

Year Book of Chiropractic®: Dr. Lawrence

Year Book of Critical Care Medicine®: Drs. Parrillo, Balk, Calvin, Franklin, and Shapiro

Year Book of Dentistry®: Drs. Meskin, Berry, Kennedy, Leinfelder, Roser, Summitt, and Zakariasen

Year Book of Dermatologic Surgery®: Drs. Greenway, Papadopoulos, and Whitaker

Year Book of Dermatology®: Drs. Sober and Fitzpatrick

Year Book of Diagnostic Radiology®: Drs. Federle, Clark, Gross, Dalinka, Maynard, Rebner, Smirniotopolous, and Young

Year Book of Digestive Diseases®: Drs. Greenberger and Moody

Year Book of Drug Therapy®: Drs. Lasagna and Weintraub

Year Book of Emergency Medicine®: Drs. Wagner, Dronen, Davidson, King, Niemann, and Roberts

Year Book of Endocrinology®: Drs. Bagdade, Braverman, Haas, Horton, Kannan, Landsberg, Molitch, Morley, Nathan, Odell, Poehlman, Rogol, and Ryan

Year Book of Family Practice®: Drs. Berg, Bowman, Davidson, Dexter, and Scherger

Year Book of Geriatrics and Gerontology®: Drs. Beck, Burton, Ostwald, Rabins, Reuben, Roth, Shapiro, and Whitehouse

Year Book of Hand Surgery®: Drs. Amadio and Hentz

Year Book of Hematology®: Drs. Spivak, Bell, Ness, Quesenberry, Wiernik, and Blume

Year Book of Infectious Diseases: Drs. Keusch, Barza, Bennish, Poutsiaka, Skolnik, and Snydman

Year Book of Medicine®: Drs. Klahr, Cline, Petty, Frishman, Greenberger, Malawista, Mandell, and O'Rourke

Year Book of Neonatal and Perinatal Medicine®: Drs. Fanaroff and Klaus

Year Book of Nephrology, Hypertension, and Mineral Metabolism: Drs. Coe, Curtis, Favus, Henderson, Kashgarian, Luke, and Myers

Year Book of Neurology and Neurosurgery®: Drs. Bradley and Wilkins

Year Book of Nuclear Medicine®: Drs. Gottschalk, Blaufox, Neumann, Strauss, and Zubal

Year Book of Obstetrics, Gynecology, and Women's Health: Drs. Mishell, Herbst, and Kirschbaum

Year Book of Occupational and Environmental Medicine®: Drs. Emmett, Frank, Gochfeld, and Hessl

Year Book of Oncology®: Drs. Ozols, Cohen, Glatstein, Loehrer, Tallman, and Wiersma

Year Book of Ophthalmology®: Drs. Wilson, Augsburger, Cohen, Eagle, Flanagan, Grossman, Laibson, Maguire, Nelson, Rapuano, Sergott, Spaeth, Tipperman, and Ms. Salmon

Year Book of Orthopedics®: Drs. Sledge, Poss, Cofield, Dobyns, Griffin, Springfield, Swiontkowski, Wiesel, and Wilson

Year Book of Otolaryngology–Head and Neck Surgery®: Drs. Paparella, and Holt

Year Book of Pain®: Drs. Gebhart, Haddox, Jacox, Janjan, Marcus, Rudy, and Shapiro

Year Book of Pathology and Laboratory Medicine: Drs. Mills, Bruns, Gaffey, and Stoler

Year Book of Pediatrics®: Dr. Stockman

Year Book of Plastic, Reconstructive, and Aesthetic Surgery®: Drs. Miller, Cohen, McKinney, Robson, Ruberg, Smith, and Whitaker

Year Book of Podiatric Medicine and Surgery®: Dr. Kominsky

Year Book of Psychiatry and Applied Mental Health®: Drs. Talbott, Ballanger, Breier, Frances, Meltzer, Schowalter, and Tasman

Year Book of Pulmonary Disease®: Dr. Petty

Year Book of Rheumatology®: Drs. Sergent, LeRoy, Meenan, Panush, and Reichlin

Year Book of Sports Medicine®: Drs. Shephard, Drinkwater, Eichner, Torg, Anderson, and Mr. George

Year Book of Surgery®: Drs. Copeland, Bland, Deitch, Eberlein, Howard, Luce, Seeger, Souba, and Sugarbaker

Year Book of Thoracic and Cardiovascular Surgery®: Drs. Ginsberg, Wechsler, and Williams

Year Book of Urology®: Drs. Andriole and Coplin

Year Book of Vascular Surgery®: Dr. Porter

1997

The Year Book of NEUROLOGY AND NEUROSURGERY®

"Published without interruption since 1902"

Neurology

Editor

Walter G. Bradley, D.M., F.R.C.P.

Professor and Chairman, Department of Neurology, University of Miami School of Medicine, Florida

Neurosurgery

Editor

Robert H. Wilkins, M.D.

Professor and Chief, Division of Neurosurgery, Duke University Medical Center, Durham, North Carolina

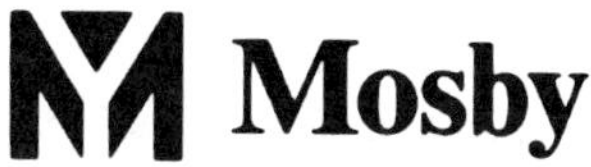

St. Louis Baltimore Boston Carlsbad Chicago Naples New York Philadelphia Portland
London Madrid Mexico City Singapore Sydney Tokyo Toronto Wiesbaden

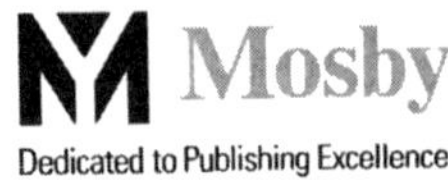
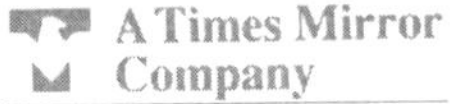

Vice President and Publisher, Continuity Publishing: Kenneth H. Killion
Director, Editorial Development: Gretchen C. Murphy
Acquisitions Editor: Li Wen Huang
Illustrations and Permissions Coordinator: Lois M. Ruebensam
Director, Continuity–EDP: Maria Nevinger
Project Manager, Editing: Jill C. Waite
Assistant Project Supervisor, Production: Laura M. Higgins
Freelance Staff Supervisor: Barbara M. Kelly
Director, Editorial Services: Edith M. Podrazik, B.S.N, R.N.
Information Specialist: Kathleen Moss, R.N.
Circulation Manager: Lynn D. Stevenson

1997 EDITION
Copyright © January 1997 by Mosby–Year Book, Inc.

Printed in the United States of America
Composition by Reed Technology and Information Services, Inc.
Printing/binding by Maple-Vail

Mosby–Year Book, Inc.
11830 Westline Industrial Drive
St. Louis, MO 63146

Editorial Office:
Mosby–Year Book, Inc.
161 North Clark Street
Chicago, IL 60601

International Standard Serial Number: 0513–5117
International Standard Book Number: 0–8151–1209–2

Associate Editors

Alan R. Berger, M.D.
Professor and Associate Chairman, Department of Neurology, University of Florida Health Sciences Center, Jacksonville, Florida

Joseph R. Berger, M.D.
Professor and Chairman, Department of Neurology, University of Kentucky College of Medicine, Lexington, Kentucky

John P. Blass, M.D., Ph.D.
Winifred Masterson Burke Professor of Neurology and Medicine; Chief, Division of Chronic and Degenerative Disease, Cornell University Medical College at Burke Medical Research Institute, White Plains, New York

Robert A. Davidoff, M.D.
Professor of Neurology, Department of Neurology, University of Miami School of Medicine, Miami, Florida

Gerald M. Fenichel, M.D.
Professor and Chairman of Neurology, Department of Neurology, Vanderbilt University School of Medicine, Nashville, Tennessee

Albert M. Galaburda, M.D.
Professor of Neurology and Neuroscience, Harvard Medical School; Director of the Division of Behavioral Neurology, Department of Neurology; Emily Fisher Landau Professor of Neurology and Neuroscience, Beth Israel Hospital, Boston, Massachusetts

Myron D. Ginsberg, M.D.
Peritz Scheinberg Professor of Neurology; Director of Cerebral Vascular Disease Research Center, University of Miami School of Medicine, Miami, Florida

Rodrigo Kuljis, M.D.
Division of Behavioral Neurology, University of Miami, Miami, Florida

Bruce Nolan, M.D.
Associate Professor of Clinical Neurology; Director of the Sleep Disorders Center; Department of Neurology, University of Miami School of Medicine, Miami, Florida

Jerome D. Posner, M.D.
Chairman and Professor of Neurology Department, Memorial Sloan-Kettering Cancer Center, New York, New York

Robert M. Quencer, M.D.
Professor of Radiology, Neurological Surgery, and Ophthalmology; Director, Division of Magnetic Resonance Imaging, University of Miami School of Medicine, Miami, Florida

Eugene R. Ramsay, M.D.
Professor of Neurology, Department of Neurology, University of Miami School of Medicine, Miami, Florida

J.R. Sanchez-Ramos, M.D., Ph.D.
Associate Professor, Department of Neurology, University of Miami School of Medicine and Miami Veterans Administration Medical Center, Miami, Florida

Norman J. Schatz, M.D.
Voluntary Professor of Clinical Neurology and Ophthalmology, University of Miami School of Medicine, Mercury Hospital, Miami, Florida

Subramaniam Sriram, M.D.
Professor of Neurology, Department of Neurology, Vanderbilt University Medical Center, Nashville, Tennessee

David Stumpf, M.D., Ph.D.
Benjamin and Virginia T. Boshes Professor of Neurology; Chairman, Department of Neurology; Professor of Pediatrics, Northwestern University Medical School, Chicago, Illinois

Ronald J. Tusa, M.D., Ph.D.
Professor of Otolaryngology and Neurology; Director of the Dizziness and Balance Center; University of Miami School of Medicine, Miami, Florida

Table of Contents

Journals Represented

Mosby and its Editors survey more than 1,000 journals for its abstract and commentary publications. From these journals, the Editors select the articles to be abstracted. Journals represented in this YEAR BOOK are listed below.

Acta Neurochirurgica
Acta Neurologica Scandinavica
Acta Oto-Laryngologica
Acta Paediatrica
Acta Radiologica
Age and Ageing
American Journal of Human Genetics
American Journal of Medicine
American Journal of Neuroradiology
American Journal of Pathology
American Journal of Public Health
American Journal of Roentgenology
American Journal of Surgery
Anaesthesia and Intensive Care
Annals of Neurology
Annals of Oncology
Annals of Otology, Rhinology and Laryngology
Archives of Disease in Childhood
Archives of Environmental Health
Archives of Neurology
Archives of Otolaryngology-Head and Neck Surgery
Archives of Pathology and Laboratory Medicine
Arthritis and Rheumatism
Brain
British Journal of Neurosurgery
British Medical Journal
Cell
Clinical Pediatrics
Clinical Radiology
Critical Care Medicine
Developmental Medicine and Child Neurology
Diabetic Medicine
Epilepsia
European Respiratory Journal
Headache
International Journal of Oral and Maxillofacial Surgery
Journal of Applied Physiology: Respiratory, Environmental and Exercise
    Physiology
Journal of Bone and Joint Surgery (American Volume)
Journal of Bone and Joint Surgery (British Volume)
Journal of Clinical Endocrinology and Metabolism
Journal of Computer Assisted Tomography
Journal of Gerontology
Journal of Hand Surgery (American)
Journal of Laryngology and Otology
Journal of Medical Genetics
Journal of Neurology

Journal of Neurology, Neurosurgery and Psychiatry
Journal of Neuropathology and Experimental Neurology
Journal of Neuropsychiatry and Clinical Neurosciences
Journal of Neurosurgery
Journal of Spinal Disorders
Journal of Trauma: Injury, Infection, and Critical Care
Journal of the American Medical Association
Journal of the Neurological Sciences
Journal of the Royal Society of Medicine
Lancet
Laryngoscope
Magnetic Resonance in Medicine
Mayo Clinic Proceedings
Metabolism: Clinical and Experimental
Minimally Invasive Neurosurgery
Muscle and Nerve
Nature
Neurology
Neuropediatrics
Neurosurgery
New England Journal of Medicine
Ophthalmology
Otolaryngology - Head and Neck Surgery
Pain
Pediatric Neurology
Pediatric Radiology
Pediatrics
Postgraduate Medical Journal
Quarterly Journal of Medicine
Radiology
Revue Neurologique
Scandinavian Journal of Rehabilitation Medicine
Science
Spine
Stroke
Surgical Neurology
Thorax

STANDARD ABBREVIATIONS

The following terms are abbreviated in this edition: acquired immunodeficiency syndrome (AIDS), cardiopulmonary resuscitation (CPR), central nervous system (CNS), cerebrospinal fluid (CSF), computed tomography (CT), deoxyribonucleic acid (DNA), electrocardiography (ECG), health maintenance organization (HMO), human immunodeficiency virus (HIV), intensive care unit (ICU), intramuscular (IM), intravenous (IV), magnetic resonance (MR) imaging (MRI), and ribonucleic acid (RNA).

NOTE

The YEAR BOOK OF NEUROLOGY AND NEUROSURGERY is a literature survey service providing abstracts of articles published in the professional literature. Every effort is made to assure the accuracy of the information presented in these pages.

Neither the editors nor the publisher of the YEAR BOOK OF NEUROLOGY AND NEUROSURGERY can be responsible for errors in the original materials. The editors' comments are their own opinions. Mention of specific products within this publication does not constitute endorsement.

To facilitate the use of the YEAR BOOK OF NEUROLOGY AND NEUROSURGERY as a reference tool, all illustrations and tables included in this publication are now identified as they appear in the original article. This change is meant to help the reader recognize that any illustration or table appearing in the YEAR BOOK OF NEUROLOGY AND NEUROSURGERY may be only one of many in the original article. For this reason, figure and table numbers will often appear to be out of sequence within the YEAR BOOK OF NEUROLOGY AND NEUROSURGERY.

Publisher's Preface

With this edition of the YEAR BOOK, we say goodbye to our esteemed colleague, Robert H. Wilkins, M.D., with whom we've worked on the YEAR BOOK for the past three editions. Throughout this time he has provided readers with insightful and thought-provoking commentary of the highest caliber. Moreover, we at Mosby–Year Book, Inc., have been treated to an enjoyable and rewarding association. We extend our deepest appreciation to Dr. Wilkins for the service he has provided and for his unending support, leadership, and enthusiasm for this publication. He will be missed by all of us here, and we wish him the very best in all his future endeavors.

We are pleased that Scott Gibbs, M.D., has agreed to take the helm as our new Editor of the "Neurosurgery" section. Please join us in welcoming him to his new role.

Mosby–Year Book, Inc.

NEUROLOGY

WALTER G. BRADLEY, D.M., F.R.C.P.

The Practicing Neurologist and Neuroscience in the Decade of the Brain

The Decade of the Brain was initiated by an act of Congress in 1990, both to bring to the public awareness of the major advances coming in the neurosciences in the 1990s and as a vehicle by which it was hoped Congress would increase research support for the neurosciences. Now, more than halfway through the decade, the first objective has clearly been achieved. Few people have not heard of the Decade of the Brain or have not heard of the great advances in our understanding of such diseases as those named after Huntington, Parkinson, and Alzheimer and also in amyotrophic lateral sclerosis (ALS) and stroke. With regard to research funding, it is a question of whether the glass is half full or half empty. The National Institute of Neurological Diseases and Stroke has done relatively well compared with some of the institutes, but there has been no major influx of new money.

The importance of the Decade of the Brain was recognized by the American Academy of Neurology with the initiation of the Decade of the Brain Symposia. These plenary symposia provide a yearly review of some of the high points in recent advances in the neurosciences and their implication for the practicing neurologist. For my sins, I find myself Chair of the Scientific Issues Committee of the American Academy of Neurology and responsible in part for the annual Decade of the Brain Symposia. These plenary sessions have proved to be highly successful, with an audience of more than 4,000. Neurologists in practice always give very high marks to the Decade of the Brain Symposia in the meeting evaluations. It is clear that though we may find ourselves in 1 subspecialty area of practice or research, we all retain the questing interest in the function of the brain and how diseases are produced. These symposia offer us vicariously the ability to feel a part of the development of our understanding in these areas.

To give a talk at the Decade of the Brain Symposia is difficult. The audience ranges from research colleagues who will critique one's presentation for accuracy to the general neurologists whose neuroscience knowledge was acquired in medical school perhaps 30 years ago. Nevertheless, good presenters can make even the most esoteric science of interest to a general audience. To prove this one has only to attend these academy plenary sessions. However, the innovations in science can sometimes be bewildering for the nonexpert. I well remember one early Decade of the Brain talk that involved the blossoming field of molecular genetics. The speaker held the audience spellbound, listening to how such leaps of knowledge of disease flowed from the ability to play with minute fragments of DNA in the laboratory. However, I remember looking around at the audience to see that many had a glazed look, the cause of which was clear. The lecturer most was most definitely speaking in English, and they knew the individual words and their meaning. However, when these words were strung together in sentences, the total meaning was unclear because they were so full of new phrases and concepts. Nevertheless, the import was clear and the message spellbinding.

By now most of us have become comfortable with the recognition of *what we need to know* and *what we can accept on faith*. For instance, we know that molecular genetics can discover the protein, abnormality of which is responsible for an inherited disease, by using the technique that used to be termed *reverse genetics* and is now called *positional cloning*. We know that from blood specimens collected from each of the members of large families with the disease, it is possible to determine chromosomal linkage, chromosomal localization, and eventually the actual gene. From this gene, the gene product, a protein, can be translated and the function eventually determined. Work of this nature led to the discovery, for instance, of mutations of the muscle sarcolemmal sodium channel responsible for hyperkalemic periodic paralysis and of the T-tubule dihydropyridine receptor, mutations of which are responsible for hypokalemic periodic paralysis. We do not feel the need to understand exactly how these discoveries were made, just as we do not need to know how the chip engineers or software designers make our personal computers work.

We are now very much into the bottom line. "Well, molecular genetics, what disease have you elucidated for me this week?" This hectic pace sometimes blinds us to how time consuming such research is and what brilliant leaps of concept development go into these breakthroughs. Several papers in this year's issue of NEUROLOGY AND NEUROSURGERY lend weight to this last statement.

It has taken 5 years to get from the discovery that the gene for infantile spinal muscular atrophy lay on the long arm of chromosome 5 to the suggestion of what gene may be responsible (Abstracts 1–14 and 1–15). This gene may be 1 coding for a protein that switches off apoptosis, which normally terminates programmed cell death, deficiency of which could allow continuing death of the motor neuron pool.

Almost 10 years have passed since the dystrophin gene was discovered as the cause of Duchenne's muscular dystrophy. We understand a great deal of the function of dystrophin, namely, to stabilize the sarcolemmal membrane as a scaffolding, which can be distorted like a chain-link fence but nevertheless allows the muscle membrane to stretch and contract easily as it must do with every twitch. However, as paper Abstract 1–22 demonstrates, we still do not understand what dystrophin does in the brain or how mental retardation is produced in Duchenne's dystrophy. We are, however, getting closer to understanding how muscle may correct for the defective protein in Duchenne's dystrophy carriers. This will be important when we can begin gene therapy with the transfection of the competent dystrophin gene (Abstract 1–23).

All this may seem a long way from the hurly-burly of everyday neurologic practice, where we may have to advise patients with optic neuritis (Abstract 8–3) or discuss the risks and management of migraine (Abstracts 5–3 and 5–7) or transient ischemic attacks and strokes (Abstracts 2–3 and 2–11). However, the substrate of what we do now and what we expect to be able to do in 1 or 2 years for the many neurologic diseases that we have to look after rests on advances in neurosciences. Molecular genetics is the marvel of the Decade of the Brain. By the end of the decade, we may hope to be able to bring work on DNA and RNA to the investigation and treatment of diseases in which genetic factors play a relatively minor role, such as stroke, Parkinson's disease, and epilepsy. It is that knowledge that keeps all of us on our toes.

Neurologic Therapy

It is probably preaching to the choir to say that neurology today is a field of active therapy. The days when journals were filled largely with descriptive papers that defined syndromes and delineated natural history and pathologic conditions are gone. We are now in the era of neurologic treatment. This message, although clear to the practicing neurologist, needs to be taken to those outside the profession. We need to get the message to health maintenance organizations and primary care physicians who consider that a specialty such as neurology, if not totally superfluous, is at least numerically so. General physicians are poorly trained in neurology, and it is frustrating to our neurologic leadership to find that the national organizations and local residency directors for family and general medicine are uninterested in receiving help from neurologists and in improving their residency training. General physicians are often not aware of the latest breakthroughs in neurologic therapy, yet they are increasingly caring for neurologic problems without the assistance of neurologic consultations.

We also need to get out the message concerning the active field of neurologic therapy to medical students. Across the United States, scheduled rotations for medical students on the neurology service are either being abandoned or moved into the fourth year to accomodate general practice training in the third year. Hence, unless we can reorganize the neuroscience curriculum to expose medical students to clinical neurology in the first and second years, most medical students will have made their career decisions before they have the benefit of a clinical neurology rotation in the fourth year. This is bound to result in fewer bright young medical students entering neurology, which in the long run is bound to be detrimental to our profession.

Many papers in this volume of the YEARBOOK OF NEUROLOGY AND NEUROSURGERY deal with exciting new therapeutic advances. Only a few can be mentioned here, but the interested reader will find many more in the body of this volume. The Phase III study of copolymer-1 in treating multiple sclerosis demonstrated a 29% reduction in relapse rate. Another study showed that low-dose oral methotrexate significantly reduced the rate of progression of multiple sclerosis.

What may be a major key to unlocking the cause of ALS, namely, the discovery by Rothstein and colleagues (Abstract 1–19) of selective loss of the glial glutamate transporter in the brain and spinal cord of ALS patients gave rise to the development of riluzole, which recently has been released in the United States for the treatment of ALS. Preliminary reports of the use of 2 other drugs to treat ALS, namely, insulin-like growth factor 1 and brain-derived neutrophic factor, indicate that these can also significantly slow the rate of the progression of the disease. None of these agents cures or arrests the disease; nevertheless, these discoveries are exciting compared with the situation only a few years ago when we had no effective treatment of any kind for ALS. It is still going to be several years before treatment protocols are fully defined. We will probably see the development of combinations of these agents and innovative ways of stimulating neurotrophin receptors on motor neurons. These may include intrathecal pumps, implantation of capsules containing genetically engineered cells synthesizing neurotrophins, or the development of a neurotrophin receptor agonist that can be administered by mouth.

Treatment of epilepsy continues to be a very active field. Pharmacologic advances in the last 2 years have been extremely vigorous. More new agents have been released in this period than in any 2-year period before. The surgical treatment of epilepsy has continued to be refined. A new nonablative treatment for intractable epilepsy is the procedure of chronic vagal nerve stimulation by an implanted stimulator that produces a reduction in seizure frequency in some patients.

Neurologists and neuroscientist are characterized by their inquisitiveness and self-motivation. Hence, I do not expect that the current problems of health care reorganization are going to severely disrupt the advances in treatment that have occurred in the last few years. Rather, they will simply slow them. It is important that we keep in the forefront of our consciousness the realization of just how far neurology has come in the last 10 years in term of treatment and how the rate of advance continues to rise exponentially. We all need a little glimmer of hope in this era of health care reorganization (for which we might read "disorganization") in the United States.

Tort Reform and No-Fault Compensation for Medical Injury

There is no doubt that the current tort system for compensating for medical injury in the United States leaves a great deal to be desired. From the point of view of the medical profession, it does nothing for our good name to see 2 so-called experts, 1 for the plaintive and 1 for the defense, arguing against each other whether black is white. As an alternative, the system that to a large extent operates in England has advantages. In this, lists of potential expert witnesses are submitted by both the plaintiff and the defense, from which a single expert is agreed on. This expert acts as a witness to the court.

No one is satisfied by the current U.S. tort system for compensating for medical injuries. Patients and relatives are alternately bemused and traumatized by the long drawn-out system that often seems like play acting. Physicians accused of "malpractice" feel personally attacked and abused, because most would be judged by an unbiased group of peers to have provided adequate care according to the community norm and certainly not guilty of heinous intentional damage to the patient. Nevertheless, to obtain compensation, lawyers have to allege "malpractice." Lawyers are happy to get large settlements but recognize that the outcome is something of a lottery. Those with real concern for their clients realize they cannot take on many a worthwhile case because the likely settlement is insufficiently high to cover costs. Hence, I have argued for tort reform and for the institution of a national medical injury insurance scheme that would compensate patients who suffer iatrogenic or even fortuitous medical injury.

Unfortunately, not even a no-fault insurance scheme makes everyone happy; witness the car insurance situation in some parts of the United States. If my insurance company has to pay for the damages to my car that result from a collision due to some other driver's negligence, I am unhappy, particularly if it results in an increase in *my* premium next year.

With this background, it is interesting to review the early experience of a piece of tort reform that does involve no-fault, namely, the system for compensating infants born with neurologic injury in the state of Florida. The first 4 years of experience of the Neurological Injury Compensation Association (NICA) are reviewed in a recent paper by Horwitz and Brennan.[1] The NICA was set up in 1988 response to the rising cost and shrinking availability of malpractice insurance for obstetricians in Florida in the late 1980s. Similar changes were occurring throughout the United States at that time. Malpractice premiums for Florida obstetricians had risen to about $175,000 per year, and the largest medical malpractice underwriter had withdrawn from the state. The NICA "spreads the load" in a way that is appropriate for an insurance scheme. Participating obstetricians pay a $5,000 yearly premium; all other physicians, excluding physicians in training, pay $250 per year, and nonpublic hospitals pay $50 per live birth. The scheme compensates only for injuries to the brain and spinal cord of a live infant weighing more than 2,500 grams at birth caused by oxygen deprivation or mechanical injury. The claim petition is relatively simple and inexpensive to file. The adjudication is nonadversarial, and hence one would expect that the process would be relatively well utilized, particularly by those families with few resources to make such claims.

The outcome has, in fact, been significantly different from that expected, though it is too early to decide if this is the final picture.

As Horwitz and Brennan[1] report, the number of claims filed is significantly less than would have been expected. The average compensation to successful claimants is somewhat less than in the previous tort system ($1.1 million compared with $1.4–$1.7 million), but when allowance is made for attorney's fees, the compensation received by the family is probably very similar.

The NICA still believes that more claims will be forthcoming and, in fact, had reverse funds of about $90 million in 1992. By the end of 1993, it had paid only about $4 million in patient compensation and administrative expenses.

The outcome from the point of view of the availability of insurance coverage for obstetricians and the retention of practicing obstetricians in the state has been good. Attorneys who "bet on the lottery" have not been happy with the cap of $100,000 on pain and suffering awards. Nevertheless, the overheads of the system as a whole have been significantly less than with the old adversarial tort system.

Can we or should we consider proposing a similar national insurance scheme for a wider range of medical injuries in the United States? The answer may come from a deeper and more long-term review of no-fault schemes such as that of Florida or a similar one in Virginia. Compensation for birth injuries is a relatively circumscribed medicolegal problem, and the broader field of medical injury would certainly be much more difficult to administer. There is still the need for a system that allows suit to be brought against those guilty of true malpractice, but exactly who should decide whether a case presents prima facie evidence of malpractice would undoubtedly provide a field day for the lawyers.

Perhaps the most important observation is that no-fault compensation for medical injury and tort reform can occur in a relatively painless fashion, and for this reason everyone interested in this field should read the paper by Horwitz and Brennan.[1]

Walter G. Bradley, D.M., F.R.C.P.

Reference

1. Horwitz J, Brennan TA: No-fault compensation for medical injury: A case study. *Health Affairs* 14:164–179, 1995.

1 Neuromuscular Disorders

Neuropathies

Guillain–Barré Syndrome in Northern China: The Spectrum of Neuropathological Changes in Clinically Defined Cases
Griffin JW, Li CY, Ho TW, et al (Johns Hopkins Univ, Baltimore, Md; Vanderbilt Univ, Nashville, Tenn; Univ of Pennsylvania, Philadelphia; et al)
Brain 118:577–595, 1995

1–1

Introduction.—The pathophysiologic changes underlying Guillain-Barré syndrome remain controversial. Neuropathologic changes were studied at autopsy of 12 patients who died at Second Teaching Hospital, Shijiazhuang, China, between 1990 and 1994. These patients included both those with primarily demyelinating neuropathy and those with primarily axonal degeneration, as well as those with and without prior *Campylobacter jejuni* infection.

Methods.—All autopsies were performed between 2 and 8 hours after death and were limited dissections. Seven of these patients were children. The majority of deaths occurred during the seasonal outbreak of this syndrome.

Findings.—Three of these 12 patients had typical acute inflammatory demyelinating polyneuropathy (AIDP) with lymphocytic infiltration and macrophage-mediated demyelination. Six had acute motor axonal neuropathy (AMAN) predominantly axonal involvement and wallerian-like nerve fiber degeneration. In 3, both sensory and motor fibers were affected (acute motor-sensory axonal neuropathy, or AMSAN). Three had only minor changes in spinal roots and sciatic nerves, although they were paralyzed at the time of death. In both AMAN and AMSAN patients, macophages were present in the periaxonal space (Figs 3 and 4), surounding or displacing the axon and surrounded by an intact myelin sheath.

Conclusion.—The results of the autopsies of 12 patients from northern China with Guillain-Barré syndrome suggest that this syndrome can be associated with diverse pathologic changes. The predominant patterns appear to differ in different regions of the world, which may reflect varying antecedent infections. At autopsy, periaxonal macrophages in patients with axonal neuropathy suggest an important epitope may be localized to

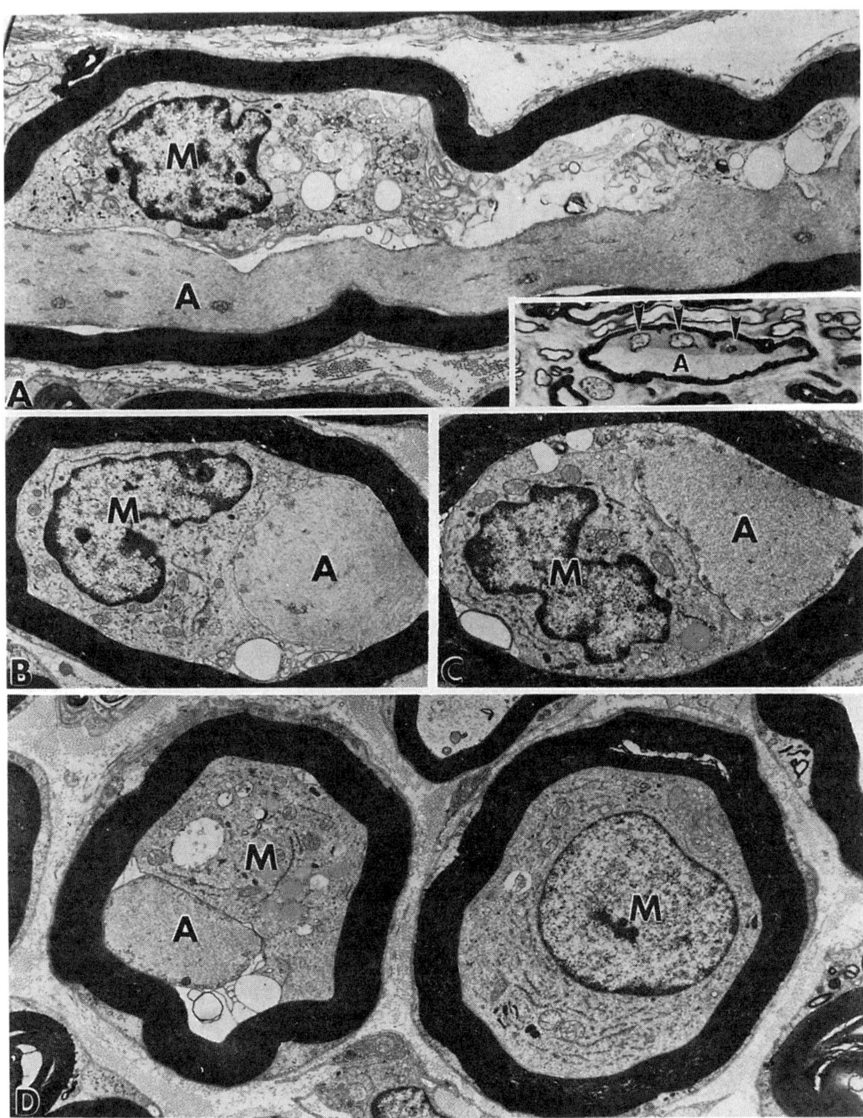

FIGURE 3.—Electron microscopy of periaxonal macrophages in the acute motor axonal neuropathy pattern case. **A,** longitudinal section of a fiber. In this internode, the axon (*A*) appears condensed. Between the axon and the myelin sheath, a macrophage (*M*) and its process are interposed. The myelin sheath appears normal; original magnification ×5,260. The inset is a light micrograph of a longitudinal section showing 3 macrophage nuclei inside the myelin sheath and above the axon (*A*); original magnification ×690. **B–D,** transverse sections from the ventral root. Note that in all of these fibers the myelin sheath appears normal, but the periaxonal space is occupied by a macrophage (*M*) that displaces the axon (*A*). In **D,** these 2 neighboring fibers illustrate different stages of axonal injury. In the fiber to the *left,* an axon (*A*) is present, and the macrophage (*M*) occupies the periaxonal space. In the fiber to the *right,* the axon has disappeared, and only the macrophage (*M*) remains; original magnification ×6,750. **B,** original magnification ×6,520. **C,** original magnification ×8,760. (By permission of Oxford University Press. Griffin JW, Li CY, Ho TW, et al: Guillain-Barré syndrome in northern China: The spectrum of neuropathological changes in clinically defined cases. *Brain* 118:577–595, 1995.)

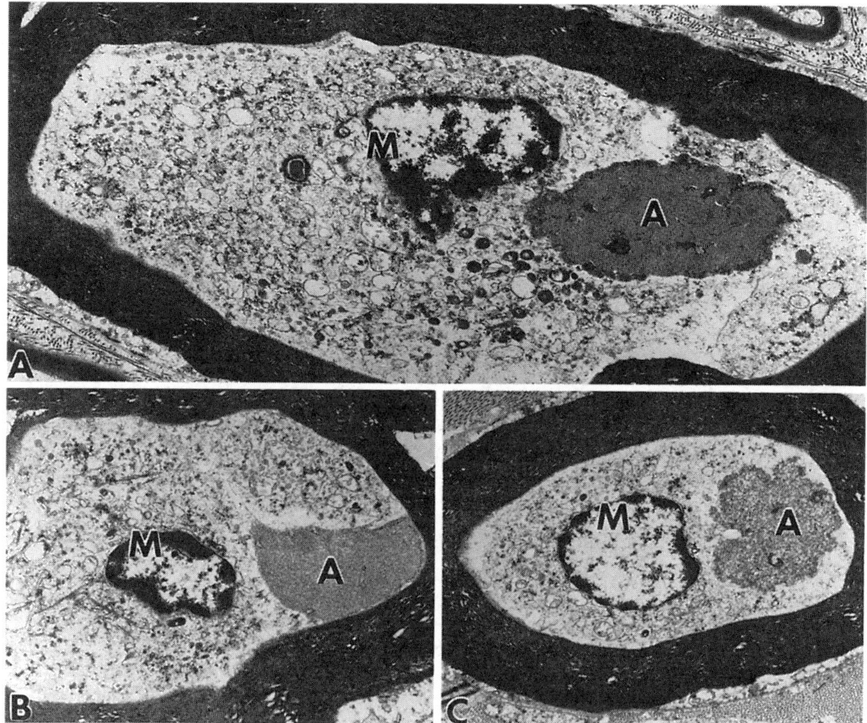

FIGURE 4.—Electron micrographs illustrating periaxonal macrophages in the acute motor axonal neuropathy pattern case. **A,** these fibers each contain a mononuclear cell (*M*) within the periaxonal space, surrounded by normal-appearing myelin and surrounding or displacing a compressed-appearing axon (*A*). **A,** original magnification ×10,000. **B,** original magnification ×9,000. **C,** original magnification ×18,000. (By permission of Oxford University Press. Griffin JW, Li CY, Ho TW, et al: Guillain-Barré syndrome in northern China: The spectrum of neuropathological changes in clinically defined cases. *Brain* 118:577–595, 1995.)

the axolemma or periaxonal space. At autopsy if patients have little apparent structural damage to the nerve, severe paralysis can occur without prominent nerve structural changes, indicating that physiologic block or nerve terminal changes may be involved in this paralysis. The different pathologic findings of patients with different subtypes of this syndrome may reflect differences in pathologenetic mechanisms.

Guillain–Barré Syndrome in Northern China: Relationship to *Campylobacter jejuni* Infection and Anti-Glycolipid Antibodies

Ho TW, Mishu B, Li CY, et al (Johns Hopkins Univ, Baltimore, Md; Vanderbilt Univ, Nashville, Tenn; Veteran Affairs Ctr, Nashville, Tenn; et al)
Brain 118:597–605, 1995

1–2

Background.—Guillain-Barré syndrome is an acute paralytic neuropathy characterized by symmetric ascending flaccid paralysis, areflexia, and an albuminocytologic dissociation in cerebrospinal fluid. In Australia, Europe, and the United States, the most common form of this syndrome is acute inflammatory demyelinating polyneuropathy (AIDP). In China and India, the most common form appears to be acute motor axonal neuropathy (AMAN). The pathogenesis of Guillain-Barré syndome was explored prospectively in patients from northern China, where seasonal epidemics are common.

Study Design.—All patients with clinically defined Guillain-Barré syndrome admitted to the Second Teaching Hospital of the Hebei Medical College at Shijiazhuang between January 1991 and December 1992 were included in the study. Of these, 129 underwent the electromyographic (EMG) studies required for classifcation. Thirty-eight of these patients also underwent an environmental exposure history, as well as serial clinical, serologic and electrodiagnostic examinations. Normal controls were derived from the same region of China.

Findings.—The AMAN pattern was present in 65% and the AIDP pattern in 24% of the 129 patients who underwent EMG testing. The AMAN form of this disease had a clear June to September peak occurrence pattern (Fig 1). The median age of AIDP patients was 6.6 years and of AMAN patients was 20 years (Fig 2). Patients were significantly more likely than controls to demonstrate evidence of exposure to *Campylobacter jejuni* infection. The frequency of exposure was greater among AMAN patients than among AIDP patients. There was no pattern to antiglycolipid serologic studies.

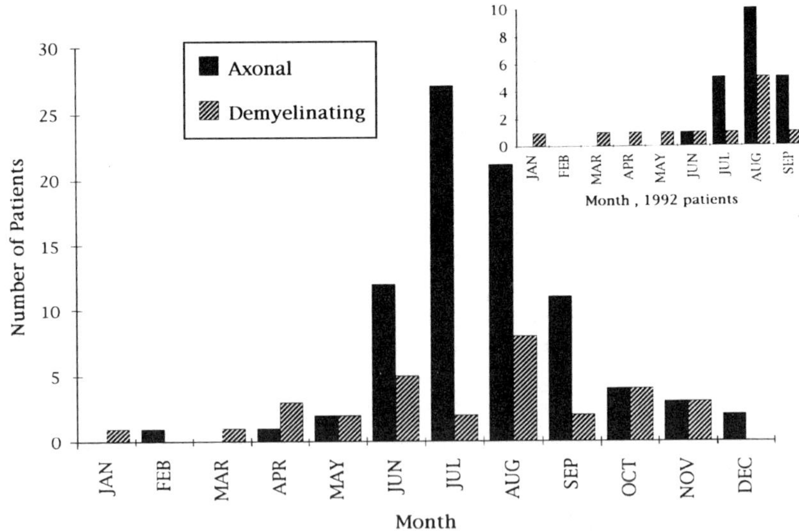

FIGURE 1.—Seasonal distribution of Guillain-Barré syndrome patients in Hebei Province from January 1991 to December 1992. *Inset,* seasonal distribution of 38 intensively studied 1992 patients. (By permission of Oxford University Press. Ho TW, Mishu B, Li CY, et al: Guillain-Barré syndrome in northern China: Relationship to *Campylobacter jejuni* infection and anti-glycolipid antibodies. *Brain* 118:597–605, 1995.)

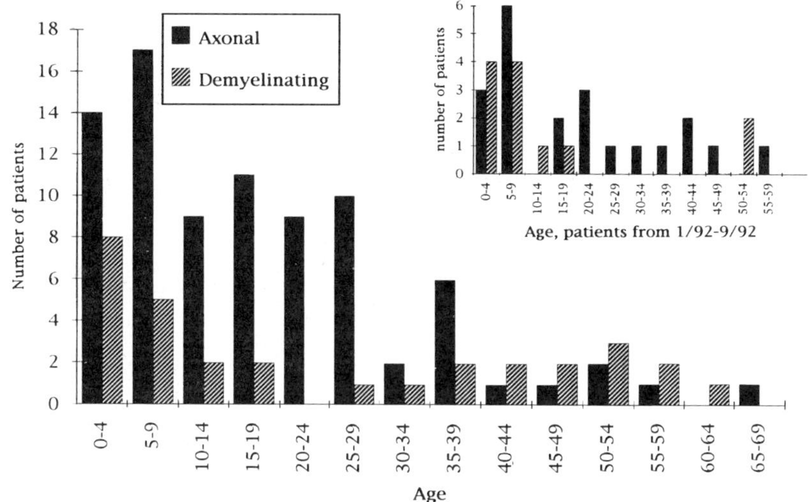

FIGURE 2.—Age distribution of the Guillain-Barré syndrome patients in Hebei Province from January 1992 to December 1992. *Inset,* age distribution of 38 intensively studied 1992 patients. (By permission of Oxford University Press. Ho TW, Mishu B, Li CY, et al: Guillain-Barré syndrome in northern China: Relationship to *Campylobacter jejuni* infection and anti-glycolipid antibodies. *Brain* 118:597–605, 1995.)

Conclusions.—Guillain-Barré syndrome occurs in yearly summer outbreaks in northern China. Based on electrophysiologic criteria, it can be divided into 2 main subtypes: AIDP and AMAN. The AMAN form is more common, particularly during the summer outbreaks. Infection with *C. jejuni* may play a role, especially in the AMAN form of this syndrome.

▶ The Chinese paralysis syndrome has caused great interest since information first started to appear in the West about 10 years ago. These 2 papers go a long way to clarifying the nature of that condition. The attacks of illness tend to occur in epidemics, particularly in summer months. Though typical Guillain-Barré syndrome (AIDP) with a typical course and predominant segmental demyelination occurs during such epidemics, almost twice as many patients have a more acute condition, with predominantly axonal degeneration (AMAN). In the United States and Europe, the death rate is higher and the prognosis worse for those with AMAN; in the Chinese paralysis syndrome, the rate of recovery and prognosis are similar to those seen in AIDP. Inflammation in the nerve roots and proximal nerves is relatively uncommon in AMAN compared with AIDP. *Campylobacter jejuni* infections are more common in AMAN (76%) than in AIDP (42%) compared with controls (about 6%). The pathologic process that appears specifically related to AMAN is macrophage infiltration of the periaxonal space, suggesting an autoimmune process directed to the axolemma. Similar cases with predominantly axonal degeneration and little inflammation have been seen in other parts of the world, and hence the Chinese paralysis syndrome is not a specific entity. It seems probable that there may be several etiologic factors, *C. jejuni* being only one that leads to a greater degree of axonal degeneration.

W.G. Bradley, D.M., F.R.C.P.

Pathology of the Motor-Sensory Axonal Guillain-Barré Syndrome
Griffin JW, Li CY, Ho TW, et al (Johns Hopkins Univ, Baltimore, Md; Second Teaching Hosp of Hebei Med College, Shijiazhuang, Hebei Province, People's Republic of China; Vanderbilt Univ, Nashville, Tenn; et al)
Ann Neurol 39:17–28, 1996   1–3

Background.—Some investigators have advanced the concept of a severe motor-sensory neuropathy of acute onset caused by an immune attack on the axon, referred to as "axonal" Guillain-Barré syndrome. However, this concept is based mostly on electrodiagnostic and limited pathologic data and remains controversial. Unusually severe inflammatory demyelinating neuropathy is found in some patients at autopsy. It is unclear whether antecedent *Campylobacter jejuni* infection is associated with this syndrome. Pathologic findings in 4 patients were described.

Patients and Findings.—The 4 patients, from Hebei Province, China, were clinically diagnosed as having Guillain-Barré syndrome. They died 7, 7, 18, and 60 days after diagnosis. The 2 patients tested had high titers of antibodies recognizing *C. jejuni*, suggesting recent infection. Autopsy findings in the 3 patients with early disease demonstrated ongoing wallerian-like degeneration of fibers in the ventral and dorsal roots and peripheral nerves. There was only minimal demyelination or lymphocytic infiltration. All 3 patients were found to have many macrophages in the periaxonal space of myelinated internodes and rare intra-axonal macrophages. In the patient who had had the syndrome for 60 days, examination showed extensive large-fiber loss in the spinal roots and nerves, as well as a paucity of demyelination and remyelination.

Conclusions.—These findings confirm that some patients with severe motor-sensory Guillain-Barré syndrome, as diagnosed clinically, have primarily axonal lesions of motor and sensory fibers, even in early disease stages. In addition, it was confirmed that axonal Guillain-Barré syndrome can follow *C. jejuni* infection. The current pathologic observations suggest that such cases of motor-sensory axonal Guillain-Barré syndrome represent the most severe end of the spectrum of immune attack on axonal epitopes.

▶ Griffin et al, made major advances in the understanding of axonal types of Guillain-Barré syndrome. In the Chinese paralysis syndrome, they demonstrated a high prevalence of *C. jejuni* antibodies and a prognosis that is generally no worse than "ordinary" Guillain-Barré syndrome with predominant demyelination. They demonstrated binding of antibodies and complement at the nodes of Ranvier and the attraction of macrophages to the nodes of Ranvier to strip myelin loops from the axolemma of the neurons. These changes occur predominantly distally in the nerves of patients with the acute motor axonal neuropathy form of Guillain-Barré syndrome. This paper described the abnormalities of the severe axonal form of motor-sensory Guillain-Barré syndrome. There was little demyelination or inflammation, but macrophages infiltrated the periaxonal space of myelinated internodes, producing axonal degeneration. This appears to be the severe form of what in the Chinese paralysis syndrome is generally a more benign acute motor axonal neuropathy.

W.G. Bradley, D.M., F.R.C.P.

Guillain-Barré Syndrome Without Sensory Loss (Acute Motor Neuropathy): A Subgroup With Specific Clinical, Electrodiagnostic and Laboratory Features

Visser LH, Van Der Meché FGA, Van Doorn PA, et al (Erasmus Univ, Rotterdam, The Netherlands)
Brain 118:841–847, 1995

1–4

Background.—Clinical variations within the classical forms of Guillain-Barré syndrome have been documented, which possibly may result from different pathogenic mechanisms. Clinical, electrodiagnostic, and laboratory characteristics, as well as response to treatment with IV immunoglobulin (IVIg) or plasma exchange, were evaluated in patients with Guillain-Barré syndrome but without sensory loss (motor Guillain-Barré syndrome).

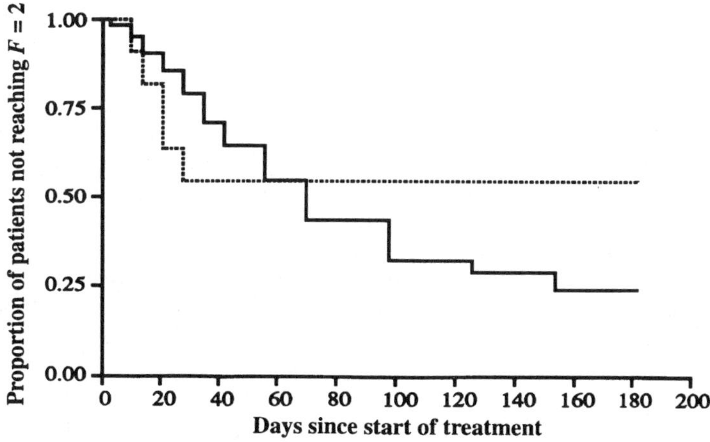

FIGURE 1.—Kaplan-Meier curves indicating the number of patients not managing to walk independently during the follow-up period of 181 days after treatment with plasma exchange (log rank test, not significant). *Broken line,* motor Guillain-Barré syndrome patients treated with plasma exchange. *Continuous line,* other Guillian-Barré syndrome patients treated with plasma exchange. (By permission of Oxford University Press. Visser LH, Van Der Meché FGA, Van Doorn PA, et al: Guillain-Barré syndrome without sensory loss (acute motor neuropathy): A subgroup with specific clinical, electrodiagnostic and laboratory features. *Brain* 118:841–847, 1995.)

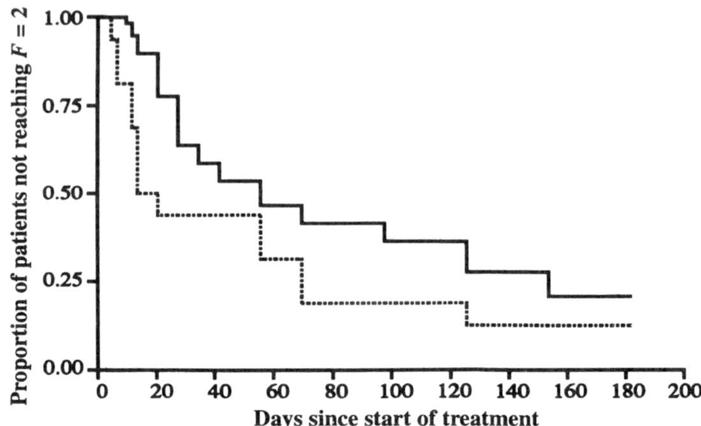

FIGURE 2.—Kaplan-Meier curves indicating the number of patients not managing to walk independently during the follow-up period of 181 days after treatment with IV immunoglobulin (log rank test, $P = 0.07$). *Broken line,* motor Guillain-Barré syndrome patients treated with IV immunoglobulin. *Continuous line,* other Guillain-Barré syndrome patients treated with IV immunoglobulin. (By permission of Oxford University Press. Visser LH, Van Der Meché FGA, Van Doorn PA, et al: Guillain-Barré syndrome without sensory loss (acute motor neuropathy): A subgroup with specific clinical, electrodiagnostic and laboratory features. *Brain* 118:841–847, 1995.)

Patients and Findings.—The study included 147 patients with Guillain-Barré syndrome, 27 of whom did not have sensory loss. All patients were followed for 6 months. Compared with the other 120 patients, the 27 patients with motor Guillain-Barré syndrome had a more rapid onset of weakness (3.9 vs. 6.1 days) and earlier nadir (6.3 vs. 9.1 days). Initially predominant distal weakness and sparing of the cranial nerves also were noted in 67% and 26% of the patients with motor Guillain-Barré syndrome, vs. 27% and 68% in the 120 patients with other Guillain-Barré syndrome. Of the patients with motor Guillain-Barré, 41% had experienced gastrointestinal illness (resulting from a *Campylobacter jejuni* infection in 67%) before onset of the syndrome. In contrast, 13% of the other patients with Guillain-Barré syndrome experienced gastrointestinal problems before disease onset, with infection caused by *C. jejuni* in 28%.

High titers of anti-GM_1 antibodies were observed more frequently in patients with motor Guillain-Barré syndrome, 42% compared with 5% among the remaining 120 patients. Limited or no indications of demyelination were noted in patients with motor Guillain-Barré syndrome on electrodiagnostic evaluation. Half of these patients did show profuse denervation activity.

Sixteen of the patients with motor Guillain-Barré syndrome were treated with IVIg and 11 with plasma exchange. Only 2 of those in the former group did not achieve independent walking compared with more than half of those in the latter treatment group (Figs 1 and 2). Median time to achieve independent walking also was less for patients receiving IVIg compared with those treated with plasma exchange. Among the patients with motor Guillain-Barré syndrome who had a *C. jejuni* infection, a

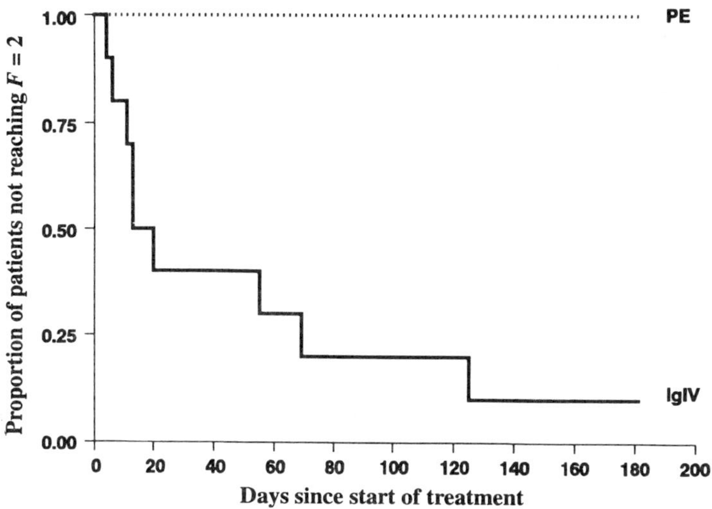

FIGURE 3.—Kaplan-Meier curves indicating the proportion of patients with an acute motor neuropathy after a *Campylobacter jejuni* infection who did not recover to independent locomotion during the 181 days of follow-up, according to treatment group (log rank test, P = 0.002). *Abbreviations*: *PE*, plasma exchange; *IgIV*, IV immunoglobulin treatment. (By permission of Oxford University Press. Visser LH, Van Der Meché FGA, Van Doorn PA, et al: Guillain-Barré syndrome without sensory loss (acute motor neuropathy): A subgroup with specific clinical, electrodiagnostic and laboratory features. *Brain* 118:841–847, 1995.)

significant difference in treatment response was noted. None of the 6 patients receiving plasma exchange achieved independent walking, whereas the mean time to this stage was 55 days among the 10 patients treated with IVIg (Fig 3).

Conclusion.—Patients with motor Guillain-Barré syndrome represent a distinct subgroup, as demonstrated by their clinical, electrophysiologic, and laboratory characteristics. Identification of subgroups, such as patients with motor Guillain-Barré syndrome, may further clarify the pathogenesis of Guillain-Barré syndrome and may have implications for treatment.

▶ Visser et al. are to be congratulated on an interesting article that clearly showed significant differences between the pure motor variant of the Guillain-Barré syndrome and that in the more typical patients—the greater frequency of *C. jejuni* and less evidence of demyelination in patients with the pure motor Guillain-Barré syndrome. It is different from the more typical syndrome and is reminiscent of the Chinese paralysis syndrome that has recently received attention. The greater response of patients with the pure motor Guillain-Barré syndrome to IVIg rather than to plasmapheresis is of considerable clinical significance, although it still remains to be proved by double-blind controlled trials. One caveat about the study is that it is not clear how frequently sensory examinations were undertaken and whether this was consistent for all patients.

W.G. Bradley, D.M., F.R.C.P.

Blocs de Conduction et Neuropathies Périphériques

Kuntzer T, Magistris MR (Ctr Hosp Univ Vaudois, Lausanne, Suisse; Hôpital Cantonal Univ de Genève, Suisse)
Rev Neurol 151:368–382, 1995

1–5

Introduction—Conduction block (CB) in the myelinated nerve fibers of a peripheral nerve causes partial or total loss of function, most commonly motor function. Conduction block results from a focal loss of electric properties in the nerve fiber. The literature was reviewed and the diagnostic criteria for CB were examined.

Methods.—Electromyographic (EMG) studies allow differentiation between nerve dysfunction resulting from axonal lesions and dysfunction that can be attributed to CB (Fig 1). The etiologies for peripheral neuropathy with CB vary greatly and include physical trauma (electric, thermal, percussion, compression, or constriction injuries), and chronic inflammatory, autoimmune, toxic, or ischemic mechanisms (Fig 2). The severity of the nerve dysfunction depends on the location and duration of the nerve entrapment. Conduction block is seen predominantly in acquired focal or multifocal neuropathies with clinical signs suggestive of segmental nerve demyelinization and in abnormal conduction patterns suggestive of non-

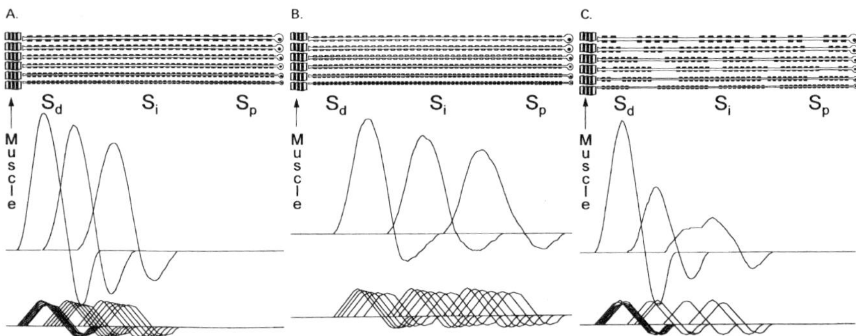

FIGURE 1.—Mathematical model of a peripheral myelinated nerve consisting of 6 motor units (MU) with different fiber diameters. Distal (S_d) intermediary (S_i), and proximal (S_p) stimulations. The evoked responses (*3 upper curves*) are produced by summation of the 6 individual MU potentials (*lower curves*). **A,** physiologic model. Individual axons are of different diameters and therefore have different conduction velocities, resulting in a progressive temporal dispersion of the evoked responses with interphase shift of the individual MU potentials. Differences between the negative peaks of the responses evoked by S_i / S_d, and then S_p / S_i, are in percent: increase in duration of 9% and 12%, reduction in amplitude of 9% and 15%, and in area of 1% and 5%. **B,** homogeneous demyelinating model. Compared with **A,** the latencies are markedly prolonged (the distal latency is increased by 220%), and the amplitudes are reduced because of desynchronization of individual MU potentials by 10% for the former and 21% for the latter. The reduction in amplitude is 14% (former) and 14% (latter) and in area 5% (former) and 1% (latter). **C,** inhomogeneous demyelinating model. There is partial distal demyelination with a concomitant prolonged distal latency of 43% compared with **A.** Between the S_i / S_d evoked responses, there is conduction block (CB) of 3 axons with reduction of 55% in amplitude and 48% in area, without increase in duration. The response evoked by proximal stimulation results from temporal dispersion of the individual MU potentials whose axons are partially demyelinated; the increase in duration is 46%, with a reduction in amplitude of 46% and area of 12%. (Courtesy of Kuntzer T, Magistris MR: Blocs de conduction et neuropathies périphériques. *Rev Neurol* 151:368–382, 1995.)

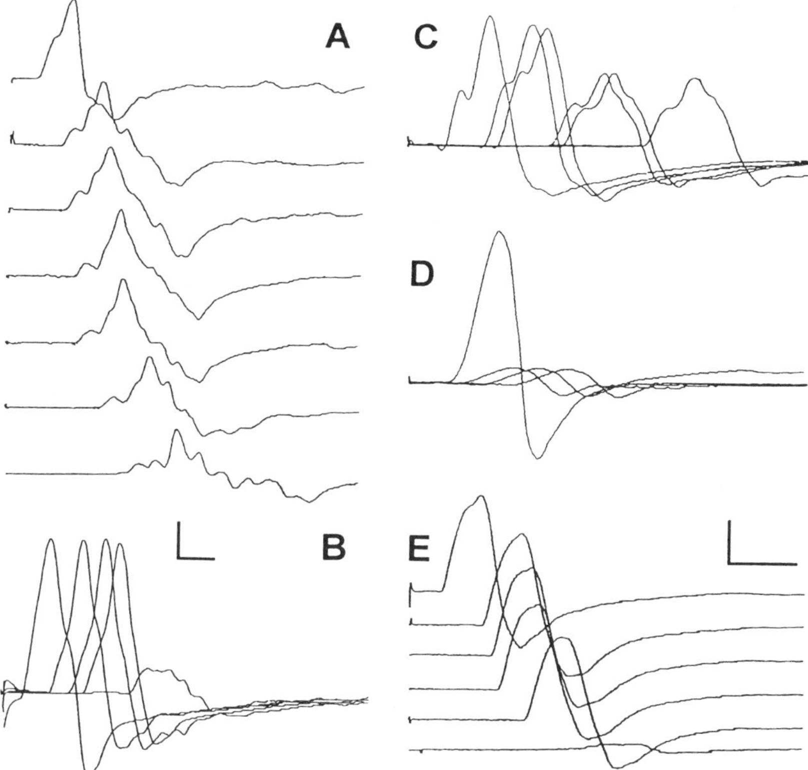

FIGURE 2.—Segmental ulnar nerve stimulation studies; abnormal temporal dispersion and conduction block (CB). Surface recording, with the active electrode placed over the abductor digit minimi muscle and the reference electrode at the base of the fifth digit. **A**, chronic inflammatory demyelinating neuropathy. Stimulation at the wrist, below the elbow, at the ulnar groove, 4 cm above the elbow, at the axilla, and at Erb's point. The distal latency is increased by 30% compared with the normal value, whereas the nerve conduction velocities are within the normal range. Temporal dispersion is abnormal with each stimulation: 56% increase in duration in the forearm, 31% in the elbow and the arm, and 26% between the Erb's point and axilla. Between the most proximal and distal stimulation sites, the total increase in duration is 230%, with reduction in amplitude of 44% and in area of 13% (2 mV, 5 mecs). **B**, multifocal motor neuropathy with persistent CB and antiganglioside GM_1 antibodies in a patient with a 3-year follow-up. Stimulation at the wrist, below the elbow, above the elbow, at the axilla, and at Erb's point. There is a proximal CB with reduction in amplitude of 83% and in area of 73%, without increase in duration (2 mV, 5 mecs). **C**, ulnar neuropathy at the elbow secondary to repeated microinjuries of 16 weeks' duration. Stimulation at the wrist, below the elbow, at the ulnar groove, above the elbow, at the axilla, and at Erb's point. Between the third and fourth responses, there is reduction in amplitude of 27% and in area of 38%. Due to an increase in duration of 16%, a CB cannot be ascertained, and a double-collision study should be carried out. It is worth noting the axonal loss with a 40% reduction in distal area compared with the normal side (2 mV, 5 mecs). **D**, Guillain-Barré syndrome 2 days after onset. Distal stimulations 1 cm apart from the canal of Guyon. There is no response with proximal (elbow) stimulation (not depicted). Early CB with a reduction in amplitude of 89% and in area of 85% and an increase in duration of 12% (2 mV, 5 mecs). **E**, radiation-induced brachial plexopathy 7 months after supraclavicular irradiation for breast carcinoma. Stimulation at the wrist, below the elbow, at the ulnar groove, above the elbow, at the axilla, and at Erb's point. There is an almost complete CB between axilla and Erb's point (5 mV, 5 mecs). (Courtesy of Kuntzer T, Magistris MR: Blocs de conduction et neuropathies périphériques. *Rev Neurol* 151:368–382, 1995.)

homogeneous demyelinization. In contrast, conduction abnormalities seen in the hereditary or congenital neuropathies are usually diffuse and homogeneous.

Conclusion.—A correct EMG diagnosis of CB in a peripheral nerve will avoid ineffective treatment. However, interpretation of the EMG requires a high degree of experience and skill.

▶ This review of publications of patients with peripheral neuropathies and multifocal conduction block highlighted the many potential underlying etiologies that can be responsible. In practice, when the causes of multiple nerve entrapments are excluded, the majority of these cases are caused by autoimmune inflammatory neuropathies. It is important, however, to remember the other etiologies and to search for them.

W.G. Bradley, D.M., F.R.C.P.

Long-Term Treatment of Chronic Inflammatory Demyelinating Polyradiculoneuropathy With Plasma Exchange or Intravenous Immunoglobulin
Choudhary PP, Hughes RAC (Guy's Hosp, London)
Q J Med 88:493–502, 1995   1–6

Background.—Patients with chronic inflammatory demyelinating polyradiculoneuropathy (CIDP) experience progressive or relapsing limb weakness and have neurophysiologic findings of multifocal demyelination affecting the peripheral nerves or spinal roots. The disorder is believed to be inflammatory—and probably immunologic—in nature and usually responds to treatment with corticosteroids and immunosuppressive drugs. Plasma exchange (PE) is reportedly helpful for some but not all patients.

Management.—The value of PE was compared with that of IV immunoglobulin (IVIg) as long-term treatment in 105 patients with CIDP who had either progressed over more than 8 weeks or followed a relapsing-remitting course. The results of treatment were evaluable in 33 patients who received PE and 22 given IVIg. Plasma exchanges began with 5 treatments over an 8- to 14-day period with a 50:50 mixture of normal saline solution and 4.5% albumin as replacement fluid. Intravenous immunoglobulin was given in a dose of either 0.4 g/kg daily for 5 days or 1 g/kg daily for 2 days.

Results.—Twenty-three of 33 patients improved after PE, 15 of them substantially. Women were more likely to respond, as were patients with a relatively short duration of CIDP. Seven of the 23 responders required long-term PE. Twelve of 305 PE sessions were attended by complications, the most serious of which was septicemia. Fourteen of 21 evaluable patients responded to treatment with IVIg. Again, women were more likely to respond. Seven patients required long-term treatment. Except for 1 patient with syncope secondary to severe hypotension, there were no serious side effects from IVIg. Four patients who required long-term PE were successfully changed to IVIg treatment; 2 of them were eventually able to cease all treatment. Two patients who initially received IVIg subsequently did well on PE treatment.

Recommendations.—Intravenous immunoglobulin is preferred as initial treatment of CIDP for both practical and economic reasons. A relatively few patients who fail to respond to IVIg may do well with PE.

▶ This is an open-label nonrandomized study, which makes it difficult to compare the efficacy of PE and IVIg. The author did not state whether the patients received prednisone or not or the reasons for using 1 or other of the trial treatments. With these reservations, it does appear that the efficacy of the 2 treatments was approximately similar in the long term. Because the complication rate is so much less for IVIg than PE and because IVIg can be given on an outpatient basis and even by a home infusion service, IVIg is preferable for patients who are "corticosteroid failures."

W.G. Bradley, D.M., F.R.C.P.

Anti-MAG Antibody-Associated Polyneuropathies: Improvement Following Immunotherapy With Monthly Plasma Exchange and IV Cyclosphosphamide
Blume G, Pestronk A, Goodnough LT (Washington Univ, St Louis)
Neurology 45:1577–1580, 1995   1–7

Introduction.—The outcome of treatment of sensory-motor polyneuropathies associated with anti–myelin-associated glycoprotein (MAG) antibodies has varied even with relatively intensive immunosuppression. Prompted by earlier encouraging results, 4 patients with anti-MAG antibody–associated polyneuropathies were treated with combined therapy using cycles of plasma exchange and cyclophosphamide.

Treatment.—Patients received plasma exchange on 2 consecutive days, followed by IV cyclophosphamide, 1 g/m². The regimen was repeated monthly for 5 to 7 months. Effects of treatment were monitored using hand-held myometer for quantitative assessment of muscle strength and clinical and electrodiagnostic studies for evaluation of sensory function.

Patients.—All 4 patients had sensory-motor polyneuropathy with disabling symptoms and high serum titers of IgM anti-MAG antibodies. Two patients had distal weakness in the upper and lower extremities, the third had a gait disorder, and the fourth had severe sensory loss. Electrodiagnostic studies showed evidence of demyelination in 3 patients and probably primary axonal disorder in 1.

Outcome.—Strength and sensation improved in the 5 to 24 months after treatment in all patients. Between 5 and 18 months after treatment was begun, quantitative muscle testing showed increased strength in all patients, averaging approximately one third of the total level of strength. Improvement correlated with a reduction of titers of serum IgM anti-MAG antibodies, falling by an average of 78% in 3 patients who completed 6 treatments. Furthermore, patients noted greater functional abilities, including improved gait and manual dexterity.

Conclusion.—Selected patients with sensory-motor polyneuropathies associated with high serum titers of IgM autoantibodies against MAG may have quantitative and useful functional improvement after immunotherapy with monthly plasma exchange and IV cyclophosphamide. These effects may persist for up to 2 years after completion of treatment.

▶ Although this study involved only a small number of patients, it is important, because it defined the extent of improvement that can be seen in patients with intensive therapy of anti-MAG antibody–associated polyneuropathies. In these 4 patients, there was an improvement averaging approximately one third of the total level of strength, which in some patients return to normal, and in all patients was associated with a reduction in fatigue and a significant functional improvement. Improvement continued for up to 2 years, though it should be noted that there was no evidence that a cure can be obtained by this treatment regimen.

W.G. Bradley, D.M., F.R.C.P.

Neuropathy Associated With "Benign" Anti-Myelin-Associated Glycoprotein IgM Gammopathy: Clinical, Immunological, Neurophysiological Pathological Findings and Response to Treatment in 33 Cases
Ellie E, Vital A, Steck A, et al (Univ Hosp of Bordeaux, Pessac, France; INSERM U 394, Bordeaux, France; Hôpital Pellegrin, Bordeaux, France; et al)
J Neurol 243:34–43, 1996   1–8

Introduction.—The association of late-onset peripheral neuropathy with monoclonal gammopathies (MGs) has received considerable attention in recent years. Thirty-three patients referred for peripheral neuropathy associated with nonmalignant anti–myelin-associated glycoprotein (MAG) IgM MG were evaluated to further describe the clinical, immunologic, electrophysiologic, and pathologic characteristics of the disorder.

Patients and Methods.—The mean age of patients (29 men and 4 women), onset of symptoms was 67 years; mean duration of symptoms at examination was 72 months. Patients were divided into 3 groups on the basis of clinical signs and symptoms. Eleven (group 1) had pure sensory neuropathy, 16 (group 2) had sensorimotor neuropathy with mild weakness, and 6 (group 3) had sensorimotor neuropathy with severe weakness and wasting. Other causes of peripheral neuropathy were excluded in all cases. Findings analyzed included immunologic studies, assays of anti-MAG and antiglycolipid sulphoglucuronyl paragloboside (SGPG) (anti-SGPG) antibodies, HLA typing, electrophysiologic studies, and pathologic conditions.

Results.—The mean age at neuropathy in group 1 patients was symmetric and slowly progressive or stable. The first symptom was paresthesia in the lower limbs, and Romberg's sign was always present. Symptoms had little effect on the activities of these patients. Group 2 patients had a longer duration of symptoms, more extensive involvement of the limbs, and a greater degree of disability. Intention tremor and marked ataxia were common. All group 3 patients had severe ataxia, a duration of symptoms between that of groups 1 and 2, and considerable limitation of mobility. Lung function test results revealed a restrictive syndrome. Overall, 45% of patients experienced severe disability, and 2 deaths appeared to be the direct result of the neuropathy.

Electrophysiologic testing showed a demyelinating process in 90% of cases. In more than 95%, nerve biopsy specimens examined by electron microscopy showed widening of the myelin lamellae. With a mean follow-up of 54 months, treatment consisting of corticosteroids and chemotherapy or plasma exchanges yielded generally poor responses; more effective was IV immunoglobulin, which led to clear improvement in 4 of 17 treated patients. There was no correlation between clinical severity of disease and the anti-SGPG antibody titers (range 1.1–355). Raised levels of CSF protein were reported in 22 of 24 cases.

Discussion.—Neuropathy associated with nonmalignant anti-MAG IgM MG typically occurs in the elderly, and most patients are men. Patients in groups 1 and 2 experience progressive weakness starting in the lower limbs. The hands are involved in a few years, motor function is affected, and tremor appears. This condition should not be considered benign, because disability can be severe, and disease-related deaths have occurred.

▶ This is a worthwhile review of a large number of patients with polyneuropathy due to anti-MAG gammopathy. It emphasized that this is not necessarily as benign a condition as hither was believed, because some of the patients became totally disabled. In this series, response to therapy was less than has been suggested in the literature, but one can always ask whether the treatment with prednisone and cyclophosphamide was as intensive and long term as necessary. Intravenous immunoglobulin seemed to be the best treatment, which would certainly fit with my experience.

W.G. Bradley, D.M., F.R.C.P.

Treatment of Multifocal Motor Neuropathy With High Dose Intravenous Immunoglobulins: A Double Blind, Placebo Controlled Study

Van den Berg LH, Kerkhoff H, Oey PL, et al (Univ Hosp Utrecht, The Netherlands; Univ Hosp, Amsterdam)
J Neurol Neurosurg Psychiatry 59:248–252, 1995   1–9

Objective.—Some patients with apparent motor neuron disease, whose test results demonstrate motor conduction block, may actually have multifocal motor neuropathy (MMN) and may respond to high-dose IV immunoglobulin (IVIg). The effect of IVIg in patients with this form of motor neuron disease was studied in a double-blind, placebo-controlled trial.

Methods.—Electrodiagnostic studies were performed to confirm demyelination, and IgM and IgG anti-GM$_1$ antibodies were measured in 6 patients with MMN before and after IVIg treatment. Four patients received 2 IVIg treatments (0.4 g/kg) for 5 days and 2 placebo treatments for 5 days, and 2 patients received 1 IVIg treatment and 1 placebo treatment in a randomized order. Patients were hospitalized during treatment and examined before and after treatment and at weekly intervals thereafter. Disability was measured before and after treatment and at day 14.

Results.—Muscle strength improved in 5 patients after IVIg treatment and declined after placebo treatment. One patient responded in the same way to both placebo and IVIg treatments.

Conclusion.—Treatment with IVIg can improve muscle strength in patients with MMN.

▶ Multifocal motor neuropathy has received considerable attention over the last few years as a treatable cause of motor neuron disease. A number of authors have suggested that IV cyclophosphamide is the therapy of choice for this condition. In my experience, this condition is rare among patients with typical amyotrophic lateral sclerosis (ALS). Most patients with MMN have features that would be atypical for ALS, including diffuse areflexia, a very slow course, relatively little atrophy despite marked weakness, and, most important of all, the absence of upper motor neuron features. I have treated these patients with IVIg and have seen moderate benefit. This clinical observation was confirmed in this careful double-blind, placebo-controlled trial by Van den Berg and his colleagues. In view of the significantly greater toxicity of IV cyclophosphamide, IVIg appears to be the treatment of choice for such patients.

W.G. Bradley, D.M., F.R.C.P.

Double-Blind, Placebo-Controlled Study of the Application of Capsaicin Cream in Chronic Distal Painful Polyneuropathy

Low PA, Opfer-Gehrking TL, Dyck PJ, et al (Mayo Found, Rochester, Minn)
Pain 62:163–168, 1995   1–10

Background.—Capsaicin, in a 0.075% cream, has been reported to show a weak beneficial effect in painful diabetic neuropathy. It is an alkaloid that depletes tissues of substance P and reduces neurogenic plasma extravasation, the flare response, and chemically induced pain. The efficacy of topical capsaicin in the treatment of chronic distal painful polyneuropathy was determined.

Study Design.—In a double-blind, placebo-controlled randomized study, the 2 limbs were assigned to capsaicin in a 0.075% cream or to placebo applied 4 times daily for 8 consecutive weeks. The first tube contained the active placebo methyl nicotinate. In the final 4-week single-blind, washout phase, the placebo was administered bilaterally. The following scales were employed to assess efficacy: investigator global, patient global, Visual Analogue Scale (VAS) of pain severity, VAS of pain relief, activities of daily living, and allodynia. Safety was assessed using a neurologic disability scale, nerve conduction studies, computer-assisted sensory examination for vibration and thermal cooling and warming, quantitative sudomotor axon reflex test (QSART), and quantitative flare response.

Patients.—Forty patients with bilateral symmetric chronic painful neuropathy of the lower extremities were studied, and 39 completed the 12-week study. All had neuropathic pain of long duration (median 56 months) and moderate, relatively nonselective impairment of large- and small-fiber function. Half of the patients had idiopathic distal small-fiber neuropathy and only 7 had diabetes.

Results.—The efficacy indices did not differ significantly between the capsaicin and placebo sides after 4 and 8 weeks of treatment, with no loss of benefit the last 4 weeks consisting of the single-blind placebo washout phase. A small number of indices favored the placebo at early time points (1–4 weeks), presumably because of hyperalgesia and intensification of burning pain that was common on the capsaicin side. At 4 weeks, 51.4% of patients reported improvement with capsaicin and 53.8% with placebo; at 8 weeks, 56.4% reported improvement with capsaicin, 64.1% with placebo; at 12 weeks, 59.0% reported improvement with capsaicin and 66.7% with placebo. All the safety indices showed no differences between sides.

Conclusion.—In patients with chronic distal painful neuropathy, a large percentage of limbs may improve after placebo use. There is no evidence of a change in neurogenic flare response, which is due primarily to substance P; in quantitative sensory test results of small-fiber function using thermal cooling and thermal warming; or in postganglionic sudomotor function measured using QSART to suggest that the effects of capsaicin sufficiently depletes substance P when capsaicin is applied to intact skin.

▶ Original reports of the therapeutic efficacy of capsaicin cream were encouraging and were based on both open label studies and double-blind controlled studies. This carefully designed study by Low et al. refuted these earlier studies. The present study treated few diabetics, which might explain the differences from earlier reports. A more likely explanation for the disparity, however, is the fact that patients with chronic pain are well-known placebo responders, a fact that was addressed by the use of methyl nicotinate in the placebo cream. This and clinical experience suggest that capsaicin is not very effective in the treatment of painful polyneuropathies.

W.G. Bradley, D.M., F.R.C.P.

Successful Treatment of Neuropathies in Patients With Diabetes Mellitus

Krendel DA, Costigan DA, Hopkins LC (Emory Univ, Atlanta, Ga)
Arch Neurol 52:1053–1061, 1995   1–11

Introduction.—Disabling, progressive neuropathies occasionally develop in patients with diabetes mellitus. A review of 21 such patients treated at the study institution over a 6-year period revealed 2 distinct forms of the neuropathies: axonal and demyelinating. Clinical data were presented for these patients, together with treatment and outcome.

Patients and Methods.—The patients (12 men and 9 women) ranged in age from 53 to 77. Non–insulin-dependent diabetes mellitus was present in 15 and IDDM in 6; all patients were disabled by progressive weakness. Based on results of electrophysiologic studies, 15 patients had evidence of axonal neuropathy and 6 had demyelinating neuropathy. Biopsies were performed on 14 patients. Treatment, given alone or in combination, consisted of IV immunoglobulin in 15 cases, prednisone in 13, cyclophosphamide in 5, plasma exchange in 3, and azathioprine in 1. Patients were interviewed and examined before the start of treatment and at regular intervals thereafter.

Results.—All NIDDM patients had axonal neuropathy. Weight loss had occurred in 10 of these patients, and 13 had involvement of the thighs, thoracic bands, or both. Seven of the 10 patients in this group who underwent biopsy exhibited perivascular or vascular inflammation. Patients who were insulin dependent had demyelinating neuropathy. None reported weight loss. The lower extremities were more severely affected than the upper extremities in 2 patients in this group, but 3 patients experienced an approximately symmetric neuropathy. All 4 patients who underwent nerve biopsy showed evidence of onion bulb formation. Occlusion of vessels and inflammatory vasculopathy were not apparent in those with demyelinating neuropathy. In both groups, anti-inflammatory treatment, anti-immune treatment, or both successfully stopped the patients' condition from worsening and brought about improvement in strength and mobility. Complications did occur, however, and included an increased or new requirement for insulin in 5 patients treated with prednisone. One patient with autonomic neuropathy experienced severe hypotension during plasma exchange.

Conclusion.—Two forms of disabling polyneuropathy were found in these patients with NIDDM and IDDM. Axonal neuropathy was caused by inflammatory vasculopathy, whereas demyelinating neuropathy was indistinguishable from chronic inflammatory demyelinating polyradiculoneuropathy. Anti-inflammatory and anti-immune therapy brought about a response and functional improvement.

▶ It is all too easy in a patient with diabetes mellitus to conclude that any neuropathic symptoms are caused by the diabetes mellitus. In fact, patients with diabetes mellitus have a higher prevalence of a number of other autoimmune diseases that affect the peripheral nervous system, including pernicious anemia, chronic inflammatory demyelinating polyneuropathy, and vasculitis. The treatment of these is somewhat counterintuitive in terms of the diabetes mellitus, because it usually requires corticosteroid therapy. Because of the problems of corticosteroid therapy in those who are diabetic, it is necessary often that patients have a failed 2-month trial of obsessive control of the diabetes mellitus before accepting that immunosuppressant therapy is required. I have been particularly interested in inflammatory lumbosacral plexopathies associated with diabetes mellitus and the response of such patients to prednisone and cyclophosphamide and in other patients IV immunoglobulin. This review by Krendall et al. emphasized that such patients are not uncommon.

W.G. Bradley, D.M., F.R.C.P.

The Aetiology of Diabetic Neuropathy: The Combined Roles of Metabolic and Vascular Defects

Stevens MJ, Feldman EL, Greene DA (Univ of Michigan, Ann Arbor)
Diabetic Med 12:566–579, 1995

1–12

Introduction.—Diabetic neuropathy is a common complication of diabetes mellitus that strongly contributes to the development of sepsis, debility, and lower limb amputations. Its importance has prompted numerous studies seeking to clarify its pathogenesis. Although its cause is not yet certain, both metabolic and vascular defects have been implicated. The current hypotheses of the pathogenesis of diabetic neuropathy were reviewed.

Metabolic Defects.—Substantial evidence suggests that diabetic patients have alterations in the polyol pathway, which metabolizes glucose to sorbitol and fructose by aldose reductase. These patients demonstrate sorbitol and fructose accumulation and *myo*-inositol depletion, which has been implicated in reduced nerve conduction velocity (NCV). These alterations in the polyol pathway may lead to reduced (Na,K)-ATPase activity and intracellular osmotic dysregulation. Increased aldose reductase activity and accumulated sorbitol dehydrogenase cause oxidation of the NADPH/NADP$^+$ (nicotinamide adenine dinucleotide phosphate) redox couple and reduces the NADH/NAD$^+$ (nicotinamide adenine dinucleotide) redox couple. Depletion of NADPH can reduce the synthesis of nitric oxide, an important vasodilator and neuromodulator.

Vascular Defects.—Considerable evidence suggests that nerve ischemia is central to the pathogenesis of diabetic neuropathy. This hypothesis is supported by the effectiveness of vasodilatory agents in improving or normalizing NCV. It has been proposed that nerve fiber degeneration may be caused by endoneurial hypoxia secondary to nerve microvessel damage. Both nerve vascular histologic abnormalities and rheologic abnormalities, which have been found in diabetic patients, can result in compromised neural blood flow.

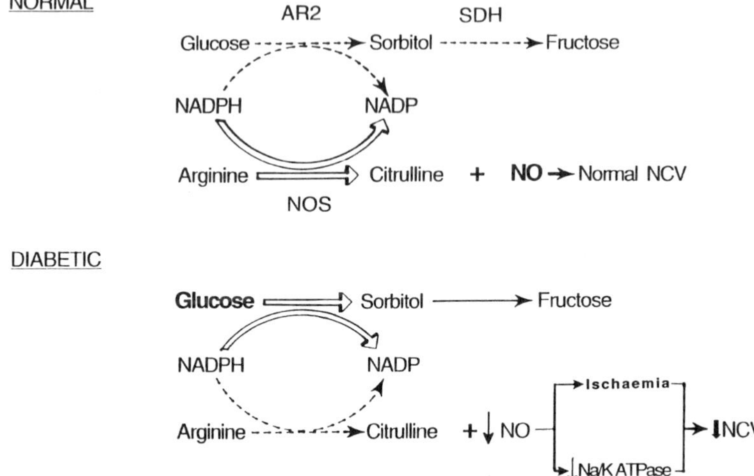

FIGURE 3.—Metabolic competition for NADPH by aldose reductase and nitric oxide synthase in normal and diabetic state. *Abbreviations: AR2,* aldose reductase; *SDH,* sorbitol dehydrogenase; *NO,* nitric oxide; *NOS,* nitric oxide synthase; *NCV,* nerve conduction velocity; *NADPH,* reduced form of nicotinamide adenine dinucleotide phosphate; *NADP,* nicotinamide adenine dinucleotide phosphate; *Na/KAT-Pase,* sodium and potassium–activated adenosine triphosphate. (The aetiology of diabetic neuropathy: The combined roles of metabolic and vascular defects; by Stevens MJ, Feldman EL, Greene DA; Copyright 1995 *Diabetic Med;* reprinted by permission of John Wiley & Sons, Ltd.)

Links.—Several mechanisms link the metabolic and vascular defect hypotheses. The depletion in nitric oxide caused by alterations in the polyol pathway can affect vascular smooth muscle and decrease (Na, K)-ATPase, thereby possibly resulting in vasoconstriction and decreased endoneurial blood flow (Fig 3). In addition, decreased prostaglandin metabolism can reduce the release of noradrenaline and modulate endoneurial blood flow. Abnormal fatty acid metabolism can disrupt membrane stability and function, thereby disrupting neural energy production. Excess protein glycosylation can damage the vascular supply or alter the composition of the extracellular matrix. Hyperglycemia-induced disruption in the synthesis, axonal transport, signal transduction, and local production of growth factors may interfere with axonal maintenance, regeneration, and remyelination.

Conclusion.—There is considerable evidence of an interdependence among the metabolic and vascular factors affecting nerve function, thus suggesting that intervention focusing on a key defect occurring early in the cascade may prevent diabetic neuropathy.

▶ When 2 good people argue, there is often right on both sides. The vascular and metabolic theories of the cause of diabetic neuropathy might be likened to those 2 good people arguing. There is good evidence in favor of both hypotheses, and the pendulum of opinion has swung back and forth between these 2 theories for many years. This is the final conclusion of this excellent review of the etiology of diabetic neuropathy. Stevens et al. concluded that many of the metabolic and vascular factors interact. They suggested that we need to look at a key factor earlier in the cascade of biochemical and vascular abnormalities, chemotherapeutic modulation of which can arrest the pathologic process. That key factor, however, still remains to be elucidated.

W.G. Bradley, D.M., F.R.C.P.

Progressive Sensory-Motor Polyneuropathy With Tomaculous Changes Is Associated to 17p11.2 Deletion

Mancardi GL, Mandich P, Nassani S, et al (Univ of Genoa, Italy; Chiavari Hosp, Italy)
J Neurol Sci 131:30–34, 1995   1–13

Introduction.—Focal thickenings of the myelin sheath (tomacula) are distinctive pathologic features of different disorders of the peripheral nerves, including hereditary neuropathy with pressure palsy (HNPP). Recently a deletion of a 1.5-Mb region on chromosome 17 (17p11.2) has been associated with HNPP, but whether different clinical phenotypes with identical pathologic change have the same genetic defect is not clear. Three patients were examined for 17p11.2 deletion.

Methods.—Three patients with progressive sensory-motor polyneuropathy were examined for the presence of 17p11.2 deletion by Southern blotting and fluorescent in situ hybridization.

Clinical Features.—Two patients had a generalized slowing evolving predominantly distal motor polyneuropathy with mild sensory disturbances. In the third patient, the onset was in the proximal part of 1 arm that subsequently affected the distal portions of all limbs. The clinical course was progressive at the onset. Neurophysiologic studies confirmed the diffuse involvement of the peripheral nervous system without conduction blocks at the common sites of nerve compression. None of the patients had clinical history of pressure palsy, transitory loss of strength, or sensory disturbances.

Results.—All patients showed prominent and numerous tomaculous changes affecting more than 15% of the examined internodes at single fibers on teased fibers examination. In all patients, Southern blotting showed a single band, and fluorescent in situ hybridization demonstrated only 1 signal at the specific 17p11.2 region.

Conclusion.—These patients showed a definitely different clinical profile from HNPP, but the pathologic changes and the genetic defect were the same. It appears that the presence of prominent tomaculous changes involving a large number of internodes is associated with the 17p11.2 deletion whatever the clinical phenotype of peripheral neuropathy. The molecular study of the 17p11.2 region should be considered as a noninvasive method for the differential diagnosis in selected patients with progressive polyneuropathy.

► This report is of interest, because it demonstrated that tomacular changes in a nerve biopsy specimen are a strong indication of the presence of the chromosome 17p11.2 deletion, even in the absence of the phenotype of hereditary neuropathy with liability to pressure palsies. All 3 patients had the clinical picture of progressive sensorimotor polyneuropathy, and only results of nerve biopsy indicated the underlying genetic abnormality. Molecular genetic screening for the chromosome 17p11.2 region may become an important initial evaluation of patients with chronic progressive sensory-motor polyneuropathies.

W.G. Bradley, D.M., F.R.C.P.

Motor Neuron Disorders

Identification and Characterization of a Spinal Muscular Atrophy-Determining Gene
Lefebvre S, Bürglen L, Reboullet S, et al (Inst Natl de la Santé et de la Recherche Médicale, Paris; Inst Necker, Paris; Genethon, Evry, France; et al)
Cell 80:155–165, 1995   1–14

Background.—Spinal muscular atrophy (SMA), a common autosomal recessively inherited disorder, is a degenerative disorder of the lower motor neurons that culminates in progressive paralysis with muscle atrophy. All 3 phenotypic forms of SMA map to chromosome 5q11.2-q13.3, where large-scale deletions have been found.

Objective.—An attempt was made to narrow the critical region of the SMA-associated gene and to characterize a small 140-kb area within the telomeric region.

Findings.—An inverted duplication of a 500-kb element was identified in normal chromosomes. The critical 140-kb interval was found to contain a 20-kb gene, the survival motor neuron (*SMN*) gene encoding a novel 294–amino acid protein. A highly homologous gene was found in the centromeric element in 95% of control individuals. The gene was absent in 93% of 229 patients with SMA and was interrupted in another 5.6%. The 3 patients retaining *SMN* had either a point mutation or short deletions in the consensus splice sites of introns 6 and 7.

Interpretation.—The *SMN* gene appears to be a determining gene for SMA, as evidenced by the presence of deleterious mutations in patients who neither lack the gene nor have an interrupted form. It is possible that regulatory elements or genes mapping near *SMN* account for the large genomic rearrangements found in type I SMA, thereby altering the clinical phenotype.

▶ This paper by Lefebvre et al. reported the finding of mutations of an alternative gene to that reported by Roy et al. (Abstract 1–15) in Werdnig-Hoffmann disease. This gene is located in the same region of chromosome 5q, and its function is yet to be determined. The finding of complete or partial deletion of gene in 98.6% of patients with SMA provides strong evidence that deficiency of the gene product may be responsible for Werdnig-Hoffmann disease. However, as this article indicated, further work is needed before the final answer is known.

W.G. Bradley, D.M., F.R.C.P.

The Gene for Neuronal Apoptosis Inhibitory Protein Is Partially Deleted in Individuals With Spinal Muscular Atrophy
Roy N, Mahadevan MS, McLean M, et al (Children's Hosp of Eastern Ontario, Ottawa, Canada; Univ of Ottawa, Ont, Canada; Roswell Park Cancer Inst, Buffalo, NY; et al)
Cell 80:167–178, 1995   1–15

Background.—The various forms of spinal muscular atrophy (SMA), caused by depletion of motor neurons in the spinal cord, are among the most frequent autosomal recessive disorders and have been linked with DNA markers in the 5q13 region of chromosome 5. Many motor neurons examined at autopsy exhibit swelling and chromatolysis, and it has been proposed that the inappropriate persistence of normally occurring apoptosis accounts for SMA.

Objective.—A novel gene for neuronal apoptosis inhibitory protein (NAIP) was mapped to the SMA region of chromosome 5q13.1, and the protein was found to contain domains having sequence homology with baculovirus proteins that inhibit virally induced insect-cell apoptosis.

Findings.—The first 2 coding exons of the gene for *NAIP* were deleted in 67% of type I SMA chromosomes and in only 2% of non-SMA chromosomes. Analysis using the reverse transcriptase polymerase chain reaction technique demonstrated internally deleted and mutated forms of the *NAIP* transcript in patients with type I SMA but not in unaffected individuals.

Interpretation.—Inhibition of apoptosis in spinal motor neurons by NAIP is consistent with the pathologic findings in SMA. The large regions of genomic DNA spanned by the various forms of *NAIP* suggest that neighboring genes may also be involved in depletion of the gene.

▶ The chromosomal localization of Werdnig-Hoffmann disease was discovered in 1990, but it was not until this year that characterization of this region of chromosome 5q13 has sufficiently advanced to identify putative genes. Of several suggested candidate genes, the *NAIP* gene appears teleologically to be the most satisfying candidate. Werdnig-Hoffmann disease frequently begins before birth, and progressive loss of motor neurons so early in life raises the possibility that there is some process inhibiting the normal programmed cell death for motor neurons, which is a feature of embryonic development. A mutation causing dysfunction of such a gene would be likely to allow continuation of programmed cell death. However, only two thirds of the cases exhibited deletions in this gene, and further studies are needed to confirm that this is *the* gene responsible for Werdnig-Hoffmann disease.

W.G. Bradley, D.M., F.R.C.P.

Autosomal Dominant Distal Spinal Muscular Atrophy in Four Generations

Boylan KB, Cornblath DR, Glass JD, et al (Johns Hopkins Univ, Baltimore, Md; VA Med Ctr, Salt Lake City, Utah; Columbia Univ, New York; et al)
Neurology 45:699–704, 1995   1–16

Background.—Distal spinal muscular atrophy (SMA) is a rare lower motor neuron disorder, with weakness predominating in the leg and foot muscles. This condition may be difficult to differentiate clinically from type II Charcot-Marie-Tooth disease. Members of a 4-generation extended family with autosomal dominant distal SMA were studied.

Patients.—Thirteen family members showed a consistent pattern of distal limb weakness that was distinct from that usually seen in peroneal muscular atrophy.

Clinical Features.—The patients had a slowly progressive distal limb amyotrophy beginning in the second to fourth decades (average age 34). Motor axon loss was manifested initially and predominantly in calf and toe flexor muscles, whereas muscles of the anterolateral compartment and toe dorsiflexors were less severely involved. Most patients had triceps weakness, even when distal upper limb muscles were only mildly affected. Electromyography was indicative of motor denervation. Sensation was preserved, and sensory nerve action potentials were normal.

Pathologic Conditions.—Muscle biopsy findings were compatible with chronic partial denervation and reinnervation similar to that reported in more proximal or generalized forms of SMA. Combined silver/cholinesterase/immunocytochemical staining of terminal intramuscular nerves in mild disease showed abundant axonal branching, segmentation of end plates, and numerous thin unmyelinated terminal motor axons, suggesting motor axon collateral reinnervation. In the most severe disease, there was marked loss of terminal motor end-plate innervation, suggesting loss of motor axon collaterals with disease progression. Multipoint linkage analysis of chromosome 5q microsatellite markers excluded the 5q11.2-13.3 region as the location of the distal SMA locus.

Summary.—It appears that the neurologic disorder in this family represents a form of distal SMA, different from that in patients with weakness involving primarily the anterolateral leg muscles. The distal SMA in the present family and childhood-onset proximal SMA (SMA 5q) may be the results of mutations at separate loci.

▶ Charcot-Marie-Tooth disease type II patients may have virtually no sensory abnormality and hence may be considered to have a distal SMA. However, by definition, they must have electrophysiologic or pathologic evidence of sensory nerve degeneration. The family described here with dominantly inherited distal spinal muscular atrophy clearly had no electrophysiologic or clinical evidence of sensory involvement, even though no nerve biopsy was performed. The sensory sparing, together with the clinical features of the "wrong way round" involvement (i.e., the posterior calf muscles being worse than the anterior shin muscles and the triceps involved even when the biceps, deltoid, and intrinsic muscles were spared), should be the pointer to this diagnosis. The disorder is not linked with the infantile/juvenile proximal pseudomyopathic *SMA* gene to the locus on chromosome 5q. This condition may well be heterogeneous, because some patients with distal SMA have autosomal-recessive inheritance or are sporadic.

W.G. Bradley, D.M., F.R.C.P.

Dynamic Electromyography and Muscle Biopsy Changes in a 4-Year Follow-Up: Study of Patients With a History of Polio

Stålberg E, Grimby G (Univ Hosp, Uppsala, Sweden; Univ of Göteborg, Sweden)

Muscle Nerve 18:699–707, 1995   1–17

Background.—Some patients with a history of poliomyelitis report progressive loss of muscular strength many years after the acute phase of the disease; this is 1 of the criteria for postpolio syndrome (PPS). Long-term follow-up data on patients with a history of polio were analyzed to determine whether and in what ways the muscular findings changed over time.

Methods.—The analysis included 18 patients with sequelae of poliomyelitis. The patients had contracted polio 29 to 56 years previously. They were studied on 2 occasions 4 years apart. Eleven patients had new symptoms consistent with PPS at the first evaluation, and 3 more had new symptoms at the second evaluation. The evaluations included clinical testing, static and dynamic knee extensor strength testing, electromyographic (EMG) studies, and, in 10 patients, muscle biopsies. Of 28 legs

TABLE 2.—Macroelectromyographic and Single Fiber–Electromyographic–Fiber Density Findings at the 2 Examinations and the Median of the Intraindividual Change (in Percent) Between the 2 Investigations (Change %)

EMG	*n*	First examination	Second examination	Change %
Macro MUP amplitude				
Stable	16	10.2 (1.4)	14.7 (2.1)	67.0*
Unstable	12	16.3 (6.4)	19.0 (4.8)	34.7
All	28	11.0 (3.1)	16.6 (2.5)	55.8*
SFEMG-FD				
Stable	16	3.0 (0.3)	3.6 (0.3)	26.0*
Unstable	12	4.9 (0.6)	4.8 (0.3)	−4.9
All	28	4.1 (0.3)	3.9 (0.2)	−1.5

Note: Macro-MUP amplitudes are normalized for age, and the values in the table are the median and standard error of the mean values of the group.

* Significant difference ($P < 0.01$).

Abbreviations: EMG, electromyogram; *MUP*, motor unit potential; *SFEMG-FD*, single fiber–electromyographic–fiber density.

(Dynamic electromyography and muscle biopsy changes in a 4-year follow-up: Study of patients with a history of polio; by Stalberg E, Grimby G; *Muscle Nerve*; Copyright 1995 *Muscle Nerve*; reprinted by permission of John Wiley & Sons, Inc.)

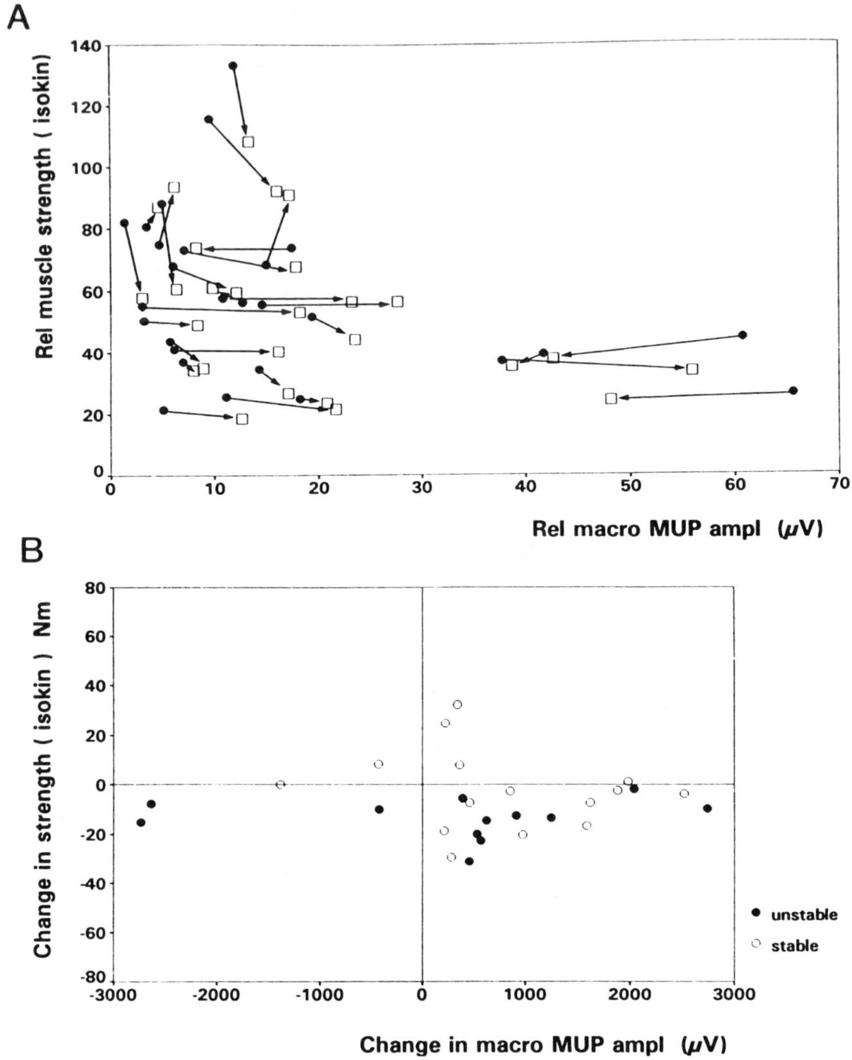

FIGURE 3.—**A,** changes in relative macro-MUP amplitude and in isokinetic strength (percent of reference values) during the 4-year period. *Arrows* link the first (*circles*) and second (*squares*) examination. Note that many legs show little change in strength but pronounced changes in macro-MUP amplitude. The initially largest macro-MUPs decreased between the 2 examinations. **B,** the same data in absolute values. An increase in macro-MUP amplitude in combination with a decrease in strength, often only slight, was the most common finding. *Abbreviations: rel,* relative; *MUP,* motor unit potential; *ampl,* amplitude. (Dynamic electromyography and muscle biopsy changes in 4-year follow-up: Study of patients with a history of polio; by Stalberg E, Grimby G; *Muscle Nerve;* Copyright 1995 *Muscle Nerve;* reprinted by permission of John Wiley & Sons, Inc.)

with EMG recordings at both examinations, 12 showed new or increased muscle weakness between examinations and 16 did not.

Results.—Isometric muscle strength, measured as peak torque for knee extension, was 56% of age-matched control levels at the first examination, with a median 8% decrease by the second examination. Isokinetic strength was 57% initially and subsequently decreased by 7%. Only patients with new weakness in the examined leg (the unstable group) had a significant decrease in torque (median, 13%). The mean muscle fiber area was about 170% of control values, with no significant changes in fiber composition or areas during follow-up.

At the initial EMG evaluation, the median macro–motor unit potential (MUP) amplitude in the polio patients was approximately 11 times higher than control levels. A further 56% increase occurred during follow-up, although the percent change was significant only in the stable group (Table 2). Macro-MUP increased in 23 of 28 legs, 15 of which had decreased strength. It decreased in 5 legs, 3 of which had decreased strength (Fig 3). The relative and absolute increases in macro-MUP amplitudes were inversely correlated with the initial macro-MUP amplitude. In most patients, a relative increase in the number of muscle fibers in a motor unit occurred during follow-up. However, this increase accounted for the increase in the raw macro-MUP data in just 1 patient. Single-fiber EMG recordings revealed a moderate number of muscle fibers with increased jitter or occasional impulse blocking at both evaluations.

Conclusion.—Patients with a history of polio have a high macro-MUP amplitude, probably as a result of reinnervation. The macro-MUP increases in amplitude over time as a compensatory response to neuronal loss, although it is not correlated with dynamic changes in muscle strength. The neuronal loss in patients without new strength loss is probably well compensated for by reinnervation and maintenance of fiber size. The complex causes of reduced muscle strength and the compensatory processes for it create difficulties in identifying predictors of new weakness.

▶ The postpolio syndrome strikes at the heart of patients who had polio 30 or more years ago. The fear is that the terrifying condition from which they recovered with such difficulty is going to return. What causes this slowly progressive weakness in patients with progressive postpolio muscular atrophy, a subgroup of the postpolio syndrome, remains something of an enigma. Some have suggested that the wasting and weakness result from gradual loss of the ability of the residual motor neurons to maintain the grossly enlarged (here, 11-fold) branching of the terminal axons or from death of some of the residual motor neurons. This study by Stålberg and Grimby is a tribute to their perseverance and that of their patients. They found that the mean macro-MUP, which provides an estimate of the size of the motor units, is often increased even though muscle strength decreases. The extent of this increase was less for initially larger macro-MUPs. The authors believed that these studies indicate that progressive motor neuron death is responsible for the progressive postpolio muscular atrophy. Unfortunately, a direct estimate of the number of motor units, although technically difficult in the quadriceps, was not performed to validate this suggestion.

W.G. Bradley, D.M., F.R.C.P.

Motor Neuron Disease (Amyotrophic Lateral Sclerosis) Arising From Longstanding Primary Lateral Sclerosis
Bruyn RPM, Koelman JHTM, Troost D, et al (Oudenryn Hosp, Utrecht, The Netherlands; Amsterdam Academic Med Ctr)
J Neurol Neurosurg Psychiatry 58:742–744, 1995   1–18

Introduction.—Primary lateral sclerosis (PLS) is a nonfamilial form of progressive spasticity. Its relationship with both the hereditary spastic paraplagias and amyotrophic lateral sclerosis (ALS) remains uncertain. Three patients, 1 of whom underwent autopsy, demonstrated that long-standing PLS may develop into ALS.

> *Typical Case Report.*—Man, 33, described heaviness in his legs and cramps in the calves and proximal leg muscles, present for the past 6 years. The family history was noncontributary. All extremities were hyperreflexic, and patellar clonus and a left extensor plantar sign were noted. The CSF was normal. Primary lateral sclerosis was diagnosed, and the patient's condition deteriorated very slowly. Both legs were moderately spastic and Babinski's signs were present 21 years after the initial diagnosis; however, there were no fasciculations or atrophy. Peroneal conduction velocities were reduced, with no evidence of denervation. The patient was lost to follow-up and died of pneumonia 32 years after first being seen.
>
> There was marked loss of anterior horn cells from the spinal cord and mild cell loss in Clarke's columns. Amylaceous bodies, occasional neuronophagia, and reactive gliosis were seen throughout the cord. The pyramidal tracks exhibited a marked myelin pallor. Macrophages and activated microglial cells in most of the spinal cord stained immunocytochemically with major histocompatibility complex common framework antigen.

Discussion.—Amyotrophic lateral sclerosis developed in these 3 patients 7½ , 9, and 27 or more years after PLS had been diagnosed. Lower motor neuron disease was recognized clinically in the first 2 patients. It is possible that PLS and nonfamilial ALS are manifestations of a single disorder.

► Amyotrophic lateral sclerosis is a pleomorphic disease with many anatomically different forms, as well as different rates of progression. One of the vexing questions has always been whether this difference from 1 group to another indicates that we are dealing with several different diseases. This description of the eventual development of lower motor neuron degeneration allowing a diagnosis of ALS in 3 patients who previously appeared to have primary lateral sclerosis for many years suggested that the 2 conditions may be the same. The strongest support for this contention comes from several examples of 1 family with the same gene causing familial ALS in whom individuals have had PLS, progressive muscular atrophy, bulbar palsy, and classic ALS.

W.G. Bradley, D.M., F.R.C.P.

Selective Loss of Glial Glutamate Transporter GLT-1 in Amyotrophic Lateral Sclerosis
Rothstein JD, Van Kammen M, Levey AI, et al (Johns Hopkins Univ, Baltimore, Md; Emory Univ, Atlanta, Ga)
Ann Neurol 38:73–84, 1995   1–19

Purpose.—Cloning studies have now identified at least 3 glutamate transporters: GLT-1 and GLAST, which are astroglial-specific proteins, and EAAC1, which is found only in neurons. Patients with amyotrophic lateral sclerosis (ALS) have abnormalities of glutamate transport. Crude synaptic membranes from the brain regions most affected by the disease, the motor cortex and spinal cord, show striking reductions of high-affinity glutamate transport. The nature of the glutamate transport defect in ALS was studied by using antipeptide antibodies specific for each of the human glutamate transporters.

Methods and Results.—Neural tissue from 22 patients with ALS and 17 controls was studied. Mean age at death was 61 for those with ALS and 64 for the controls. Immunoblots of all brain and spinal cord regions studied showed detectable immunoreactive protein for EAAC1, GLT-1, and GLAST. However, GLT-1 immunoreactive protein was decreased 71% in the motor cortex of subjects with ALS and 57% in the lumbar spinal cord. About onefourth of motor cortex specimens from subjects with ALS consistently showed more than a 90% loss of GLT-1 immunoreactive protein. In contrast, frontal cortex specimens from subjects with ALS showed no differences in immunoreactive protein compared with control specimens. Other brain regions from subjects with ALS, such as the striatum, hippocampus, and sensory cortex, did not demonstrate the GLT-1 abnormality (Fig 4). One of 3 subjects with familial ALS showed more than an 80% loss of GLT-1 protein in all brain regions studied.

Immunoblots for the neuronal synaptic membrane protein synaptophysin demonstrated no significant change in the mean immunoreactive levels in any brain region. In a few cases, a small loss of synaptophysin was observed along with loss of the neuronal marker EAAC1. Immunohistochemical studies showed that GLT-1 immunoreactive protein was essentially absent in motor cortex layers 2 through 5 from subjects with ALS. Immunoreactivity of GLT-1 was noted only in occasional astroglial cells from layers 1 and 6. Although GLAST immunoreactivity was less homo-

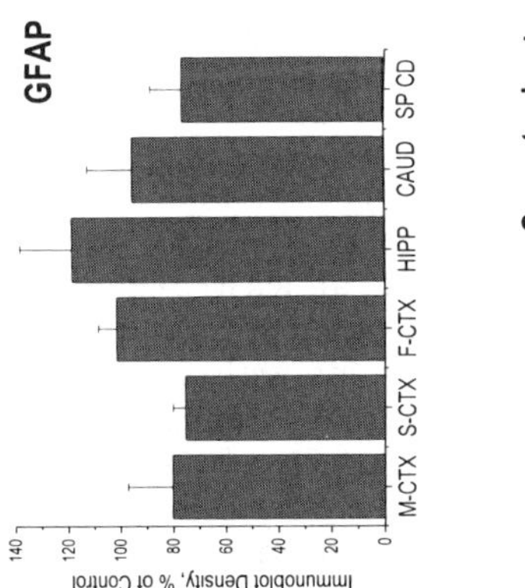
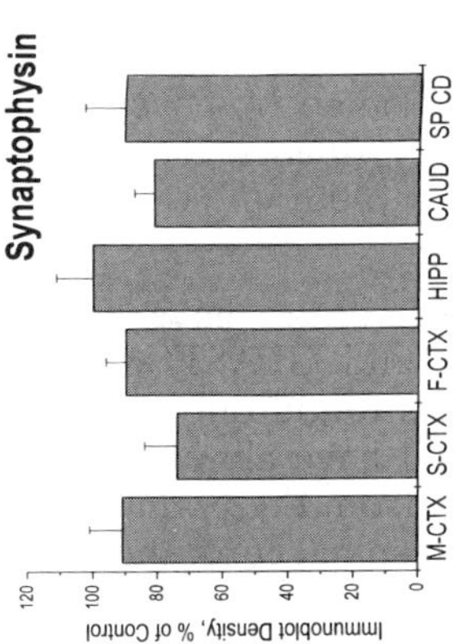
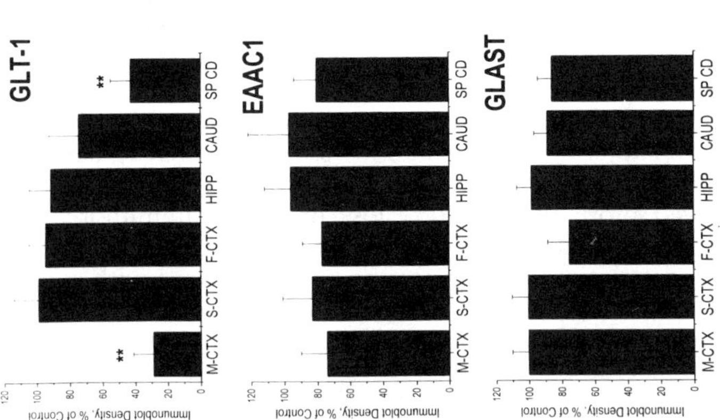

FIGURE 4.—Summary of analyses from immunoblots performed on *GLT-1, GLAST, EAAC1, GFAP,* and *synaptophysin* in amyotrophic lateral sclerosis (ALS) and control brain regions and spinal cord. Immunoblots were performed using equal amounts of protein from ALS and control specimens. Each column represents the mean ± standard error of 8 to 20 patient specimens. There were 8 to 16 control specimens studied for each tissue region. Values in parentheses are the number of individual ALS specimens studied for each tissue region. Each specimen was also evaluated in duplicate or triplicate. There was a significant loss of GLT-1–immunoreactive protein in motor cortex and spinal cord, whereas there were no significant changes in the other transporters from ALS specimens in the tissue regions studied. *Double asterisk* indicates statistically significant (*P* < 0.01) differences compared with matched control tissue region (independent *t* test). *Abbreviations: GFAP,* glial fibrillary acidic protein; *M-CTX,* precentral motor cortex; *S-CTX,* postcentral somatosensory cortex; *F-CTX,* frontal cortex; *HIPP,* hippocampus; *CAUD,* caudate; *SP CD,* spinal cord (lumbar). (Reprinted from *Annals of Neurology* volume, 38:73–84, 1995; by permission of Little, Brown and Company [Inc].)

geneous in subjects with ALS than in controls, GLAST and EAAC-1 immunoreactivity was unchanged for the most part.

Conclusion.—Immunoblotting and immunohistochemical studies of brain tissue suggest that patients with ALS have substantial loss of the glutamate transporter GLT-1. Transporter protein loss is observed mainly in the motor cortex and spinal cord. Astroglial GLT-1 immunoreactive protein in the motor cortex is lost from layer 2 through layer 5, even though astroglia are not decreased in patients with ALS. Thus, the observed GLT-1 loss could reflect selective loss of the protein from astroglia or loss of a subset of GLT–1 positive astroglia in affected regions. The mechanism of selective GLT-1 loss is unknown but may reflect selective damage of the GLT-1 protein by other cellular events. Loss of glial glutamate transport could play a key role in the loss of upper and lower motor neurons in patients with ALS.

▶ This is a key paper that appears to provide the final link in the chain demonstrating excess glutamate activity as the pathogenetic mechanism in at least a major proportion of patients with ALS. However, the cause of the loss of the glial glutamate transporter GLT-1 remained undiscovered. Glutamate transport is very sensitive to oxidative damage, and hence this defect in GLT-1 could still be secondary. Even so, it may be the final common path that leads directly to neuronal damage. Study of the gene for GLT-1 and its messenger RNA may help resolve this question. This paper comes at a particularly opportune time because of the recent report of the multicenter phase III trial of riluzole in almost 1,000 patients with ALS that confirmed and extended the results of a smaller study published earlier.[1] Riluzole extended survival in ALS patients with both bulbar and limb onset. Publication of the full results of this study are awaited, but it appears likely that riluzole will be released shortly for distribution in the United States.

W.G. Bradley, D.M., F.R.C.P.

Reference

1. Bensimon G: Proceedings of the 6th Annual Symposium on ALS/MND, Dublin, 1995.

Muscular Disorders

Inclusion Body Myositis and Myopathies

Griggs RC, Askanas V, DiMauro S, et al (Univ of Rochester, New York; Univ of Southern California, Los Angeles; College of Physicians and Surgeons, New York; et al)
Ann Neurol 38:705–713, 1995   1–20

Background.—Inclusion body myositis (IBM) appears to be distinct from the other major idiopathic inflammatory myopathies, namely, dermatomyositis and polymyositis. Inflammation is rarely encountered in a familial or hereditary form of IBMs (h-IBM) but is almost always observed in the sporadic form (s-IBM). Diagnostic criteria for IBM were proposed, and immune considerations, myonuclear alterations, mitochondrial abnormalities, treatment, and avenues of future research were discussed.

Diagnostic Criteria.—Clinical features characteristic of IBM include onset (age ≥30) of muscle weakness that persists for at least 6 months. Muscle weakness must affect proximal and distal muscles of the arms and legs, and other features are required as well. Laboratory findings include serum creatine kinase levels less than 12 times normal and a muscle biopsy specimen demonstrating intracellular amyloid deposits or 15- to 18-nm tubulofilaments. Electromyography is consistent with features of an inflammatory myopathy. In rare cases IBM with inflammation may be familial, and this condition differs from h-IBM. A number of other conditions, especially those that are immune mediated, can occur with IBM. Patients who meet other criteria but show only muscle inflammation may receive a diagnosis of possible IBM.

Treatment and Research Targets.—No established treatment exists for s-IBM, and little is known of the natural history of the disorder. Although immunosuppressive drugs are used because of the inflammatory abnormality of IBM, these agents have not been effective. Some trials report better results from treatment with IV immunoglobulin (IVIg). Several research strategies are suggested by the demonstration of amyloid in muscle in s-IBM. Identification of amyloidogenic proteins, determination of the origin of prion proteins, and investigation of the role of apolipoprotein E may be promising avenues of study. A cause for the lack of effectiveness of immunosuppressive therapies might also be pursued. One theory proposes that a nuclear abnormality causes s-IBM and that inflammatory exudates are a secondary reaction.

Conclusion.—No effective treatment has been developed for s-IBM, nor has the natural history of the disorder been determined. Immune suppressant treatment and IVIg therapy need further study. Clues to the pathogenesis of s-IBM may be found in the specific ultrastructural abnormalities of myonuclei. Evidence also supports T cell–mediated myocytotoxicity in the development of the disorder.

▶ It is my impression and that of a number of other "gray beards" that we are seeing something of an epidemic of IBM. These cases occur predominantly in the elderly, and hence the increased problems could be caused by increasing aging of the population. However, the clinical features of a slowly progressive myopathy with a rather curious distribution of muscle involvement, particularly involving the quadriceps and the long flexors of the fingers, make it likely that these cases were not missed in earlier studies. The observation by Griggs et al. of the deposition within the muscle fibers of amyloid and amyloid precursor proteins, prion proteins, and so forth raised the possibility that this could be a prion disease. To date, no positive evidence of transmission has been reported, but the definitive long-term primate inoculations have yet to be investigated. This paper resulted from an international workshop. Research is very active in this field at present. A few patients show a moderate response to immunosuppressant therapy, though this is less than in typical polymyositis-dermatomyosis. The trials of IVIg sadly fail to show marked benefit.

W.G. Bradley, M.D., F.R.C.P.

Common Variable Immunodeficiency and Inclusion Body Myositis: A Distinct Myopathy Mediated by Natural Killer Cells

Dalakas MC, Illa I (Natl Inst of Neurological Disorders and Stroke, Bethesda, Md)
Ann Neurol 37:806–810, 1995

1–21

Objective.—The cause of inclusion body myositis (IBM) is not known. The cases of 2 patients with long-standing common variable immunodeficiency, in whom IBM developed, were used to provide evidence, for the first time, that natural killer (NK) cells participate in the myocytotoxic process.

Case Reports.—Two men, 36 and 48, had atrophy and weakness in the muscle groups selectively affected in IBM, which had been present for 5 years in the 36-year-old and for 4 years in the 48-year-old. At age 13 years, common variable immunodeficiency, a disorder marked by agammaglobulinemia and immunologic abnormalities, was diagnosed in both men. Muscle biopsy specimen showed typical features of IBM. Immunophenotypic analysis of the endomysial cells showed increased number of NK cells, defined as $CD57^+$, $CD56^+$, $CD3^-$, $CD8^-$, and $CD68^-$, accounting for 8.5% to 9.5% of the total cells. The other endomysial cells included macrophages, $CD8^+$ cells, and $CD4^+$ T cells. The NK cells expressed intercellular cell adhesion molecule-1 and were the only cells that invaded muscle fibers negative for major histocompatibility (MHC) class I. The MHC class I antigen was absent or weakly expressed in only some of the muscle fibers surrounded by $CD8^+$ cells. Enteroviral or retroviral sequences were not amplified. In contrast, in sporadic IBM, NK cells accounted for less than 1% of the total cells and all muscle fibers expressed MHC class I. Both patients were treated with IV immunoglobulin, and 1 showed improved strength with normalization of NK cells on repeat muscle biopsy.

Conclusion.—Inclusion body myositis can develop in patients with common variable immunodeficiency. The combination of these 2 rare diseases is unexpected but important because of their capacity to mediate muscle fiber injury through a dual mechanism: 1 non–MHC-restricted mediated by NK cells and other MHC class I–restricted mediated by $CD8^+$ cells.

These cases represent an immune myopathy in which NK cells participate in the myocytotoxic process.

▶ I believe we are seeing an epidemic of IBM. We have recognized the existence of the condition for more than 20 years but are now seeing so many cases that we can recognize them clinically even before biopsy. The chronic lower limb to upper limb progression of the predominantly proximal myopathy, together with the characteristic finger flexion weakness, is the clue to the clinical diagnosis. The possibility of an "epidemic" and the findings of amyloid-like proteins and prion proteins in the muscle biopsy specimen raise thoughts of a slow virus infection. So far no positive transmission studies have been reported. This paper of IBM in patients with common variable immunodeficiency syndrome might support the hypothesis of a nonconventional viral infection resulting from diminished immunocompetence of the host.

W.G. Bradley, D.M., F.R.C.P.

Deletion Status and Intellectual Impairment in Duchenne Muscular Dystrophy
Bushby KMD, Appleton R, Anderson LVB, et al (Univ of Newcastle Upon Tyne, England; Royal Liverpool Children's Hosp, England; Newcastle Gen Hosp, Newcastle Upon Tyne, England)
Dev Med Child Neurol 37:260–269, 1995   1–22

Background.—A survey of 721 patients with Duchenne muscular dystrophy (DMD) showed that approximately one fifth had an intelligence quotient (IQ) less than 70 and that 3% had an IQ less than 50. The deficit is limited to verbal IQ and is not progressive. The high level of concordance in IQ between affected brothers and the lack of disability in those with other degenerative neuromuscular disorders suggest that the deficit is a direct effect of the mutation causing muscle weakness. The protein product of the *DMD* gene, dystrophin, is present in brain, as well as in muscle, and appears to be localized to the neocortex, hippocampus, and cerebellum.

Objective.—Abnormalities in the dystrophin gene were related to intellectual function in 74 patients with a diagnosis of DMD or intermediate DMD/Becker muscular dystrophy.

Findings.—Fourteen patients (18%) had a full-scale IQ of 70 or less, and 3 (4%) had an IQ less than 50. A complementary DNA (cDNA) deletion was found in 57 patients (77%), as was a duplication in 1 patient. Full-scale IQ scores did not relate to the presence or absence of a deletion or to the number of exons deleted. Boys whose deletion breakpoint was distal to exon 30 were more often intellectually deficient. The 7 deletions that were shared between 2 or more unrelated patients were associated with a wide range of IQ scores. An especially low verbal IQ score was not associated with any particular deletion.

Implications.—The presence or absence of a cDNA deletion does not in itself influence IQ in patients with DMD. Deletions in the distal region of the gene are likelier than more proximal deletions to be associated with retardation. That the intellectual deficit associated with DMD is a general result of a malfunctioning dystrophin molecule is likely.

▶ One of the puzzling features of DMD that is still awaiting explanation 8 years after the discovery of the gene is the mental retardation present in approximately 25% of patients. The IQ distribution of patients with DMD is shifted about 15 points to the left compared with the normal population. With the discovery that dystrophin deficiency is responsible for the muscle degeneration, it was hoped that an understanding of the basis for the intellectual impairment would follow. An alternative splicing form of dystrophin is present in the brain, although its function is, as yet, undetermined. This study showed that the details of the gene deletions do not explain the degree of intellectual impairment. It will take a more detailed understanding of the functional defects in the dystrophin of the brain and muscle in these patients to clarify our understanding.

W.G. Bradley, D.M., F.R.C.P.

Genetic and Biochemical Normalization in Female Carriers of Duchenne Muscular Dystrophy: Evidence for Failure of Dystrophin Production in Dystrophin-Competent Myonuclei

Pegoraro E, Schimke RN, Garcia C, et al (Univ of Pittsburgh, Pa; Kansas Univ Med Ctr; Kansas City; Louisiana State Univ, New Orleans; et al)
Neurology 45:677–690, 1995   1–23

Background.—Females related to boys with Duchenne muscular dystrophy (DMD) may be heterozygous carriers of the mutated dystrophin gene. Carriers have a mixture of dystrophin-positive and dystrophin-negative myonuclei in their skeletal muscle fibers. As many as 10% of carriers have muscle weakness.

Objective.—Nineteen female carriers of the DMD gene, all of whom had a mosaic dystrophin immunofluorescence pattern, were studied. The dystrophin protein content of muscle tissue was determined, and patterns of X-chromosome inactivation in DNA samples from blood and muscle were studied. Six of the patients had symptoms of progressive myopathy.

Findings.—Five patients had equal numbers of normal and mutant dystrophin genes in their peripheral blood, reflecting random X-chromosome inactivation. None of them had more than mild disability. Their muscle tissue had at least 60% of the normal dystrophin content, and no more than minor histopathologic abnormalities were present. Fourteen carriers had a skewed X-inactivation pattern of their peripheral-blood DNA, with one X chromosome active in 75% or more of the nuclei. Clinical involvement was more severe in these patients; those with mild disease were only 5 to 10 years old. Dystrophin levels averaged less than

30% of normal in older patients, all of whom had dystrophic changes in their muscle biopsy specimens. Nearly 80% of patients with a skewed X-inactivation pattern had more dystrophin-positive nuclei in muscle than in blood, evidencing genetic "normalization." In 65% of these patients, however, the dystrophin-positive nuclei did not produce dystrophin. In contrast, the patients with a random inactivation pattern exhibited biochemical "normalization."

Implications.—Biochemical normalization appears to take place in most or all asymptomatic carriers of the DMD gene. Older boys may not recover full dystrophin function when given gene therapy, because either production of dystrophin protein is deficient or an unstable protein is produced.

▶ For 20 years, it has been recognized that some, but not all, female carriers of DMD have clinical and laboratory changes indicating manifestation of the mutant dystrophin gene. The serum creatine kinase level is highest in the first 1 or 2 decades, but clinical signs of a proximal myopathy rarely appear until the fourth to seventh decade, when some cases have been diagnosed as limb-girdle muscular dystrophy. This variability was thought to be explained by variable lyonization (inactivation) of the X chromosome bearing the mutant dystrophin gene. This elegant paper confirmed and expanded this concept, but it did not answer all the questions. In the random inactivation patients, although they had mild symptoms of myopathy, the normal myonuclei worked overtime to produce an amount of dystrophin greater that 60% of normal (biochemical normalization). In the skewed inactivation patients with preferential inactivation of the normal X chromosome, segmental necrosis in areas of predominantly mutant myonuclei presumably led to preferential loss of these mutant nuclei, and hence the muscle moved toward genetic normalization. Strangely these normal myonuclei were incapable of producing biochemical normalization; this still needs explanation. Note that there may be a group of DMD carriers who have skewed inactivation of the mutant myonuclei, who would be expected to have normal clinical and serum creatine kinase findings, and who might have been missed in this study. However, Matthews et al.[1] found that 5 nonmanifesting carriers had random inactivation.

W.G. Bradley, D.M., F.R.C.P.

Reference

1. Matthews PM, Benjamin D, van Bakel I, et al: Muscle X-inactivation patterns and dystrophia expression in Duchenne muscular dystrophy carriers. *Neuromuscul Disord* 5:209–220, 1995.

Diagnosis of Malignant Hyperthermia: A Comparison of the in Vitro Contracture Test With the Molecular Genetic Diagnosis in a Large Pedigree

Healy JMS, Quane KA, Keating KE, et al (Univ College, Cork, Ireland; Cork Univ, Ireland)
J Med Genet 33:18–24, 1996

1–24

Purpose.—The inherited skeletal muscle disorder malignant hyperthermia (MH) is one of the main causes of anesthesia-related death. The standard diagnostic test for MH is an in vitro contracture test (IVCT) performed on a muscle biopsy specimen; in the European protocol, the results are reported as MH susceptible (MHS), MH normal (MHN), and MH equivocal (MHE). This system has been validated by genetic linkage studies and by the identification of causative MH mutations in the *RYR1* gene. Linkage studies were performed in an Irish MH pedigree using markers linked to the *MHS* locus on chromosome 19, including a search for known *RYR1* mutations.

Methods and Findings.—In this pedigree, using the European protocol for MHS diagnosis excluded a link between the MHS phenotype and the *RYR1* locus. In subsequent analyses, the cutoff point for MHS status was increased, and a diagnosis of MHN was assumed in subjects who did not reach this threshold. The results suggested close linkage between MHS status and the *RYR1* locus. All MHS subjects in the study pedigree who met the raised cutoff point had the previously described *MHS Gly341Arg RYR1* mutation.

Conclusion.—Tight linkage between *MHS* and *RYR1* markers is demonstrated in an Irish family with malignant hyperthermia. This condition may be caused by a number of different mutations, however. The results suggest that all patients diagnosed as being MHS or MHE on the basis of the European protocol should be considered MHS for clinical purposes. It remains to be seen why some family members will show an MHE or MHS response in the absence of any demonstrable mutation.

▶ Malignant hyperthermia is an important condition not only to anesthesiologists but also to neuromuscular specialists; it has been reported in a number of disorders, including Duchenne's dystrophy, myotonias, and other myopathies. The dominantly inherited MH causes problems in genetic counseling, because screening tests for susceptibility are notoriously fallible. Despite attempts at standardizing the caffeine and halothane contracture tests, there are a good number of equivocal results, as this paper pointed out. Having had experience with these susceptibility tests, I adopted the pragmatic approach of advising all first-degree relatives of the possibility that they might have an anesthetic hyperthermic reaction. The discovery that mutations of the ryanodine receptor (*RYR*) underlie a high proportion of patients with dominant MH allows us to advance the screening of at-risk patients. This paper confirmed that a high threshold in the caffeine-halothane contracture studies is required to establish the presence of an *RYR1* mutation. Unfortunately, several different mutations can cause MH, and at present no commercially available genetic screening test is available.

W.G. Bradley, D.M., F.R.C.P.

2 Cerebrovascular Disease

Diagnosis and Prognosis

Frequency and Accuracy of Prehospital Diagnosis of Acute Stroke

Kothari R, Barsan W, Brott T, et al (Univ of Cincinnati, Ohio; Univ of Michigan, Ann Arbor; Reading Fire Dept, Ohio)
Stroke 26:937–941, 1995

2–1

Introduction.—The various experimental treatments for acute ischemic stroke all must be given within a few hours after the onset of stroke to be effective. This raises important questions about how well prehospital and emergency department personnel can make the diagnosis of acute stroke. The frequency and accuracy of the prehospital diagnosis of stroke were assessed in 1 emergency medical service (EMS) system.

TABLE 1.—Accuracy of Emergency Medical Technician or Paramedic Diagnosis of Stroke or Transient Ischemic Attack

Diagnosis	No.	%
Total	86	
Prehospital diagnosis in agreement with final diagnosis	62	72
TIA	15	
Brain infarction	35	
Intracerebral hemorrhage	10	
Subarachnoid hemorrhage	2	
False-positive final diagnosis, not stroke or TIA	24	28
Infection/sepsis*	8	
Syncope	5	
Cardiac disease*	2	
Seizure*	2	
Brain metastasis*	1	
Drug overdose*	2	
Hyponatremia*	1	
Arthritis	1	
Global amnestic syndrome	1	
Radial nerve palsy	1	

*Effective emergency department treatment available.
Abbreviation: TIA, transient ischemic attack.
(Kothari R, Barsan W, Brott T, et al: Frequency and accuracy of prehospital diagnosis of acute stroke; *Stroke;* 1995; 26:937–941; reproduced with permission of *Stroke;* Copyright 1995 American Heart Association.)

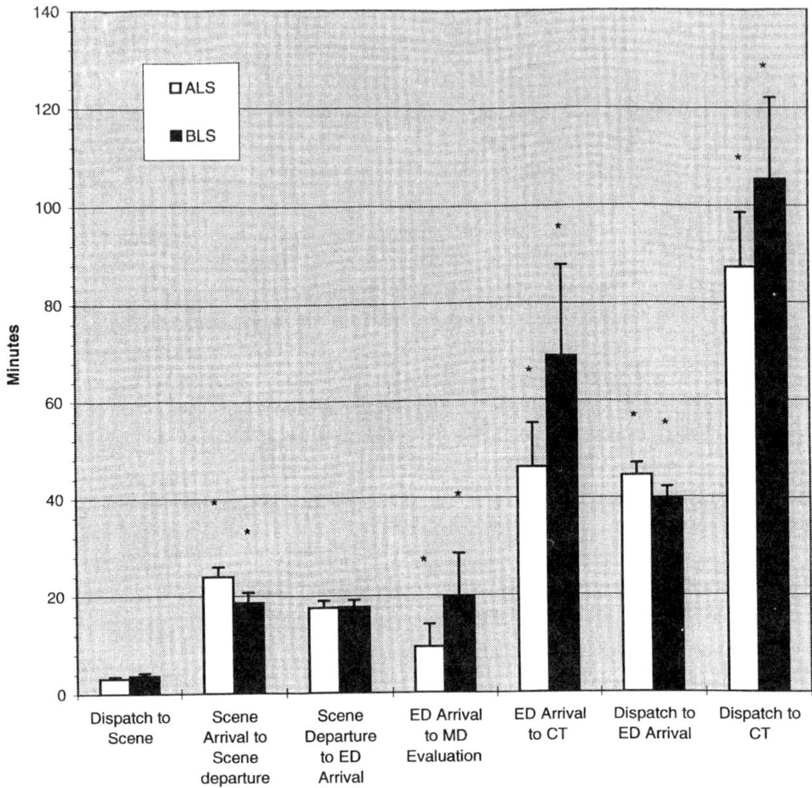

FIGURE.—Prehospital and emergency department time intervals for patients with possible stroke who were transported by advanced life support and basic life support units. *Asterisk* refers to the advanced life support time intervals significantly different from basic life support time intervals (*P* <0.05; 95% confidence interval). *Abbreviations: ALS*, advanced life support; *BLS*, basic life support; *ED*, emergency department. (Kothari R, Barsan W, Brott T, et al: Frequency and accuracy of prehospital diagnosis of acute stroke; *Stroke*; 1995; 26:937–941; reproduced with permission of *Stroke*; Copyright 1995 American Heart Association.)

Methods.—The study was performed in a 2-tiered EMS system serving a suburban community of 13,000 people. The prehospital records of 4,413 consecutive patients were reviewed to identify those with potential stroke based on the diagnosis of transient ischemic attack (TIA) or stroke made by an EMS dispatcher, emergency medical technician (EMT), or paramedic. In addition to assessing the accuracy of these diagnoses, the study looked at the patient prehospital triage times and the time intervals in patient transport and evaluation.

Results.—In 2% of the patients, an EMT or paramedic made a diagnosis of stroke or TIA on the scene. Of 86 patients meeting the study inclusion criteria, 72% had a final hospital discharge diagnosis of stroke or TIA. The rate of correct identification was 52% for EMS dispatchers and 72% for paramedics. Paramedic-level interventions were needed by 22 of 86 patients, including airway intubation in 3 patients.

Paramedics made an incorrect diagnosis of TIA or stroke in 24 patients, 16 of whom proved to have acute conditions for which effective treatments are available (Table 1). The mean time from the emergency call to arrival on the scene was 3 minutes. The time to arrival at the hospital was 40 minutes for patients transported by basic life support units vs. 45 minutes for those transported by advanced life support units. However, the latter group of patients were seen by a physician and underwent CT of the brain more quickly after arrival (Fig).

Conclusion.—Preliminary data suggest that the EMS system can carry out prompt prehospital evaluation of patients with possible stroke or TIA. The findings suggest that these patients need urgent evaluation and transport; many of them need paramedic-level interventions, and many have acute medical conditions for which specific therapies are available. A prospective study of the prehospital management of stroke in the entire Cincinnati metropolitan area is currently in progress.

▶ The subject of this report is of considerable current interest in that the rapid and accurate recognition of stroke by prehospital personnel is crucial if acute stroke patients are to receive urgent hospital attention and be given the benefits of acute pharmacologic neuroprotectant therapy or thrombolysis once these therapeutic modalities (now in the testing phase) become implemented in clinical practice. The fact that 28% of this patient cohort thought to have stroke by EMTs or paramedics failed to have this diagnosis would indicate the need for an enhanced level of community and paramedical training. Nonetheless, the authors stated that the majority of these misdiagnosed patients had acute conditions for which effective therapies were available.

M.D. Ginsberg, M.D.

The Effect of a Stroke Unit: Reductions in Mortality, Discharge Rate to Nursing Home, Length of Hospital Stay, and Cost: A Community-Based Study
Jørgensen HS, Nakayama H, Raaschou HO, et al (Bispebjerg Hosp, Copenhagen; Frederiksberg Hosp, Copenhagen)
Stroke 26:1178–1182, 1995   2–2

Objective.—Increasing evidence favors treatment of stroke patients in specialized stroke care units. The effect of stroke unit treatment on unselected patients with acute stroke was assessed.

Setting.—A community-based, prospective, and consecutive study of 1,241 unselected stroke patients was conducted in 2 neighboring communities within Greater Copenhagen. In the Bispebjerg community, all acute stroke patients were treated and rehabilitated on a stroke unit. Management included a standardized evaluation program, a goal-oriented treatment program that was initiated as soon as the patient arrived in the unit and performed within the frame of a multidisciplinary integrated approach guided by weekly multidisciplinary sessions and weekly assessments of neurologic deficits and functional disabilities. In the community of Frederiksberg, acute treatment and rehabilitation were performed exclusively on a general neurologic or medical ward. Except for this difference in stroke treatment, the 2 communities and patient groups were comparable, particularly in age, sex, marital status, cardiac disease, previous stroke, stroke severity, and type. Hypertension and diabetes mellitus were more common in the stroke unit patients.

Outcome.—Treatment of acute stroke patients in the stroke unit significantly reduced in-hospital mortality by 21% and lowered case fatality by 20% at 6 months and 18% at 1 year compared with treatment on the general wards. In addition, treatment on the stroke care unit markedly reduced discharge rate to a nursing home by 20% and increased discharge rate to a patient's home by 16%. Furthermore, patients treated on the stroke unit spent, on average, 13 fewer days in the hospital, reducing the average length of hospital stay by 30%. These beneficial effects were incurred independent of whether patients not treated in the stroke unit were treated in neurologic or medical wards.

Conclusion.—Treatment of unselected patients with acute stroke on the dedicated stroke care unit reduces the relative risk of death by approximately 50%, reduces the relative risk of discharge to a nursing home by approximately 40%, and almost doubles the relative chance of discharge to a home compared with treatment on the general wards. The reduction in length of hospital stay translates to considerable savings of 1,313 bed-days and 3 places at a nursing home per 100 stroke patients.

▶ Although this was not a double-blind, controlled trial of treatment of patients with acute strokes in a stroke unit compared with a general hospital ward, this study has some advantages over such previously reported studies. All severities of stroke were included in this study, because no informed consent was required in this 2-hospital comparison. It seems unlikely that any systematic difference between the patients admitted to the 2 hospitals could have explained the findings. The therapeutic benefit of the stroke unit is quite dramatic. It must be assumed that the results of this study from Denmark would translate into similar findings in other developed countries in the world.

W.G. Bradley, D.M., F.R.C.P.

Prognosis for Patients Following a Transient Ischemic Attack With and Without a Cerebral Infarction on Brain CT
Eliasziw M, for the North American Symptomatic Carotid Endarterectomy Trial (NASCET) Group (Univ of Western Ontario, Canada; John P Robarts Research Inst, London, Ont, Canada; Victoria Hosp, London, Ont, Canada)
Neurology 45:428–431, 1995   2–3

Introduction.—The prognostic importance of cerebral infarctions observed on brain CTs of patients with transient ischemic attacks (TIAs) has not been determined. A group of patients with TIAs and severe angiographically defined carotid artery stenosis (70%–99%) was assessed for the relationship between the finding of a cerebral infarction on brain CT and outcome.

Patients and Methods.—The study patients had been recruited by the North American Symptomatic Carotid Endarterectomy Trial (NASCET). Those selected for the present analysis had a TIA as their latest ischemic event. At a median of 10 days after the last TIA, patients underwent CT of the head. Scans were evaluated for the presence of brain infarctions located in the anterior circulation of the brain and ipsilateral to the symptomatic stenosed carotid artery. These lesions were classified according to size (small, medium, and large) and location (cortical, deep, and subcortical).

Results.—Findings on brain CTs were negative in 114 (64.8%) patients and positive in 62. Twelve patients with positive findings had infarcts inappropriate to the stenosed carotid artery. Eighteen of the 50 patients with appropriate brain infarctions had bilateral lesions. Most of the lesions were small (<1 cm) and none were large (>4 cm). Approximately half were subcortical infarcts and half either cortical or deep infarcts. Patients with infarctions were somewhat older than those with negative CTs (mean ages, 66.6 vs. 63.1). The 2 groups were similar in risk factors for stroke and dose of aspirin, but those with CT-verified brain lesions had a longer duration of symptoms and were more likely to have higher degrees of carotid stenosis and carotid plaque ulceration, as well as a history of hypertension. During a mean follow-up of 16 months, 12 patients with and 12 patients without cerebral infarctions had ipsilateral strokes. Six patients died, 4 from the group with infarction and 2 from the group without infarction. Regression analysis with adjustment for all known risk factors yielded no increased risk of ipsilateral stroke at 2 years for the patients with infarctions on CT.

Conclusion.—Cerebral infarctions on the brain CTs of patients with severe carotid artery stenosis and TIAs are common, but their presence, whether unilateral or bilateral, was not found to increase the risk of subsequent ipsilateral stroke. Thus, the finding of infarctions in this setting should not alter prognosis or treatment.

▶ This interesting report dealt with a question of ongoing concern to cerebrovascular clinicians: Under what circumstances are apparent TIAs accompanied by ipsilateral cerebral infarction on CT scan? This careful analysis of patients from the NASCET study suggested that older age, higher blood pressure, diabetes mellitus, and ipsilateral plaque ulceration are significantly higher in incidence in the group showing appropriate brain infarctions. However, after adjustments for other patient characteristic factors were made, the presence of brain infarction on CT appeared not to influence the risk of ipsilateral stroke at 2 years; however, other factors (notably, duration of TIA, hypertension, and contralateral carotid occlusion) did. The authors' conclusion is thus worth emphasizing: The presence of appropriate infarction after TIA should not, of itself, be a reason for altering treatment or reassessing prognosis.

M.D. Ginsberg, M.D.

Mitral Valve Prolapse and the Risk of Stroke After Initial Cerebral Ischemia

Orencia AJ, Petty GW, Khandheria BK, et al (Mayo Clin and Mayo Found, Rochester, Minn)
Neurology 45:1083–1086, 1995   2–4

Objective.—Mitral valve prolapse has been linked to cerebral ischemia in young adults in referral-based studies. However, little is known about the risk of subsequent stroke or transient ischemic attack (TIA) for patients with mitral valve prolapse who have had an initial ischemic event. The risk of recurrent cerebral ischemia among patients with mitral valve prolapse was investigated in a community-based study.

Methods.—The analysis included 49 residents of 1 Minnesota county who had an initial ischemic stroke or TIA and an echocardiographic diagnosis of mitral valve prolapse. The cerebral events occurred from 1975 through 1990; the patients were followed through 1991 for the occurrence of a subsequent stroke. The diagnosis of mitral valve prolapse was made before that of the initial ischemic stroke or TIA in 27 patients and afterward in 22. The patients' risk of later stroke was compared with the age- and sex-adjusted rates of recurrent cerebral ischemia in the population of Rochester, Minnesota.

Results.—Patients consisted of 31 women and 18 men, with a mean age of 72. Subsequent stroke occurred in 9 patients, for a rate of 5.5/100 person-years. The number of expected recurrent strokes in Rochester patients experiencing their first initial stroke from 1975 through 1984 was 10.72, for a relative risk of 0.84. Rochester patients having their initial ischemic stroke or TIA from 1975 to 1979 were expected to have 12.31 recurrent strokes, for a relative risk of 0.73. When compared with these rates, the risk of recurrent stroke was not increased for patients with mitral valve prolapse and initial cerebral ischemic events.

Conclusion.—For patients with documented mitral valve prolapse and an initial episode of cerebral ischemia, the risk of subsequent stroke does not appear to be any greater than the age- and sex-adjusted rates of recurrent stroke in the general population. Thus, patients with mitral valve prolapse do not need any revised treatment for the prevention of recurrent cerebral ischemia. There is no need to test the clinical safety and efficacy of anticoagulant therapy for patients with mitral valve prolapse.

▶ This community-based study of a small cohort of patients with initial ischemic stroke or TIA and evidence of mitral valve prolapse concluded that this underlying condition appears not to confer increased risk of subsequent stroke when compared with the expected local population incidence in general. Two different analytic methods were used that employed stroke population statistics over 2 different epochs. Both methods yielded the same results. Intriguingly, 30 of the 49 patients with mitral prolapse had received anticoagulants at some period. Although statistical analysis was unable to show an effect of this anticoagulation on subsequent stroke occurrence, one wonders whether differences in the use of this or other medications in the prolapse population vs. the general stroke population might be a confounding factor in this type of analysis.

M.D. Ginsberg, M.D.

Diagnostic Techniques

Asymptomatic Cerebral Embolic Signals in Patients With Carotid Stenosis: Correlation With Appearance of Plaque Ulceration on Angiography

Valton L, Larrue V, Arrué P, et al (Rangueil Univ Hosp, Toulouse, France)
Stroke 26:813–815, 1995   2–5

Background.—Patients with greater than 70% narrowing or an angiographically defined ulceration of the internal carotid artery have an increased risk of stroke. Abnormal high-intensity transient signals (HITSs) indicating cerebral emboli can be seen on transcranial Doppler ultrasonograms of the middle cerebral arteries (MCAs) of even asymptomatic patients. The association between these embolic signals and carotid angiographic findings was investigated.

Methods.—The 40-minute recordings of transcranial Doppler monitoring for embolism in 26 patients were reviewed, as were the bilateral carotid angiograms. Of the 26 patients, 10 had experienced a cerebral transient ischemic attack, 1 had experienced a retinal transient ischemic attack, 9 had had an ischemic stroke, and 6 were asymptomatic. The angiograms and Doppler recordings were reviewed by independent neuroradiologists blinded to the findings of the other examination and the clinical data.

Results.—High-intensity transient signals were identified in 8 MCAs in 7 patients. Of these, 4 (50%) MCAs were symptomatic, as were 16 (40%) of the MCAs without HITSs. The internal carotid artery was narrowed by an average of 67% in patients with HITSs and 55% in patients without HITSs, a nonsignificant difference. Ipsilateral carotid angiograms identified ulceration in 63% of the patients with HITSs and only 23% of the patients without HITSs.

Conclusion.—Neither a history of clinical symptoms nor the degree of carotid stenosis was significantly predictive of embolic ultrasonographic signals. However, angiographic evidence of ulceration was significantly associated with embolic signals. Therefore, transcranial Doppler ultrasonographic monitoring may have clinical utility as a noninvasive assessment tool for evaluating the thromboembolic risk of carotid plaques.

▶ This report continues to increase our awareness that abnormal HITSs, which many previous studies have rather convincingly shown correspond in all probability to solid emboli, are a rather frequent occurrence by transcranial Doppler ultrasonography in the MCAs of patients with both asymptomatic and symptomatic carotid stenosis. This report made the additional point that the odds ratio of observing angiographic evidence of carotid ulceration is increased 5.7-fold in patients with embolic signals compared with patients without such signals. The full significance of these presumed embolic events is not known. Despite the fact that the majority are "asymptomatic" in the conventional sense, we still have no firm idea of more subtle ways in which these recurrent embolic events might induce cumulative injury. The latter topic should receive attention in future studies.

M.D. Ginsberg, M.D.

Transcranial Doppler–Detected Microemboli in Patients With Acute Stroke

Tong DC, Albers GW (Stanford Univ, Palo Alto, Calif)
Stroke 26:1588–1592, 1995   2–6

Background.—Transcranial Doppler sonography (TCD) can detect microembolic signals in various clinical conditions, including experimental

TABLE 2.—Embolic Sources by Subgroup

Group 1: High-risk embolic source (n = 18)	
Prosthetic valve (all aortic)	
Bioprosthetic	1
Mechanical	2
AF (11 chronic, 2 paroxysmal)	13
Carotid stenosis	2
Group 2: Embolic source of uncertain risk (n = 10)	
Internal carotid occlusion	2
Carotid siphon occlusion	1
Left ventricular thrombus (old)	2
Myocardial infarction (old)	2
PFO	2
Mitral strands and PFO	1
Group 3: Nonembolic source (n = 10)	
Vasculitis	2
Nonembolic	8

Abbreviations: AF, atrial fibrillation; *PFO,* patent foramen ovale.
(Tong DC, Albers GW: Transcranial Doppler–detected microemboli in patients with acute stroke; *Stroke;* 1995; 26:1588–1592; reproduced with permission of *Stroke;* Copyright 1995 American Heart Association.)

TABLE 4.—History of Prior Stroke or Transient Ischemic Attack Versus Presence of Embolic Phenomena

	Embolic-Positive Patients	Embolic-Negative Patients	Total
Prior stroke or TIA	4/4 (100)*	14/34 (41)	18/38 (47)
Stroke or TIA within 3 months	2/4 (50)*	1/34 (3)	3/38 (8)

Note: Values in parentheses are percentages.
* $P < 0.05$ for emboli-positive vs. emboli-negative subgroups.
Abbreviation: TIA, transient ischemic attack.
(Tong DC, Albers GW: Transcranial Doppler–detected microemboli in patients with acute stroke; *Stroke*; 1995; 26:1588–1592; reproduced with permission of *Stroke*; Copyright 1995 American Heart Association.)

models of embolization. Although the significance of these microemboli are not yet clear, several lines of evidence point to an association with increased risk of embolic stroke. The prevalence of TCD-detected microemboli and their relationship to risk of cerebral embolism was investigated in patients with acute stroke.

Patients and Findings.—Thirty-eight patients (mean age 70) with acute anterior circulation stroke were placed in 1 of 3 groups based on presumed mechanism of stroke. There were 18 patients in the high-risk group (group 1), 10 in the medium-risk group (group 2), and 10 in the low-risk group (group 3). All patients underwent TCD within 48 hours of admission.

No significant association between the prevalence of selected stroke factors and detection of microemboli was observed. Overall, microemboli were detected in 4 of the 38 patients, 3 of whom were in group 1. The remaining patient was in group 2 (Tables 2 and 4). Mechanical prosthetic valves were noted in 2 of the emboli-positive patients. High-grade carotid stenosis and a small patent foramen ovale associated with mitral valve strands also were observed in 1 patient each. No other source of embolization was identified in these patients after appropriate diagnostic evaluations were completed. In patients with microemboli, a history of cerebral ischemia and more recent symptoms (< 3 months) were more frequently noted compared with patients without microemboli. The number of microemboli was directly related to the acuity of previous symptoms among patients with a cardiac source of embolization.

Conclusion.—Microemboli detected on TCD were associated with an increased prevalence of previous cerebrovascular ischemia and may represent a risk factor for this condition. Transcranial Doppler sonography may help identify patients at higher risk for cerebrovascular ischemia, although further prospective studies using large numbers of patients are needed to better define this role.

▶ This useful study employing TCD sonography contributes to a rapidly accruing body of evidence that microemboli detected by TCD are indeed associated with increased prevalence of ischemic vascular events in the brain.

M.D. Ginsberg, M.D.

Asymptomatic Cerebral Embolic Signals in Symptomatic and Asymptomatic Carotid Artery Disease

Markus HS, Thomson ND, Brown MM (St George's Hosp, London)
Brain 118:1005–1011, 1995   2–7

Objective.—Transcranial Doppler ultrasonography was performed in a prospective study on patients with carotid stenosis, some of whom were asymptomatic, to detect embolic signals in the middle cerebral arteries (MCAs).

Study Design.—Thirty-seven patients with 38 symptomatic internal carotid artery stenoses of 30% or greater were studied within 6 months after transient ischemic attacks or a minor stroke. Twenty-one asymptomatic patients with carotid stenosis and 26 normal participants were examined. The average age of all participants was in the 60-year-old range. Each MCA was examined for 20 minutes using the same transcranial pulsed Doppler unit and a 2-MHz probe.

Findings.—Initial recordings demonstrated embolic signals in 21% of MCAs ipsilateral to symptomatic carotid stenosis, 4% of vessels ipsilateral to asymptomatic stenosis, and 1 of 52 MCAs in control participants. When all recordings, including 1-hour studies, were considered, half of 15 arteries with 80% stenosis yielded embolic signals. There was, however, no significant overall correlation between the presence or number of embolic signals and the degree of internal carotid stenosis. In 10 patients restudied 1 month after carotid endarterectomy, embolic signals were detected only in 1 patient who continued to have frequent amaurosis fugax; both the patient's symptoms and the embolic signals were eliminated by ingestion of aspirin.

Conclusion.—High-intensity embolic signals, resembling those produced by solid emboli in animal studies, are detected by transcranial Doppler ultrasonography in some patients having a potential source of cerebral embolism. This method may prove to be a useful means of estimating the risk of stroke and the need for endarterectomy or other treatment.

▶ This is an important prospective study that clearly established the high frequency of embolic phenomena in carotid arterial disease. The striking rank order of embolic signal frequency (normal vessels << asymptomatic vessels << symptomatic vessels), the extraordinary frequency in arteries with high-grade stenosis, and the subsidence of embolic signals after endarterectomy constitute powerful evidence indeed as to the symptomatic relevance of embolic events. As the authors suggested, transcranial Doppler ultrasonography may well prove to be a useful measure of stroke risk in this setting.

M.D. Ginsberg, M.D.

Ultrasound Findings in Carotid Artery Dissection: Analysis of 43 Patients
Sturzenegger M, Mattle HP, Rivoir A, et al (Univ of Bern, Switzerland)
Neurology 45:691–698, 1995   2–8

Introduction.—The use of ultrasound (US) holds promise as a noninvasive method of early diagnosis and follow-up of patients with internal carotid artery dissection (ICD). Although MRI can prove dissection, stenosis is difficult to grade with this imaging technique, and arteriopathies and tortuosities may not be detected. Because of these and other limitations of MRI, 43 consecutive patients were evaluated with US.

Patients and Methods.—The patients consisted of 28 men and 15 women (mean age 47). All had an extracranial ICD proved by angiography, MRI, or both at an average of 4.4 days after US was performed. Data were available on findings of complete physical and neurologic examinations, blood and blood chemistry, ECG, chest x-ray film, and x-ray examination of the cervical spine. All patients had Doppler sonography performed, and 39 patients had extracranial duplex scanning. Ultrasound examinations were performed at an average of 7.7 days after the onset of symptoms.

Results.—In 53% of patients, warning symptoms preceded the stroke. Intense unilateral headache occurred in 47%, as did a transient ischemic attack in 21%. Sensitivity in the detection of ICD was 93% for extracranial Doppler sonography, 86% for transcranial Doppler sonography, and 79% for duplex sonography, for an overall sensitivity of 95%. All occlusions and high-grade stenoses were detected by the 3 methods. The combined methods had an 80% detection rate in patients with moderate- or low-grade stenoses. Extracranial Doppler was more successful (70%) in these cases than were transcranial Doppler (40%) and duplex sonography (20%). The US findings in the 33 patients with occlusion or high-grade stenosis included absent flow signal in the internal carotid artery (100%) and biphasic flow in its bulb (86%), a high-resistance flow pattern of the ipsilateral common carotid artery (91%), signs of collateral flow across the circle of Willis (97%), and low flow in the middle cerebral artery on transcranial insonation (79%). Duplex examination confirmed absent internal carotid artery flow or stump flow in occlusion or high-grade stenosis (100%), and excluded an atherosclerotic origin by revealing a patent bulb (100%) and the absence of plaques (95%). Forty patients had US follow-up at 6- to 8-week intervals; 63% had recanalization that occurred at variable intervals of up to 6 months.

Conclusions.—Diagnosis of ICD cannot be made on clinical grounds because findings are variable. In this group of patients with suspected ICD, hemodynamic findings at US were abnormal in 95% for the 3 techniques combined. Diagnostic sensitivity was decreased in cases of low-grade stenosis. The combination of Doppler and duplex examination offers a sensitive screening method and a powerful diagnostic tool for ICD.

▶ This rather sizable series of consecutive patients with carotid dissection used both extracranial and transcranial Doppler and duplex sonography. Despite the nearly 100% diagnostic sensitivity when all 3 US methods were used in combination in patients who had either an occlusion or a high-grade stenosis, the authors themselves noted that neither of these findings in combination nor any single finding was pathognomonic for ICD. Furthermore, the specificity of these methods could not be assessed, because the patient group was thought to be biased toward those at greater risk of developing cerebral ischemia resulting from more severe stenosis.

M.D. Ginsberg, M.D.

Treatment

Intravenous Thrombolysis With Recombinant Tissue Plasminogen Activator for Acute Hemispheric Stroke: The European Cooperative Acute Stroke Study (ECASS)
Hacke W, for the ECASS Study Group (Univ of Heidelberg, Germany; Univ of Helsinki; Univ of Rome; et al)
JAMA 274:1017–1025, 1995   2–9

Objective.—The safety and efficacy of IV thrombolysis in patients with acute ischemic stroke were examined in a prospective, randomized, double-blind, placebo-controlled trial entitled the European Cooperative Acute Stroke Study. A total of 620 adult patients with at least moderate neurologic deficit from hemispheric stroke but no major early signs of infarction on CT examination were recruited at 75 hospitals in 14 European countries. Patients with existing neurologic conditions causing disability or concomitant medical disorders were not included.

Treatment.—Patients were randomized to receive either recombinant tissue plasminogen activator (rt-PA) or placebo intravenously. The dose of rt-PA was 1.1 mg/kg up to 100 mg. A bolus consisting of 10% of the total dose was given over 1 to 2 minutes, followed by a 1-hour infusion of the rest of the dose. Data were available for 247 actively treated patients and 264 placebo recipients.

Efficacy.—After 3 months, no significant difference was evident in Barthel Index scores between the patients given rt-PA and those given placebo. Rankin Scale scores were somewhat better in actively treated patients in an intention-to-treat (ITT) analysis. Mortality 1 month after stroke was greater in the actively treated patients, but not significantly so. Neurologic scores did not improve significantly in the rt-PA group within the first week after stroke. Surviving patients who received active treatment spent less time in the hospital than those assigned to receive placebo.

Survival and Safety.—In the ITT analysis and the target population, case fatality rates were consistently higher in patients given rt-PA (Fig). Intra-

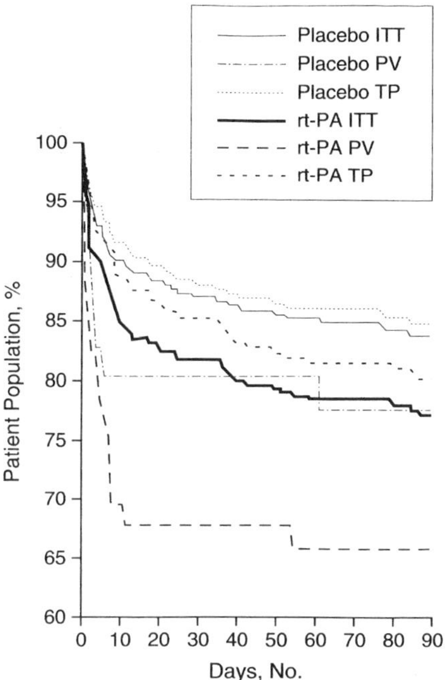

FIGURE.—Kaplan-Meier survival curve depicted for the different patient cohorts. Seven-day survival is lowest in the group of patients with protocol violations treated with recombinant tissue-type plasminogen activator. Highest survival rates are found in the target population placebo group and the intention-to-treat placebo groups. Differences in survival between recombinant tissue-type plasminogen activator–treated patients and placebo groups reach significance only after 90 days in both the target population and the intention-to-treat group. Among the patients with protocol violations, the difference is significant after 7 days. Note that the *y* axis begins at 60%. *Abbreviations: ITT,* intention-to-treat; *PV,* protocol violations; *TP,* target population; *rt-PA,* recombinant tissue-type plasminogen activator. (*JAMA;* October 4, 1995; 274:1017–1025; Copyright 1995, American Medical Association.)

cranial hemorrhage was comparably frequent in the 2 groups. In the ITT analysis, 40% of patients had some degree of intracranial bleeding.

Implications.—Although IV rt-PA provides for neurologic improvement in some patients with acute ischemic stroke, it is difficult to determine the patients who are likely to respond. Because ineligible patients who are treated have an unacceptably increased risk of hemorrhagic complications and death, this treatment cannot be recommended for an unselected patient population.

▶ This was an ambitious multicenter study, and its results are of interest but must be interpreted with considerable caution. Not emphasized in the abstract is the fact that patients were randomized to treatment with rt-PA or placebo within *6 hours* from the onset of symptoms, and the mean or median time to treatment (not clear from Table 2 of the original article) from the onset of symptoms was 4.3 to 4.4 hours. In fact, the majority of patients were entered in the *4- to 6-hour* time window. There is reason to believe that the 4- to 6-hour window is possibly too late for the efficacious application of rt-PA. The recently published results of the National Institutes of Health

(NIH) trial clearly indicate that rt-PA administered *within 3 hours* of stroke onset and at a dose of 0.9 mg/kg was convincingly demonstrated to improve neurologic outcome (as measured by a variety of outcome scales) at 3 months and that mortality was comparable in treated vs. untreated patients. Thus, the major suggestion of the ECASS, that thrombolysis may be effective in a subgroup of patients "with moderate to severe neurologic deficit and without extended infarct signs on the initial CT scan" may be a finding applicable only to patients entered in the relatively late (4- to 6-hour) time window after stroke onset (and treated at the dose level used in that study). The NIH study results, by contrast, suggest that earlier onset of systemic rt-PA therapy is, in fact, efficacious in all ischemic stroke subgroups.

M.D. Ginsberg, M.D.

Reference

1. NINDS and Stroke rt-PA Stroke Study Group: Tissue plasminogen activates for acute ischemic stroke. *N Engl J Med* 333:1581–1587, 1995.

ECASS: Lessons for Future Thrombolytic Stroke Trials
Fisher M, Pessin MS, Furian AJ (Univ of Massachusetts, Worcester; Tufts Univ, Boston; Cleveland Clinic Found, Ohio)
JAMA 274:1058–1059, 1995   2–10

The Trial.—The European Cooperative Acute Stroke Study (ECASS) was the first large-scale randomized, blinded study of high-dose IV recombinant tissue-type plasminogen activator (rt-PA) treatment for acute stroke. More than 600 patients, seen within 6 hours of the onset, were recruited by 75 centers in 14 countries. An intention-to-treat analysis failed to show that rt-PA was beneficial. There were, however, indications that patients with stroke might benefit from thrombolysis provided that more refined selection criteria are used and treatment is administered more effectively.

Diagnosis.—Inexplicably, experienced investigators misinterpreted a number of the initial CT studies. Whether this reflected inadequate education or overlooking subtle abnormalities in the hyperacute setting is not clear. When CT "violators" were removed, a greater proportion of patients made an excellent recovery, but the rate of cerebral hemorrhage did not change significantly. It may be feasible to identify those patients with unsalvageable ischemia through the presence of CT hypodensity shortly after the onset of stroke. Compromised arterial blood flow may be detected by single-photon emission CT, MR angiography, or perfusion MRI. A lack of vascular imaging in the ECASS meant that lesions that might not require thrombolysis and those not expected to respond optimally were not identified.

Treatment.—Recanalization may be more consistently achieved by supraselective catheterization, allowing thrombolytic agents to be administered directly into the thrombus or proximal to it. This does not seem to entail an increased risk of parenchymal brain hemorrhage. Optimally, rt-PA will be administered after an imaging study but within 3 hours after the onset of stroke.

▶ This is an editorial comment on the ECASS study (see Abstract 2–9). The ECASS and this editorial comment were both published before the National Institutes of Health multicenter study that convincingly established the efficacy of rt-PA in ischemic stroke when used up to 3 hours after stroke onset. The issues raised in this editorial comment, including the possible "more consistent" recanalization achieved by the use of supraselective arterial catheterization with local delivery of thrombolytic agents, await the results of further study.

M.D. Ginsberg, M.D.

Clinical Features and Pathogenesis of Intracerebral Hemorrhage After rt-PA and Heparin Therapy for Acute Myocardial Infarction: The Thrombolysis in Myocardial Infarction (TIMI) II Pilot and Randomized Clinical Trial Combined Experience
Sloan MA, for the TIMI Investigators (Maryland Med Research Inst, Baltimore; Univ of Maryland, Baltimore; Univ of Miami, Fla; et al)
Neurology 45:649–658, 1995   2–11

Introduction.—Intracranial hemorrhage (ICH) occurring as a complication of thrombolytic therapy for acute myocardial infarction (MI) has reported frequencies ranging from 0.1% to 0.9%, depending on the agent administered. The nature of ICH in this setting was studied in the Thrombolysis in Myocardial Infarction (TIMI) II Pilot and Randomized Clinical Trial involving 23 participants.

Methods.—Patients eligible for TIMI II were seen within the first 4 hours of MI with ST-segment elevation and treated with recombinant tissue-type plasminogen activator (rt-PA), heparin, and aspirin. The dose of rt-PA was reduced from 150 to 100 mg after an unexpected number of ICHs occurred with the higher dose. Overall, 23 of 56 cerebrovascular complications were primary parenchymatous ICHs. These 23 cases were reviewed for clinical and radiologic features, type of manifestation, associated factors, and temporal course.

Results.—Fourteen of the patients were men, and 9 were women. Most (87%) were white, and the mean age of the group was 63.3. Three of 10 patients given 150 mg of rt-PA and 6 of 11 in the 100-mg group had low body weight (weight was not reported for 2 patients). A history of hypertension was present in 61%, and 56.5% developed or maintained systolic blood pressure of 160 mm Hg or more or diastolic blood pressure of 90 mm Hg or more during the rt-PA infusion and before onset of neurologic symptoms. The most common initial finding (82%) was a decreased level of consciousness. Although onset was usually gradual, 61% of patients exhibited a maximal deficit within 6 hours of onset. The site of the primary hemorrhage was lobar in 16, thalamic in 4, and brain stem–cerebellum in 3 patients. Six patients had multiple lobar hemorrhages. The mean size of the primary ICHs was 35.8 mL, and size did not differ in the 100-mg and 150-mg rt-PA groups. Hypofibrinogenemia was present in 4 patients and was profound in 3. Three of the 5 patients who died as a result of ICH were found to have had cerebral amyloid angiopathy. The overall case fatality rate within 1 month was 48%.

Conclusions.—A temporal relationship was observed between rt-PA administration and ICH. Hemorrhage was initiated and enlarged during the period of active fibrinolysis and may have been potentiated by concomitant antithrombotic therapy. Factors that may contribute to ICH in this setting are acute or persistent hypertension before or during rt-PA infusion, life-threatening ventricular arrhythmias, cerebral amyloid angiopathy and other vascular lesions, and hypofibrinogenemia.

▶ In the large TIMI II trial of thrombolytic therapy for acute MI, primary intraparenchymal brain hemorrhages accounted for half of all cerebrovascular complications and occurred in 1.3% of patients treated with the higher (150-mg) dose of rt-PA and in 0.4% treated with the 100-mg dose. This report, a retrospective analysis of these patients, called attention to a number of possible risk factors for ICH, including higher rt-PA dose, lower body weight, presence of hypertension, ventricular arrhythmias, hypofibrinogenemia, underlying cerebral amyloid angiopathy, and concomitant heparin therapy. Unfortunately, the retrospective, non–case-control nature of this report makes it impossible to know the relative importance of any of these factors. The predominantly lobar distribution of many of these hemorrhages would suggest that hypertension, by itself, may not be the primary risk factor in these patients. In general, the presence of underlying cerebral abnormalities that might predispose to ICH with rt-PA needs to be kept in mind, but, from the data of this report, it can only be speculated.

M.D. Ginsberg, M.D.

Does Arterial Recanalization Improve Outcome in Carotid Territory Stroke?
von Kummer R, Holle R, Rosin L, et al (Univ of Heidelberg, Germany)
Stroke 26:581–587, 1995   2–12

Objective.—Acute stroke patients with occlusion of the middle cerebral artery were prospectively studied by repeated CT, angiography, and transcranial Doppler ultrasound (TCD) before and after thrombolytic therapy to determine whether arterial recanalization can independently influence clinical course after stroke.

Subjects.—From February 1988 to October 1993, 77 consecutive patients with acute hemispheric stroke were entered in this study.

Methods.—Patients were examined by combined Scandinavian Stroke Score and neurologic status at admission, CT and angiography before and after thrombolytic treatment, and TCD 24 hours after thrombolytic therapy.

Results.—Recanalization rates at 8 and 24 hours after stroke correlated with occlusion site, collateral blood supply, and Scandinavian Stroke Score at admission. The middle cerebral artery branch had a good recanalization rate, whereas the intracranial internal carotid artery bifurcation had a low rate of recanalization. Six of 7 patients with delayed recanalization had good outcomes. Recanalization less than 8 hours after symptom onset had no independent predictive value. Recanalization at 24 hours was associated with a favorable outcome. Recanalization had no independent effect on mortality in this group of stroke patients.

Conclusion.—In this group of patients with occlusion of the middle cerebral artery, arterial recanalization was difficult to achieve within 8 hours of stroke onset, especially when collaterals were scarce and the occlusion occurred in an adverse site such as the intracranial internal carotid bifurcation. When conditions were more favorable, arterial recanalization improved clinical outcome even if it occurred more than 8 hours after symptom onset. The site of arterial occlusion, state of collaterals, and extent of parenchymal hypodensity should be considered when trials are designed to assess the effect of recanalizing therapies for acute stroke.

▶ This is an interesting study, but it is important to note that although prospective, it was not randomized and, in fact, incorporated a variety of treatments (intra-arterial urokinase, intra-arterial recombinant tissue-type plasminogen activator, and IV tissue plasminogen activator). Treatment was initiated within 6 hours, and, in fact, the interval to treatment appears to have averaged around 4 to 4½ hours. Nonetheless, recanalization in some patients occurred in a delayed fashion. The fact that recanalization observed at 24 hours was associated with an increased proportion of good outcomes (23%–75%) does not imply a cause and effect relationship because these data cannot be compared within the study to a *comparable* group of patients who did not show this effect. It is interesting that the middle cerebral artery trunk occlusion was the predominant occlusion site in patients with recanalization between 8 and 24 hours. To recapitulate, this study should not be construed as showing a potential benefit of delayed recanalization, because this may represent merely an epiphenomenon in a more favorable patient subgroup. Experimental and clinical evidence strongly favors the initiation of thrombolytic therapy as early as possible after ischemic stroke.

M.D. Ginsberg, M.D.

Treatment of Dural Sinus Thrombosis Using Selective Catheterization and Urokinase

Horowitz M, Purdy P, Unwin H, et al (Univ of Texas Southwestern Med Ctr, Dallas; Children's Hosp of Dallas; Scott and White Clinic, Temple, Tex)
Ann Neurol 38:58–67, 1995
2–13

Objective.—Experience with 12 patients with thrombosed cerebral dural venous sinuses who underwent transvenous catheterization and urokinase infusion was added to the 13 cases previously reported in the English literature.

Patients.—The study consisted of 5 males and 7 females aged 6 weeks to 65 years with thrombosis involving the sagittal sinus and at least 1 transverse sinus. All patients were fully heparinized; the partial thromboplastin times were 1.5 to 2 times control.

Management.—A No. 6 French sheath was placed in a femoral vein (preferably the right-sided femoral vein) and another in the contralateral femoral artery. A complete cerebral angiographic study was done, extending imaging into the late venous phase. A catheter and wire were advanced via the femoral vein through the right atrium and into the superior cava. If feasible, the right internal jugular vein was catheterized, and a microcatheter was advanced coaxially over a guide wire into the involved sinus or sinuses. A number of back and forth rotary motions were necessary at times. Urokinase was instilled at 15-minute intervals in aliquots of 50,000 IU to bathe the thrombus. The total dose ranged from 250,000 to 500,000 IU. The system was secured to the thigh, and patients received a continuous infusion at a rate of 60,000 to 100,000 units/hour. Venography was repeated 18 to 24 hours later, and an arteriogram was obtained if the sinuses appeared to be patent.

Results.—There were no major complications of treatment despite the fact that 5 patients had preinfusion infarcts, 4 of which were hemorrhagic. The treated sinus was functionally patent in all but 1 of the 12 patients. The only failure was in 1 patient who had been symptomatic for at least 2 months. Ten of the 11 patients followed had good to excellent clinical outcomes.

Conclusion.—Selective catheterization of the thrombosed dural venous sinus with instillation of urokinase is a safe and effective approach. Further work is needed to identify those patients whose conditions can be managed by systemic heparinization or merely observed.

▶ This encouraging series showed that of 12 patients treated with urokinase delivered via transfemoral catheter directly into thrombosed cerebral dural sinuses, 11 patients showed reestablishment of venous sinus drainage or complete resolution of the thrombus with neurologic improvement. Treatment durations of 36 hours to several days were necessary to achieve this result. A large spectrum of presumed etiologies was represented (dehydration, oral contraceptives, tumor, systemic lupus erythematosus, sinusitis, mastoiditis, etc.). It is unlikely that controlled studies of thrombolytic therapy in this condition will ever be undertaken because of the rarity of the condition and its multiple etiologies. The impressive clinical outcome in these patients and the absence of major therapeutic morbidity argue strongly for thrombolytic treatment, particularly when it can be instituted early in the course of the disease. The previous literature in this condition supports a beneficial therapeutic effect of heparin as well, though of less striking benefit than thrombolysis in the present study. It should be noted that all patients of this series were receiving warfarin at the time of discharge.

M.D. Ginsberg, M.D.

Early Anticoagulation After Large Cerebral Embolic Infarction: A Safety Study

Chamorro A, Vila N, Saiz A, et al (Hosp Clin i Provincial, Barcelona, Spain)
Neurology 45:861–865, 1995   2–14

Background.—The safety of early anticoagulation after embolic stroke has been questioned, particularly in patients with severe strokes and large infarctions. However, there are no clearly established definitions of severity, infarction size, or timing. The relationship between admission clinical indices of severity, infarction size, and the occurrence of hemorrhagic complications was evaluated prospectively in patients with nonseptic cerebral embolic infarctions who were given early anticoagulation treatment.

Methods.—Over a 5-month period, 83 patients with cerebral infarctions were given anticoagulants within 72 hours of the onset of symptoms. On admission, the patients were classified into either the high-risk group (stroke symptoms indicating involvement of 3 or more CNS domains, a Mathew Scale score of 74 or less, or CT evidence of hemorrhagic infarction) or the low-risk group (stroke symptoms indicating involvement of fewer than 3 domains, a Mathew Scale score of greater than 74, and no CT evidence of blood). Infarction size was calculated from CT images. Changes in hemorrhagic status based on clinical and radiologic assessment were noted in each group.

Results.—There were 46 patients in the high-risk group and 37 patients in the low-risk group. The 2 groups did not demonstrate significantly different trends for hemorrhagic transformation (occurring in 26% of the high-risk group and 22% of the low-risk group) or for hemorrhagic worsening (occurring in 4% of the high-risk group and 14% of the low-risk group). Hemorrhagic worsening was significantly associated only with a mean activated partial thromboplastin time (aPTT) more than twice as high as control values. The timing of heparin administration was similar in patients in whom hemorrhagic worsening did or did not develop.

Conclusion.—The development of hemorrhagic complications was not related to either the neurologic deficit or the size of the infarction. Therefore, a delay in heparin administration when clinically indicated is not justified in alert patients. However, the level of anticoagulation should be carefully monitored to maintain the aPTT at less than twice the control value.

▶ The risk of recurrent embolization in the first days or weeks after an embolic cerebral infarct is substantial, yet clinicians are hesitant to institute prompt anticoagulation for fear of precipitating hemorrhagic transformation or frank intracerebral hemorrhage. This report is important in that it showed that anticoagulation with heparin within the first 72 hours is safe provided that the aPTT is rigorously monitored and kept at about 1.5 times control. These data clearly show that patients who experienced clinical hemorrhagic worsening had a mean aPTTs of 2.9 ± 0.8 compared with an aPPT of 1.6 ± 0.4 in patients not showing such worsening—a highly significant difference. Thus, prompt but judiciously regulated heparinization appears appropriate in the management of large cerebral embolic infarction.

M.D. Ginsberg, M.D.

The Warfarin-Aspirin Symptomatic Intracranial Disease Study
Chimowitz MI, for the Warfarin-Aspirin Symptomatic Intracranial Disease Study Group (Univ of Michigan Med Ctr, Ann Arbor; Henry Ford Hosp and Health Science Ctr, Detroit; Tufts–New England Med Ctr, Boston; et al)
Neurology 45:1488–1493, 1995   2–15

Objective.—The effectiveness of warfarin was compared with that of aspirin for preventing ischemic stroke, myocardial infarction, and sudden death in patients having symptomatic stenosis of a major intracranial artery in a retrospective multicenter study.

Patients.—Seven centers enrolled 151 patients in the study, all of whom had at least 50% stenosis of the carotid, vertebral, or basilar artery or 1 of the major cerebral vessels. In addition, all patients had transient ischemic attacks (62 patients) or stroke (89) in the territory of the stenotic artery. Patients with occlusion of an intracranial vessel or extracranial internal carotid stenosis of 50% or greater proximal to an intracranial stenosis were excluded.

Treatment.—The local physician selected treatment with either 325 mg of aspirin daily or warfarin, the latter adjusted to maintain the prothrombin time at 1.2 to 1.6 of control. Eighty-eight patients received warfarin, and 63 received aspirin. The 2 groups were comparable with respect to age, degree of stenosis, and vascular risk factors.

Results.—Major vascular events occurred at a rate of 18 per 100 patient-years of follow-up in aspirin-treated patients and at a rate of 8 per 100 patient-years in the warfarin group. The relative risk of stroke, myocardial infarction, or sudden death in warfarin-treated patients was 0.46. There were no major hemorrhagic complications in the aspirin group, but 3 warfarin-treated patients had such complications and 2 of them died.

Conclusion.—Warfarin may prevent major vascular events more effectively than aspirin in patients with symptomatic stenosis of a major intracranial artery. The present findings warrant a prospective randomized trial.

▶ This intriguing study was designed to provide pilot data comparing the efficacy of warfarin and aspirin in preventing recurrent ischemic stroke, myocardial infarction, or sudden death in patients with clinically symptomatic stenoses of an intracranial artery. This multicenter effort, which was intended to serve as a prelude to a randomized study, was retrospective, was nonrandomized, and considered only 151 patients (of whom 89 had had a prior stroke and 62 had had transient ischemic attacks as qualifying events). The decision as to whether to treat with aspirin or warfarin was made by the local treating physicians, a possible source of considerable intergroup bias. The outcome of the study is nonetheless intriguing: compared with aspirin, warfarin-treated patients had more than a 50% reduction in major outcome events. As the authors noted, the high incidence of stroke in patients who were switched from warfarin to aspirin after an asymptomatic period of 3 to 6 months on warfarin calls into question the common current clinical practice of a several-month period of anticoagulation followed by aspirin therapy. One awaits with interest the outcome of a prospective randomized trial to compare these 2 widely used agents.

M.D. Ginsberg, M.D.

Hemorrhage

Neurosurgical Management of Cerebellar Haematoma and Infarct

Mathew P, Teasdale G, Bannan A, et al (Inst of Neurological Sciences, Glasgow, Scotland)
J Neurol Neurosurg Psychiatry 59:287–292, 1995　　　　　　　　2–16

Objective.—The efficacy of nonoperative management of 39 patients having cerebellar hematoma and 50 others with an infarct was examined. The clinical features overlapped substantially between these groups. Compression of the brain stem and fourth ventricle was more prevalent than hydrocephalus.

Management.—Fifty-four patients were treated conservatively at the outset, whereas 35 underwent external ventricular drainage or craniectomy. In 6 of the latter, the decision to operate was made secondarily. Eight patients had craniectomy after a trial of drainage failed. The patients who were successfully managed conservatively tended to be younger, their symptoms manifested earlier, and they had a higher level of consciousness. Initial surgery was selected more often for patients with hematoma than for those with cerebellar infarction.

Outcome.—All but 3 of the 39 patients with a cerebellar hematoma recovered independent function. Four patients remained moderately disabled. In all 3 fatal cases a treatment-limiting decision was made at the outset. Forty-three of 50 patients with infarcts recovered, 2 with moderate disability. All 3 patients who died were elderly and in deep coma. All but 1 of the 34 infarct patients whose conditions were managed conservatively made a good recovery.

Recommendations.—A patient with cerebellar hematoma or infarction who secondarily becomes comatose should undergo evacuation on an urgent basis. If coma is present from the outset or a patient secondarily becomes deeply comatose and has hydrocephalus, external drainage is indicated. Evacuation follows if the patient improves, but otherwise a treatment-limiting decision is appropriate.

▶ These authors reported their impressive experience in managing cerebellar hematomas and infarcts, conditions that share in common their life-threatening mass effects in the posterior fossa. The article contained useful flow diagrams depicting the authors' recommendations for neurosurgical management of these 2 similar conditions. For cerebellar hematoma, craniectomy with evacuation of the lesion was undertaken in patients who were conscious on admission to hospital but who later deteriorated to coma or develop acute hydrocephalus and in initially comatose patients with hydrocephalus who improved with external ventricular drainage. By contrast, in the management of cerebellar infarct, the authors chose external ventricular drainage as the initial procedure in both initially conscious and initially comatose patients showing acute hydrocephalus, but chose craniectomy as the initial procedure in patients conscious on admission to hospital who deteriorated to coma. Thus, only 2 patients of 50 with cerebral infarct were managed with craniectomy, 7 with external ventricular drainage, and 34 patients were managed conservatively, of whom 33 had a good outcome. These are useful guidelines for clinicians confronting these conditions.

M.D. Ginsberg, M.D.

Recurrence of Bleeding in Patients With Primary Intracerebral Hemorrhage

Passero S, Burgalassi L, D'Andrea P, et al (Univ di Siena, Italy)
Stroke 26:1189–1192, 1995   2–17

Background.—Recurrent bleeding in patients with primary intracerebral hemorrhage has not been thoroughly studied. The frequency of rebleeding was determined to help clarify the natural course of this subtype of stroke, and risk factors were identified to improve secondary prevention.

Methods.—One hundred twelve survivors of a first primary intracerebral hemorrhage were followed prospectively for a mean 84 months after hospital discharge. Several demographic variables, medical history, and clinical and laboratory findings were analyzed to determine possible risk factors for rebleeding.

Findings.—Twenty-seven survivors (24%) had 1 or more rebleedings during follow-up. Eight recurrences (30%) happened in the first year of follow-up, the remainder occurring up to 11.5 years later. The mortality associated with rebleeding was high. Seventy percent of the patients died of their second or third hemorrhage. In univariate and multivariate analyses, the only significant predictor of rebleeding was lobar location of the first hemorrhage. Patients with rebleeding tended to be older and to have a history of previous transient ischemic attack or ischemic stroke than patients without rebleeding. The former also had hyperlipidemia less often than the latter. However, these associations were nonsignificant. Poor control of arterial hypertension during follow-up was documented in 7% of hypertensive patients without rebleeding and in 47% of hypertensive patients with rebleeding.

Conclusion.—Rebleeding after a first primary intracerebral hemorrhage is not as uncommon as generally believed. The risk of rebleeding is apparently high after hemorrhage at the junction of the gray and white matter, a site considered typical of hemorrhages caused by amyloid angiopathy, and when control of arterial hypertension is poor.

▶ This useful survey pointed out that rebleeding after a primary intracerebral hemorrhage is more common than might be expected at first glance. Interestingly, poor control of hypertension after the first bleed was 7 times more common in patients who underwent subsequent rebleeding than in those who did not. Patients whose first intracerebral hemorrhage was in a lobar location had a higher proportion of rebleeding than did patients with hemorrhages in other locations, a finding that, as the authors noted, may implicate amyloid angiopathy as an underlying condition particularly predisposing toward recurrent hemorrhage. It is of note, however, that only approximately one third of patients with rebleeds had identical loci for the first and second hemorrhages. This may also suggest that certain etiologies of primary hemorrhage predispose to recurrent hemorrhage at multifocal sites.

M.D. Ginsberg, M.D.

Vasculopathies

Clinical Characteristics of Rapidly Progressive Leuko-Araiosis
Tarvonen-Schröder S, Räihä I, Kurki T, et al (Univ of Turku, Finland; Turku Univ Hosp, Finland)
Acta Neurol Scand 91:399–404, 1995   2–18

Introduction.—When periventricular white matter hypodensity is noted on CT scans in the absence of hydrocephalus or known white matter disease, it is termed leukoaraiosis (LA). No studies have been published describing the progression of the LA finding on CT. The progression of LA and its clinical relevance were examined in prospective follow-up study of patients with CT-defined LA.

Study Population.—Computed tomography brain scans were performed for 252 patients from January to December 1989 in Turku City Hospital. Of these, 111 had a finding of LA. From September to December 1992, 40 of these patients were reassessed. Two were excluded from the study due to hydrocephalus. The remaining 38 patients comprised the study group.

Findings.—During follow-up CT, 11 of the 38 patients had rapid progression of LA. There were no differences in the number of infarctions at baseline or the number of cortical or central infarctions between the progressing LA (prLA) and the nonprogressing LA (nprLA) group of patients. At follow-up, the number of infarctions had increased in both groups. In the prLA groups, this was caused by an increase in cortical infarctions, whereas in the nprLA group it was caused by an increase in central infarctions. Whereas prLA was associated with heart failure and atrial fibrillation, nprLA was associated with sudden onset of symptoms.

Conclusion.—These results suggest that there are different subgroups within a population of patients with LA findings on CT. Rapid progression of LA was found in one third of a series of 38 patients. There was no difference in the number or type of infarctions between these 2 groups at baseline. At follow-up, prLA was associated with cortical infarctions, heart failure, and atrial fibrillation, whereas nprLA was associated with central infarctions and sudden onset of symptoms. The occurrence of LA was not related to infarction distribution, and the progression of LA was not related to the number of brain infarctions. Other cardiovascular risk factors did not differentiate between these 2 groups.

▶ This interesting study reported progression of LA (over a follow-up averaging 3.2 years) in almost one third of a series of 38 patients. The latter can be regarded as representative of the 111 patients initially studied by CT; this study is thus an important reminder that LA may progress over a short period. The increasing number of cortical infarcts in the prLA patients, contrasting with a slight increase in central (i.e., lacunar) infarcts in nprLA patients, defied a facile explanation but may hint at differences in underlying vascular mechanisms in these 2 subgroups. More interesting is the significantly higher incidence of heart failure (82% vs. 37%) and of atrial fibrillation (55% vs. 19%) in the prLA group. It seems reasonable to regard these as potential risk factors for progression of LA, providing another rationale for therapeutic intervention in these states.

M.D. Ginsberg, M.D.

Cerebral Autosomal Dominant Arteriopathy With Subcortical Infarcts and Leukoencephalopathy: A Clinicopathological and Genetic Study of a Swiss Family

Jung HH, Bassetti C, Tournier-Lasserve E, et al (Univ Hosp Bern, Switzerland; INSERM U25, Paris; Univ Hosp Zürich, Switzerland)
J Neurol Neurosurg Psychiatry 59:138–143, 1995   2–19

Background.—Various causes have been identified for familial stroke. In the past 20 years, several clinical reports have discussed familial disorders with an autosomal dominant pattern of inheritance consisting of recurrent strokelike episodes and the development of subcortical dementia in the absence of major vascular risk factors, particularly hypertension. A Swiss family with autosomal dominant disease characterized by recurrent strokelike episodes and the development of subcortical dementia with genetic linkage to chromosome 19 was described.

Methods and Findings.—The family was affected by cerebral autosomal dominant arteriopathy with subcortical infarcts and leukoencephalopathy (CADASIL) linked to chromosome 19q12. Several members in 3 generations had recurrent strokelike episodes. In some, subcortical dementia, migrainelike headaches, and depression developed. Clinically affected members had multiple subcortical infarcts and diffuse leukoencephalopathy on MRI. In 1 family member, necropsy demonstrated a distinctive nonamyloid and nonatherosclerotic angiopathy or small cerebral and leptomeningeal arteries with concentric depositions of a basophilic granular material replacing the smooth muscle cells of the media. Linkage analysis was done with 6 chromosome 19 markers spanning the estimated CADASIL interval. There were no recombinant or positive lod scores, which strongly suggested linkage of this condition to the CADASIL locus.

Conclusion.—Cerebral autosomal dominant arteriopathy with subcortical infarcts and leukoencephalopathy is a syndrome with distinctive clinical, neuroradiologic, and histopathologic characteristics linked to a specific chromosomal locus. Its occurrence in several unrelated families suggests a genetic homogeneity. The current findings suggest that CADASIL is a type of hereditary stroke that is more common than believed. It should be considered in the differential diagnosis of hereditary stroke.

▶ This report rather thoroughly investigated a Swiss family with the CADASIL syndrome, an entity emerging as an intriguing cause of recurrent familial stroke. The 1 necropsy case in this series supported the notion that this syndrome is produced by an unusual vasculopathy, distinct from atherosclerosis and amyloid angiopathy, characterized by granular degeneration of the media and loss of smooth muscle cell actin. One awaits with interest the eventual identification of the abnormal gene product in this condition.

M.D. Ginsberg M.D.

Vascular Malformations of the Central Nervous System

Challa VR, Moody DM, Brown WR (Wake Forest Univ, Winston-Salem, NC)
J Neuropathol Exp Neurol 54:609–621, 1995   2–20

Objective.—Vascular malformations of the brain and spinal cord remain clinically dangerous lesions, despite advances in diagnostic and interventional neuroradiology and surgical techniques. Staining and radiographic techniques were investigated to better understand the nature and structure of and damage done by these malformations.

Discussion.—Calcifications were frequently observed in vascular malformations and occasionally were seen on plain radiographs. At times differentiation from tumor calcifications was difficult. Intravenous contrast material considerably enhanced the visibility of these malformations on CT scans, although cerebral or spinal cord angiography was sometimes required to evaluate vascular nature and differentiate from tumor. Parenchymal and subarachnoid hemorrhages were seen clearly on contrast-enhanced CT. Magnetic resonance angiography and flow analysis, in addition to MRI, provided essential information in instances of angiographically occult malformations with profuse hemosiderin and blood breakdown products.

On CT, cavernous angiomas were visualized as hyperdense, well-defined lesions. In cases of arteriovenous malformations (AVMs), vascular nature, as well as size, site, and origin and number of the feeding vessels, could be identified on cerebral angiography. Typically AVMs were wedge shaped, with the base situated toward the leptomeninges and the apex directed toward the center of the brain. With venous angiomas, a system of venules ending in a collecting vein was a common finding. The collecting vein emptied into a subependymal vein or a transcerebral vein that entered the subarachnoid space.

Conclusion.—The possibility of missed multiple malformations can be eliminated by performing 4-vessel angiography. However, 15% of vascular malformations, particularly cavernous angiomas and small AVMs, may go undetected on angiography, and some may be missed on CT examination as well. In such instances, the MRI may be abnormal, thereby improving sensitivity and specificity of radiologic diagnoses of lesions. There is, at present, no reliable radiologic method to visualize capillary telangiectases.

▶ This useful review article discussed the classification of CNS vascular malformations, their modes of clinical manifestation, radiologic appearances, and neuropathologic conditions. The article was beautifully illustrated with representative cerebral arteriograms, CT scans, MR images, and gross and microscopic histopathologic material. It is recommended to the general reader as a superb and succinct compendium of information on this important area of cerebrovascular abnormalities.

M.D. Ginsberg, M.D.

3 Epilepsy and Electroencephalography

Diagnosis for True Seizures and Pseudoseizures

Clinical Utility of Video-EEG Monitoring

Chen LS, Mitchell WG, Horton EJ, et al (Childrens Hosp Los Angeles; Univ of Southern California, Los Angeles)
Pediatr Neurol 12:220–224, 1995   3–1

Objective.—Split-screen video electroencephalography (EEG) permits a correlation of paroxysmal behavior with EEG findings. This technique has proved useful in the diagnosis of a number of different conditions such as pseudoseizures, staring episodes, head drops, and shuddering attacks. However, video-EEG is very expensive, so its diagnostic value must be carefully defined. The general usefulness of continuous video-EEG monitoring in children was retrospectively assessed.

Methods.—Video-EEG was used in the evaluation of 230 children over a 3-year period. The baseline frequency of events ranged from multiple events per day to less than 1 per week, and the duration of monitoring ranged from 8 hours to 2 to 5 days. These variables were assessed for their impact on event detection rates in patients with and without gradual withdrawal of antiepileptic drugs before monitoring.

Results.—Video-EEG was significantly less likely to capture events if they occurred less often. Detection rates were 85% in patients with daily events compared with 63% in those with at least weekly events and 50% for those with events less frequent than weekly. The duration of monitoring and the withdrawal of antiepileptic drugs did not significantly affect event detection rates. Video-EEG had high diagnostic rates in the differentiation of seizure and nonseizure events (70%), in the classification of seizure types (88%), and in the evaluation of candidates for epilepsy surgery (64%). Overall, the diagnostic information provided by video-EEG changed clinical management for 45% of the patients.

Conclusion.—Continuous video-EEG monitoring is an efficient and valuable diagnostic tool in pediatric neurology. It can help in determining the nature of paroxysmal disorders and in making management decisions in patients with epilepsy. The technique is cost-effective for children with daily events. Further study is needed to determine whether increasing the duration of monitoring or withdrawing antiepileptic drug therapy can make video-EEG more efficient in patients with less frequent events.

▶ Long-term video-EEG monitoring has generally been accepted as a useful tool in the diagnosis of patients with presumed epilepsy. This articles supported this belief and added some important observations. A positive yield from the procedure was realized in more than 80% of the patients and was enhanced with recordings of greater than 24 hours and when anticonvulsant medications were discontinued. In 70% of the patients the diagnosis was altered. When properly done, this is a very effective method of confirming or establishing a diagnosis and should be considered in patients who are not responding adequately to therapy.

E.R. Ramsay, M.D.

Induction of Pseudoseizures With Intravenous Saline Placebo
Slater JD, Brown MC, Jacobs W, et al (Univ of Miami, Fla)
Epilepsia 36:580–585, 1995

3–2

Background.—Patients with so-called nonepileptic seizures (NESs) undergo a paroxysmal experience that is interpreted by an observer as resembling epilepsy. Possibilities include migraine, syncope, hypoglycemia, and cardiac arrhythmia. Pseudoseizures, in contrast, are a symptom of an underlying psychopathologic condition resulting not from excessive neuronal discharge but from an abnormal emotional state. A failure to recognize pseudoseizures for what they are may entail considerable cost, both

TABLE 3.—Ictal Characteristics of Pseudoseizures and Epilepsy

Characteristics	Pseudoseizures % (n)	Epilepsy, % (n)	P Value
Positive induction	90.63 (29/32)*	0.0 (0/42)*	≤.00005*
Change in seizure frequency with medication change	18.75 (6/32)*	71.43 (30/42)*	≤.00005*
Generalized	40.63 (13/32)	40.48 (17/42)	.9897
Partial	84.38 (27/32)	83.33 (35/42)	.9041
Increased seizure frequency with stress	28.13 (9/32)	21.43 (9/42)	.4774
Postictal behavior†	15.63 (5/32)*	66.67 (28/42)*	≤.00005*
Incontinence	0.0 (0/32)*	26.19 (11/42)*	.001*
Self-injury	3.13 (1/32)	19.05 (8/42)	.0382
Combativeness	0.0 (0/32)	2.38 (1/42)	.5676
Crying/yelling	12.5 (4/32)	0.0 (0/42)	.0413
Vulgar language	0.0 (0/32)	0.0 (0/42)	—

* Statistical significance.
† Defined as postevent confusion/disorientation clearly distinguishable from the ictus.
(Courtesy of Slater JD, Brown MC, Jacobs W, et al: Induction of pseudoseizures with intravenous saline placebo. *Epilepsia* 36:580–585, 1995.)

TABLE 4.—Classification of Pseudoseizures

Pseudoseizures alone
    Pseudoseizures, no previous history of
        epilepsy
    Pseudoseizures, previous history of epilepsy
        Documented true epilepsy
        History inadequate to determine previous
           epilepsy vs. pseudoseizures
        Probable long-term pseudoseizures
           (probable previous misdiagnosis of
           epilepsy)
Pseudoseizures and concurrent epilepsy

(Courtesy of Slater JD, Brown MC, Jacobs W, et al: Induction of pseudoseizures with intravenous saline placebo. *Epilepsia* 36:580–585, 1995.)

---

financial and psychosocial. Attempts have been made to use various placebos to "activate" the events so that they can be recorded.

Objective and Methods.—The effects of injecting normal saline solution intravenously were examined in a prospective series of 101 adult patients referred in a recent 2-year period with paroxysmal clinical phenomena thought to be epilepsy but that resisted standard antiepileptic drug treatment. Comprehensive evaluation included videotaping, brain imaging, ictal and interictal electroencephalographic recordings, single photon emission CT, and extensive psychological and neuropsychological evaluation. When given the injection, patients were told that they were receiving 2 different concentrations of a drug designed to lower the seizure threshold.

Results.—Events were not induced in any of 41 patients who had a final diagnosis of epilepsy alone. In contrast, events were inducible in all but 3 of 32 patients in whom pseudoseizures were diagnosed. One of the 29 inducible patients with pseudoseizures also received a diagnosis of epilepsy. Epileptic patients were likelier to have a change in seizure frequency when medication was changed. They were also likelier than those with pseudoseizures to be incontinent and to exhibit postictal behavior (Table 3).

Discussion.—Injecting a saline placebo is a reliable and safe means of distinguishing between true epilepsy and pseudoseizures. The distinction may otherwise be difficult to make, in part because pseudoseizures are not a unitary disorder (Table 4).

▶ The incidence of pseudoseizures may be as much as one third that of epilepsy. Thus, a significant number of patients have NESs. Differentiating epilepsy from NES is often difficult. This paper demonstrated that the use of suggestion and IV saline solution is highly effective and selective in precipitating pseudoseizures. This is a very helpful tool in the evaluation of patients with unusual or refractory seizures. The authors also suggested a classification of pseudoseizures that would be helpful in comparing diagnostic and therapeutic outcomes in these patients.

E.R. Ramsay, M.D.

Self-Injury and Incontinence in Psychogenic Seizures

Peguero E, Abou-Khalil B, Fakhoury T, et al (Vanderbilt Univ, Nashville, Tenn)
Epilepsia 36:586–591, 1995   3–3

Objective.—As many as 30% of patients with psychogenic seizures may injure themselves, typically by biting their tongues or lips or bruising their limbs. Seeing 2 patients who incurred significant injury that required emergency care prompted a survey of 102 consecutive patients in whom electroencephalography (EEG) and closed-circuit TV monitoring had led to a diagnosis of psychogenic seizures. Seventy-three patients (or a close relative or friend) were available for a semistructured telephone interview.

Study Population.—The ages of the 56 females and 17 males with psychogenic seizures ranged from 9 to 52 years, with an average of 32. Thirty epileptic patients with an average age of 29 served as a control group. The majority of these patients had partial epilepsy.

Findings.—Forty percent of the patients with psychogenic seizures and 27 of the 60 patients without coexisting epilepsy reported having incurred injury during a seizure (Table 2). Five of the 13 patients who also had epilepsy were easily able to distinguish between epileptic and psychogenic seizures. Thirty-two patients reported bladder incontinence, and 5 of them had bowel incontinence as well. A history of injury was twice as frequent in patients with psychogenic seizures who had attempted suicide than in those who had not. About three fourths of the control patients with epilepsy had sustained injuries during seizures, and about half had had significant injuries, including burns and fractures. More than half of the epileptic patients reported incontinence.

TABLE 2.—Comparison of Psychogenic Seizures and Epilepsy Control Groups for
Self-Injury, Related Features, and Iatrogenic Complications

	Psychogenic, n = 73 (%)	Epileptic n = 30 (%)	P Value
Injuries	29 (40)	23 (77)	.001
Type of injury			
Lacerations sutured	4 (5)	7 (23)	<.05
Burns	0	10 (33)	<.000001
Fractures	3 (4)	8 (27)	<.005
Bruises/minor wounds	23 (31)	19 (63)	<.01
Tongue biting	32 (44)	18 (60)	NS
Tongue bleeding	20 (27)	12 (40)	NS
Urinary incontinence	32 (44)	17 (57)	NS
Status epilepticus (or pseudostatus)	37 (51)	16 (53)	NS
Endotracheal intubation	5 (7)	0	NS
Allergic reactions to AEDs	12 (16)	5 (17)	NS
Suicide attempts	23 (31)	3 (10)	<.05

Abbreviations: AEDs, antiepileptic drugs.
(Courtesy of Peguero E, Abou-Khalil B, Fakhoury T, et al: Self-injury and incontinence in psychogenic seizures. *Epilepsia* 36:586–591, 1995.)

Conclusion.—Neither a history of self-injury nor incontinence should eliminate the diagnosis of psychogenic seizures.

▶ The diagnosis of epilepsy is usually based on the history. Components usually viewed as indicating an organic (epileptic) process include self-injury, tongue biting, and incontinence. This article clearly illustrated how frequently these items are reported in patients with nonepileptic seizures (NESs). In my experience, these items are frequently reported in patients with NESs. The treating physician must always be skeptical of the historical details obtained unless observed and documented by a physician or appropriate health care worker.

E.R. Ramsay, M.D.

Outcome After Diagnosis of Psychogenic Nonepileptic Seizures
Walczak TS, Papacostas S, Williams DT, et al (Helen Hayes Hosp, New York; Columbia Presbyterian Med Ctr, New York)
Epilepsia 36:1131–1137, 1995   3–4

Objective.—The diagnosis and treatment of psychogenic nonepileptic seizures (PNESs) are not well defined. Follow-up studies were carried out on a large series of video-EEG–confirmed PNES patients to clarify this area.

Study Design.—The study group consisted of 72 consecutive, video-EEG–confirmed PNES patients who had received counseling and had been referred for psychotherapy. These patients were contacted from 12 to 27 months after diagnosis and asked to respond to a structured telephone questionnaire. The questionnaire examined PNES frequency, antiepileptic drug (AED) use, occupational status, global self-rating, and psychotherapeutic treatment.

Findings.—In this large series of PNES patients, PNESs had stopped in 35%, decreased by more than 80% in 41%, and decreased by less than 80% in 24%. The majority were no longer taking AEDs. Occupational status improvement had occurred in only 20%. In the group overall, 57% rated themselves significantly improved since diagnosis. Persistence of PNESs was significantly associated with longer duration before diagnosis and the presence of additional psychiatric disease. Persistence was not associated with gender, epilepsy, the use of placebo activation during diagnosis, or the extent of psychotherapy.

Conclusion.—After diagnosis, PNESs disappeared or decreased in most patients in this large series, and most were able to stop taking AEDs. The majority of patients believed that their overall status was improved. Improvement appeared to be associated with earlier diagnosis. The improvement of the patients in other measures did not usually translate into improvement in occupational status.

▶ Increasingly we are recognizing that some patients diagnosed as having epilepsy may have other causes for their symptoms. Psychogenic NESs, or pseudoseizures, are an important component of these patients. Because of our lack of experience, patients with NESs would often be left untreated after the diagnosis was made. The authors of this paper looked at the outcome of a group of patients with NESs who were referred after diagnosis for psychiatric care. Because the correct diagnosis was addressed, two thirds of the patients discontinued the use of anticonvulsant medications with improvement or resolution of their symptoms. This underscores both the need for correct diagnosis and the good outcome that can be realized with proper therapy.

E.R. Ramsay, M.D.

Prolactin Secretion Following Repetitive Seizures
Malkowicz DE, Legido A, Jackel RA, et al (Med College of Pennsylvania, Philadelphia; St Christopher's Hosp for Children, Philadelphia; Bristol-Meyers Squibb, Wallingford, Conn; et al)
Neurology 45:448–452, 1995   3–5

Background.—Elevated levels of PRL occur after various types of seizures. In generalized tonic-clonic (GTC) and partial seizures, PRL levels peak within 15 to 20 minutes of onset and decline to baseline values by 60 minutes postictus. The release of PRL can be affected by a number of factors, including the time between seizures. The effect of repetitive seizures and the relationship between the seizure-free interval (SFI) and PRL response were determined by examining PRL levels in 8 patients.

Methods.—Study participants had medically intractable partial seizures and were undergoing video-EEG monitoring as inpatients before epilepsy surgery. An indwelling IV catheter was used for blood sampling. Seizure data collected included type, focus, spread, duration, and SFI. Postictal serum PRL levels were sampled at 15, 30, and 60 minutes.

Results.—The 8 patients ranged from 12 to 44 years. One had simple partial (SP) seizures and complex partial (CP) seizures only; the remaining 7 patients had GTC seizures in addition to CP seizures, SP seizures, or both. Postictal PRL levels were studied for 24 seizures. In 17 seizures (71%), there was a significant postictal PRL release, resulting in at least a threefold increase in the 15-minute postictal PRL level over the average baseline value. The 15-minute postictal PRL levels showed considerable reductions after shorter SFIs, whereas seizures occurring after longer SFIs had more robust PRL responses (Fig). Shorter SFIs ranged from approximately 1 to 25 hours; longer SFIs recorded in this patient group ranged from 32 to 240 hours. Elevations in serum PRL showed no correlation with seizure type, focus, or duration or with type of antiepilepsy drug.

Conclusions.—The release of PRL after seizures appears to be affected by the interval between seizures. Reduced PRL responses were observed after shorter SFIs, and more substantial PRL responses were seen after longer SFIs. The amount of releasable PRL may be depleted by seizures or inhibited by PRL feedback, and the hypothalamic-pituitary axis acts to

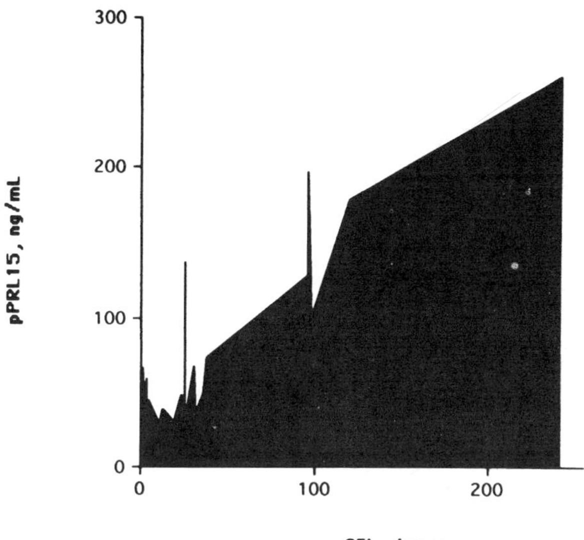

FIGURE.—Graph showing the 15-minute postictal serum PRL levels in nanograms per milliter vs. seizure-free interval in hours for all 8 subjects combined. *Abbreviations: pPRL 15*, 15-minute postictal serum PRL levels; *SFI*, seizure-free interval. (Reprinted from *Neurology*; 45:448–452, 1995; by permission of Little, Brown and Company [Inc].)

recover or restore PRL. Measurements of postictal PRL levels may be more accurate when obtained after an SFI of at least 32 hours.

▶ One clinical marker after a seizure is significant elevation of the plasma PRL level. However, increased plasma levels are not always observed after a seizure, which raises the question as to the specificity and sensitivity of this test. This paper showed that frequent seizures may deplete the PRL stores, and after several seizures, postictal elevation of PRL may not be observed. In assessing the results of a PRL level, the clinician must have information regarding the number of seizures the patient has had in the preceding 24 hours.

E.R. Ramsay, M.D.

Seizures in Women

A Comparison of Magnesium Sulfate With Phenytoin for the Prevention of Eclampsia

Lucas MJ, Leveno KJ, Cunningham FG (Univ of Texas Southwestern Med Ctr, Dallas)
N Engl J Med 333:201–205, 1995

3–6

Introduction.—In pregnant women with hypertension, magnesium sulfate is widely used to prevent eclamptic seizures. However, few studies have compared the efficacy of magnesium sulfate with other drugs such as the conventional antiepileptic drugs diazepam or phenytoin, which are more commonly used in England. Magnesium sulfate was compared with phenytoin in preventing seizures in hypertensive women during labor.

Methods.—Women with hypertension were randomly assigned to receive magnesium sulfate or phenytoin during delivery. The regimen was 10g of a 50% solution of magnesium sulfate in divided doses in the upper outer quadrant of each buttock. Thereafter, every 4 hours, 5 g of a 50% solution was injected. For severe pre-eclampsia, a loading dose of 4 mg of magnesium sulfate was given intravenously as a 20% solution. The phenytoin regimen was 1,000 mg of phenytoin in saline solution infused over a 1-hour period. Ten hours later a maintenance dose of 500 mg of phenytoin was given in a delayed-release capsule. Anticonvulsant therapy was continued for 24 hours postpartum for both regimens.

Results.—Eclamptic convulsions occurred in 10 of 1,089 women assigned to the phenytoin regimen, whereas none of the 1,049 women assigned to magnesium sulfate treatment had eclamptic convulsions. Between the 2 study groups, there were no significant differences in any risk factors for eclampsia. Maternal and infant outcomes were also similar in the 2 groups. In the 10 women with eclampsia, despite phenytoin prophylaxis, a number of peripartum complications were seen, including cesarean section, low–birth weight infants, partial abruptio placentae, and blood transfusions.

Conclusion.—For the prevention of eclampsia in hypertensive pregnant women, magnesium sulfate is superior. The long-practiced use of magnesium sulfate in the prevention of eclampsia is validated by these results. Until now, the effectiveness of phenytoin as prophylaxis against eclampsia has been studied in only small groups.

▶ Neurologists are often critical of obstetricians who use magnesium sulfate to treat pre-eclampsia, believing that modern anticonvulsants would be more effective. This study from the Obstetrics Department of the University of Texas Southwestern Medical Center at first glance refuted this opinion because the frequency of seizures was dramatically less in those receiving magnesium sulfate than in those receiving phenytoin. However, it is important to look at the study carefully. The reduction in eclamptic seizures was from 1% to 0%, and all pregnant women admitted for delivery with blood pressures greater than 140/90 mm Hg were accepted into the protocol. Pre-eclampsia was present in only a minority; only 18% had significant proteinuria, and 4% required hydralazine treatment for diastolic blood pressure of greater than 110 mm Hg. I am uncertain whether it is standard obstetric practice to administer magnesium sulfate to patients with blood pressure of only 140/90 mm Hg. Neurologists generally see peripartum patients only when they have had a seizure, and by that time they are usually receiving magnesium sulfate. Although it is possible that in such circumstances established anticonvulsants might be more effective than magnesium sulfate, this question was not answered by this study. Nevertheless, this study should certainly make neurologists more circumspect in their criticism.

W.G. Bradley, D.M., F.R.C.P.

Which Anticonvulsant for Women With Eclampsia? Evidence From the Collaborative Eclampsia Trial
Duley L, and the Eclampsia Trial Collaborative Group (Radcliffe Infirmary, Oxford, England)
Lancet 345:1455–1463, 1995   3–7

Background.—Eclampsia-related maternal deaths become proportionally more common in countries with better control of infection and hemorrhage. Because prevention of eclampsia is difficult, effective treatment is important. Anticonvulsants are typically used in the management of patients with eclampsia, but there is considerable controversy about the optimal choice of anticonvulsant. The effectiveness of magnesium sulfate, diazepam, and phenytoin was compared in a multicenter randomized trial.

Methods.—Each of 23 centers in 8 countries chose to compare either magnesium sulfate with diazepam or magnesium sulfate with phenytoin in a total of 1,687 randomly assigned women. The occurrence of recurrent convulsions, maternal death, and potentially life-threatening events were noted as outcome measures.

Results.—Of the 905 evaluable women enrolled in the comparison of magnesium sulfate and diazepam, the magnesium sulfate group had significantly fewer recurrent convulsions and a nonsignificantly lower rate of maternal mortality. There were no other significant differences between these 2 treatment groups in other measures of maternal morbidity. Perinatal mortality was nonsignificantly higher, but Apgar scores at 1 minute were significantly higher in the magnesium sulfate group. In the comparison of magnesium sulfate and phenytoin (775 women), the magnesium sulfate group had significantly fewer recurrent convulsions, a nonsignificantly lower maternal mortality, less need for ventilation, a lower incidence of pneumonia, and less use of intensive care facilities. Perinatal mortality was nonsignificantly lower, and perinatal morbidity was significantly lower in the magnesium sulfate group.

Conclusion.—Magnesium sulfate should be the therapy of choice for women with eclampsia. Other anticonvulsant drugs should be used only in randomized trials, and their efficacy should be compared with that of magnesium sulfate.

▶ This trial addressed the question as to the best treatment for patients with eclampsia. Two comparisons were made: magnesium sulfate vs. diazepam and magnesium sulfate vs. phenytoin. The study concluded that magnesium sulfate was better than either diazepam or phenytoin to control recurrent seizures but that it did not improve maternal mortality. Methodological problems limit the interpretation from these 2 trials. The results between trials cannot be compared because the patient demographics (e.g., number of pretreatment convulsions) were different. The most significant limitation is that the dose of diazepam and phenytoin given were considerably below what is used by neurologists for the treatment of acute seizures. This latter fact seriously compromises any conclusions that can be drawn from the trial. Control of blood pressure and results of other treatments were not analyzed in this report.

E.R. Ramsay, M.D.

Menstrual Disorders in Women With Epilepsy Receiving Carbamazepine

Isojärvi JIT, Laatikainen TJ, Pakarinen AJ, et al (Univ of Oulu, Finland)
Epilepsia 36:676–681, 1995   3–8

Purpose.—Among women with epilepsy, it is not uncommon to find reproductive endocrine disorders, but the pathogenesis of these conditions has not been well defined. The effects of the antiepileptic drug (AED) carbamazepine (CBZ) on reproductive endocrine function and menstrual cycling were examined prospectively in a group of 8 women beginning CBZ therapy, who were followed for 5 years. An additional group of 56 women who had undergone CBZ therapy for longer than 5 years were also examined to determine long-term effects.

Study Group.—Eight women with either idiopathic or cryptogenic epilepsy who had never previously taken AEDs participated in the prospective part of this study. Average age at the start of the study period was 29. The cross-sectional study group consisted of 56 women with epilepsy who had received CBZ monotherapy for at least 5 years. The average age of this group was 33, and they had taken CBZ for 6 to 20 years.

Findings.—In the prospective study group, serum sex hormone–binding globulin (SHBG) levels increased, serum estradiol levels decreased, and the estradiol/SHBG ratio decreased after CBZ therapy (Fig 2). Menstrual

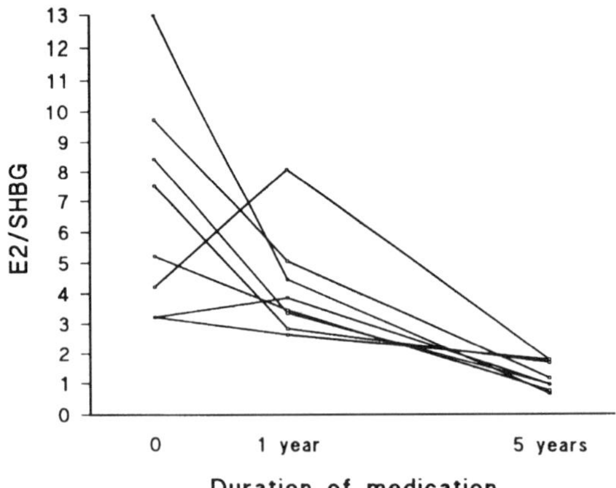

FIGURE 2.—Estradiol (pmol/L)/sex hormone–binding globulin (nmol/L) ratios in 8 women with epilepsy before medication and after 1 and 5 years of carbamazepine medication. The values of the 2 women with menstrual disorders after 5 years are presented as *solid squares*. *P* < 0.001 after 5 years; repeated measures analysis of variance and Fisher's least significant difference test. *Abbreviations: E2*, estradiol; *SHBG*, sex hormone–binding globulin. (Courtesy of Isojärvi JIT, Laatikainen TJ, Pakarinen AJ, et al: *Epilepsia* 36:676–681, 1995.)

irregularities developed during therapy in 25% of these women. In the cross-sectional study group, the frequency of menstrual disturbance was also 25%. In these patients, menstrual disorders were associated with increased serum SHBG levels, decreased serum estradiol levels, and low estradiol/SHBG ratios.

Conclusion.—Administration of the AED carbamazine was associated with an increase in serum SHBG levels, a decrease in serum estradiol levels, and low estradiol/SHBG ratios. Menstrual disorders in female epileptics receiving CBZ were associated with these changes.

▶ This study clearly demonstrated the hormonal changes that can occur with chronic use of CBZ. An increased incidence of menstrual disorders from polycystic ovarian disease and hypogonadotrophic hypogonadism has been reported in epilepsy. Part of the cause for this has been attributed to the epilepsy and uncontrolled seizures. However, these authors showed that CBZ induces chronic changes in SHBG levels and secondarily in estrogen levels, resulting in menstrual irregularities. The use of anticonvulsant drugs that are not metabolized in the liver likely will eliminate the hormonal changes seen with the older anticonvulsant drugs such as CBZ.

E.R. Ramsay, M.D.

Other Seizure Matters

Secular Trends and Birth Cohort Effects in Unprovoked Seizures: Rochester, Minnesota 1935–1984
Annegers JF, Hauser WA, Lee JR-J, et al (Univ of Texas, Houston; Columbia Med School, New York; Mayo Clinic and Mayo Found, Rochester, Minn)
Epilepsia 36:575–579, 1995   3–9

Background.—The incidence of epilepsy and unprovoked seizure for the population of Rochester, Minnesota from 1935 through 1984, was described and trends and birth cohort effects were evaluated.

Study Design.—Cases were derived from all Rochester, Minnesota, residents with a diagnosis of a potential seizure disorder. Seizures due to an acute cerebral nervous system assault or other known antecedent causes were excluded.

Findings.—A total of 806 Rochester residents from 1935 to 1984 met the criterion of having an initial diagnosis of cryptogenic unprovoked seizure. Overall, the age-adjusted incidence was approximately 40/100,000 person-years. The rates for males and females were similar from 1935 to 1964 but higher for males in the last 2 decades of the study period due to a decrease in the rate for females. The incidence rates decreased progressively from the first decade of life to age 40 to 59 but then increased after age 60, to describe a characteristic U-shaped lifetime incidence curve. From 1965 through 1984, incidence rates decreased progressively for each group older than 50. There was a significant protective effect of the 1930 to 1934 birth cohort.

Conclusion.—The incidence of unprovoked seizures was examined for the population of Rochester, Minnesota, from 1935 to 1984. During this period, the incidence of unprovoked seizure was relatively stable, with a consistent U-shaped incidence over the lifetime and a slightly higher rate in males than females. Incidence progressively decreased in those older than 50 from 1965 to 1984. This incidence decrease paralleled a decrease in cerebrovascular disease within this community.

▶ Epilepsy has previously been considered to have the highest occurrence in infancy and childhood. The authors looked at the long-term results from the community around Rochester, Minnesota. This paper showed that the highest incidence is in the older patient groups, perhaps evident now as more people are living into their seventies and eighties. Epilepsy in the elderly patient is becoming recognized as an important medical problem. The authors also suggested that 1 risk factor is nonstroke-related cerebral vascular disease. Careful medical monitoring and early treatment may ultimately reduce the occurrence of seizures in older patients.

E.R. Ramsay, M.D.

Risk of Recurrence After First Unprovoked Tonic-Clonic Seizure in Adults

Bora I, Seçkin B, Zarifoglu M, et al (Uludag Univ, Bursa, Turkey)
J Neurol 242:157–163, 1995   3–10

Background.—The likelihood of recurrence after an initial unprovoked seizure has profound implications for patient lifestyle. The management of these patients remains controversial. The influence of age, sex, family history, seizure type, electroencephalographic (EEG) patterns, and anticonvulsive drug (ACD) therapy on seizure recurrence after an initial unprovoked seizure was examined prospectively.

Study Group.—The study group consisted of 147 adult outpatients who had experienced an initial seizure between October 1988 and January 1991 and were followed until June 1993. Patients with simple or complex partial seizures and those with proven structural lesions were excluded. The follow-up period ranged from 27 to 54 months.

Findings.—The overall recurrence rate was 14% by 1 month, 22% by 3 months, 32% by 6 months, and 41% by 1 year. After this time the rate remained relatively stable. The rate of recurrence was highest in the first year and declined with increasing time after first seizure. Age, sex, family history, EEG results, and ACD therapy had no significant influence on recurrence rate. Risk of recurrence was significantly higher if the first seizure was nocturnal than if it was during the daytime.

Conclusion.—The influence of several factors on the rate of recurrence after first unprovoked seizure was explored. The majorty of recurrences were observed within the first year after initial seizure. The only significant predictor of seizure recurrence in this patient group was the time of day at which the initial seizure occurred.

▶ Whether to treat patients after they experience a first seizure continues to be a dilemma. In this article, the recurrence rate was low (31.8%), with most becoming evident within 6 months. Factors not affecting outcome were age, sex, and EEG findings. Of interest was the difference in outcome according to time that a seizure occurred. Seizures occurring between midnight and 9 AM had a significantly higher rate of recurrence. Anticonvulsant treatment reduced the recurrence rate but with the number of patients studied, the difference in outcome did not reach statistical significance. This study suggested that in general treatment is not warranted after the first unprovoked seizure in the absence of risk factors.

E.R. Ramsay, M.D.

Late-Onset Drop Attacks in Temporal Lobe Epilepsy: A Reevaluation of the Concept of Temporal Lobe Syncope
Gambardella A, Reutens DC, Andermann F, et al (McGill Univ, Montreal; Montreal Neurological Hosp and Inst)
Neurology 44:1074–1078, 1994   3–11

Background.—The atonic seizure is a form of epileptic "drop" attack in which the patient, without convulsing, abruptly falls from a standing or sitting position but fully recovers within seconds or, at most, a few minutes. Patients with secondary generalized epilepsy or partial epilepsy involving the mesial frontal or rolandic region of the cortex are most often affected, but patients with temporal lobe epilepsy also may exhibit drop attacks.

Objective.—The clinical findings of 6 patients with temporal lobe drop attacks (TLDAs) who underwent either anterior temporal resection or selective resection of the amygdala and hippocampus were reviewed. All patients were followed for 1 year or longer.

Findings.—Most patients began having habitual seizures in the second or third decade of life, but 2 had earlier involvement. In no case were TLDAs the initial manifestation. The average interval from the onset of epilepsy to TLDAs was 24.4 years. A unilateral temporal origin of seizures in the dominant left hemisphere was documented in all but 1 of the 6 patients. The exceptional patient had limbic seizures. Postoperatively 3 patients were free of seizures while receiving antiepileptic drug treatment. One patient had had episodes of dizziness and lip smacking but no drop attacks. Two patients continued to have seizures but less frequently than before.

Discussion.—Patients with temporal lobe epilepsy occasionally have drop attacks some time after the onset of epilepsy. These do not always represent bitemporal or extratemporal seizure foci but instead are probably related to the rapid spread of ictal discharge and involvement of the pontine reticular formation. Drop attacks increase the patient's disability, and it is important to distinguish them from both loss of balance and secondary convulsions.

▶ Episodes of loss of consciousness that resemble syncope have been described to occur during temporal lobe complex partial seizures. Some have debated whether this is produced directly by the seizure. This paper clearly demonstrated the ictal origin for "temporal lobe syncope" with scalp and depth electrode recordings, with further support being the resolution of symptoms after temporal lobectomy. Some important facts to appreciate are that temporal lobe syncope does not occur without prior manifestation of typical temporal lobe complex partial seizures and that temporal lobe syncope begins after the patient has had epilepsy for several years.

E.R. Ramsay, M.D.

A Randomized Controlled Trial of Chronic Vagus Nerve Stimulation for Treatment of Medically Intractable Seizures

The Vagus Nerve Stimulation Study Group (Oregon Health Sciences Univ Epilepsy Ctr, Portland)
Neurology 45:224–230, 1995

3–12

Background.—From 10% to 20% of patients in whom epilepsy develops are resistant to medical treatment, and some of these patients are not candidates for surgical treatment. Animal studies demonstrated an antiseizure effect of acute vagus nerve stimulation (VNS), and chronic stimulation has proved effective in monkeys with recurrent seizures from alumina gel foci. Pilot clinical studies have shown an implanted pacemaker-like stimulator to effectively reduce seizures both acutely and over the long term.

Objective.—Chronic intermittent VNS was evaluated in a randomized multicenter study of 114 patients with common types of epilepsy resistant to medical measures.

Study Design.—A programmable generator was implanted subcutaneously in the left subclavicular fossa and connected to 2 stimulating electrodes wrapped about the vagus nerve in the carotid sheath. The patients were randomized in a blinded manner to receive either high-level stimulation at what was presumed to be a therapeutic level or low-level, subtherapeutic stimulation. The response was compared with what was observed during a 12-week baseline period.

Results.—Seizure frequency was reduced by one fourth in patients given high-level stimulation and by 6% in the low-stimulation group. Nearly one third of the former patients and 13% of the latter had their seizure frequency reduced by 50% or more. Just more than one third of the patients in the high-level stimulation group had a hoarse or tremulous voice during stimulus delivery. Patients in both groups occasionally coughed or noted throat pain. One patient assigned to high-level stimulation had a myocardial infarction. There was no overall effect on cardiac function or the frequency of ectopic beats and no significant increase in gastric acid output.

Conclusion.—Some patients with common forms of medically intractable seizures may benefit from VNS.

▶ This study reported the results of VNS, which is a novel approach to the treatment of epilepsy. Early basic research suggested that vagal stimulation modulated and reduced the frequency of seizures. This article reported the first well-controlled trial on the use of VNS. Patients receiving "high-dose" stimulation had a very significant reduction in seizure frequency. Although we do not understand the mechanism of effect, for patients with refractory epilepsy, VNS provides a very reasonable option for control of their seizures.

E.R. Ramsay, M.D.

4 Pediatric Neurology

Epilepsy

Risk Factors for a First Febrile Seizure: A Matched Case-Control Study
Berg AT, Shinnar S, Shapiro ED, et al (Northern Illinois Univ, DeKalb; Albert Einstein College, Bronx, NY; Montefiore Epilepsy Management Ctr, Bronx, NY; et al)
Epilepsia 36:334–341, 1995   4–1

Background.—Recent studies of the risk factors for a febrile seizure have focused mostly on family history and perinatal factors. There is little information on the features of the acute illnesses during which febrile seizures occur. The risk factors for a first febrile seizure were identified in a matched case-control study, with special emphasis on the characteristics of the acute illness.

Methods.—Case patients were identified through hospital emergency departments (EDs), and control patients were identified through outpatient clinics and EDs. The patients, 69 children with first febrile seizures and no history of previous unprovoked seizures, were matched for age, site of routine pediatric care, and date of visit. Each patient was matched with 1 or 2 febrile control subjects with no history of previous febrile or unprovoked seizures.

Findings.—Multivariate analysis indicated that the degree of temperature and a history of febrile seziures in a first-degree or higher relative were significant independent risk factors. Gastroenteritis as the underlying illness was significantly inversely related to febrile seizures. Maternal smoking during pregnancy had marginal significance as a predictor of febrile seizures.

Conclusion.—Several factors, especially the degree of fever, appear to be associated with a first febrile seizure. Also, the risk of a febrile seizure may vary depending on the type of underlying illness.

▶ It is not surprising that body temperature elevations greater than 38.3°C correlated with the occurrence of simple febrile seizures. However, this does not mean that the seizures always occur when the temperature is rapidly rising. Febrile seizures can occur anytime during a febrile illness in a genetically predisposed child, and the diagnosis does not depend on the time relationship between seizure onset and height of the fever.

G.M. Fenichel, M.D.

Long Term Outcome of Prophylaxis for Febrile Convulsions
Knudsen FU, Paerregaard A, Andersen R, et al (Glostrup Univ, Denmark)
Arch Dis Child 74:13–18, 1996   4–2

Background.—Major cohort studies have shown that long-term ou t-comes are normal for most children with febrile convulsions. As a result, long-term prophylaxis with antiepileptic agents has been abandoned for the most part. However, febrile convulsions may be associated with more subtle adverse outcomes in motor, neurologic, intellectual, or cognitive functions. In addition, it is unknown whether medical intervention in early childhood affects long-term prognosis, including the occurrence of subsequent epilepsy. These questions were investigated in a randomized, controlled, long-term follow-up study.

Methods and Findings.—Follow-up data were collected from 289 children 12 years after randomization to intermittent prophylaxis (group 1) or no prophylaxis (group 2). All had had febrile convulsions in early childhood. At follow-up mean age in group 1 was 14 years and in group 2 was 14.1 years. Body weight, height, and head circumference were also comparable between groups. The groups also had very similar findings on neurologic assessment, the Stott motor test of fine and gross motor development, the Wechsler Intelligence Scale for children (including verbal intelligence quotient [IQ], performance IQ, and full-scale IQ), a neuropsychologic test battery (including short- and long-term, auditory, and visual memory), and visuomotor tempo, computer reaction time, and reading tests. Scholastic achievement was also comparable between groups. The incidence of epilepsy in 0.7% in group 1 and 0.8% in group 2.

Conclusion.—Type of treatment of febrile convulsions in early childhood did not affect the occurrence of subsequent epilepsy or long-term neurologic, motor, intellectual, cognitive, and scholastic abilities. Thus, in the long term, preventing new febrile convulsions appears to be no better than abbreviating them.

▶ Epileptologists, who see adults with refractory seizures, often elicit a history of febrile seizures during infancy and believe that a causal relationship exists. Child neurologists, who see children with febrile seizures, know that they are rarely a precursor of epilepsy. This is 1 of the few prospective long-term (12 years) follow-up studies of febrile convulsions. It confirmed that febrile seizures have a benign outcome whether they are simple or complex (prolonged, multiple, partial) or whether or not they are prevented with diazepam. Febrile seizures do not beget afebrile seizures unless both are caused by an underlying brain disorder.

G.M. Fenichel, M.D.

Low Risk of Seizure Recurrence After Early Withdrawal of Antiepileptic Treatment in the Neonatal Period
Hellström-Westas L, Blennow G, Lindroth M, et al (Univ Hosp, Lund, Sweden)
Arch Dis Child 72:F97–F101, 1995
4–3

Introduction.—Neonatal seizures often indicate severely disordered brain function, but occasionally a transient functional disturbance related to hypoxia, infection, or other transient factors may be responsible. The use of prophylaxis for several months was studied to determine whether the risks exceed the benefits.

Patients.—The risk of seizures recurring in the first year of life in infants with neonatal seizures was studied in 1,283 infants in tertiary neonatal intensive care, 58 (4.5%) of whom had neonatal seizures at up to 46 weeks of postconceptional age. The chief causes were hemorrhage, ischemia, and birth asphyxia. All infants had some form of neonatal distress. The median duration of amplitude-integrated electroencephalographic (EEG) monitoring was 67.5 hours.

Management.—Phenobarbital in an initial dose of 10 to 20 mg/kg was used most often. If seizures did not cease, repeated doses of 0.5 mg of diazepam/kg were given, and lidocaine was added if necessary. If seizures persisted, phenytoin and, in some cases, pyridoxine were given. Treatment was phased out when seizures ceased and no EEG seizure pattern was evident (Fig 2).

Results.—All but 3 of the 36 surviving infants received antiepileptic treatment, but only 2 of them were treated for longer than 20 days. The median duration of treatment was 4½ days. Only 2 infants had recurrent seizures in the first year of life when not receiving prophylaxis. The outlook for infants having 10 or fewer neonatal seizures was comparatively good. All 3 surviving infants with postneonatal seizures had initially had more than 10 seizures. Recurrent seizures could not be related to the early EEG findings or to the presence of structural abnormalities in the brain.

Recommendations.—It seems feasible to withdraw antiepileptic drug treatment shortly after neonatal seizures are controlled. When there are more than 10 neonatal seizures, treatment may be withdrawn before discharge if the EEG findings are normal. Ongoing treatment may be required for those few infants who have frequent, severe seizures and markedly abnormal EEG findings.

▶ Seizures that occur during an acute self-limited encephalopathy (hypoxia, infection) almost always subside when the encephalopathy resolves. Only a small percentage of newborns who have such seizures will continue to have seizures later on, and keeping them on anticonvulsant medication therapy is not known to prevent later epilepsy. It is reasonable to discontinue medicine as soon as possible after the encephalopathy has resolved.

G.M. Fenichel, M.D.

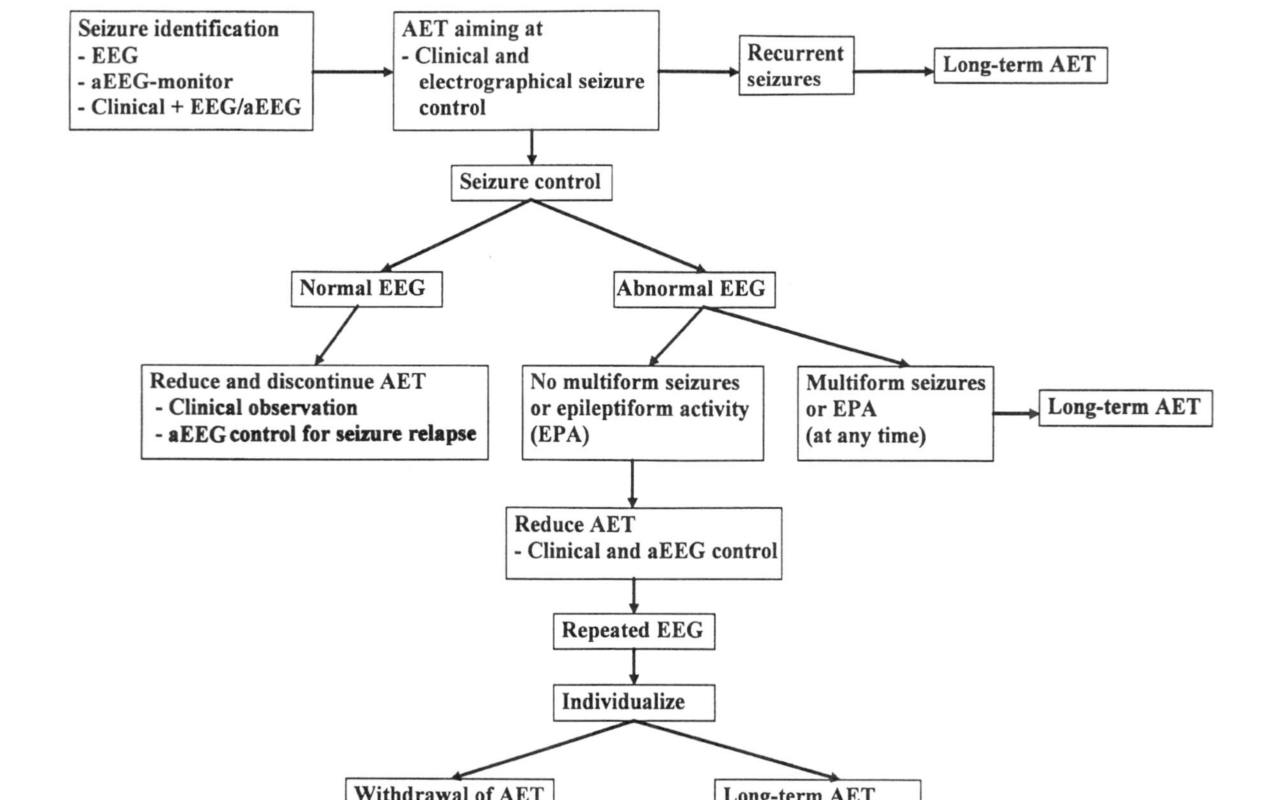

FIGURE 2.—Diagnostic criteria and management of neonatal seizures, including antiepileptic treatment drug withdrawal procedures as applied in this study. *Abbreviations: EEG, electroencephalogram; aEEG, amplitude-integrated electroencephalogram; AET, etiology; EPA, interictal epileptiform activity.* (Courtesy of Hellström-Westas L, Blennow G, Lindroth M, et al: Low risk of seizure recurrence after early withdrawal of antiepileptic treatment in the neonatal period. *Arch Dis Child* 72:F97–F101, 1995.)

Intractable Epilepsy in Children: The Efficacy of Lamotrigine Treatment, Including Non–Seizure-Related Benefits
Uvebrant P, Bauzienè R (Östra Hosp, Gothenburg, Sweden; Vilnius Univ Children's Hosp, Lithuania)
Neuropediatrics 25:284–289, 1994   4–4

Background.—Although most children with epilepsy respond to therapy, 1 in 5 has intractable seizures. Two of 3 of these patients are also sensitive to the side effects of antiepileptic drugs (AEDs). Lamotrigine (LTG), a medication chemically unrelated to AEDs, was used to treat patients refractive to standard AED therapy who also had additional neuroimpairments to determine its efficacy in this patient population.

Methods.—Fifty treatment-refractory children and adolescents with epilepsy formed the study cohort. Lamotrigine was given as add-on therapy to all but 6 patients whose AED treatment had been discontinued. A baseline seizure history was obtained with the use of a diary before treatment was begun. Demographic and medical data including an electroencephalogram, laboratory tests, CT, MR and single photon emission CT imaging, and a baseline Visual Analogue Scale score were recorded. The initial dose of LTG ranged from 0.3 to 2.2 mg/kg per 24 hours, depending on the dosage of AEDs already given. Patient response was identified as excellent, markedly improved, or having no or doubtful effect.

Results.—Treatment with LTG ranged from 4 to 35 months. In 24 children (53%), LTG had no effect on seizure control. Five patients had excellent results (seizure free), and 16 improved markedly (30% reduction in seizures). The response was comparable in children with different types of seizures and in those with and without normal neuroanatomy. Nonseizure results also occurred; in some children, autistic symptoms decreased; in others, mental state improved; and symptoms improved in 2 of 3 children with attention deficit hyperactivity disorder. Side effects were common, occurring in 42% of patients.

Conclusions.—Lamotrigine had both psychotropic and anticonvulsive effects in a group of children with intractable seizures. It is a useful adjunctive therapy for individuals who are treatment refractive.

▶ Lamotrigine appears to have a wide spectrum of antiepileptic activity and is useful in both partial and generalized seizures. It has established benefit in treating children with absence epilepsy, atonic seizures, and the Lennox-Gastaut syndrome. This article suggested that it may have some benefit as a psychotropic agent as well, especially in children with hyperactive behavior. If this is true, it would be welcome news, because most other AEDs tend to increase hyperactivity.

G.M. Fenichel, M.D.

Neonatal Neurology

Hypoxic Ischaemic Encephalopathy: Early Magnetic Resonance Imaging Findings and Their Evolution

Rutherford MA, Pennock JM, Schwieso JE, et al (Hammersmith Hosp, London)
Neuropediatrics 26:183–191, 1995

4–5

Objective.—Eighteen infants with hypoxic ischemic encephalopathy (HIE) were studied with MRI to document early imaging findings, to follow their evolution over the first 8 weeks of life, and to determine which acute signs are associated with the development of structural brain lesions.

Patients and Methods.—Eligible infants were born at term, exhibited neurologic abnormalities within the first 48 hours of life, and showed signs of fetal distress. Excluded were infants with an infectious or metabolic cause for encephalopathy. The 18 infants who entered the study had a total of 51 MRI scans. Using Sarnat's classification, 1 infant had grade I, 10 had grade II, and 4 had grade III HIE. Scans were obtained as soon as possible after birth, then repeatedly over the next 8 weeks. Three observers scored the images and reached a consensus.

Results.—Seven control infants scanned during the acute phase (days 1–5 of life) showed no brain swelling after the third day of life. All appeared to have normal myelination. The posterior part of the posterior limb of the internal capsule (PLIC) was seen as low signal intensity with T2-weighted spin-echo sequences. All but 1 infant with HIE showed signs of brain swelling in the acute phase, and 2 of 12 with marked brain swelling died. Brain swelling was seen in only 1 infant with HIE during the subacute phase (day 6–20) and in none during the chronic phase (day 1–56). Two of 6 infants with highlighting of the cortex during the acute phase died. Cortical highlighting was present in the 4 survivors and in 2 additional infants during the subacute phase; all 6 had this finding in the chronic phase. Other important findings in infants with HIE were a diffuse loss of gray/white differentiation, loss of signal in the PLIC, and high signal in the basal ganglia and hippocampus. T1-weighted spin-echo or inversion recovery sequences were better than T2-weighted spin-echo sequences in identifying these signs.

Conclusion.—Signs of brain swelling clear after the first week of life in infants with HIE, allowing the exact pattern of injury to be identified. Infants whose scores were initially high ($\geq$7) in the acute phase continued to have high scores, reflecting the development of permanent structural changes in the brain. Only infants in whom structural brain lesions developed exhibited loss of signal from within the PLIC, cortical highlighting, or loss of gray/matter differentiation.

▶ Serial cranial MRI of term newborns documents the severity and course of HIE. Brain swelling occurs in all newborns with HIE during the first week, including those with mild HIE. Brain swelling in isolation does not predict neurologic morbidity. However, the combination of marked brain swelling, loss of signal in the posterior limb of the internal capsule, cortical highlighting, and diffuse loss of gray/white matter differentiation accurately predicts mortality and chronic morbidity in survivors.

G.M. Fenichel, M.D.

Rapidly Progressive Enlargement of the Fourth Ventricle in the Preterm Infant With Post-Haemorrhagic Ventricular Dilatation
Rademaker KJ, Govaert P, Vandertop WP, et al (Wilhelmina Children's Hosp, Utrecht, The Netherlands; Univ Hosp, Gent, Belgium; Univ Hosp Utrecht, The Netherlands)
Acta Paediatr 84:1193–1196, 1995   4–6

Introduction.—Periventricular-intraventricular hemorrhage (PVH-IVH) is the most common ultrasound abnormality detected during the neonatal period in preterm infants with a gestational age of less than 32 weeks. Six patients who developed a rapid enlargement of the fourth ventricle after PVH-IVH were described.

Study Group.—Six preterm infants at 2 regional neonatal ICUs from 1990 to 1995 were diagnosed with a rapidly enlarging fourth ventricle by cranial ultrasound.

Findings.—Six preterm infants developed rapid enlargement of the lateral and fourth ventricles. Lumbar puncture was ineffective in all cases. In 5 of the 6 infants, bradycardia and cyanosis occurred while the infants were on ventilation therapy. Shunting of CSF from the lateral ventricle resolved these symptoms in 2 of the 3 survivors, suggesting panhydrocephaly. In the other survivor, an isolated fourth ventricle was diagnosed and a separate drain was installed. In all cases, there was extensive damage to the brain.

Conclusion.—Rapid enlargement of the fourth ventricle is a rare complication that can follow PVH-IVH. A combination of ultrasound recognition and cyanotic spells or bradycardia should indicate the need for a rapid relief of pressure. These infants require close follow-up because they can go on to develop fourth ventricle isolation without clinical symptoms.

▶ Posthemorrhagic hydrocephalus remains a difficult management problem in premature newborns who have sustained intraventricular hemorrhage. A permanent shunt cannot be placed until the blood has reabsorbed. This article brought attention to a syndrome of fourth ventricular dilatation that causes apnea, bradycardia, and potentially death from increased pressure in the posterior fossa. The diagnosis is made by routine serial ultrasonography. The ventricle must be drained once the diagnosis is established.

G.M. Fenichel, M.D.

Neurological Correlates of Fetal Cocaine Exposure: Transient Hypertonia of Infancy and Early Childhood

Chiriboga CA, Vibbert M, Malouf R, et al (Columbia Univ, New York; Harlem Hosp, New York)
Pediatrics 96:1070–1077, 1995

4–7

Introduction.—There have been few controlled studies of neurologic function among cocaine-exposed infants beyond the neonatal period. The results of neurologic and developmental assessments of 119 cocaine-positive and cocaine-negative infants followed for up to age 24 months were compared in a prospective cohort study.

Methods.—Eligibility was based on the presence of maternal risk factors: a history of IV drug use or of sexual contact with a high-risk partner. Infants were evaluated every 3 months in the first year and every 6 months in the second year of life. Examiners were blinded to drug exposure and HIV status. On the basis of infant urine toxicology, 51 infants tested positive and 68 were negative for cocaine and its metabolites. Neurologic diagnoses were classified as hypertonic and nonhypertonic.

Results.—Newborns who were cocaine positive had significantly lower mean birth weights and higher rates of small for gestational age status than cocaine-negative infants. Cocaine positivity was not associated with withdrawal symptoms or seizures but was significantly associated with all types of hypertonia at age 6 months (41% vs. 25% in cocaine-negative infants). Hypertonic tetraparesis (HTP) was 4 times more likely to be seen in cocaine-positive infants, and these associations remained significant when adjusted for perinatal variables. The rates of hypotonia were similar for cocaine-positive and cocaine-negative groups. Hypertonia had resolved in 97% of affected infants by 24 months. Leg hypertonia tended to be more persistent than arm hypertonia. Developmental scores were similar for cocaine-negative and cocaine-positive groups at all assessment periods. Infants who were cocaine positive and showed early HTP had significantly lower mean developmental scores at 6 and 12 months than those without HTP.

Conclusion.—Infants with cocaine-positive urine toxicology are significantly more likely to have hypertonia than are similarly high-risk infants who are cocaine negative. Most affected children outgrow hypertonia between 18 and 24 months. Cocaine-related hypertonia resembles hereditary stiff baby syndrome and may involve alterations in α-butyric acid or dopaminergic systems. Infants with the more extreme form of cocaine-related hypertonia appear to be at increased risk for subsequent neurodevelopmental problems.

▶ Children exposed to cocaine in utero are often exposed to other substances of abuse and sexually transmitted diseases and may have had inadequate intrauterine nutrition. They are at risk for cerebral palsy, mental and growth retardation, and seizures. In a large cohort of children being followed because they were at risk for HIV infection, a syndrome of transitory "cerebral palsy," characterized mainly by HTP, was identified in children exposed to cocaine in utero. The later consequences of this transitory hypertonia are unknown, and predicting long-term outcome is difficult.

G.M. Fenichel, M.D.

Other Pediatric Neurology Matters

Neurologic Manifestations of Pediatric Systemic Lupus Erythematosus
Steinlin MI, Blaser SI, Gilday DL, et al (Univ of Toronto; Hosp for Sick Children, Toronto)
Pediatr Neurol 13:191–197, 1995   4–8

Introduction.—Systemic lupus erythematosus (SLE) is an autoimmune disease with multisystem involvement. Pediatric SLE patients in a large series were reviewed to determine the frequency of CNS manifestations.

Study Group.—The study group consisted of 91 juveniles with SLE seen at 1 institution between 1976 and 1992. Average age of SLE onset was 13 years.

Findings.—Of the 91 patients, 40 had CNS involvement. In 19, the CNS manifestation was a presenting symptom, in 12 patients it occurred within the first year, and in 9 patients it occurred up to 7 years after diagnosis. Neuropsychiatric SLE was present in 19 children. This syndrome included depression, concentration or memory problems, and psychosis. Seizures occurred in 8, cerebral ischemia in 6, chorea in 1, papilledema in 2, and peripheral neuropathy in 2 patients. Nine patients had severe headache. More than 1 CNS manifestation was present in 7 children in this series. Computed tomography or MRI was helpful in diagnosing patients with focal ischemic lesions or venous sinus thrombosis. Electroencephalography was not useful in patients with diffuse symptoms and detected abnormality in only 33% of patients with seizures. Single-photon emission CT was abnormal in most patients with neuropsychiatric SLE. The lupus anticoagulant was present in the patient with chorea and in most of the patients with cerebral vascular events. The long-term outcome was good, with only 1 death and 3 children with persistent CNS deficits.

Conclusion.—In a historical series of 91 patients with pediatric SLE, CNS involvement was detected in 44%, with diverse manifestations. Investigations and treatment must be suited to the presenting symptoms. The overall prognosis was good, with only 1 death and excellent recovery in the majority of patients.

Neurologic Characteristics of Childhood Lupus Erythematosus
Parikh S, Swaiman KF, Kim Y (Univ of Minnesota, Minneapolis)
Pediatr Neurol 13:198–201, 1995   4–9

Objective.—The incidence of CNS manifestations in pediatric SLE patients was documented in a large series.

Study Group.—The study group consisted of 108 pediatric SLE patients seen at 1 institution between 1953 and 1990. Of the 108 pediatric SLE patients, CNS involvement was documented in 25. Average age at diagnosis was 13 years, and there were 22 girls and 3 boys. The diagnosis was established by both clinical and laboratory criteria.

Findings.—In 4 of the 25 patients, the neurologic symptoms preceded the diagnosis. Four patients had neurologic symptoms as presenting symptoms. The most frequent neurologic symptoms were headache and behavioral problems, especially depression, followed by chorea, hemiplegia or diplegia, seizures, visual loss, and cranial neuropathy. Vertigo and myelopathy each occurred in 1 patient. All patients were treated with corticosteroids and azathioprine. Dosages were increased until neurologic symptoms improved. The longest period of treatment before symptomatic improvement was 3 to 4 months.

Conclusion.—A large retrospective series of pediatric SLE patients was reviewed and CNS manifestations were determined to be common. Neurologic symptoms should be treated as disease exacerbations and respond well to immunosuppressive therapy.

▶ These 2 articles together comprise the largest series of children with neurologic manifestations of SLE. Both made the point that CNS disturbances are the initial feature in almost 20% of cases. Psychiatric disturbances, including frank psychoses, seizures, and chorea, are the most common early CNS manifestations. These are not usually associated with focal disturbances on imaging studies and are more likely to be caused by immune complex deposition than by ischemia. Central nervous system lupus should not be thought of as only a vascular disease. When stroke does occur, it is often associated with the presence of the lupus anticoagulant. Long-term prognosis for children with CNS lupus has improved by the judicious use of immunosuppressive therapy.

G.M. Fenichel, M.D.

Rett Syndrome: Clinical Peculiarities and Biological Mysteries
Hagberg B (East Hosp, Gothenburg, Sweden)
Acta Paediatr 84:971–976, 1995   4–10

Introduction.—Rett syndrome (RS), a disorder that nearly exclusively affects girls, has been clinically recognized only since the middle 1980s. Although apparently normal at birth, patients with RS generally cease to develop by 2 years and end up with severe multiple impairments. The clinical and genetic characteristics of this poorly understood neurodevelopmental deficiency were examined.

History and Diagnostic Criteria.—Andreas Rett, a University of Vienna pediatrician, first reported RS in a 1966 study of 31 female patients. The girls exhibited mental regression, abnormal neurology, and peculiar behavioral symptoms. Similarly impaired girls were reported in Japan and

Sweden. Those affected showed head circumference stagnation, a loss of purposeful hand skill followed by development of stereotypic hand movements, psychomotor regression, and gait ataxia. Four clinical stages have been described: early-onset stagnation, rapid developmental regression, a pseudostationary period, and late motor deterioration. Duration of the latter 2 stages may be decades. Variant cases of RS have also appeared; some show a milder degree of impairment, whereas others appear severely damaged from birth. Infantile seizures herald onset in up to 10% of cases of RS.

Swedish Series.—A group of 170 Swedish females with RS were studied. These patients ranged in age from 2 to 52 and were diagnosed from 1960 through 1994. Classic RS was present in 75% and variant forms in 25%.

Clinical and Neurologic Characteristics.—There may be many mildly impaired patients in whom RS has not been diagnosed. Clinical peculiarities include hand clapping or wringing, hyperventilation and breath-holding episodes, air swallowing, night laughing, bruxism, screaming attacks, and scoliosis. Intensive eye communication often appears after the regression period. Patients do not have traditional neurodegenerative abnormalities. In some young girls single-photon emission CT reveals an immature type of hypoperfusion in both the prefrontal and midbrain–upper brainstem areas. Laboratory testing is helpful only in excluding other disorders.

Genetics.—Although the genetic basis for RS is acknowledged, the mode of transmission is unclear. The X chromosome is not likely to be primarily involved; recent data suggest a gene locus for RS on the p-arm of chromosome 11. Deceleration of skull growth and brain hypoplasia point to a defect in the arrest of programmed normal neuronal cell death or lack of a specific brain growth factor.

▶ Rett syndrome occurs only in girls and the prevalence is estimated to be 1:10,000. Most cases are sporadic, but X-linked dominant inheritance with lethality in male fetuses is suspected. One study has suggested a candidate gene on chromosome 11.

Most affected girls have a typical clinical course. Developmental arrest usually begins at 12 months and is followed within a few months by rapid loss of language skills, decreased use of the hands, gait ataxia, and autistic behavior. Typical tonic-clonic seizures, partial complex seizures, or myoclonic seizures occur in most children between the ages of 2 and 4 years. Atypical variants are now recognized in which the degree of mental retardation may be mild. However, the full spectrum of phenotypes associated with RS cannot be delineated until a biological marker of the disease is established.

G.M. Fenichel, M.D

Prognostic Factors in Childhood Bacterial Meningitis

Kaaresen PI, Flægstad T (Univ Hosp of Tromsø, Norway)
Acta Paediatr 84:873–878, 1995   4–11

Background.—Despite better antibiotic therapy and intensive care, bacterial meningitis continues to be a major cause of mortality and morbidity among children. The associated mortality is about 5%, and permanent neurologic sequelae occur in 10% to 20%. The findings of previous studies on the association between symptom duration and outcome in patients with bacterial meningitis have been conflicting. The influence of symptom duration and prehospital antibiotic treatments and possible risk factors related to poor prognosis in childhood bacterial meningitis were investigated in the current study.

Methods and Findings.—Ninety-two children aged 1 month to 13.8 years were studied. Four children died, for a mortality of 4.3%. Permanent neurologic complications occurred in 14 (15.2%). The most common sequela was hearing impairment, which was strongly correlated with the length of symptom duration. In a multiple logistic regression analysis, risk factors independently related to subsequent death or sequelae were symptom duration of more than 48 hours, prehospital seizures, peripheral vasoconstriction, fewer than $1,000 \times 10^6$ leukocytes in CSF, and a temperature of 38.5°C or greater on admission. Prehospital antibiotic treatment, given orally or parenterally, was unrelated to outcome.

Conclusion.—Until effective prophylaxis against bacterial meningitis is available, early recognition of high-risk patients plus new treatment strategies such as dexamethasone and anticytokine therapy may help improve prognosis. The risk factors identified may be useful in determining who is at high risk for death or morbidity. Further research is needed to examine the impact of length or prediagnostic history.

▶ This study confirmed the previous impression that early treatment is the most important factor in determining outcome in children with bacterial meningitis. A delay of 48 hours greatly increases the risk of hearing loss. Peripheral vasoconstriction and a low body temperature at the time of initial examination are particularly ominous signs that correlate with neurologic morbidity and mortality. Intravenous antibiotic therapy must be started at the first suggestion of bacterial meningitis in a child.

G.M. Fenichel, M.D.

Outcome of Children With Opsoclonus-Myoclonus Regardless of Etiology

Hammer MS, Larsen MB, Stack CV (Children's Mem Hosp, Chicago)
Pediatr Neurol 13:21–24, 1995   4–12

Background.—Myoclonic encephalopathy of infancy (MEI) is characterized by acute or subacute onset of opsoclonus and frequent, irregular myoclonic limb jerking. Myoclonic encephalopathy of infancy has been associated with occult neuroblastoma. Bolthauser et al.[1] has specified 4 criteria for diagnosing MEI: the presence of marked motor incapacitation from myoclonic jerking, cerebellar ataxia, or both; opsoclonus; acute or subacute onset; and no evidence of infectious CNS disease. One series of patients with MEI as diagnosed by these criteria was presented.

Patients and Findings.—Eleven patients with opsoclonus and myoclonus, with or without a history of neuroblastoma, were admitted to 1 center in the past 11 years. Occult neuroblastoma was found in 8. Seven children with neuroblastoma and 1 without had subsequent delayed development with motor incoordination and speech delay. Initial treatment consisted of ACTH for 9 children and prednisone for 1. One child was not treated. Nine treated children had symptom recurrences during the gradual withdrawal or discontinuation of ACTH. The ACTH often had to be started again or increased, though several episodes were self-limiting and did not require treatment after ACTH withdrawal. Prednisone was ineffective in controlling opsoclonus-myoclonus, regardless of its cause. Most children with opsoclonus-myoclonus of any etiology had developmental delays that were more severe at a higher rate than previously reported. In children with neuroblastoma, symptoms were unaffected by tumor removal.

Conclusion.—Patients with opsoclonus-myoclonus without neuroblastoma have a better chance for normal neurologic development than children with MEI and neuroblastoma. Compared with ACTH, prednisone is ineffective in controlling opsoclonus-myoclonus of any etiology for any significant length of time.

Reference

1. Boltshauser E, Deonna TH, Hirt HR: Myoclonic encephalopathy of infants or "dancing eyes syndrome." *Helv Paediatr Acta* 34:119–133, 1979.

▶ Among children with the opsoclonus-myoclonus syndrome (MEI), some have neuroblastoma and some do not. The neuroblastoma is often occult and found only after searching several times. It seems likely that all children with MEI have a neuroblastoma. The response to treatment and the outcome are the same whether or not 1 is found. Compared with prednisone, ACTH is a better choice.

G.M. Fenichel, M.D.

Incidence of Neurological Complications of Surgery for Congenital Heart Disease

Fallon P, Aparício JM, Elliott MJ, et al (Inst of Child Health, London; Hosp for Sick Children, London)
Arch Dis Child 72:418–422, 1995   4–13

Introduction.—As the mortality associated with surgical repair of congenital heart defects has fallen, concerns have been raised about the extent of associated neurologic morbidity. The frequency of neurologic events after cardiac surgery was determined in a consecutive series of 523 patients undergoing cardiac surgery at the Hospital for Sick Children, London.

Study Design.—From November 1990 to October 1991, there were 523 surgical discharge summaries at this hospital, which were examined for adverse neurologic events occurring between operation and discharge.

Findings.—Adverse neurologic events were recorded in 31 of 523 cardiac surgery cases and included 16 seizures, 11 pyramidal signs, 8 extrapyramidal signs, 6 comas, and 6 neuro-ophthalmic deficits. There were significantly more adverse neurologic events after repairs for arch anomalies. There was an association between adverse neurologic events and the duration of cardiopulmonary bypass, as well as with a period of low-perfusion pressure. Of the 31 patients with adverse neurologic events, 8 died and 4 were lost to follow-up. Of the remaining 19 patients with long-term data available, 9 had preoperative neurodevelopmental abnormalities, 6 had persisting neurologic problems that could be traced directly to the perioperative period, and 4 were normal.

Conclusion.—In a series of 523 patients undergoing surgery to correct congenital cardiac defects, 31 had adverse neurologic events. Of these, 19 had long-term follow-up available. Ten of these patients had persisting neurologic deficit. In 4 of these patients it was difficult to determine the amount of deficit due to perioperative events, but in 6 patients their deficit could be directly related to their cardiac surgery. This represents a significant proportion of young patients whose lives remain impaired despite correction of their cardiac abnormality. Further research is necessary to limit this neurologic damage associated with surgery to repair congenital cardiac defects.

▶ Cyanotic congenital heart disease is associated with an increased incidence of delayed psychomotor development, especially when surgical repair is delayed until late childhood. Surgical repair during infancy reduces the incidence of developmental delay by preventing chronic hypoxia. The incidence of permanent neurologic disorders attributed to surgery is relatively small, and the main risk factor is prolonged cardiopulmonary bypass. In assessing neurologic function after surgery, one must also consider that many children with congenital heart disease also have cerebral anomalies.

G.M. Fenichel, M.D.

5 Headache and Pain

Oral Sumatriptan for the Long-Term Treatment of Migraine: Clinical Findings
Rederich G, Rapoport A, Cutler N, et al (Hawthorne Community Med Group, Calif; New England Ctr for Headache, Stamford, Conn; California Clinical Trials Group, Beverly Hills, Calif; et al)
Neurology 45 (suppl 7):15S–20S, 1995   5–1

Introduction.—Migraine is typically a recurrent condition. Therefore, patients may use acute therapy repeatedly, which may result in diminished therapeutic efficacy and increased drug-related side effects. Sumatriptan, a selective serotonin receptor agonist, has proved effective for the acute treatment of migraine. The efficacy of oral sumatriptan for long-term acute treatment for separate migraine attacks over the course of 1 year was evaluated in a randomized, double-blind, placebo-controlled, crossover study.

Methods.—Adults with at least a 1-year history of migraine with or without aura and 2 to 6 migraine attacks monthly during the preceding 60 days were given randomly ordered oral sumatriptan (100 mg) and placebo in a 3:1 ratio for 3 blocks of 4 migraine attacks. The patients were instructed to take no other medication for at least 2 hours after taking the study medication. Up to 650 mg of acetaminophen could be taken as rescue medication 2 to 4 hours after taking the study medication, and patients' usual migraine treatment could be taken 4 hours after the study medication. Patients rated headache severity, clinical disability, and nausea and vomiting on diary cards before taking the study medication, hourly for 12 hours, and every 6 hours for 48 hours. They also documented their use of rescue medication. After each migraine attack, the patients returned their diary cards to the clinic and obtained the study medication to be used for the next attack.

Results.—A significantly greater proportion of the patients obtained headache relief using sumatriptan than using placebo. Complete headache relief occurred at 2 hours in 25% to 28% of those taking sumatriptan and in 4% to 8% of those taking placebo and at 4 hours in 43% to 48% of those taking sumatriptan and in 4% to 15% of those taking placebo. The differences in relief rates were significant beginning 1 hour after taking the study drug. Clinical disability was reported by 91% of the patients at baseline and was significantly more effectively relieved by sumatriptan than by placebo. Nausea was reported by 57% to 60% of the patients at baseline and was relieved at 2 hours in 66% and at 4 hours in 83% of those taking sumatriptan and at 2 hours in 55% and at 4 hours in 63% of those taking placebo. The first use of rescue medication was reported at 18 to 38 hours after sumatriptan use and at 4 hours after placebo use. Although there were more reports of drug-related adverse events after sumatriptan treatment, there was no difference in the incidence of adverse events in the 2 groups after adjustment for the number of administrations.

Conclusion.—The therapeutic efficacy of 100 mg of oral sumatriptan, in the treatment of migraine attacks remained consistent for up to 1 year. Repeated administration was not associated with changes in the type or severity of adverse events.

▶ By now neurologic clinicians are well aware of the efficacy of subcutaneous sumatriptan and know that it constitutes a major therapeutic addition to the abortive treatment of migraine. The recent introduction of the oral preparation of the medication has been welcomed largely because of convenience for patients. The present study indicated that oral sumatriptan is efficacious in a substantial proportion of patients and that, even with continued use, it retains its efficacy for an extended period. Not surprisingly, the oral preparation does not relieve symptoms in as many patients as the parenteral medication. Clinicians must determine in individual patients which form of the drug to prescribe, and individual patients must decide, on the basis of their experience, which form is best for individual headaches.

R.A. Davidoff, M.D.

Transnasal Butorphanol in the Treatment of Acute Migraine
Hoffert MJ, Couch JR, Diamond S, et al (John R Graham Headache Ctr, Boston; Univ of Oklahoma, Norman; San Francisco Headache Clinic, Calif; et al)
Headache 35:65–69, 1995   5–2

Introduction.—Headache specialists have not agreed on whether it is appropriate to use narcotic analgesics to treat migraine. Butorphanol, which may be administered transnasally and was recently approved by the Food and Drug Administration, has comparatively low abuse potential and is a potent analgesic with a rapid onset of action. The risk of regurgitating medication is eliminated. Butorphanol is not a federally controlled substance.

Study Design.—Adult patients at 10 headache centers who were diagnosed as having migraine with or without aura volunteered to participate in a randomized double-blind, placebo-controlled trial of butorphanol. Patients (ages 21–63) had had 2 to 8 migraine attacks per month but were in good general health. They were assigned to receive butorphanol or placebo in a 2:1 ratio. Active treatment consisted of 1 mg of butorphanol per spray. Prophylactic agents were allowed during the trial.

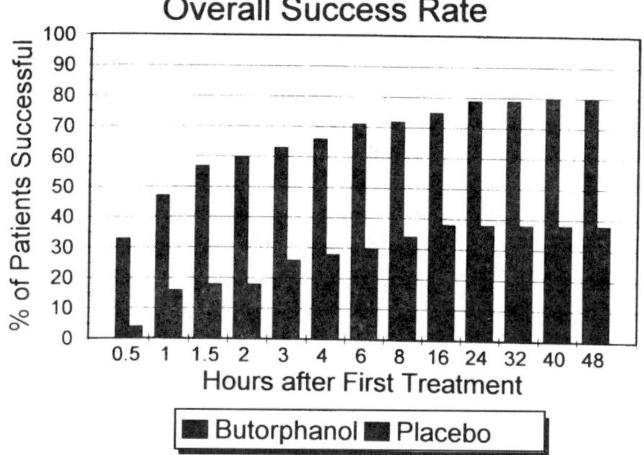

FIGURE 1.—Percent of subjects in butorphanol and placebo groups who experienced treatment success over time. Success is defined as decrease in headache pain intensity rating from moderate, severe, or incapacitating to none or slight ($P < 0.05$ at each time point, χ^2 test). (Courtesy of Hoffert MJ, Couch JR, Diamond S, et al: Transnasal butorphanol in the treatment of acute migraine. *Headache* 35:65–69, 1995.)

Results.—Eighty percent of the 107 actively treated patients and 38% of the 50 placebo recipients achieved success by 40 hours (Fig 1). More than half the butorphanol-treated patients who responded did so within 1 hour of receiving the first dose, and nearly all of them had responded by 6 hours. The difference in response was significant at 90 minutes and thereafter. Fewer actively treated patients required rescue medication. Side effects were frequent (Table 3) and often intense. One fourth of patients chose not to receive butorphanol after the first dose. Side effects were not dose dependent.

Recommendations.—The best approach to patients with frequent migraine attacks is to attempt to reduce the risk of headache by prophylactic medication and other measures. If an opioid analgesic is to be used to

TABLE 3.—Side Effects Occurring With an Incidence Greater Than 5%

Side Effect	Butorphanol (%)	Placebo (%)
Dizziness	58	4
Nausea and/or vomiting	38	18
Drowsiness	29	0
Unpleasant taste	17	0
Paresthesias	13	2
Sweating	12	0
Confusion	9	4
Nasal irritation	8	2
Tremor	8	0
Euphoria	7	0
Nervousness	7	7

(Courtesy of Hoffert MJ, Couch JR, Diamond S, et al: Transnasal butorphanol in the treatment of acute migraine. *Headache* 35:65–69, 1995.)

relieve symptoms when primary measures fail, transnasal butorphanol is an effective choice.

▶ Butorphanol is a mixed agonist-antagonist opioid analgesic. Such drugs act as partial agonists and antagonists at separate opioid receptors. Many clinicians prefer to use such medication because they believe they have a lower potential for abuse and addiction. These medications do, however, have such potential and must not be overprescribed. Patients must be warned about the capability of the drug to produce dependency when abused. However, for patients who do not have severe or disabling side effects, intranasal butorphanol is often a valuable adjunct for those who require abortive or symptomatic therapy for their acute migraine attacks.

R.A. Davidoff, M.D.

Efficacy, Safety, and Tolerability of Dihydroergotamine Nasal Spray as Monotherapy in the Treatment of Acute Migraine
The Dihydroergotamine Nasal Spray Multicenter Investigators (New England Ctr for Headache, Stamford, Conn; Univ of Oklahoma, Oklahoma City; San Francisco Headache Clinic, Calif; et al)
Headache 35:177–184, 1995   5–3

Background.—Dihydroergotamine (DHE) has many advantages as a treatment for migraine. It is less likely than ergotamine to produce vomiting, and it is able to rapidly end acute attacks, even at their peak. Physical dependence has not been noted with DHE, in contrast to ergotamine. The drug appears to selectively constrict capacitance vessels, altering resistance vessels less than ergotamine in equivalent dosage. For this reason, DHE may have less potential for causing coronary vasospasm. Nasally administered DHE is rapidly absorbed. The most common adverse effects have included local reactions of the nasal mucosa, nasal obstruction, and congestion.

Study Population.—The safety and tolerance of DHE nasal spray were examined in 206 patients enrolled in 2 double-blind, placebo-controlled trials. Active medication was used by 102 patients and a placebo spray by 104. Twenty-four patients treated a single headache, whereas 182 treated 2 episodes. Most patients were women aged 18 to 62 with a history of common migraine and a family history of migraine. All participants were in good general health.

Observations.—Patients receiving active medication had significantly less pain than placebo recipients within 4 hours after treatment. In 1 study, DHE proved better than placebo in relieving nausea. In both studies, DHE-treated patients rated themselves as being symptomatic for a shorter time than those given placebo. Physicians confirmed that the DHE spray was significantly better than placebo in relieving headache pain in both studies. More placebo patients required rescue medication. Active treatment was safe and well tolerated. Only 2 patients withdrew because of side effects, and there were no serious lasting effects. The most common side effects of DHE were nasal congestion, nasal irritation, and throat discomfort. There were no important laboratory abnormalities.

Conclusion.—The self-administered DHE nasal spray is effective and safe when used as monotherapy for migraine.

▶ All of us who treat patients with migraine headaches are confronted with individuals who do not respond to conventional abortive therapy, who should not receive medications that are potentially addictive (e.g., narcotics, sedative/hypnotic combinations, caffergot) because of the frequency of their headaches, or who will not give themselves injections at home. Intranasally administered DHE represents a major addition to our ability to treat such patients with acute migraine. Intranasal DHE is safer than caffergot, has few serious side effects, is easily administered, and is effective in a substantial number of patients. Of great importance is that it causes very little physical dependency. Nasal DHE is readily compounded by some local pharmacists.

R.A. Davidoff, M.D.

Headache and Neck Pain in Spontaneous Internal Carotid and Vertebral Artery Dissections

Silbert PL, Mokri B, Schievink WI (Mayo Clinic and Mayo Found, Rochester, Minn)
Neurology 45:1517–1522, 1995

5–4

Background.—Early identification of arterial dissection may enable early treatment, possibly preventing a more serious cerebral ischemic complication. Headache and neck pain in patients with internal carotid artery dissection (ICAD) or vertebral artery dissection (VAD) were studied to determine the patterns of headache and clinical manifestations that should raise early suspicion of the presence of dissection.

Patients and Findings.—One hundred sixty-one consecutive symptomatic patients were included. One hundred thirty-five had spontaneous dissections of the internal carotid artery and 26 of the vertebral artery. Mean age in the former group was 47 and in the latter group was 40.7. Eighteen percent of those with ICAD and 23% with VAD had a history of migraine. Sixty-eight percent with ICAD and 69% with VAD reported headache. When present, headache was the initial manifestation in 47% of those with ICAD and in 33% of those with VAD. Eye, facial, or ear pain but no headache was present in 10% of the patients with ICAD. Median time from headache onset to the development of other neurologic manifestations was 4 days for patients with ICAD and 14.5 hours for those with VAD. Headache was usually ipsilateral to the side of dissection in both groups. Among patients with ICAD, headaches were distributed posteriorly in 83%. They were steady in 73% and pulsating in 25%. Twenty-six percent of the patients with ICAD had neck pain compared with 46% of those with VAD. Median headache duration in patients in both groups was 72 hours. However, in 4 patients with ICAD, headaches were prolonged, persisting for months to years.

Conclusion.—Headache is the most common clinical manifestation in patients with symptomatic ICAD and VAD, occurring in more than two thirds of patients with each type of dissection. Headache was the first symptom in nearly half of those with ICAD and in one third of those with VAD. Neck pain occurred more commonly in patients with VAD than in those with ICAD. The pain in ICAD was usually ipsilateral and distributed over the anterior head. In VAD, the pain was either ipsilateral or bilateral and usually distributed over the posterior head region. Pain was constant more often than pulsating. Sixty-two percent of the patients with ICAD and 60% with VAD said that the headache was unique.

▶ Any new-onset head or neck pain must be considered suspect because it may herald a CAD or VAD that can result in stroke with permanent neurologic deficits or even death. A high index of suspicion is necessary because, as noted in the article, a substantial minority of the patients have a history of migraine headaches. Importantly, the head pain frequently precedes the neurologic deficit and can do so by as much as 1 or 2 weeks. The syndrome develops as a result of tearing of the arterial wall, and ischemia arises either because of occlusion of the lumen at the site of the dissection or from embolization from the torn edge of the intima. Treatment with antiplatelet or anticoagulant medication must be instituted as rapidly as possible.

R.A. Davidoff, M.D.

Extratrigeminal Ice-Pick Status

Martins IP, Parreira E, Costa I (Inst Portugês de Oncologia, Lisboa)
Headache 35:107–110, 1995   5–5

Background.—Idiopathic stabbing headache is a brief and sharp stabbing head pain felt predominantly in the distribution of the first division of the trigeminal nerve and occurs mainly in individuals with migraine. Six patients with an identical type of headache but with an extratrigeminal location were described.

Findings.—Over a 7-year period, 5 women and 1 man aged 33 to 65 were seen in the emergency department for daily attacks of very intense, ice pick–like pain that recurred every minute in a "statuslike" fashion in the same points of the scalp. The pain was self-limited, lasting from 16 hours to 9 days, and felt outside the cutaneous area of the trigeminal nerve, mainly in the retroauricular, parietal, and occipital regions. The attacks occurred suddenly with no evident trigger factors. The pain occurred independent of movements of the head and neck and was not modified by palpation of the occipital nerve trunks or the neck. Two patients had recurrent episodes. None of the patients had migraine. The headache responded to oral indomethacin. In 1 patient, the pain changed site after a local infiltration with procaine.

Conclusion.—This unusual headache may be a variant of idiopathic stabbing headache, but it differs from it by its temporal profile (in "status"), its posterior (extratrigeminal) location, and its lack of association with migraine. The headache is usually severe but remits spontaneously and responds promptly to indomethacin.

▶ Ice pick–like pains (also called idiopathic stabbing headaches, jabs and jolts, or needle-in-the-eye syndrome) characteristically occur around the orbit or the temple, and many patients feel the pains at the site or side of their customary migraine headache. Phenomena that appear identical to ice pick–like pains have also been reported by patients with cluster headaches and temporal arteritis. The authors described a similar syndrome but 1 located in a different location that may have a different temporal pattern. It is responsive to indomethacin in a manner similar to that of ice pick–like headaches associated with migraine.

R.A. Davidoff, M.D.

Prevalence and Clinical Features of Abdominal Migraine Compared With Those of Migraine Headache
Abu-Arafeh I, Russell G (Royal Aberdeen Children's Hosp, Scotland)
Arch Dis Child 72:413–417, 1995   5–6

Objective.—Increasing evidence suggests that abdominal migraine is a separate entity that can be distinguished from other causes of recurrent abdominal pain. The epidemiology of recurrent abdominal pain was assessed in schoolchildren in the city of Aberdeen, with special emphasis on headache migraine and abdominal migraine.

Methods.—In a random manner, 10% of schoolchildren aged 5 to 15 years were selected from the schools' lists and given a questionnaire inquiring, among other symptoms, about the history of headache and abdominal pain over the past year. Children with at least 2 episodes of severe headache pain, severe abdominal pain, or both, attributed by their parents to either unknown causes or migraine, were invited for clinical interview and examination. The diagnosis of abdominal migraine was based on criteria adopted by Symon and Russell[1] that included dull or colicky pain severe enough to interfere with normal daily activities; periumbilical or poorly localized pain; pain associated with any 2 of the following—anorexia, nausea, vomiting, or pallor; attack lasting for at least 1 hour; and complete resolution of symptoms between attacks.

Results.—A total of 1,754 (81%) children responded. The prevalence of headache and abdominal pain was high, with 72% of children having at least 1 episode of abdominal pain over the past year and 66% having at least 1 episode of abdominal pain over the past year. In addition, 32% with headache pain and 22% with abdominal pain had pain severe enough to interfere with normal activities. After interview, 159 fulfilled the International Headache Society's diagnostic criteria for migraine headache; 58 children had abdominal migraine, and 44 children had both migraine and abdominal migraine. The estimated prevalence rate was 10.6% for migraine headache and 4.1% for abdominal migraine.

Abdominal migraine was more common in girls than in boys. The pain started at a mean age of 7.0 years with 2 distinct peaks at the ages of 5 and 10 years. Attacks occurred at a mean of 14 times yearly, with each attack lasting for a mean of 17 hours. About one third of the children had first-degree relatives with migraine headache. These children lost a mean of 3.7 school days each year because of abdominal pain. Children with migraine headache and children with abdominal migraine had similar demographic and social characteristics, patterns of associated recurrent painful conditions, trigger and relieving factors, and associated symptoms during attacks.

Conclusion.—With a prevalence of 4.1% in children 5 to 15 years old, abdominal migraine is clearly a sizeable clinical problem and a significant cause of recurrent abdominal pain. It appears that abdominal migraine and migraine headache may have a common pathogenesis given the similarities between the 2 conditions.

Reference

1. Symon DNK, Russell G: Abdominal migraine: A syndrome defined. *Cephalalgia* 6:223–228, 1986.

▶ A great deal of debate surrounds the idea of abdominal migraine, and many consider it an ill-defined entity. Some investigators challenge its reality; others believe the origin of the syndrome to be epileptic or psychogenic. The International Headache Society declined to include abdominal migraine in its classification. Few controlled data about these problems exist. Drs. Abu-Arafeh and Russell studied a large number of children with recurrent abdominal pain by questionnaire and defined a group who have certain characteristics commonly seen in children with migraine. However, only a prospective study combined with therapeutic intervention using medication that we know work as preventives for migraine will answer remaining questions regarding the migrainous causation of recurrent abdominal pain in children.

R.A. Davidoff, M.D.

Case-Control Study of Migraine and Risk of Ischaemic Stroke in Young Women

Tzourio C, Tehindrazanarivelo A, Iglésias S, et al (INSERM U360, Villejuif, France; Hôpital Saint-Antoine, Paris; Hôpital de Meaux, France; et al)
BMJ 310:830–833, 1995   5–7

Introduction.—The relation between migraine and ischemic stroke has been little studied. Some association has been found in women younger than 45, but the sample size was small. The association between migraine and ischemic stroke was further studied in a larger group of young women, with consideration of 2 other known vascular risk factors: oral contraceptive use and cigarette smoking.

Methods.—A case-control study was designed that included 72 women younger than 45 who had a first ischemic stroke and 173 randomly chosen controls who were hospitalized for acute orthopedic or benign rheumatologic illness. All patients were interviewed with the use of a structured questionnaire that probed their history of headaches, migraine features, and other vascular risk factors.

Results.—Case and control patients were similar in mean age, body mass index, history of diabetes, and educational background but differed in the use of oral contraceptives, smoking, and history of hypertension and hypercholesterolemia. The risk of stroke in current users of oral contraceptives varied with the estrogen dose, from an odds ratio of 4.8 for pills with 50 µg of estrogen to 1.7 for pills with 20 µg of estrogen and 1.0 for pills with progestogen. Only current heavy smokers had an elevated risk of ischemic stroke (odds ratio 2.4). There was no association between migraine and either smoking or use of oral contraceptives in either case or control patients. However, migraine was strongly associated with ischemic stroke, because 60% of case patients and only 30% of control patients had migraine. The risk of stroke was higher in association with migraine with aura than with migraine without aura (odds ratio 6.2 vs. 3.0). Among women with a history of migraine, the risk of ischemic stroke rose to 13.9 in patients who used oral contraceptives and to 10.2 in heavy smokers compared with women who had no migraine and no history of oral contraceptive use or smoking.

Discussion.—Analysis showed that history of migraine, oral contraceptive use, and current heavy cigarette smoking all were strong, independent risk factors for ischemic stroke in women younger than 45. The presence of more than 1 of these factors substantially increased risk. Contrary to other controlled studies, migraine both with and without aura was associated with increased risk. More research is needed to determine the nature of this association, because it is possible that risk may be elevated only in migrainous women who have a condition predisposing to ischemic stroke. It is suggested that migrainous women be advised not to smoke and to use only low-dose pills if they use oral contraceptives.

▶ This investigation was a continuation of the authors' studies of ischemic stroke in patients with migraine. Their conclusion that ischemic infarction is strongly associated with migraine both with and without aura was buttressed, by convincing data. The risk was greatest, however, in patients with classic migraine. Most important, their data indicated that the risk for stroke was considerably increased in migrainous women who use contraceptive pills or who heavily smoke. Although the absolute risk of stroke is low, these 2 risk factors must be discussed with all young female migraineurs.

R.A. Davidoff, M.D.

The Management of Central Post-Stroke Pain

Bowsher D (Walton Hosp, Liverpool, England)
Postgrad Med J 71:598–604, 1995

5–8

Background.—Central post-stroke pain (CPSP), originally called thalamic syndrome, was first described in 1906. Many authors have noted the lack of response of central pain to conventional analgesic therapy. In the past, the "pain pathways" were cut to relieve pain in patients in whom the pain was present primarily or entirely in a body region below a surgically accessible spinal level. Many of the proponents of this ineffective procedure apparently did not notice the pathophysiologic similarity between thalamic syndrome and spontaneously painful postcordotomy dysesthesia. Present management of CPSP was discussed.

Management.—Central post-stroke pain is characterized by frequently burning or freezing pain; an onset usually occurring months after stroke; difficulty distinguishing sharp sensations from blunt and warm from cool in the affected area; exacerbation by stress, with alleviation with relaxation; and little or no difficulty falling asleep. Allodynia is present in 60% of the patients and is pathognomonic. In treating CPSP, physicians should not waste time trying conventional analgesics. Adrenergically active antidepressants should be initiated as soon as possible after the onset of pain. Mexiletine can be added if pain is not relieved by the tolerated antidepressant. Before mexiletine treatment is initiated, all hypotensive drugs should be stopped for 48 hours. Other drugs, especially tricyclics, should be continued. Blood pressure and Visual Analogue Scale scores should be obtained before mexiletine treatment commences. The recommended dosage is 400 mg orally, followed by 200 mg every 6 hours. Blood pressure is determined every hour for the first 24 hours. If blood pressure declines significantly, mexiletine should be stopped and attempts made to increase blood pressure. If pain is successfully relieved after 2 or 3 days, the patient is discharged on a dose that does not cause dizziness. Patients unresponsive to antidepressants with mexiletine should be referred to a pain clinic.

Conclusion.—Originally called thalamic syndrome, CPSP was renamed because many patients have infarcts that are not in the thalamus. Pain is located in an area of sensory deficit and characterized by increased thresholds for temperature and pinprick. Initial treatment consists of adrenergically active antidepressants. Time should not be wasted trying conventional analgesics, because response to these drugs is slight at best.

▶ The problem of treating CPSP still frustrates clinicians because the responses to conventional treatment have been limited. In addition, many clinicians find the diagnosis difficult because objective findings may be subtle in patients who complain of severe and unremitting pain. As stressed by the author, the cornerstone of achieving intractable pain reduction is pharmacologic treatment, with an emphasis on the use of tricyclic antidepressants often combined with anticonvulsants. The use of mexiletine was emphasized, but others[1] have found it less efficacious. The use of physical therapy and relaxation techniques is typically helpful. Early treatment improves the prognosis considerably.

R.A. Davidoff, M.D.

Reference

1. Gonzales GR: Central pain: Diagnosis and treatment strategies. *Neurology* 45(suppl 9):S11–S16, 1995.

6 Behavioral Neurology

Alzheimer's Disease

Apolipoprotein E and Alzheimer's Disease: The Implications of Progress in Molecular Medicine
Mayeux R, Schupf N (Columbia Univ, New York; New York State Inst for Basic Research in Developmental Disabilities, Staten Island)
Am J Public Health 85:1280–1284, 1995   6–1

Objective.—Because progress in molecular genetics now makes it possible to determine the future risk of many diseases, the tests raise scientific, social, legal, and ethical questions. A newly developed test for Alzheimer's disease (AD) was reviewed.

Public Health Burden of Alzheimer's Disease.—By the year 2000 about 10 million Americans will have AD and require expensive care for as long as 10 to 15 years. Late-onset disease has been linked to the ϵ4-type allele of apolipoprotein E. Although the presence of the ϵ4 allele is neither necessary nor sufficient to cause AD, this finding may be confounded by the genotypic distributions of age at onset or by a disequilibrium with another as yet unidentified susceptibility gene. Those who agree with the multiple-gene theory view apolipoprotein genotypes as risk factors rather than genetic markers of AD.

Screening and Testing.—Screening large populations is not practical, particularly because half of the patients with AD do not have the ϵ4 allele. It is doubtful that prevention based on apolipoprotein E or on the ϵ2 or ϵ3 alleles would be beneficial. Diagnostic testing would not lower the costs of evaluation for most patients because most do not have the ϵ4 allele. Those who do represent only 2% to 3% of the population. Early detection provides ambiguous prognostic implications and does not consider morbidity and mortality of other diseases.

Consequences of Testing.—Testing should be accompanied by pretest and posttest counseling that may have to include a large number of risk factors, particularly because no treatment exists for AD.

Privacy and Confidentiality.—Policies must be established that regulate access to genetic information to prevent discrimination in employment and insurance and access to stored DNA to circumvent unauthorized use of samples from identified individuals.

Conclusion.—Molecular approaches will be incorporated into the study of public health problems. The ethical, legal, and social implications of these new methods must be carefully considered.

▶ The authors provided an illuminating review of the ongoing controversy about the role of apolipoprotein genotyping in clinical practice and in neuroepidemiologic research. Furthermore, they offered a cogent and sensible assessment of the present value of this information and pointed to the unresolved issues of the protection and disclosure of the increasing volume of this and related genetic information. Because some apolipoprotein genotypes are risk factors and not inevitable predictors of AD, the article emphasized the need for further understanding of (1) associated risk factors, (2) actual causative factors, and (3) their precise interactions to begin to interpret the significance of their combined risks in individuals and for the statistical study of populations.

R. Kuljis, M.D.

LDL Receptor-Related Protein, a Multifunctional ApoE Receptor, Binds Secreted β-Amyloid Precursor Protein and Mediates Its Degradation
Kounnas MZ, Moir RD, Rebeck GW, et al (American Red Cross, Rockville, Md; Massachusetts Gen Hosp, Boston)
Cell 82:331–340, 1995   6–2

Background.—In Alzheimer's disease (AD) there are extracellular deposits of insoluble aggregates of Aβ peptide in the brain, derived from the membrane protein β-amyloid precursor protein (APP). The secreted form of APP, which contains the Kunitz proteinase inhibitor (KPI) domain, is generated by proteolytic cleavage within its extracellular domain and is internalized and degraded by cells. This process may well involve the low-density lipoprotein receptor–related protein (LRP), which promotes the catabolism of tissue factor pathway inhibitor, another Kunitz-type inhibitor.

Objective.—β-Amyloid precursor protein was studied to determine its susceptibility to catabolism by LRP. The isoforms APP770 and APP695 (which lack the KPI domain) were purified from cell cultures transfected by the respective complementary DNAs.

Findings.—Receptor-associated protein, which antagonizes LRP, suppressed the degradation of secreted APP770. Antibody against LRP had the same effect. Degradation was much reduced in fibroblasts that were genetically deficient in LRP. In contrast, secreted APP695 was a poor ligand for LRP.

Discussion.—Inheritance of the ε4 allele of the *apoE* gene increases the risk of AD. The present finding that secreted APP770 is a novel LRP ligand indicates that LRP is a receptor for both APP and apoE. Genetic variants of both of these molecules are genetically linked with or closely related to familial and sporadic AD.

▶ This receptor mediates the metabolism of the precursor of the amyloid protein deposits present in AD lesions and of the only molecular risk factor for the disease identified so far. It may therefore prove to be 1 of the key mechanisms in the pathophysiology of AD, and, thus, a putative site for pharmacologic palliative and preventive interventions.

R. Kuljis, M.D.

Do Nonsteroidal Anti-Inflammatory Drugs Decrease the Risk for Alzheimer's Disease?: The Rotterdam Study

Andersen K, Launer LJ, Ott A, et al (Erasmus Univ, Rotterdam, The Netherlands)
Neurology 45:1441–1445, 1995   6–3

Objective.—Because studies have reported the presence of immune processes in the brains of patients with Alzheimer's disease (AD), some investigators have postulated that nonsteroidal anti-inflammatory drugs (NSAIDs) may lower the risk of the disease. A cross-sectional study of the relationship between NSAID use, the risk of AD, and cognitive function was conducted.

Methods.—The study included 6,258 community-dwelling or institutionalized individuals older than 55 with 228 individuals with dementia, 155 of whom had AD. A total of 365 used prescription NSAIDs and 365 used topical drugs.

Results.—Persons who used NSAIDs tended to be women, older, less well educated, and to use more benzodiazepines than all nonusers of NSAIDs. There was no difference in aspirin use between individuals with or without AD. Significantly more individuals with AD used benzodiazepines. The risk of AD for NSAID users was 0.38. The risk for topical medication users was comparable at 0.54, although the confidence interval was larger and the relation was significant.

Conclusion.—There is a possibility that NSAIDs lower the risk of AD. Additional studies must be conducted to determine the role of inflammation in the neurodegenerative process.

▶ The Rotterdam Study is a helpful contribution to the debate about the presumed inflammation-mediated pathophysiologic changes of AD. Most previous studies have used small samples and have had difficulties with the assessment of multiple variables that can confound interpretation of outcomes. Many of these problems were substantially addressed in this study, which supported the hypothesis that anti-inflammatory therapy may reduce the risk of AD. This study and previous work in this field underscored the need for additional investigation to verify more rigorously the effect of this intervention, to identify the best drugs, and to determine the ideal tempo of drug administration.

R. Kuljis, M.D.

Familial Alzheimer's Disease in Kindreds With Missense Mutations in a Gene on Chromosome 1 Related to the Alzheimer's Disease Type 3 Gene
Rogaev EI, Sherrington R, Rogaeva EA, et al (Univ of Toronto; Hosp for Sick Children, Toronto; Univ of Florence, Italy; et al)
Nature 376:775–778, 1995   6–4

Background.—Initial studies of the *S182* gene on chromosome 14q24.3—also known as the Alzheimer's disease (AD) type 3 gene—suggested that there might be other genes with similar sequences. A new gene that has substantial nucleotide and amino acid sequence similarity to the *S182* gene was reported.

Findings.—The newly cloned gene, designated *E5-1*, is encoded on chromosome 1. The study also identified mutations, including 3 new missense mutations of the *S182* gene, associated with the *AD3* subtype of early-onset familial AD, which starts between the ages of 30 and 60. The *E5-1* and *S182* proteins were predicted to be integral membrane proteins with 7 membrane-spanning domains, including a large exposed loop between the sixth and seventh domains (Fig 3). Nucleotide sequence analysis of the open reading frame of *E5-1* revealed 2 missense mutations at conserved amino acid residues in patients with a type of familial AD with a later age at onset (50–70) than the *AD3* subtype.

Conclusion.—A new gene and its association with early AD were reported. The *E5-1* and *S182* genes seem to be members of a *presenilins* family of related genes, and mutations in conserved residues of E5-1 could play a role in the development of AD. Further research into the biochemical functions of *E5-1* and *S182* may aid in determining the causative processes of AD. There may also be other AD susceptibility genes.

▶ This is an important study in the rapidly growing field of mutations associated with AD in a familial pattern (FAD). The work centered on a novel gene in chromosome 1, whereas previous candidates or confirmed loci are in chromosomes 21, 14, and 19. This novel gene (*E5-1*) has sequence homologies with the recently identified gene in chromosome 14 and belongs to the family of genes known as *presenilins.* This work may lead to the identification of common mechanisms by which the mutations in the various *presenilins* result in FAD, which may in turn help to identify and understand the mechanisms implicated in the far more common sporadic AD.

R. Kuljis, M.D.

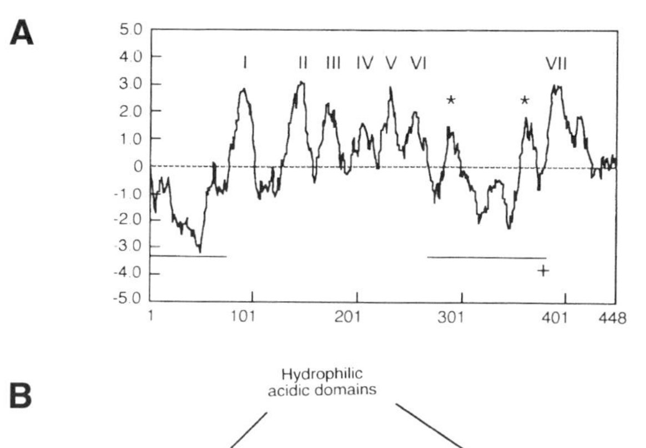

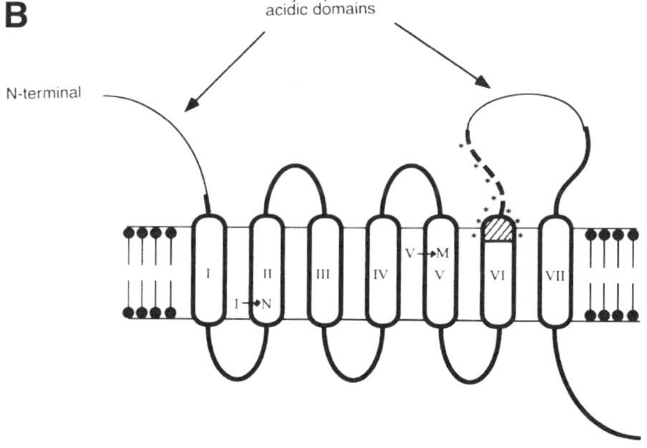

FIGURE 3.—**A**, hydrophobicity plot for the putative E5-1 polypeptide using the hydrophobicity indices of Kyte and Doolittle (see original article for complete reference information) with a calculation window of 15 residues. The 7 putative TM domains are numbered I to VII (*top*). The 2 apolar domains within the TM6→TM7 loop, which could be either TM domains or membrane-associated structural components of the TM6→TM7 loop, are noted by *asterisks*. Hydrophilic domains are *underlined*. A single putative *N*-linked glycosylation site is indicated by a *cross* at residue 405. The Thr 281 in S182 is changed to Pro 287 in E5-1, which obliterates the first putative glycosylation sequence observed in S182. Comparison with the same plot for the putative S182 protein shows virtual overlap if allowances are made for the differences in the sizes of the acidic hydrophilic domains at the N terminus and between TM6 and TM7. **B**, predicted structure of the E5-1 polypeptide. Sequences conserved between E5-1 and S182 are depicted by *thick lines* and divergent sequences by *thin lines*. The location of the alternatively spliced domain is depicted by a *broken line with asterisks*. In the sorter isoform, the hatched space within TM6 would be removed at residue Asp 263 and spliced to residue Ser 296, thereby reconstituting TM6. The approximate locations of the mutations are noted by single-letter amino acid codes, with the wild-type sequence on the *right*. (Reprinted with permission from *Nature*; Rogaev EI, Sherrington R, Rogaeva EA, et al: Familial Alzheimer's disease in kindreds with missense mutations in a gene on chromosome 1 related to the Alzheimer's disease type 3 gene. *Nature* 376:775–778; Copyright 1995; Macmillan Magazines Limited.)

Increased Risk of Mortality in Alzheimer's Disease Patients With More Advanced Educational and Occupational Attainment

Stern Y, Tang MX, Denaro J, et al (Columbia Univ, New York; Gertrude H Sergievsky Ctr, New York)
Ann Neurol 37:590–595, 1995   6–5

Background.—This study was designed to assess the influence of educational and occupational attainment (EOA) on the clinical manifestations of Alzheimer's disease (AD). Educational and occupational attainment may provide a protective reserve against dementia, so patients with greater EOA would be more capable of coping with this disease. This implies that at every level of clinical severity, AD pathologic changes would be more advanced in patients with higher EOA. This issue was examined by studying the rates of mortality of patients with probable AD as a function of their EOA.

Study Group.—A registry of patients with AD was established based on data from a dementia study in the Washington Heights and Inwood communities of New York City. Persons were eligible if they met criteria for probable AD, did not have Parkinson's disease, had not had a stroke, and had at least 1 yearly follow-up or reliable information about the date of death. Elderly people without dementia were recruited from the same communities as controls.

Study Design.—All participants received a standardized diagnostic evaluation in either English or Spanish. By using the criteria of the *Diagnostic and Statistical Manual* (edition 3, revised),[1] a group of physicians and neuropsychologists at a diagnostic conference reached consensus for the diagnosis of dementia. The participant's primary occupation was also recorded.

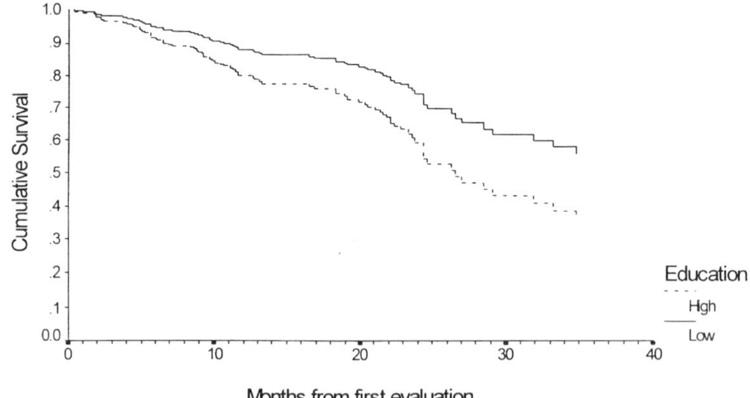

FIGURE 1.—Survival curve comparing cumulative survival in Alzheimer's disease patients with high (> 8 years) and low (≤ 8 years) of education. Curves are based on Cox's analyses, which control for age, gender, and clinical dementia rating. (Reprinted from *Annals of Neurology* 37:590–595, 1995; by permission of Little, Brown and Company [Inc.].)

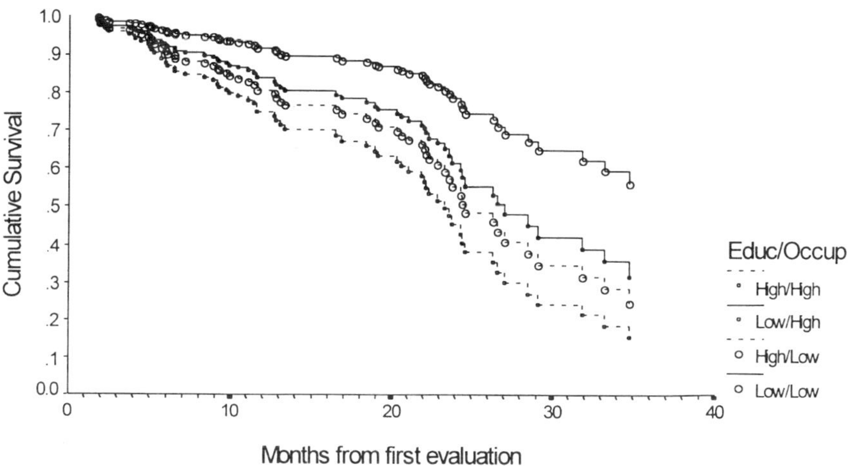

FIGURE 3.—Survival curve comparing cumulative survival in Alzheimer's disease patients classified into 4 groups based on Cox's analyses, which control for age, gender, and clinical dementia rating. (Reprinted from *Annals of Neurology* 37:590–595, 1995; by permission of Little, Brown and Company [Inc.].)

Findings.—At baseline evaluation, 448 people met the criteria for probable AD. Sufficient follow-up was available for 246 of these people to be included in the study population. Among this group, there were 78 deaths. The predictive effects of gender, clinical dementia rating (CDR), education, and occupation were assessed separately by the Cox proportional hazards modeling. A higher relative mortality rate was associated with male gender, CDR greater than 1, increased education, and higher occupational attainment. When CDR, education, gender, and age were included simultaneously in 1 Cox model, all were significant except age (Fig 1). Patients were separated into 4 education and occupation groups. There were 113 in the low education and low occupation group, 50 in the high education and low occupation group, 5 in the low education and high occupation group, and 17 in the high education and high occupation group. Compared with those with low education and occupation, participants with high education and occupation had a significantly increased mortality risk (Fig 3), as did those with high education and low occupation ratings. There were 292 people in the control group. There were 37 deaths in this group. There was no significant effect of higher educational or occupational attainment on survival in the control group.

Conclusion.—In this study of patients with probable AD, both educational and occupational attainment were associated with an increased risk of mortality. These results suggest that at any level of assessed clinical severity, the underlying AD pathologic changes are more advanced in those with more education, leading to a shorter duration between disease diagnosis and death. This implies that either education systematically influences global ratings of disease severity or that education provides a protective reserve against the clinical manifestations of AD.

Reference

1. American Psychiatric Association: *Diagnostic and Statistical Manual of Mental Disorders*, ed 3, revised. Washington, DC, American Psychiatric Association.

▶ This study evaluated the theory that higher educational and occupational achievement exerts a protective effect against AD. This effect was supported by the study, and it may take place at the level of the disease process itself. Alternatively it may reflect an improved ability of patients with higher levels of achievement to perform better cognitively well into biologically advanced stages of the disease. The observation of a higher mortality rate in the more accomplished group supports the latter possibility. The work also provides an impetus for future studies using quantitative histopathology, which will help to test more directly and rigorously the 2 competing but not mutually excluding possibilities.

R. Kuljis, M.D.

Cortical Lewy Bodies in Alzheimer's Disease

Kazee AM, Han LY (Univ of Rochester, New York)
Arch Pathol Lab Med 119:448–453, 1995

6–6

Background.—Cortical Lewy bodies (CLBs) are frequently present in the brains of patients with Alzheimer's disease (AD). The relationship of CLBs to dementia or other hallmarks of this disease are not known. This relationship was investigated.

Materials.—Postmortem examinations were performed on 48 patients with pathologically verified AD and 18 cognitively normal elderly patients from 1984 to 1991. Disease controls, 9 with Parkinson's disease without AD pathologic changes and 10 with multi-infarct dementia, were obtained from files for the same period. All brains were dissected fresh within 18 hours of death and then fixed, embedded, and sectioned. Areas involved in CLB degeneration were examined by anti-ubiquitin immunocytochemistry. Neurofibrillary tangles (NFTs) and senile plaques (SPs) were counted manually in a blinded manner.

Findings.—There were no significant differences in age or sex among these 4 groups of patients. Cortical Lewy bodies were detected in the brains as follows: 71% of the AD group, 44% of the Parkinson's group, 20% of the multi-infarct group, and none of the cognitively intact elderly. Anti-ubiquitin immunocytochemistry revealed CLBs as discrete homogenously positively staining entities (Fig 2, B). Patients with AD with detectable CLBs were different from those without CLBs; they had had their disease longer, were more likely to use psychotropic drugs, were more likely to have extrapyramidal symptoms, and had more severe brain atrophy and more degeneration in the substantia nigra. Cortical Lewy bodies were not associated with SPs or NFTs.

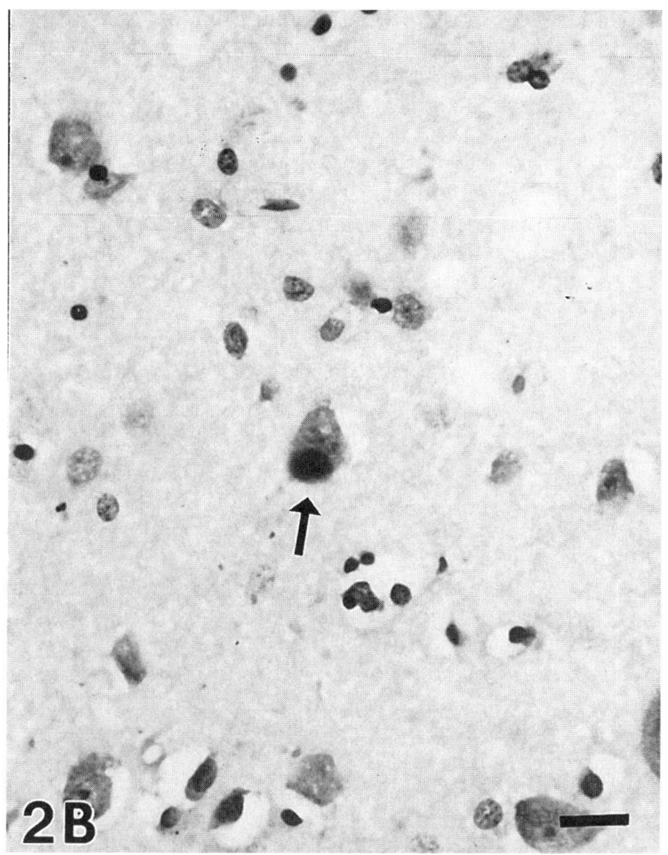

FIGURE 2.—B, cortical Lewy bodies are round, dense, homogeneously positive inclusions filling the cytoplasm of involved neurons (rabbit anti-ubiquitin antibody; calibration bar = 20 μm). (Courtesy of Kazee AM, Han LY: Cortical Lewy bodies in Alzheimer's disease. *Arch Pathol Lab Med* 119:448–453, 1995.)

Conclusion.—Patients with AD were more likely than those with Parkinson's disease, multi-infarct dementia, or those without mental impairment to have detectable CLBs in their brains. Patients with AD and CLBs had more severe symptoms than those without detectable CLBs. The incidence of CLBs was high in the brains of patients with pathologically verified AD in this series.

▶ This study indicated that the incidence of CLBs is higher in patients with AD than was suspected previously. The lesions seem not to be associated, however, with SPs or NFTs. There are some indications that their presence might parallel a higher incidence of parkinsonism and more severe cognitive impairment, among other manifestations. These results emphasized the need to search for CLBs in patients with histopathologically typical AD, and to try to ascertain the clinical manifestations that may identify patients with these lesions. It is likely that the latter may respond differently to certain drugs than patients without CLBs.

R. Kuljis, M.D.

Prospective Study of Relations Between Cortical Lewy Bodies, Poor Eyesight, and Hallucinations in Alzheimer's Disease

McShane R, Gedling K, Reading M, et al (Radcliffe Infirmary, Oxford, England; Warneford Hosp, Oxford, England)
J Neurol Neurosurg Psychiatry 59:185–188, 1995   6–7

Introduction.—Patients with dementia who have cortical Lewy bodies (CLBs) tend to have florid visual hallucinations, according to previous reports. However, given that half of patients with Alzheimer's disease (AD) may have hallucinations at some time and that many patients with CLBs have other neuropathologic changes of AD, the specificity of this connection is uncertain. Clinical factors associated with CLB disease were sought in a longitudinal study of patients with dementia.

Methods.—The study was based on a series of 98 patients who met the criteria of the *Diagnostic and Statistical Manual* (3rd edition, revised)[1] for dementia and were assessed every 4 months for up to 5 years until they died. All were initially living at home with a care giver who could provide a clear description of the patient's behavior and mental health. These assessments, which included questions about hallucinations, continued for a mean of almost 3 years. After the patients died, necropsy material was obtained for examination and clinicopathologic correlations were sought.

Results.—Fixed neocortical and limbic tissue was obtained after death from 44 of the 86 patients who died. Of 41 patients who met neuropathologic criteria for probable or definite AD, 8 also met the study criteria for CLBs. Although patients with CLBs were more likely to have had hallucinations, the trend was not significant. However, patients with CLBs were likely to have had more severe and persistent hallucinations than the patients with dementia who did not have CLBs. These associations were independent of the severity of cognitive decline. Although poor eyesight was related to the severity of hallucinations, it was not related to their persistence.

Conclusion.—Patients with CLBs have more persistent and severe hallucinations than other patients with dementia. Significant interactions were noted between the presence of CLBs, poor eyesight, and the severity of hallucinations, so poor eyesight is a potentially treatable factor in the severity of hallucinations in patients with dementia. Although confirmation by prospective studies is needed, persistent hallucinations seem to be an important diagnostic criterion for dementia associated with CLBs.

Reference

1. American Psychiatric Association: *Diagnostic and Statistical Manual of Mental Disorders,* ed 3, revised. Washington, DC, American Psychiatric Association.

▶ This study attempted to define some of the clinical features that permit the identification of dementia with CLBs. This is a difficult task, because the condition can have quite variable clinical manifestations among histopathologically verified cases. The authors focused on visual hallucinations and found some support for the hypothesis that they are more vivid and persistent in patients with dementia and CLBs than in patients with "typical" AD. The persistence of hallucinations, in particular, seems not to be influenced primarily by poor eyesight. Because only patients with dementia and CLBs and AD were studied, it remains to be determined whether patients with dementia and CLBs but without Alzheimer's lesions exhibit similar phenomena and whether they can be identified clinically by a different array of manifestations.

R. Kuljis, M.D.

Valproate in the Treatment of Behavioral Agitation in Elderly Patients With Dementia

Lott AD, McElroy SL, Keys MA (Univ of Cincinnati, Ohio)
J Neuropsychiatry Clin Neurosci 7:314–319, 1995   6–8

Background.—Behavioral agitation is a common problem among patients with dementia in long-term care facilities. No medication is approved for the treatment of this condition by the U.S. Food and Drug Administration. The epilepsy medication valproate could be useful in the treatment of dementia-related behavioral agitation. The safety and efficacy of this drug were investigated in an open-label prospective trial involving 10 elderly patients with dementia who were referred for treatment of behavioral agitation.

Study Group.—Patients were eligible if they were 65 or older, had a diagnosis of dementia according to the *Diagnostic and Statistical Manual* (edition 3, revised),[1] were referred for treatment of behavioral agitation, and were living in a long-term care facility. Patients with symptoms of psychosis were excluded.

Methods.—A baseline assessment of agitation was made by nursing personnel during the 2 weeks before initiation of medication therapy. Valproate, 125 mg twice daily, was begun in all patients except 1, who began with 125 mg once daily at bedtime. Based on response, side effects, and weekly serum trough evaluations, valproate concentrations were increased. A subjective global rating scale was used by nursing personnel to evaluate improvement in the patients' conditions.

Results.—The age of the 10 patients ranged from 71 to 94. Of these patients, 4 met the criteria for uncomplicated AD, 1 for AD with delusions,

2 for multi-infarct dementia, and 3 for unspecified senile dementia. Symptoms of agitation included striking the staff, cursing and insulting staff and residents, continuously screaming or babbling, wandering, and attempting to leave. All patients had significant comorbid medical conditions. After treatment with valproate, 80% of the patients had at least a 50% reduction in behavioral agitation. The response to valproate was maintained up to 34 weeks. The effective serum concentration was 13 to 52 µg/mL, with an average dosage of 500 mg/day. Valproate was well tolerated, and no abnormal laboratory values were associated with its use.

Conclusion.—Despite the small size and open-label character of this study, it suggests that valproate may be an effective and safe treatment for behavioral agitation in elderly patients with dementia. Controlled clinical trials of valproate as a treatment for behavioral agitation associated with dementia seem to be justified.

Reference

1. American Psychiatric Association: *Diagnostic and Statistical Manual of Mental Disorders*, ed 3, revised. Washington, DC, American Psychiatric Association.

▶ This is a potentially important contribution to the difficult problem of managing behavioral manifestations in patients with dementia. Should the findings be upheld in studies with larger numbers of patients, valproate might have a legitimate and useful place in this situation.

R. Kuljis, M.D.

Other Behavioral Neurology Matters

Transient Global Amnesia and Transient Ischemic Attack: Natural History, Vascular Risk Factors, and Associated Conditions
Zorzon M, Antonutti L, Masè G, et al (Univ of Trieste, Italy)
Stroke 26:1536–1542, 1995   6–9

Objective.—Transient global amnesia (TGA) is not rare in the general population and is relatively common in patients older than 50. Onset of symptoms, typically inability to recall or retain information, is sudden and lasts only a few hours, leaving the patient with amnesia about the events that occurred. The cause of the condition is unknown, although some favor a vascular basis. The results of a prospective longitudinal study of cardiovascular risk factors, associated conditions, and outcome of a group of patients with TGA were compared with patients with transient ischemic attack (TIA).

Methods.—Laboratory examinations were performed on 64 patients (28 men) aged 47 to 70 with documented episodes of TGA. Patients were prospectively reviewed annually and compared with 64 individuals with a first TIA. The control group consisted of 108 age- and sex-matched individuals. Survival rates were determined.

TABLE 2.—Number of Vascular Events, Transient Global Amnesia Recurrences, and Deaths During the Follow-Up in the Transient Global Amnesia and Transient Ischemic Attack Groups

Events	TGA Group (n=64)	TIA Group (n=64)
Stroke, fatal and not fatal	0	5 (7.8%)
TIA and stroke	0	10 (15.6%)
MI, fatal and not fatal	0	3 (4.7%)
TIA and stroke and MI	0	13 (20.3%)
TGA recurrence	6 (9.4%)	0
Deaths		
All causes	3 (4.7%)	6 (9.4%)
Vascular	0	3 (4.7%)
Not vascular	3 (4.7%)	3 (4.7%)

Abbreviations: TGA, transient global amnesia; *TIA*, transient ischemic attack; *MI*, myocardial infarction.

(Zorzon M, Antonutti L, Masè G, et al: Transient global amnesia and transient ischemic attack: Natural history, vascular risk factors, and associated conditions. *Stroke* 1995, 26:1536–1542; reproduced with permission of *Stroke*; Copyright 1995 American Heart Association.)

Results.—Attacks of TGA occurred most frequently in the group aged 50 to 60 and lasted 20 minutes to 20 hours, with a mean of 5.7 hours. In half of the patients, attacks were preceded by exercise in 18, sexual intercourse in 7, emotional stress in 4, and a hot bath in 3. During the attacks, 5 patients had a headache, 7 had high blood pressure, and 1 had paresthesia in the left arm. Interictal electroencephalogram was abnormal in 19 patients, and CT showed abnormalities in 11. When cerebrovascular risk factors were examined, only migraine was found to be significantly associated with increased risk of TGA. Otherwise no differences were found between groups. There were 3 deaths in the TGA group and 6 in the TIA group during the follow-up period. Vascular causes were responsible

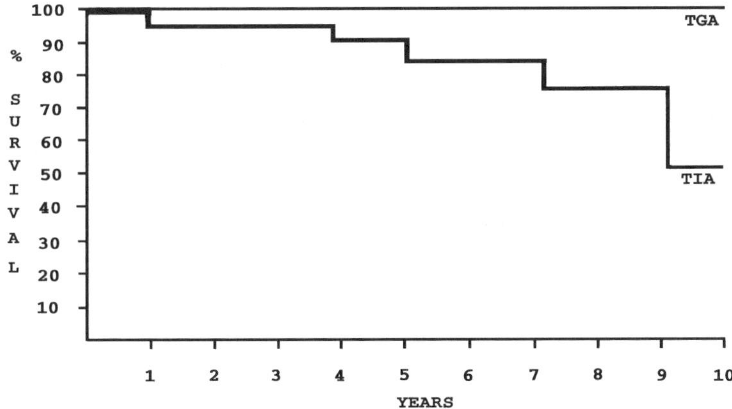

FIGURE 2.—Graph shows comparison of survival free from stroke, myocardial infarction, and vascular death in the transient global amnesia case patients and in the transient ischemic attack control subjects ($P = 0.0317$). (Zorzon M, Antonutti L, Masè G, et al: Transient global amnesia and transient ischemic attack: Natural history, vascular risk factors, and associated conditions. *Stroke* 1995, 26:1536–1542; reproduced with permission of *Stroke*; Copyright 1995 American Heart Association.)

for 3 of the TIA deaths. (Table 2). The TIA group had a significantly higher incidence of major vascular events than did the TGA group (Fig 2). There was recurrence of TGA in only 6 patients.

Conclusion.—The prevalence of vascular risk factor is similar in the TGA and control groups but significantly higher in the TIA group. The mortality rate is low and similar for all groups. Transient global amnesia and TIA do not have the same cause, spreading depression may precipitate TGA, the association between migraine and TGA is significant, and epilepsy can mimic TGA.

▶ This is a useful study of a clinical entity with an obscure cause, which may be precipitated by more than 1 condition. The results fail to support cerebrovascular disease as a causative factor, although it cannot be ruled out conclusively in at least some cases of TGA. The correlation of TGA with probable epilepsy and with migraine supports previous claims, as well as the view that TGA is etiologically heterogeneous.

R. Kuljis, M.D.

Increased Cortical Representation of the Fingers of the Left Hand in String Players

Elbert T, Pantev C, Wienbruch C, et al (Univ of Konstanz, Germany; Univ of Münster, Germany; Univ of Alabama, Birmingham)
Science 270:305–307, 1995

6–10

Background.—Changes in afferent input apparently induce plastic reorganizational changes in the adult mammalian CNS. String musicians were used as a model to study the effects of differential afferent input to the 2 sides of the human brain.

Methods.—Six violinists, 2 cellists, and 1 guitarist were studied. These 9 musicians had been playing for a mean 11.7 years. Six nonmusicians comprised a control group. In both groups, mean age was 24.

Findings.—On MR images, the cortical representation of the left hand digits was larger in the musicians than in the control subjects. The effect was smallest for the left thumb. No differences were seen among representations of the right-hand digits. There was a correlation between the amount of cortical reorganization in the representation of the fingering digits and the age at which the musicians had begun playing.

Conclusion.—The cerebral cortices of string musicians differed significantly from those of nonmusicians. The representation of the left-hand digits was greatly enlarged in the cortices of the string players. Thus, representations of different body parts in the primary somatosensory cortex depends on use and changes to conform to an individual's current needs and experiences.

▶ This imaginative study indicated that repetitive, highly skilled motor tasks are associated with an enlargement of the cortical representation of the body parts involved. The phenomenon is therefore 1 of the mechanisms involved in the learning and refinement of skilled motor acts and reflects the capability for large-scale morphologic modifications of the brain in response to experience. Similar changes may occur in cortices involved in mental imagery and other tasks that are not expressible in terms of relatively simple motor acts. However, this will be more difficult to demonstrate experimentally. Further understanding of this phenomenon may allow its exploitation for the rehabilitation and recovery of neurologic function after brain lesions.

R. Kuljis M.D.

"Hyperneglect," a Sequential Hemispheric Stroke Syndrome

Ghika J, Bogousslavsky J, Regli F (Ctr Hosp Univ Vaudois, Lausanne, Switzerland)
J Neurol Sci 132:233–238, 1995   6–11

Background.—Eight patients with hemineglect who transiently responded in an unusual way to lateralized stimuli were described. These patients had a dramatically exaggerated form of perceptual neglect, with marked movement in the direction opposite to stimulus in the neglected hemispace.

Study Group.—After an acute stroke, 8 patients with hemineglect, who were part of the Lausanne Stroke Registry, had unusual transient active orienting and explorative behavior diametrically opposite to all stimuli in the neglected hemispace. All 8 patients were examined by the same physician within 6 hours of the onset of this symptom and retested several times during a 1-week period. The responses of 3 patients were recorded on videotape. All patients were older than 65, were right handed, and had an acute sensorimotor stroke with hemianopia, multimodal hemineglect, and tonic conjugated eye and head deviation toward the side of the lesion. Two patients had an acute left hemispheric stroke, whereas 6 had a right cerebrovascular lesion.

Findings.—All patients had CT performed within 24 hours of their first symptoms. In 6 cases, at least 2 lesions were detected by CT. In the other 2 patients, there was a single large infarct associated with either hypertensive leukoencephalopathy or contralateral brain edema. The acute stroke was frontal in 4 patients, parietal in 1, parieto-occipital in 1, and subcortical in 1 patient. Five patients had infarction and 3 had cerebral hemorrhage. The time between the occurrence of the 2 lesions ranged from 1 hour to 7 years. The unusual behavior after occurrence of the acute lesion was transient, disappearing after a few days, in all 8 cases.

Conclusion.—The hyperneglect behavior observed in this small series of patients seems to be a transient response after sequential strokes in patients with preexisting hemineglect. It may represent active motor neglect with release of repulsive behaviors, with a further field of hemineglect in the nonneglected hemispace.

▶ This exaggerated form of neglect is clearly distinct to most classical descriptions, from which it differs dramatically. Its association with more than 1 lesion in the same hemisphere carries an important implication regarding localization and is an important contribution to the understanding of mechanisms engaged in the perception of extrapersonal space and in building our body image. Its transient nature requires awareness of the phenomenon by clinicians to detect it, which may explain in part why it seems not to have been recognized previously.

R. Kuljis, M.D.

7 Movement Disorders

Bilateral Fetal Nigral Transplantation Into the Postcommissural Putamen in Parkinson's Disease
Freeman TB, Olanow CW, Hauser RA, et al (Univ of South Florida, Tampa; Mount Sinai Med Ctr, New York; Woman's Ctr, Tampa, Fla; et al)
Ann Neurol 38:379–388, 1995   7–1

Background.—For several reasons, neuronal grafting is a rational investigative approach to therapy for Parkinson's disease (PD). Intrastriatal grafts of embryonic dopaminergic neurons gave promising results in animal studies, but fetal nigral transplantation has yielded inconsistent benefits in clinical trials. Many different transplant variables may affect the final results. A fetal nigral transplantation protocol designed to maximize the likelihood of graft survival and dopamine reinnervation of the target site was implemented in 4 patients.

Methods.—The experience included 4 PD patients, all with a stable levodopa-carbidopa dose for at least 3 months, a Hoehn-Yahr state of III or less during the "on" state, substantial disability during the "off" state, and predictable fluctuations in motor function. Preoperative drug manipulation did not improve their conditions. All patients received bilateral implantation of solid grafts into the postcommissural putamen. Tissue was derived from 3 to 4 donors per side; donor age was 6.5 to 9 weeks postconception. The tissues were placed at intervals of about 5 mm throughout the 3-dimensional configuration of the postcommissural putamen. The patients received a total of 6 months of cyclosporine immunosuppression. Evaluations were performed at baseline and at 1, 3, and 6 months postoperatively. Positron emission tomography was also performed at baseline and at 6 months to assess striatal uptake of 18-fluorodopa.

Results.—All patients tolerated the surgery well and were discharged within 48 to 72 hours. Complications included an asymptomatic superficial cortical hemorrhage along the needle pathway in 1 patient and transient postoperative confusion and hallucinations in another. Clinical benefits were apparent in all patients, as reflected by significant improvements in total Unified Parkinson's Disease Rating Scale scores during the "off" state, Schwab-England disability scores during the "off" state, percent "off" time, and percent "on" time with dyskinesia (Fig 1). The patients

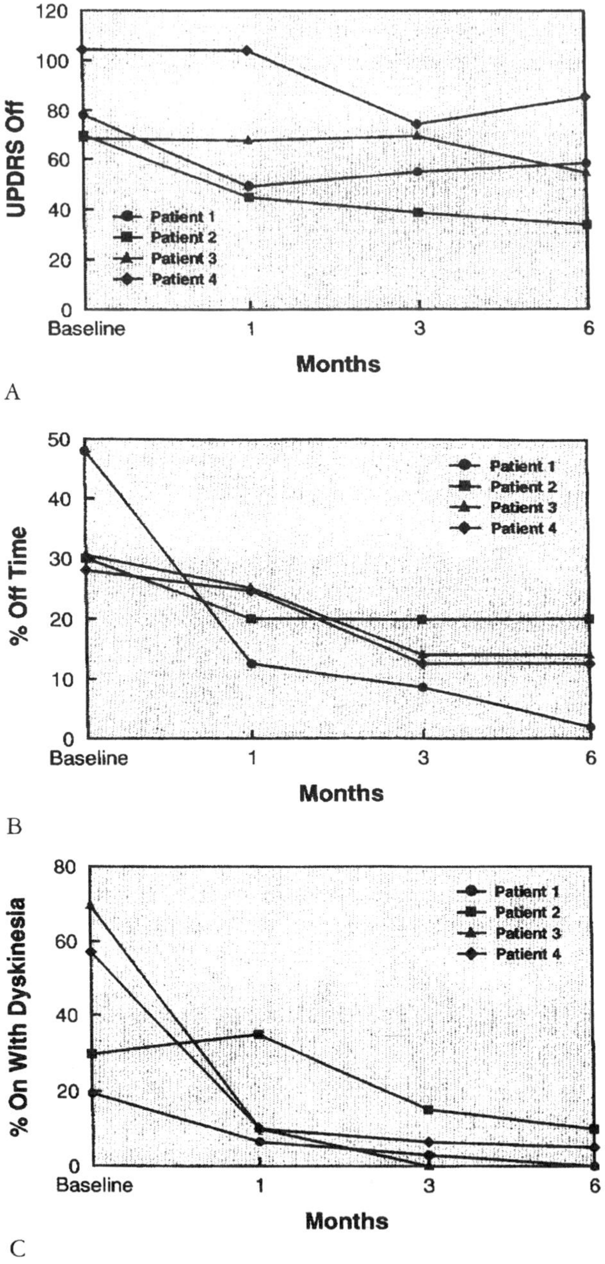

FIGURE 1.—Score of each patient at baseline and postoperative months 1, 3, and 6 for (A) UPDRS "off," (B) percent "off" time, and (C) percent "on" time with dyskinesia. *Abbreviation: UPDRS*, Unified Parkinson's Disease Rating Scale. (Courtesy of Freeman TB, Olanow CW, Hauser RA, et al: Bilateral fetal nigral transplantation into the postcommissural putamen in Parkinson's disease. *Ann Neurol* 38:379–388, 1995.)

had a mean 53% increase in striatal fluorodopa on the right side and a 33% increase on the left; all patients showed bilateral improvements.

Conclusion.—The described technique of fetal nigral transplantation produces consistent improvement, both clinically and on positron emission tomography, in patients with PD. The results support the continued investigation of fetal tissue transplantation for treatment of PD. Further research is needed to define the long-term benefits of this procedure and to define the transplant variables associated with optimal clinical response.

▶ This report summarized the results of fetal nigral grafting in 4 patients with PD 6 months after the procedure. The work is commendable for attempting to address many of the practical questions raised since the inception of fetal cell grafting in human subjects: Who should receive the implants, patients with advanced disease or young patients early in the illness? What age of fetal mesencephalon should be used? How much tissue and how many fetuses are needed for implants? Should cell suspensions be used or solid tissue? Where should the implant be made—putamen, caudate, or both? One side or both sides? During 1 procedure or staged? Should immunosuppression be used? For how long? How can we determine the survival of the fetal tissue? This excellent article provided a carefully thought-out rationale (based on animal work and review of others' experiences) for making the optimal choices, given the available limited knowledge. Time will tell if they made the right choices. Fetal tissue grafting is clearly in an experimental phase paving the way for innovative regenerative treatments of neurodegenerative disease.

J.R. Sanchez-Ramos, M.D., Ph.D.

Pen Injected Apomorphine Against Off Phenomena in Late Parkinson's Disease: A Double Blind, Placebo Controlled Study
Østergaard L, Werdelin L, Odin P, et al (Univ of Copenhagen; Aarhus Univ Hosp, Denmark; Sønderborg Hosp, Denmark; et al)
J Neurol Neurosurg Psychiatry 58:681–687, 1995   7–2

Introduction.—Apomorphine is a dopamine agonist that has effectively countered parkinsonian symptoms and "on-off" phenomena. The nephrotoxicity resulting from orally effective doses has made subcutaneous treatment preferable. The dopaminergic effects and safety of subcutaneous apomorpine were examined in 22 patients with idiopathic Parkinson's disease whose clinical history averaged nearly 10 years.

Study Plan.—Patients had received levodopa for 8 years on average. All the patients had disabling off periods on a daily basis, but none had diphasic dyskinesia. After individually titrating the dose of apomorphine, patients received apomorphine and placebo for 4-day periods in a double-blind crossover design. Apomorphine was injected subcutaneously in the anterolateral femoral area or abdominal wall by using a prefilled single-use pen. Oral antiparkinsonism drug treatment was optimized at least 1 month before the study began. Patients also received domperidone, a peripheral dopamine antagonist, to avoid nausea and vomiting and orthostatic hypotension.

Results.—The optimal dose of apomorphine averaged 3.4 mg. All 21 evaluable patients responded satisfactorily. The daily duration of off periods declined by more than half. Staff believed that off periods were more frequent during apomorphine therapy, but patients did not share this belief. Twelve of 14 patients who completed maintenance treatment improved substantially. Most patients found the injection pen quite easy to use. Involuntary movements were more prominent but not more severe during apomorphine treatment. A majority of the patients had nausea, with or without vomiting. Blood pressure changes were infrequent.

Conclusion.—Subcutaneously injected apomorphine is a useful adjunctive treatment for patients with advanced Parkinson's disease and on-off phenomena.

▶ Self-injection of apomorphine provides a time-limited solution for selected patients with frequent sudden "off" episodes. A number of factors are likely to limit the long-term usefulness of this modality of treatment. These include an increasing frequency of "off" periods, the difficulty of self-injection by a patient in the "off" state, the tendency for dyskinesias to worsen, and the development of nodules at the sites of injection. Those patients who balk at the thought of frequent self-injection with a drug that commonly produces nausea (despite the use of domperidone) or who can no longer tolerate frequent apomorphine injections might be candidates for pallidotomy, which smooths out clinical fluctuations and dyskinesias associated with chronic levodopa therapy. The long-term effects of pallidotomy on freezing and sudden "off" episodes need to be studied and compared with the benefits and limitations of apomorphine self-injection.

J.R. Sanchez-Ramos, M.D., Ph.D.

Fluctuating Parkinson's Disease: Treatment With the Long-Acting Dopamine Agonist Cabergoline

Ahlskog JE, Muenter MD, Maraganore DM, et al (Mayo Clinic, Rochester, Minn; Scottsdale, Ariz; Barrow Neurologic Inst, Phoenix, Ariz)
Arch Neurol 51:1236–1241, 1994   7–3

Background.—Long-term treatment of Parkinson's disease with levodopa commonly results in clinical fluctuations and variations in treatment response. Cabergoline is a long-acting medication that has a longer half-life than any drug currently used in the treatment of Parkinson's disease. The efficacy of cabergoline as an adjunctive medication was evaluated in 41 patients having short-duration responses to levodopa therapy.

Methods.—Forty-one patients treated with levodopa for a mean of 7.5 years formed the study cohort. Complete physical examinations including blood studies and urinalyses were performed before and after the trial was

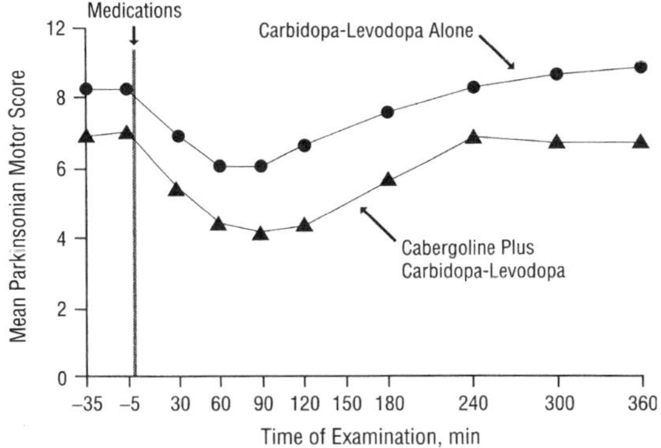

FIGURE 1.—Serial measurement of parkinsonian motor scores: the Unified Parkinson's Disease Rating Scale (UPDRS) motor battery was serially scored at defined times before and after the administration of single test doses of medications. The averages of 2 baseline trials, performed on 2 separate days, were compared with those of 2 trials during adjunctive cabergoline therapy. Testing began before the administration of each patient's first levodopa-carbidopa dose for that day; levodopa-carbidopa had been withheld for an average of 12 hours and cabergoline for approximately 24 hours. The UPDRS motor items were weighted before they were summed. For each pair of data points shown at each examination time, the mean score from the prestudy baseline trials was significantly different from the score obtained with cabergoline therapy ($P \leq 0.001$). The areas under the 2 curves were also significantly different ($P \leq 0.001$). Patients were given less levodopa (mean 135 mg) for the end of study assessments compared with the baseline trials (mean 153 mg). The mean cabergoline test dose was 2.8 mg. (*Arch Neurol*; December 1994; 51:1236–1241; Copyright 1994; American Medical Association.)

completed. Differing dosages of cabergoline were randomly assigned to 5 subgroups of patients who were treated for 13 weeks. The initial dose of 0.5 mg was increased incrementally. Primary efficacy was measured according to the Unified Parkinson's Disease Rating Scale (UPDRS), finger-tapping rate, a timed walking test, and dyskinesia scores. Secondary measures of efficacy included patient diary card ratings, activities of daily

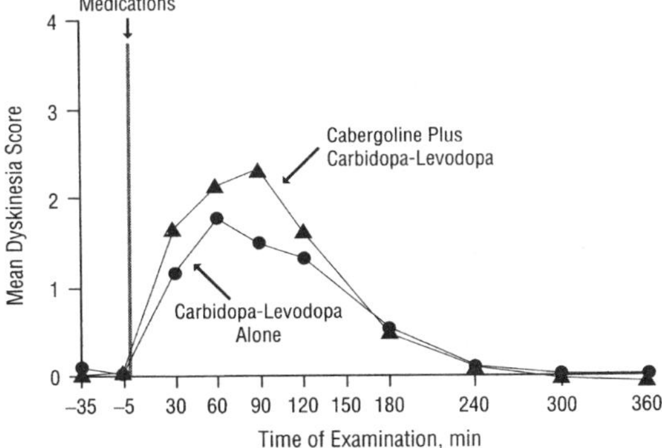

FIGURE 4.—Dyskinesias. Hyperkinetic dyskinesias were serially rated on a 4-point scale for each body part: all 4 limbs, trunk, and head/neck (maximum possible score 24). The scoring, before and after test doses of medications were administered, was conducted in conjunction with the parkinsonian motor score measurements, as described in Figure 1. No significant differences were detected between the 2 mean scores at any of the given examination times. Similarly, the areas under the 2 curves at the time of peak medication effect (30–180 minutes) were not significantly different. (*Arch Neurol*; December 1994; 51:1236–1241; Copyright 1994; American Medical Association.)

living scales, global assessments, and reduction of levodopa dosage. Data were interpreted using Student's *t* tests and the Wilcoxon signed-rank test.

Results.—The mean daily adjunctive maintenance dose of cabergoline was 2.8 mg, which allowed a reduction in the dose of levodopa from 891 to 733 mg (18%). With cabergoline therapy, there was a longer response duration (Fig 1), finger-tapping scores improved, and measures such as rising from a chair and walking times improved. The scores of dyskinesia increased slightly but were not significant (Fig 4). According to patient self-ratings, all but 1 patient reported improvement. Most patients described the change as moderate or marked. Most side effects were mild or transient.

Discussion.—Cabergoline was well tolerated by patients, showed efficacy in countering fluctuations in levodopa therapy, and had mild side effects. One major advantage of this therapy is its once-daily dosage schedule and simple instructions that are easy for patients with Parkinson's disease to interpret.

▶ Dealing with clinical fluctuations in response to levodopa is probably the most challenging aspect in the current management of advancing Parkinson's disease. The introduction of a long-acting agonist such as cabergoline to smooth out fluctuations is a natural solution to the problem. The long duration of action, however, is a double-edged sword. Adverse effects such as dyskinesias and psychiatric reactions are bound to also be of long duration, and attention must be paid to concomitant downward adjustments of levodopa dosage. It should be interesting to see whether early monotherapy with cabergoline will prevent the development of motor fluctuations and dyskinesias.

J.R. Sanchez-Ramos, M.D., Ph.D.

Widespread Cytoskeletal Pathology Characterizes Corticobasal Degeneration
Feany MB, Dickson DW (Albert Einstein College, Bronx, NY)
Am J Pathol 146:1388–1396, 1995   7–4

Introduction.—Corticobasal degeneration (CBD) is a rare, progressive neurologic disorder that is difficult to diagnose antemortem. This study further examined the pathologic changes in CBD using immunohistochemistry and laser confocal microscopy.

Materials.—Brain tissue from 11 patients with CBD were examined. The diagnosis of CBD was made based on pathologic findings of neuronal loss in cortex, basal ganglia, and brain stem, as well as astrocytic plaques and characteristic tau-positive neuronal and glial inclusions. For control, brain tissue from a patient with Alzheimer's disease was examined.

Findings.—Neuronal and glial pathologic changes were widespread. In addition to the hallmark feature of CBD consisting of swollen or ballooned achromatic neurons, numerous pyramidal and small nonpyramidal neurons throughout the affected cortical gray matter contained tau-positive neuronal inclusions. In contrast to AD, CBD showed extensive white matter abnormalities. There was marked myelin pallor with marked gliosis, and the tau-positive white matter represented axonal threads and oligodendroglial inclusions. The most intriguing feature of CBD was the presence of amyloid-negative cortical plaque. These structures actually represented abnormal tau accumulations in distal processes of astrocytes. These glial cells expressed the astrocyte markers glial fibrillary acidic protein, vimentin, and CD44, and optical sectioning with confocal microscopy localized the antigen precisely in focal dilatations of distal astrocyte processes. Numerous glial cytoplasmic inclusions were also present in the white matter and were localized to Leu 7–expressing oligodendrocytes.

Conclusion.—Abnormal tau deposition appears to be widespread in CBD, and corresponding cellular dysfunction is suggested by extensive neuronal cell loss, white matter gliosis, and astrocyte abnormalities. These findings expand the scope of abnormalities in CBD and help to understand the pathogenesis in other neurodegenerative diseases such as Alzheimer's disease that are characterized by abnormal tau deposition.

▶ Clinical manifestation of CBD, also known as corticobasal ganglionic degeneration, is varied but most often appears as a rigid-akinetic syndrome with marked asymmetry, ideomotor apraxia, and problems with voluntary gaze. Rapid progression and poor response to dopamine replacement therapy mark this neurodegenerative condition as another of the rare "parkinson plus" syndromes. Cytoskeletal pathologic findings provide an important pathogenetic clue to a common molecular mechanism for Pick's disease, Alzheimer's disease, progressive supranuclear palsy, and CBD, but explanation for the variable phenotypes remains a formidable challenge. Detailed studies of cognitive and motor decline in a series of CBD patients that can be correlated with results of postmortem neuropathologic investigation are needed.

J.R. Sanchez-Ramos, M.D., Ph.D.

The Clinical and Pathological Spectrum of Steele–Richardson–Olszewski Syndrome (Progressive Supranuclear Palsy): A Reappraisal
Daniel SE, de Bruin VMS, Lees AJ (Parkinson's Disease Society Brain Tissue Bank, London; Inst of Neurology, London; Escola Paulista de Medicina, Sao Paulo, Brazil)
Brain 118:759–770, 1995   7–5

Background.—There are no agreed-on criteria for the histologic diagnosis of Steele-Richardson-Olszewski (SRO) syndrome. Several variants have been reported. Recently, researchers have proposed dividing the neuropathology of progressive supranuclear palsy into typical, atypical, and combined types. The value of such subclassification, however, has not been established. The clinicopathologic spectrum of SRO syndrome was clarified.

Methods.—A total of 17 patients were investigated. All had a progressive bradykinetic syndrome and postmortem findings of neurofibrillary degeneration in the cerebral cortex, subcortical nuclei, and brain stem.

Findings.—Seven patients met currently accepted clinical criteria for SRO syndrome. The other 10, who did not have supranuclear gaze palsy (SGP), had alternative clinical diagnoses: 6 with idiopathic Parkinson's disease, 2 with cerebrovascular disease, and 1 each with Parkinson's syndrome and Alzheimer's disease. These 2 groups differed in clinical features. The most common complaints in patients with SRO and SGP were gait problems with falls, bradykinesia, axial dystonia, dysarthria, dysphagia, and rigidity. In patients with SRO but not SGP, bradykinesia was prominent, and falls, axial dystonia, dysarthria, dysphagia, and rigidity were less common. In patients with SRO and SGP, the onset of dementia usually occurred within a few years of manifestation. Only 3 of the 10 patients with SRO but not SGP were demented. However, 7 of these 10 patients were depressed. There were no distinct neuropathologic differences between the 2 groups.

Conclusion.—The clinicopathologic spectrum of SRO is diverse. This syndrome can be subclassified only by clinical findings. There are no apparent qualitative or quantitative morphologic distinctions. Patients without SGP may have better compensatory mechanisms, resulting in a more benign condition.

▶ This series of 17 postmortem cases was selected based on morphologic findings of cortical and subcortical neurofibrillary degeneration similar to the original description by Steele, Richardson, and Olszewski[1] and the presence of a bradykinetic syndrome in life. Histopathologic features were so variable that it was not possible to classify cases according to pathologic criteria. Even when the presence or absence of SGP was chosen as the basis for clinical classification, there were no distinct qualitative histopathologic differences between these 2 groups of cases. To underscore the lack of clinicopathologic correlation, blinded researchers could not predict the presence of SGP in life based on the presence of tangles in nuclei controlling eye movements. Clearly classification of SRO syndrome must await the development of new molecular biological markers.

J.R. Sanchez-Ramos, M.D., Ph.D.

Reference

1. Steele JC, Richardson JC, Olszewski J: Progressive supranuclear palsy. *Arch Neurol* 10:333–359, 1964.

Emotional and Functional Impact of DNA Testing on Patients With Symptoms of Huntington's Disease
Jankovic J, Beach J, Ashizawa T (Parkinson's Disease Ctr and Movement Disorders Clinic, Houston; Baylor College of Medicine, Houston)
J Med Genet 32:516–518, 1995   7–6

Background.—Many researchers have studied the potential impact of DNA testing on asymptomatic subjects at risk for Huntington's disease (HD). However, the effect of communicating the genetic findings to patients with a previous clinical diagnosis of HD has not been reported. Whether genetic confirmation of a clinical diagnosis of HD has a negative impact on mood and coping strategies was investigated.

Methods.—Thirty-six patients (18 women and 18 men) with a mean age of 53.9 had clinical diagnoses of HD confirmed by expanded CAG repeats. The mean symptom duration was 11.2 years. Coping strategies and levels of depression were evaluated before the DNA test results were disclosed and again 2 weeks and 3 months later. Ten patients with similar symptoms but in whom HD was excluded by normal CAG repeats served as a comparison group.

Findings.—Six patients in the HD group reported a subjective reaction to the positive test result. However, psychological scores, including those on the Beck Depression Inventory, functional capacity, symptom interference, independence scale, and other measures of mood and behavior, did not differ from baseline at 2 weeks or 3 months. There were no changes in these measures in the control group.

Conclusion.—Mood and coping strategies seem to be unaffected by DNA confirmation of the diagnosis of HD in symptomatic patients. Thus, extensive psychological testing and counseling do not appear to be needed for most of these patients. None of the patients in this series showed evidence of serious depression when the DNA results were disclosed, however. In patients who are depressed before DNA testing, a positive result may worsen the depression. Communication of DNA findings should be individualized and done with compassion.

▶ Although the authors suggested that extensive psychological testing and counseling do not appear necessary in most symptomatic patients, they did recognize that it is wise to exercise caution when results are conveyed to symptomatic patients who are in a state of denial. One important caveat neglected in this paper relates to the issue that HD is a family disease. Family members, who automatically are confirmed to be at 50% risk by the test results, need as much, if not more, counseling than the affected patient. Formal studies of the effects of confirmatory testing on family members need to be undertaken.

J.R. Sanchez-Ramos, M.D., Ph.D.

Striatal D₁ and D₂ Receptor Binding in Patients With Huntington's Disease and Other Choreas: A PET Study

Turjanski N, Weeks R, Dolan R, et al (Hammersmith Hosp, London; Inst of Neurology, London; Royal Free Hosp, London)
Brain 118:689–696, 1995

7–7

Background.—Previous research combined with current concepts of basal ganglia connectivity suggests that patients with the choreic variant of Huntington's disease may have a preferential loss of striatal D_2-bearing neurons, whereas patients with the akinetic-rigid variant may have a nonselective loss of striatal D_1- and D_2-bearing neurons. With positron emission tomography (PET), the neuropharmacology of the brain can be explored in vivo. This technique was used to investigate striatal D_1 and D_2 receptor binding in patients with these variants of Huntington's disease and other causes of chorea.

Methods.—Ten patients with Huntington's disease and 3 with other causes of chorea were included. Background rigidity and bradykinesia were scored on a 4-point scale.

Findings.—A severe, parallel decrease in both striatal D_1 and D_2 receptor binding was noted in patients with Huntington's disease, regardless of the predominant phenotype. The mean reduction was 60%. Patients with rigidity associated with Huntington's disease had a more marked decrease in striatal D_1 and D_2 binding compared with patients with no rigidity. Normal D_2 binding was documented in a patient with chorea associated with systemic lupus erythematosus (Figs 1 and 4).

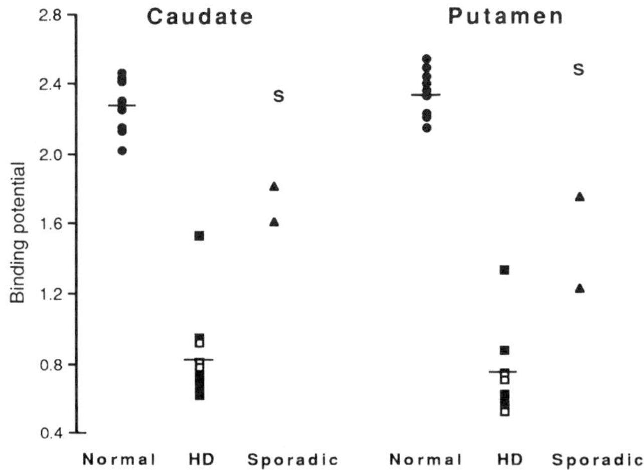

FIGURE 1.—Scatter diagram showing individual striatal ^{11}C-raclopride D_2-binding potentials of control subjects, patients with HD, patients with sporadic chorea, and a patient with systemic lupus erythematosus. *Closed squares*, choreic; *open squares*, akinetic-rigid. *Abbreviations: HD,* Huntington's disease; *S,* systemic lupus erythematosus. (Turjanski N, Weeks R, Dolan R, et al: Striatal D_1 and D_2 receptor binding in patients with Huntington's disease and other choreas: A PET study. *Brain* 118:689–696, 1995; by permission of Oxford University Press.)

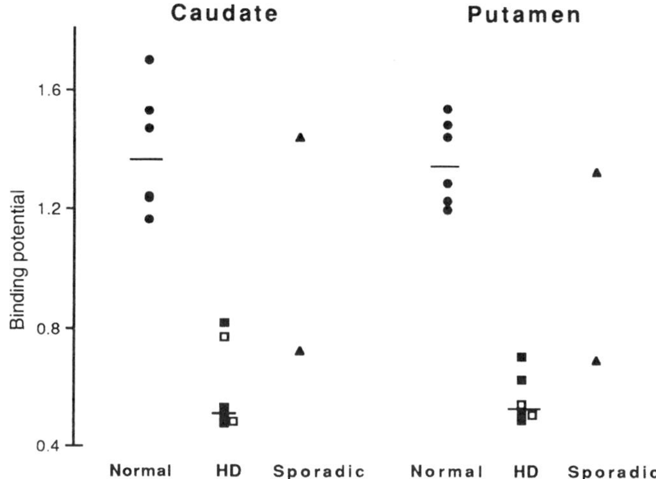

FIGURE 4.—Scatter diagram showing individual caudate and putamen ^{11}C-SCH23390 D_1-binding potentials for HD, sporadic chorea, and normal controls. *Closed squares,* choreic; *open squares,* akinetic-rigid. *Abbreviation: HD,* Huntington's disease. (Turjanski N, Weeks R, Dolan R, et al: Striatal D_1 and D_2 receptor binding in patients with Huntington's disease and other choreas: A PET study. *Brain* 118:689–696, 1995; by permission of Oxford University Press.)

Conclusion.—Untreated patients with Huntington's disease have a severe parallel decrease in striatal D_1 and D_2 receptor binding, regardless of whether chorea or rigidity predominates. However, a greater loss of mean striatal D_1 and D_2 binding occurs in those with rigidity than in choreic patients without rigidity. Though the presence of chorea may not be determined by changes in dopamine receptor binding, rigidity in Huntington's disease is correlated with striatal dopamine D_1 and D_2 receptor loss.

▶ The PET data reported here confirmed several postmortem investigations showing reduction in striatal binding of both D_1 and D_2 receptors, but unlike the postmortem work, the pattern of loss in this in vivo study did not correlate with clinical phenotype (choreic vs. rigid-akinetic). This is contrary to postmortem studies showing a preferential loss, in early choreic patients, of indirect striatal efferents indicated by loss of enkephalinergic neurons that bear D_2 receptors.[1] Consistent with the present PET study, patients with more advanced disease or the severe rigid-akinetic variant did show additional loss of the direct striatal substance P–containing projections (presumably bearing D_1 receptors) to internal segment of the globus pallidus.[2] However, striatal D_1 and D_2 receptors were reported in the normal range in a case of lupus chorea, underscoring our spotty understanding of mechanisms of chorea. Apart from the obvious differences in the selection of cases and in methodology for estimating dopamine receptor densities using in vivo PET rather than postmortem techniques, it may well be that the current model of striatal connectivity, used to explain the pathophysiology of chorea, needs revision.

J.R. Sanchez-Ramos, M.D., Ph.D.

References

1. Albin RL, Reiner A, Anderson KD, et al: Striatal and nigral neurol subpopulations in rigid Huntington's disease: Implications for the functional anatomy of chorea and rigidity-akinesia. *Ann Neurol* 27:357–365, 1990.
2. Reiner A, Albin RL, Anderson KD, et al: Differential loss of striatal projection neurons in Huntington's disease. *Proc Natl Acad Sci USA* 85:5733–5737, 1988.

Late-Onset Huntington's Disease: A Clinical and Molecular Study

James CM, Houlihan GD, Snell RG, et al (Univ of Wales, Cardiff)
Age Ageing 23:445–448, 1994   7–8

Background.—Late-onset Huntington's disease (HD) presents disease management problems that differ from those occurring in younger patients. Patients with late-onset HD in South Wales were studied for symptom and molecular identification that characterize this subset of patients.

Methods.—Demographic information was collected on patients with a diagnosis of late-onset HD. The symptoms and time of first awareness of a physical abnormality were noted. Blood was drawn from 10 individuals for measure of the expanded CAG repeat sequence.

Results.—The prevalence of HD in this community was 6.2 per 100,000. Huntington's disease had been diagnosed in 33 individuals older than 60; the oldest living patient was 86. The range of disease duration was between 0.5 and 24 years in the 9 patients who were still alive. The other 24 patients died; their ages ranged from 60 to 72 at disease onset.

TABLE 3.—Age at Onset and Size of the Expanded CAG Repeat Sequence
in the *HD* Gene in Late-Onset Huntington's Disease

Sex	Age at onset (years)	Repeat Size Disease in allele	Normal allele
F	60	39	16
F	65	38	16
F	64	39	20
F	67	39	24
F	60	39	19
M	65	38	15
M	77	38	19
M	66	39	16
M	67	38	15
F	61	39	16

(James CM, Houlihan GD, Snell RG, et al: Late-onset Huntington's disease: A clinical and molecular study. *Age Ageing* 23:445–448, 1994: by permission of Oxford University Press.)

Symptoms of movement disorder, which occurred in 32 patients (97%), were first noted by relatives, medical persons, or the patient. Gait disturbance occurred in all 32 of these patients. Impairment in cognitive ability as an initial symptom occurred in 30% of patients. Analysis of the CAG repeat sequence showed a mean value of 38.6 repeats and expansion in all patients (Table 3).

Discussion.—Elderly patients are likely to have gait disturbances develop as the first symptom of HD. Late-onset HD has no worse a prognosis than HD that develops in patients at a younger age. Despite a median age of onset of 65, these patients have a life expectancy of 13 years from diagnosis. When an older individual has symptoms of a movement disorder, HD should be included in the differential diagnosis.

▶ Most (58%) of the late-onset patients who exhibited obvious signs of HD died unaware of symptoms, and mental impairment was not prominent compared with motor disturbances. Thus, late-onset HD appears to be a less serious disorder for the individual patient but a more involved problem for the younger generations who are unaware of the potential severity of the disease. This state of affairs poses problems for genetic counseling, with the gene already having been transmitted to grandchildren by the time the genetic implications are recognized by the younger offspring of the late-onset HD patient.

J.R. Sanchez-Ramos, M.D., Ph.D.

8 Multiple Sclerosis

Copolymer 1 Reduces Relapse Rate and Improves Disability in Relapsing-Remitting Multiple Sclerosis: Results of a Phase III Multicenter, Double-Blind, Placebo-Controlled Trial
Johnson KP, Brooks BR, Cohen JA, et al (Univ of Maryland, Baltimore; Univ of Wisconsin, Madison; Univ of Pennsylvania, Philadelphia; et al)
Neurology 45:1268–1276, 1995   8–1

Background.—The identification of pathogenic factors active in multiple sclerosis (MS) has enabled advances in effective treatment for this disease. The efficacy of copolymer 1 therapy was further assessed in a large, placebo-controlled, multicenter trial.

Methods.—Two hundred fifty-one patients were enrolled in this phase III trial conducted by 11 universities. All had relapsing-remitting MS. One hundred twenty-five patients were assigned to copolymer 1 treatment and 126 to placebo at a dosage of 20 mg/day in subcutaneous injections for 2 years.

Findings.—The final 2-year relapse rates for those in the active treatment and placebo groups were 1.19 and 1.68—a 29% decrease favoring copolymer 1. Active treatment was also associated with positive trends in the proportion of relapse-free patients and median time to first relapse. Significantly more patients given copolymer 1 had an improved disability status, and more patients receiving placebo worsened. Copolymer 1 therapy was well tolerated, the most common adverse effect being an injection-site reaction. A transient self-limited systemic reaction characterized by flushing or chest tightness with palpitations, anxiety, or dyspnea followed injection in 15.2% of those receiving active treatment and 3.2% of those receiving placebo. This reaction usually lasted for 30 sec to 30 minutes.

Conclusion.—This large series confirmed the findings of an earlier pilot study demonstrating that daily subcutaneous injections of 20 mg of copolymer 1 significantly decrease the relapse rate in patients with relapsing-remitting MS. Differences in disability between the placebo and active treatment groups were also significant. Copolymer 1 was also well tolerated.

▶ The efficacy of copolymer 1 in relapsing-remitting MS was confirmed by this large study. While we await the MRI findings of the study, neurologists will be able to offer 2 equally efficacious drugs for the treatment of relapsing-remitting MS, interferon-β or copolymer 1. Because the mechanism of action of copolymer 1 appears to be quite distinct from that of interferon-β, we may also potentially see the use of these drugs in combination. By analogy to chemotherapy for neoplastic diseases, management of MS may have to rely on drugs that act at different levels and sites of the immune system.

S. Sriram, M.D.

Low-Dose (7.5 mg) Oral Methotrexate Reduces the Rate of Progression in Chronic Progressive Multiple Sclerosis

Goodkin DE, Rudick RA, Medendorp SV, et al (Univ of California, San Francisco; Cleveland Clin Found, Ohio)
Ann Neurol 37:30–40, 1995   8–2

Background.—Mounting evidence suggests that multiple sclerosis (MS) is an autoimmune disease with heightened immune activity against CNS antigens. Although immune suppression has been shown to have therapeutic benefit in patients with MS, most treatments of this sort have had limited duration of efficacy and significant toxicity. Previous studies have suggested that low-dose weekly oral methotrexate (MTX), which is an effective treatment for rheumatoid arthritis, may be clinically beneficial in patients with relapsing-remitting MS. Clinical results of low-dose oral MTX treatment in patients with chronic progressive MS were reported.

Methods.—The randomized, double-blind, placebo-controlled trial included 60 patients with clinically definite chronic progressive MS. They ranged in age from 21 to 60, and all had had MS for more than 1 year. Their Expanded Disability Status Scale (EDSS) scores ranged from 3.0 to

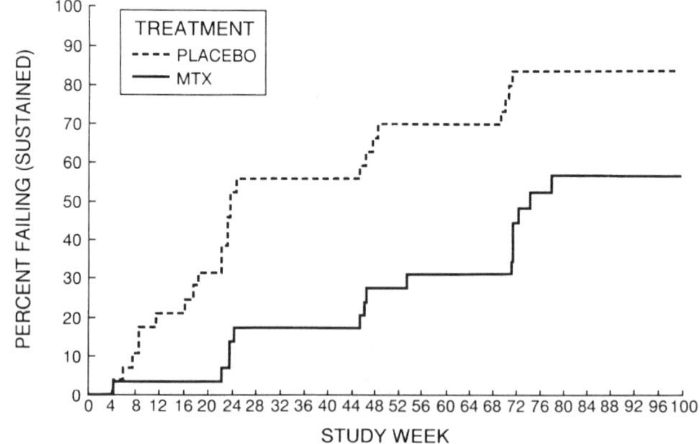

FIGURE 1.—Probability of sustained treatment failure by study week. See the original article for details regarding the required duration and magnitude of change using the composite outcome measure. *Abbreviation: MTX,* methotrexate. (Reprinted from *Annals of Neurology* volume 37:30–40, 1995; by permission of Little, Brown and Company [Inc.].)

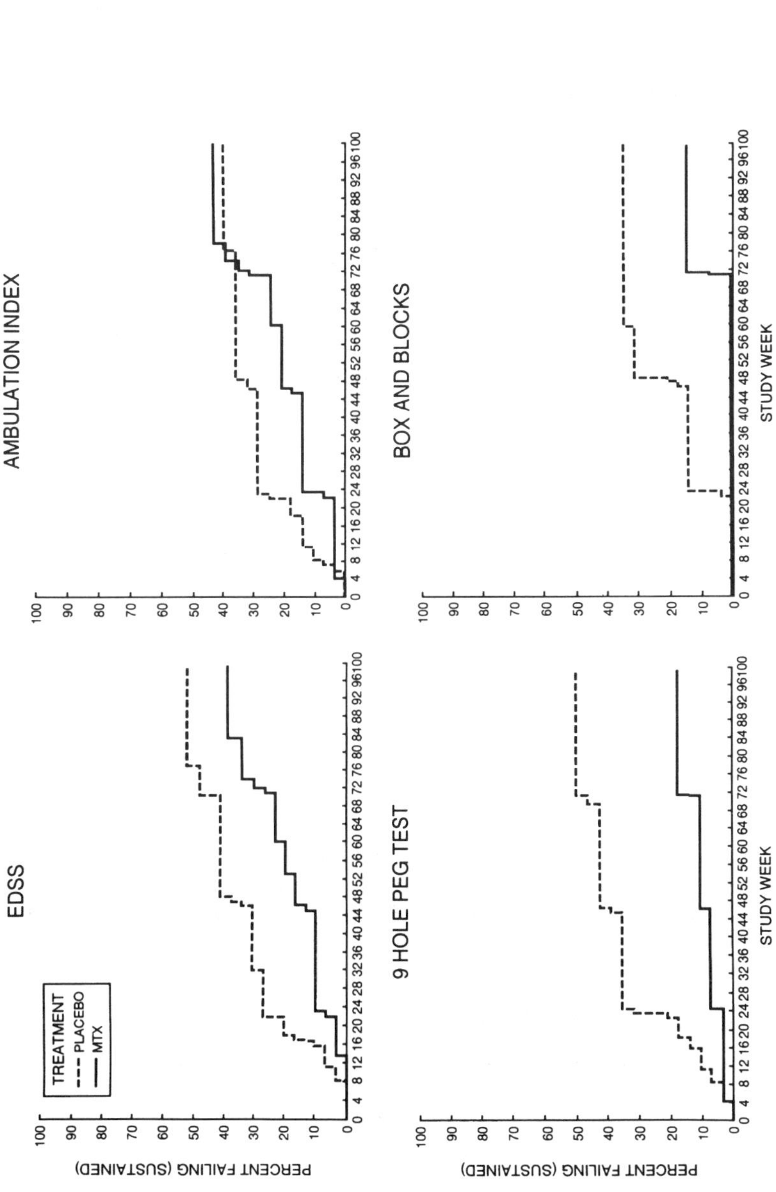

FIGURE 2.—Probability of sustained treatment failure by each of the components of the composite outcome measure by study week. See original article for details regarding the required duration and magnitude of change for each component. *Abbreviations: EDSS,* Expanded Disability Status Scale; *MTX,* methotrexate. (Reprinted from *Annals of Neurology* volume 37:30–40, 1995; by permission of Little, Brown and Company [Inc.].)

6.5, which corresponds to ambulatory status with moderate disability. After stratification for EDSS scores, the patients were randomized to receive either oral methotrexate (7.5 mg once weekly) or placebo. Treatment continued for 2 years, after which the patients were observed for up to 1 year. The clinical results were assessed by using a composite outcome measure composed of the EDSS, ambulation index, Box and Block Test, and 9-Hole Peg Test. Patients with more than a 2-month change in 1 or more of these measures were considered to be treatment failures.

Results.—Sustained progression was significantly more likely to occur in patients receiving placebo (83%) than MTX (52%). The mean time to treatment failure for 50% of the patients in each group was 74 weeks for MTX and 23 weeks for placebo (Fig 1). Methotrexate had its strongest favorable effect on the 9-Hole Peg Test, with lesser effects on the Box and Block Test and EDSS (Fig 2). Treatment group was the strongest predictor of sustained treatment failure on Cox proportional hazard modeling; secondary progressive disease was the only other significant predictor. The 2 groups showed a similar distribution of adverse experiences. At the end of treatment, 68% of the patients in both groups thought that they were in worse condition than at baseline.

Conclusion.—For patients with chronic progressive MS, low-dose weekly oral MTX therapy appears to reduce the progression of impairment on validated tests of upper extremity function. There is no clinically significant toxicity. Additional trials of this new form of therapy are needed. A forthcoming report will describe the effects of MTX on MRI findings, neuropsychological test results, and quality of life measures.

▶ Neurologists have been borrowing from the drug armamentarium of rheumatologists to treat immune-mediated disorders of the CNS. This study showed a mild but clear decrease in the rate of progression of disease severity in patients treated with MTX; the benefit was seen more in patients who had secondary progressive MS. Although the improvement seen was mild—a delay in the rate of progression of upper extremity function—the relative safety of MTX offers another choice in the treatment of secondary progressive MS.

S. Sriram, M.D.

Optic Neuritis: A Population-Based Study in Olmsted County, Minnesota
Rodriguez M, Siva A, Cross SA, et al (Mayo Clinic and Found, Rochester, Minn)
Neurology 45:244–250, 1995   8–3

Objective.—The records of all 156 patients residing in Olmsted County, Minnesota who, from 1935 through 1991, received a diagnosis of optic neuritis (ON) were reviewed.

Definition.—Incidence cases of idiopathic ON were diagnosed from a relatively rapid onset of visual failure for which no specific cause was apparent. Local retinal lesions were ruled out. In addition, at least 2 of these features were required: a cecocentral field defect with or without peripheral extension, an afferent pupillary defect, impaired color vision, pain on eye movement, and an abnormal visual evoked response.

Epidemiology.—The 156 incidence cases represented an annual age- and sex-adjusted incidence rate of 5.1 per 100,000 person-years from 1985 through 1991. The adjusted prevalence rate at the end of 1991 was 115 per 100,000. The prevalence of ON was significantly associated with both age (nonlinearly) and gender. Women had a relative risk of 2.5.

Clinical Aspects.—Nearly half the patients had ocular pain. Only 16% of patients had more than a single attack; 7% had a recurrence in the same eye. Approximately three fourths of acute episodes of ON were accompanied by impaired visual acuity on the side of the attack. In 10% of cases, acuity was impaired contralaterally as well. A central scotoma without peripheral extension was found in just more than half of patients.

Course.—During an average follow-up of 13 years, 39% of 95 patients with isolated ON in the incidence cohort progressed to clinically definite multiple sclerosis (MS) within the first 10 years (Fig 2). The rate was 49% after 20 years, 54% by 30 years, and 60% by 40 years. The risk of MS was similar in men and women. Both recurrent ON and perivenous sheathing were risk factors for MS development. The estimated 25-year survival rate for incidence cases of isolated ON was 88% compared with 84% for the general population adjusted for age and gender (Fig 3).

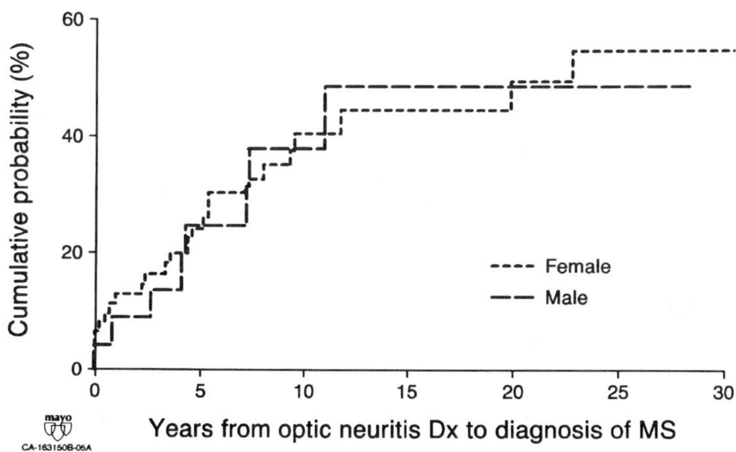

FIGURE 2.—Kaplan-Meier curves for the optic neuritis incidence cohort without previous evidence of neurologic symptoms or signs (n = 95). Percent cumulative probability of the development of clinically definite MS for women (n = 67) and men (n = 28). Ten years after the diagnosis of optic neuritis, there were 25 women and 8 men at risk for subsequent development of MS. *Abbreviations: MS*, multiple sclerosis; *Dx*, diagnosis. (Reprinted from *Neurology* volume 45:244–250, 1995; by permission of Little, Brown and Company [Inc.].)

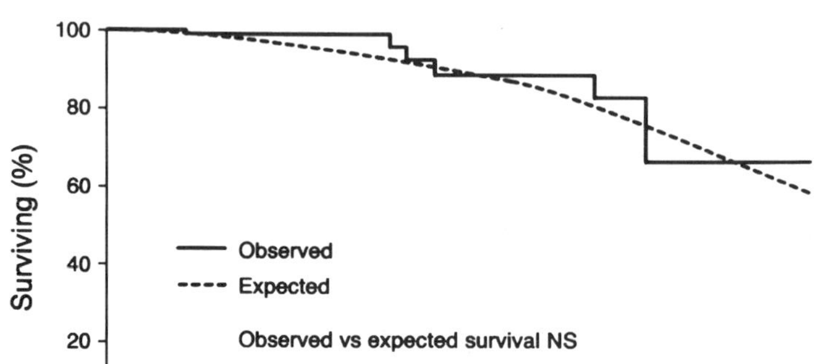

FIGURE 3.—Kaplan-Meier survival curves for the optic neuritis incidence cohort without previous evidence of neurologic symptoms or signs (n = 95) compared with an age- and sex-matched cohort from the U.S. white population. *Abbreviations: Dx*, diagnosis; *LFU*, last follow-up; *NS*, not significant. (Reprinted from *Neurology* volume 45:244–250, 1995; by permission of Little, Brown and Company [Inc.].)

▶ Advising what the future holds for patients who are seen with a first episode of ON is a clinician's dilemma. Population-based research is a powerful tool to understand the natural history of ON. This study gave firm statistical likelihood as to the future, with 40% of patients not having MS develop when observed over 40 years. This 40–40 rule could be useful for advising patients.

S. Sriram, M.D.

Prognostic Factors for Survival in Multiple Sclerosis: A Longitudinal, Population Based Study in Møre and Romsdal, Norway

Midgard R, Albrektsen G, Riise T, et al (Molde Hosp, Norway; Univ of Bergen, Norway)
J Neurol Neurosurg Psychiatry 58:417–421, 1995   8–4

Objective.—Factors influencing how long patients with multiple sclerosis (MS) live were sought in the course of a longitudinal population-based study of life expectancy, carried out in 2 Norwegian counties from 1950 to 1984.

Study Population.—The 141 women and 110 men in the study included 142 with definite MS, 43 with probable, and 66 with possible disease. Average age at the outset was 33½ years.

Observations.—Women survived longer than men. In addition to male gender, patients who were older at the onset of illness and those following a progressive clinical course also were at higher risk (Table 1). Other adverse prognostic factors included ataxia and a lack of paresthesias at the outset. Similar results were obtained when only definite and probable cases

TABLE 1.—Univariate Survival Analysis of Multiple Sclerosis in Møre and Romsdal, Norway, 1950–1984

Variable	Total No.	No. dead Total*	Multiple sclerosis†	75% survival (y) Total*	Multiple sclerosis†	P Value (Mantel-Cox) Total*	Multiple sclerosis†
Sex:							
Men	110	41	28	15.5	21.3	0.003	0.09
Women	141	29	26	24.1	24.5		
Age at onset (y):							
< 30	101	14	13	34.3	34.3	< 0.0001	0.002
30–39	79	26	22	19.4	23.0		
40–49	41	13	10	17.0	19.9		
≥ 50	30	17	9	12.1	18.0		
Year of onset:							
1950–9	49	31	26	21.3	22.6	0.07	0.31
1960–9	59	17	14	23.7	24.5		
1970–84	143	22	14	16.5	18.2		
Diagnosis:							
definite	142	37	36	21.3	23.0	0.48	0.55
probable	43	13	8	16.9	22.6		
possible	66	20	10	18.0	24.5		
Clinical course:							
Remitting + remitting progressive	214	48	40	22.6	23.7	0.0004	0.05
Primary progressive	37	22	14	13.1	17.0		

Note: Univariate survival analysis includes definite, probable, and possible multiple sclerosis.
*All causes of death.
†Multiple sclerosis as underlying and contributing cause of death.
(Courtesy of Midgard R, Albrektsen G, Riise T, et al: Prognostic factors for survival in multiple sclerosis: A longitudinal, population based study in Møre and Romsdal, Norway. *J Neurol Neurosurg Psychiatry* 58:417–421, 1995.)

were analyzed. On multivariate analysis, patients who were relatively young at the onset of illness, those following a remitting course, and those with paresthesias survived the longest.

Conclusion.—Studies such as this may help in advising patients with newly diagnosed MS as to what they can expect.

▶ This study is unique in that none of the patients were taking any long-term immunosuppressive drugs at any time during their disease. Although it should be noted that actuarial studies have not shown a significant decrease in the longevity of MS patients, certain biological markers such as age of onset, gender, and type of MS affect longevity. Counseling patients on these issues at the time of initial diagnosis is an important aspect of patient education.

S. Sriram, M.D.

Urinary Myelin Basic Protein–like Material as a Correlate of the Progression of Multiple Sclerosis
Whitaker JN, Kachelhofer RD, Bradley EL, et al (Univ of Alabama, Birmingham; Birmingham Veterans Med Ctr, Ala; Univ of Chicago; et al)
Ann Neurol 38:625–632, 1995   8–5

Introduction.—Clinical scales can help in predicting the course of multiple sclerosis (MS), but they are imprecise. Laboratory indicators of the course of MS have therefore been sought. Myelin basic protein (MBP) accounts for about 30% of CNS myelin proteins, and a material designated MBP-like material (MBPLM) can be found in elevated levels in the urine of some patients with MS. Urinary MBPLM level was examined as a possible predictor of clinical course in patients with MS.

Methods.—The study included 105 patients with relapsing-remitting MS who were participating in a multicenter, randomized trial of recombinant interferon beta-1b treatment. At 2 study centers, urine specimens were collected periodically over the 2-year study period. At a third center, urine collections were made over 2 consecutive days. All specimens were tested for their content of MBPLM by a double-antibody radioimmunoassay. The findings were correlated with the patients' clinical changes, cranial MRI findings, and development of progressive disease.

Results.—Urinary MBPLM level was significantly related to a chronic progressive course of MS, as well as with the number of lesions and the total lesional area on cranial MRI scanning (Fig 1). An increasing level of urinary MBPLM often preceded the transition from relapsing-remitting to chronic progressive MS. The urinary MBPLM levels in the different treatment groups varied by chance, precluding evaluation of the effects of treatment on urinary MBPLM. However, the 24-hour urine studies suggested that urinary MBPLM values were highest in patients changing from a relapsing-remitting to a chronic progressive course, especially those with

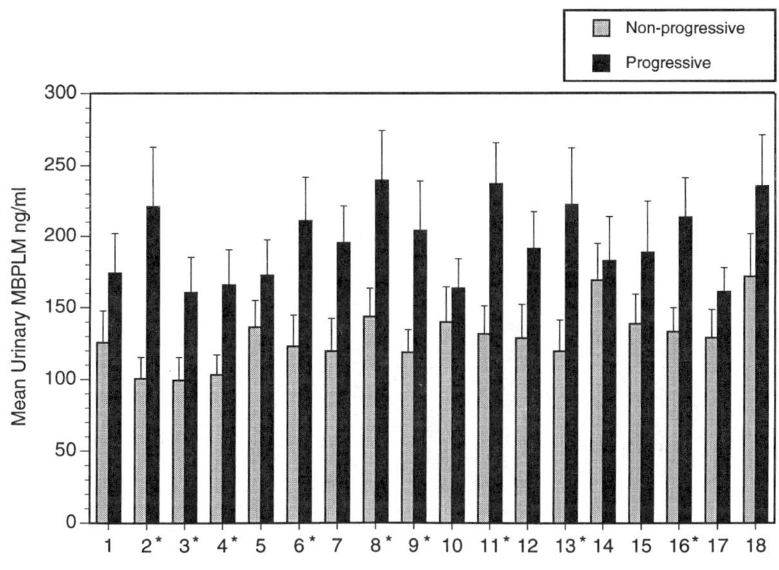

FIGURE 1.—Changes in urinary MBPLM (ng/mL) plus standard error of the mean at 6-week intervals in progressive (n = 15) and nonprogressive (n = 37) multiple sclerosis patients in group 2. Significant differences (*P* < 0.05) in mean values were noted (*asterisks*) at weeks 2 to 4, 6, 8, 9, 11, 13, and 16 and approached significance (*P* = 0.0558) at week 7 for those who remained with the relapsing-remitting form compared with those in whom multiple sclerosis became chronic progressive. *Abbreviation: MBPLM,* myelin basic protein–like material. (Reprinted from *Annals of Neurology* volume 38:625–632, 1995; by permission of Little, Brown and Company [Inc.].)

chronic progressive disease who were receiving placebo (Fig 2). Some of the correlations with MBPLM were affected by concordant changes in creatinine values.

Conclusion.—In patients with MS, measurement of urinary MBPLM may provide a useful maker of disease status. This laboratory value could serve as a surrogate marker for the failure of remission or of the transition from relapsing-remitting to chronic progressive MS. With further study, urinary MBPLM measurement could increase the accuracy and shorten the time needed to conduct clinical trials of MS treatment.

▶ Myelin basic protein is the most intensely studied neural autoantigen in MS. However, direct evidence that MBP is involved in MS is lacking. Presence of MBPLM in the urine in patients with MS strengthens the argument that MBP may be causal in MS. At present there are no satisfactory surrogate markers for disease progression in MS. Estimation of urinary MBP may serve as a surrogate marker for disease severity and also help stratify patients for entry into clinical trials.

S. Sriram, M.D.

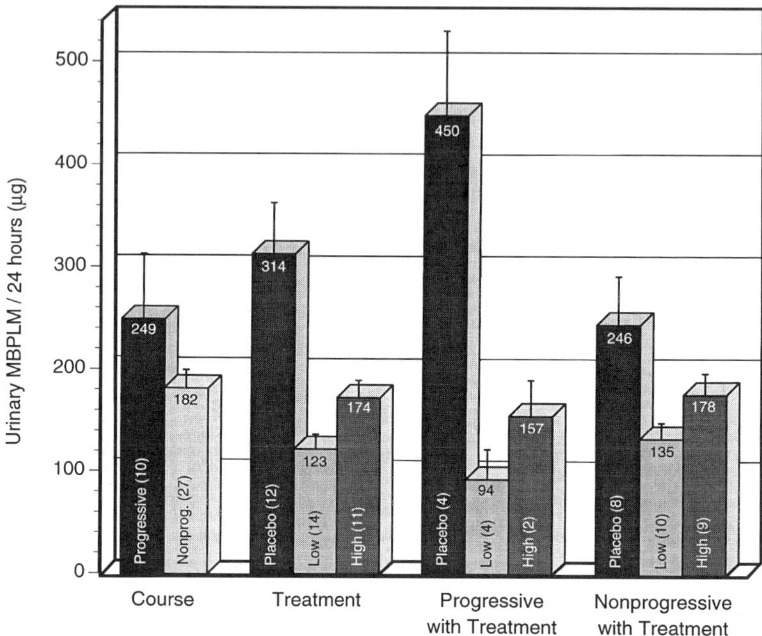

FIGURE 2.—Values of MBPLM (µg/24 hours) of group 3 patients in regard to course, treatment, and both. The mean value of urinary MBPLM is indicated for each subgroup along with the *vertical bar* for the standard error of the mean. *Numbers inside parentheses* denote the number of patients in each of the subgroups. The placebo-treated patients whose multiple sclerosis changed from relapsing-remitting to chronic progressive showed the highest values. *Abbreviation: MBPLM,* myelin basic protein–like material. (Reprinted from *Annals of Neurology* volume 38:625–632, 1995; by permission of Little, Brown and Company [Inc.].)

9 Neuroradiology

Proton MRS of Gadolinium-Enhancing MS Plaques and Metabolic Changes in Normal-Appearing White Matter

Roser W, Hagberg G, Mader I, et al (Univ of Basel, Switzerland)
Magn Reson Med 33:811–817, 1995   9–1

Background.—In multiple sclerosis (MS) patients, the appearance of an acute plaque is accompanied or preceded by blood-brain barrier disturbances. Acute plaques demonstrate gadolinium enhancement over a few weeks (Fig 1). Gadolinium-enhancing acute plaques were studied in a group of 22 MS patients.

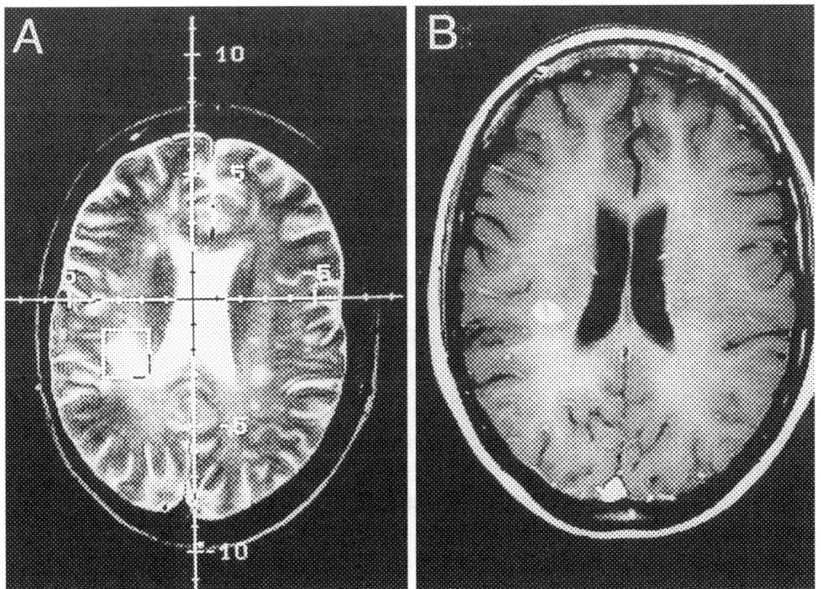

FIGURE 1.—**A,** T2-weighted (TE = 90 msec; TR = 2,500 msec) axial image of a 26-year-old patient with multiple sclerosis. The investigated plaque within the volumes of interest is indicated. **B,** T1-weighted image (TE = 15 msec; TR = 600 msec) of the same slice after application of contrast agent. The gadolinium enhancement of the indicated plaque within the white matter is evident. (Roser W, Hagberg G, Mader I, et al: Proton MRS of gadolinium-enhancing MS plaques and metabolic changes in normal-appearing white matter. *Magn Reson Med* 33:811–817, 1995.)

Subjects.—All patients included in this study were between ages 18 and 50, had clinically definite MS, had clinically active disease, had no relapses within 30 days of study entry, were taking no corticosteroids or immuno-suppressive therapy, and had at least 1 Gd-enhancing lesion on MRI. Localized short-echo time, stimulated echo acquisition mode, and double spin-echo proton spectroscopy were performed on their acute Gd-enhancing MS plaques. The resonances of *N*-acetylated metabolites (NA), creatine/phosphocreatine (Cr), choline compounds (Cho), glycine/*myo*-inositol (Ino), and lactate were assessed.

Results.—Examination of Gd-enhancing acute MS plaques revealed that the ratios of NA/Cr and NA/Cho were significantly decreased, the ratio of Cho/Cr increased, and the Ino/Cr ratio remained unchanged. No marker peaks or elevated lactate levels were detected. These metabolic changes were independent of the relative plaque size within the volume of interest.

Conclusion.—Acute Gd-enhancing MS plaques had significant metabolic changes compared with brain tissue from healthy volunteers. These changes were independent of the plaque size within the volume of interest. This indicates that these metabolic changes are found not only in the MRI-detectable lesion but also in the surrounding normal-appearing white matter. Longitudinal studies in 16 of these patients are underway to determine if the pathologic changes in normal-appearing white matter can be detected by imaging methodology.

▶ Papers dealing with MR spectroscopy in MS are potentially important and clinically relevant for 2 reasons. First, distinguishing single, large, enhancing plaques that can mimic intracerebral tumors (i.e., the pseudotumor of MS) is obviously critical. Second, the diffuse nature of MS may be determined even in the face of normal-appearing white matter on T2-weighted spin-echo images. Although decreases in *N*-acetyl-aspartate levels are a nearly ubiquitous finding in a wide range of intracerebral lesions, other chemical changes such as a significant rise in Cho levels may point to a process with predominate myelin breakdown. Although MR spectroscopy in MS has not now reached the point of sufficient diagnostic specificity to be applied with confidence to various brain lesions, it is probable that in the future MR spectroscopy may be commonly used in clinical brain imaging.

R.M. Quencer, M.D.

Multiple Sclerosis in the Spinal Cord: MR Appearance and Correlation With Clinical Parameters

Tartaglino LM, Friedman DP, Flanders AE, et al (Thomas Jefferson Univ Hosp, Philadelphia; Radiology Associates of Sarasota, Fla)
Radiology 195:725–732, 1995

9–2

Introduction.—In patients who meet the clinical criteria for multiple sclerosis (MS), 12% have plaques identified only in the spinal cord. The specific MRI features of spinal cord MS were examined.

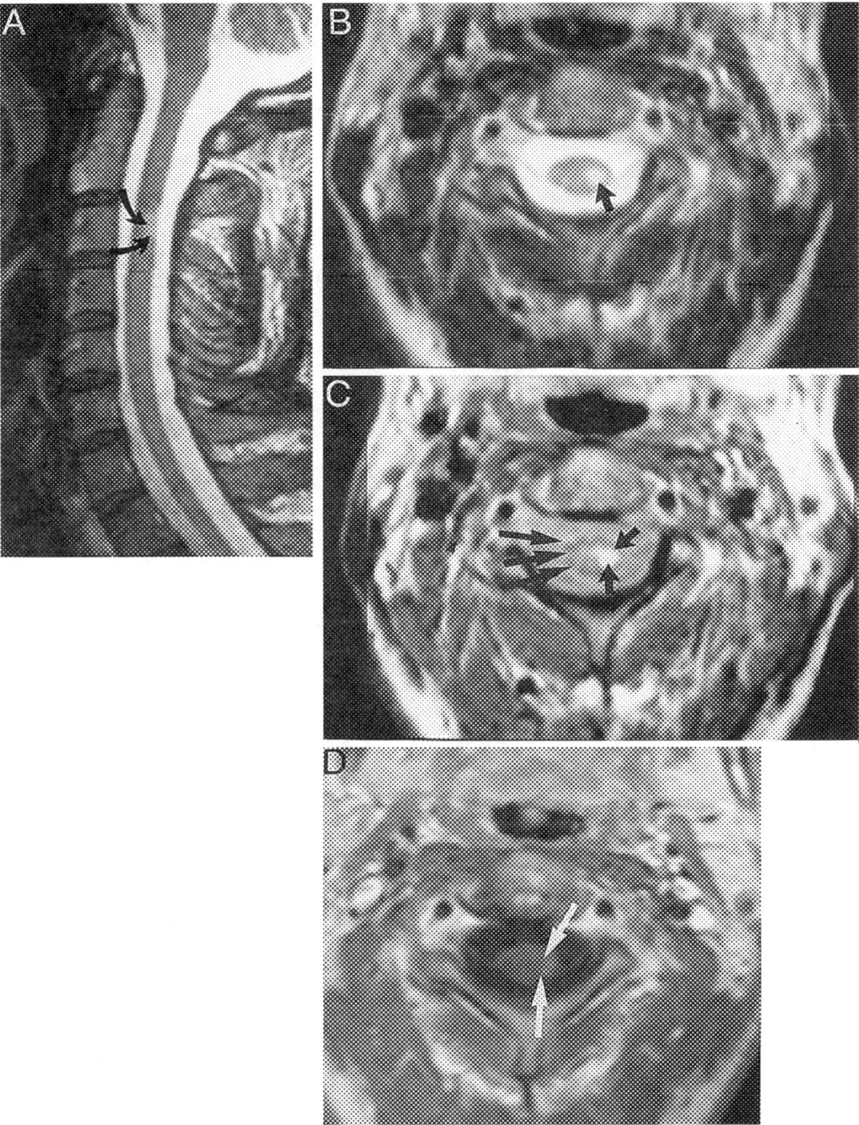

FIGURE 4.—Magnetic resonance images of the cervical spine in a 46-year-old woman with typical imaging characteristics seen in multiple sclerosis. **A,** sagittal T2-weighted fast spin-echo image (TR = 2,500 msec; TE = 102 msec; echo train length of 8) shows focal increased signal intensity posteriorly (*arrows*) at the level of C3 in a normal-sized spinal cord. The plaque is approximately half a vertebral segment long and is longer than it is wide. **B,** axial T2-weighted fast spin-echo image (TR = 3,000 msec; TE = 85 msec; echo train length of 8) through the plaque shows the typical peripheral posterolateral location in cross section (*arrow*). Note that the plaque involves less than half the cross-sectional area of the cord. **C,** axial proton-density–weighted fast spin-echo image (TR = 3,000 msec; TE = 17 msec; echo train length of 4) at the same level as **B** shows clear involvement of the left dorsal and lateral horns of the central gray matter (*large arrows*) compared with that seen in the normal right dorsal and lateral horns (*small arrows*). **D,** axial T1-weighted postcontrast image (TR = 400 msec; TE = 11 msec) at the same level as **B** and **C** demonstrates minimal enhancement at the margin of the plaque (*arrows*). (Courtesy of Tartaglino LM, Friedman DP, Flanders AE, et al: Multiple sclerosis in the spinal cord: MR appearance and correlation with clinical parameters. *Radiology* 195:725–732, 1995, Radiological Society of North America.)

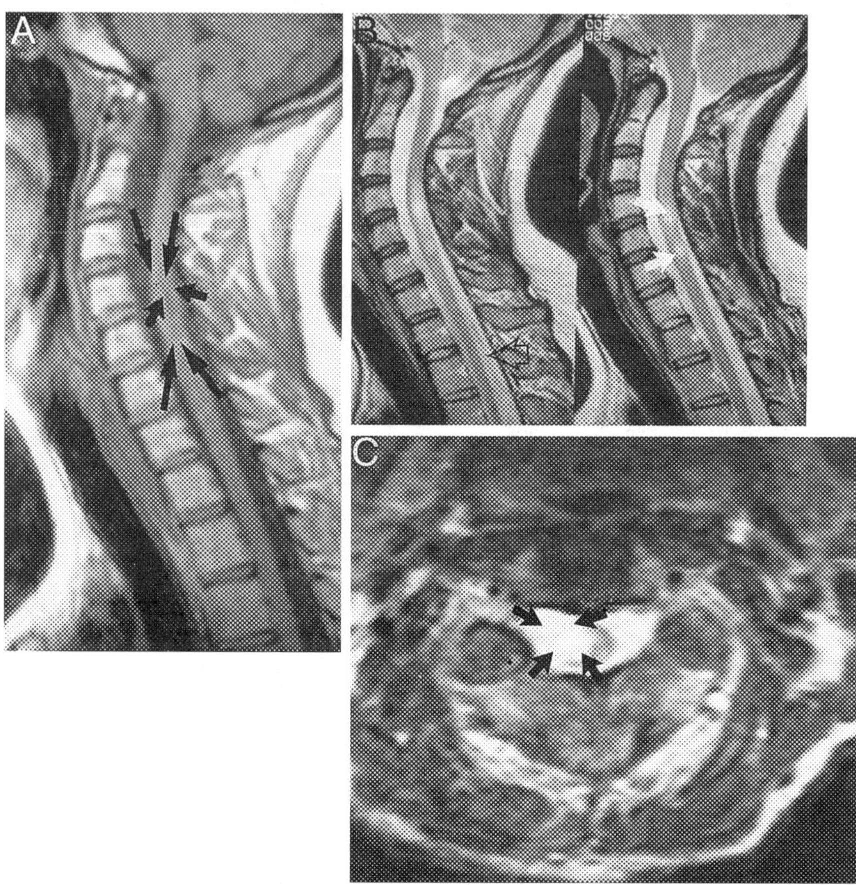

FIGURE 6.—Magnetic resonance images of the cervical spine in a 25-year-old woman with an acute episode of multiple sclerosis. A, sagittal T1-weighted image (TR = 600 msec; TE = 11 msec) shows focal swelling at C4 and C5. Focal hypointensity is seen centrally, consistent with edema and plaque (*arrows*). B, sagittal T2-weighted fast spin-echo images (TR = 2,200 msec; TE = 85 msec; echo train length of 8) show 2 plaques close together at C4 and C6. Note the different signal intensities within the more superior demyelinating plaque. It is likely that the more central hyperintensity represents the plaque (*solid curved arrows*) and the more peripheral halo of less intense signal represents edema (*solid straight arrows*). A probable third plaque is seen incidentally on the adjacent image at the upper margin of T1 (*open arrow*). C, axial T2-weighted image (TR = 2,500 msec; TE = 80 msec) shows that the plaque with cord enlargement is eccentric to the right but occupies more than half the cross-sectional area of the cord (*arrows*). (Courtesy of Tartaglino LM, Friedman DP, Flanders AE, et al: Multiple sclerosis in the spinal cord: MR appearance and correlation with clinical parameters. *Radiology* 195:725–732, 1995, Radiological Society of North America.)

Methods.—Sixty-eight consecutive patients with clinically definite or clinically probable MS and with documented spinal cord lesions on cervical or thoracic MR images (or both) were examined retrospectively. Plaques were analyzed for lesion length, cross-sectional area and location, signal intensity, and morphology, and these findings were correlated with clinical parameters such as type of MS, duration of disease, sex, and age.

The duration of MS ranged from 0 to 25 years, but on initial examination, all patients had new signs or symptoms that were referable to the spinal axis.

Findings.—In 68 patients, 124 demyelinating plaques were identified in the cervical cord, thoracic cord, or both on T2-weighted spin-echo or fast spin-echo sagittal or axial images; 58% had more than 1 plaque (mean 1.9). Majority of the plaques were less than 2 vertebral body segments long and occupied less than half the cross-sectional area of the cord (Fig 4). Most plaques were peripherally located, consistent with the anatomical location of the white matter in the cord. Although most plaques were located in the lateral and posterior aspects of the cord, involvement of the dorsal horns in the adjacent gray matter was common. Atrophy or swelling of the cord occurred significantly more often in plaques greater than 2 vertebral segments long and those that occupied more than half the cross-sectional area of the cord (Fig 6). All 7 plaques associated with swelling of the cord were seen in patients with relapsing-remitting form of MS, whereas plaques associated with cord atrophy were more likely to occur with the relapsing-progressive form of MS. There was no correlation between disease duration and number or length of plaques.

Conclusion.—The majority of MS plaques in the spinal cord are peripherally located, are less than 2 vertebral body segments long, and involve less than half the cross-sectional area of the cord. Spinal cord MS plaques should be differentiated from neoplasm, arterial or venous cord infarct, acute transverse myelitis, and various infections. In addition, the edema present with cord swelling can extend beyond the margin of the demyelinating plaque and may be difficult to differentiate from other disease entities.

▶ To those who have evaluated a large number of patients with MS involving the spinal cord, the findings described in this article are not surprising. Nonetheless, the large number of patients evaluated by Tartaglino et al. serves to confirm features important in interpreting spinal MRI. The critical observation is the location on axial sections of either the high signal on T2-weighted image or the contrast-enhanced area on T1-weighted images. Relatively short cord segment involvement (compared with spinal cord tumors) and selective involvement of the periphery of the cord (location of white matter tracts) is highly suggestive of a disease process that is demyelinating. In MS, the reason for predominate involvement of the dorsal column as seen on MRI remains uncertain but could relate to the size of the myelin sheaths in those tracts. Keeping these MR features in mind may help to prevent unwarranted cord biopsy even in the face of cord enlargement.

R.M. Quencer, M.D.

Magnetic Resonance Versus Computed Tomographic Imaging in Acute Stroke

Mohr JP, Biller J, Hilal SK, et al (Neurological Inst, New York; Univ of Iowa, Iowa City; KAI, Rockville, Md; et al)
Stroke 26:807–812, 1995   9–3

Objective.—Computed tomography and MRI were studied to determine which is preferable for the early detection of ischemic stroke or hematoma.

Subjects.—Eighty patients with acute stroke, seen at either Columbia University or the University of Iowa, participated in this study. Participants were eligible if they were between ages 18 and 90, had clinical evidence of stroke due to ischemia or intracerebral hemorrhage, and had symptom onset less than 180 minutes before hospital admission.

Study Design.—After an initial examination, the patient underwent either a CT or MR scan. Whenever possible, the patient immediately underwent the other scan as well. Follow-up images were undertaken at 24 hours, 3 to 5 days, 7 to 10 days, and 3 months. Clinical assessments were made at these times.

Findings.—The stroke was caused by hemorrhage in 5 patients and infarction in 75 patients. There were 45 CT scans performed first and 35 MR scans performed first. The median time from onset to first scan was 132 minutes. The median time from the start of the first scan to the start of the second scan was 72 minutes. For all patients with infarction, the fraction of positive first scans was greatest between 2 and 3 hours after the stroke occurred. For the 61 patients with infarction who successfully underwent both CT and MR scans at baseline, neither CT nor MRI was superior. Among those patients whose symptoms returned to normal within 24 hours, baseline CT was negative for 81% and baseline MRI was negative for 55%. When MRI and CT were performed at 24 hours after stroke onset, findings were similar for both types of scan. Both MRI and CT were better able to define lesions at 24 hours than at baseline.

Conclusion.—With the use of technology widely available in 1991, there were no significant differences between MR and CT scans for the early detection of ischemic lesions in this large cohort of stroke patients.

▶ This important article addressed an issue that will assume increasing importance as more centers are established to treat acute stroke with thrombolytic agents. The results of this study indicate that when *routine* MRI (T2, proton density, and T1) is done on conventional midfield (0.5-tesla) and high-field (1.5-tesla) scanners, MRI offers no advantages over CT in acute stroke detection. It must be emphasized that only 5 of 8 patients had hematomas, so greater numbers in this patient category need analysis. Experience has shown that CT has some advantages over MRI in the detection of blood whether it is in the subarachnoid space or in the brain parenchyma. The real test of MRI vs. CT in the clinical setting of acute stroke will be more apparent when diffusion-weighted MRI is compared with CT.

Here it is likely that MRI will be more sensitive to the changes of acute stroke and hence will be the primary noninvasive imaging modality.

R.M. Quencer, M.D.

New Magnetic Resonance Techniques for Acute Ischemic Stroke

Fisher M, Prichard JW, Warach S (Univ of Massachusetts, Worcester; Yale Univ, New Haven, Conn; Harvard Med School, Boston; et al)
JAMA 274:908–911, 1995   9–4

Objective.—Computed tomography and standard MRI can detect, localize, and assess the extent of subacute stroke 1 to 7 days after onset. However, they cannot depict the full extent of brain ischemia in the first 12 to 24 hours after the stroke. The ability to determine the location, extent, and severity of focal ischemia at this time would make a major contribution to the development of various therapies for acute stroke. Three new techniques for the acute evaluation of ischemic stroke—diffusion-weighted MRI, perfusion imaging, and MR spectroscopy—were reviewed.

Diffusion-Weighted Imaging.—When 2 strong, rapidly switched gradient pulses are used with routine MRI pulse sequences, diffusion-weighted MRI is sensitive to random movement of water molecules. Substances with greater movement of water molecules, such as CSF, look darker than brain parenchyma on diffusion-weighted images. The apparent diffusion coefficient (ADC) of water can be calculated for each pixel in the image, and multiple images with different levels of diffusion weighting can be obtained to make the absolute ADC measurement more accurate. In the new "trace mapping" technique, averaged ADCs are obtained from all 3 orthogonal planes.

Diffusion-weighted imaging with echo planar imaging (EPI) substantially reduced the time needed to perform the examination, providing all of the echoes needed to make a single brain slice during an acquisition period of 25 to 100 msec. Initial declines in ADCs and hyperintensity can be detected within minutes after arteries are blocked in stroke. The postischemic decline in ADC values may result from reduced extracellular water, which accompanies the intracellular influx of sodium, calcium, and chloride ions from the extracellular space after hypoxic ischemia. The ADC values may be heterogeneous because of the variability in ischemic injury, and the differences could aid in distinguishing the core of the infarct from its potentially reversible penumbra of surrounding tissue.

Perfusion Imaging.—Perfusion imaging can be based on the magnetic susceptibility effect of gadolinium-containing contrast agents or on noninvasive magnetic labeling of arterial blood. In the former technique, a rapid IV bolus of MRI contrast agent is given, then ultrafast imaging of the brain is performed to show dynamic changes in regional blood volume. Images are taken every 1 to 2 sec to monitor the passage of the contrast agent; the amount of signal loss is proportional to the cerebral blood volume in normal brain tissue. Qualitative mapping of cerebral blood flow can be performed using EPI, a single inversion pulse to inflowing arterial spins, and subtraction of tagged and untagged EPI images. Blood flow can also be imaged by spin labeling of arterial input.

Advances in Magnetic Resonance Spectroscopy.—The lactate elevation that occurs with stroke can easily be detected by MR spectroscopy in the acute period and after several months. Although stroke is probably associated with an immediate increase in lactate as a result of anaerobic glycolysis, the later elevations must reflect a tissue injury response, perhaps involving macrophage infiltration. A large ^{1}H signal from the *N*-acetyl group—mainly *N*-acetyl-aspartate—follows stroke, and signals from choline-containing compounds may be elevated.

Discussion.—Recent advances in the imaging of stroke include diffusion-weighted imaging, which can show the location and extent of the ischemic lesion as soon as the patient can be examined; perfusion imaging, which can evaluate microvascular flow and demonstrate regions of perfusion deficits corresponding to major vascular territories; and MR spectroscopy, which uses biochemical measurements to assess the metabolic abnormalities associated with focal brain ischemia.

▶ The MR-based imaging techniques of diffusion and perfusion MR and MR spectroscopy allow the acquisition of anatomical and metabolic information previously unavailable for acute stroke. Early in the course of an acute ischemic stroke, conventional MR may be normal but diffusion and perfusion images are abnormal. Because diffusion and perfusion can be implemented on conventional MR systems, it would be most valuable if acute MRI were integrated within or directly adjacent to an angiographic suite. Swift documentation of a lack of hemorrhage, loss of normal anisotropic water diffusion, and diminished cerebral perfusion could precede angiography. The angiogram then is used to demonstrate the presence or absence of an intravascular clot. The challenge now is to develop centers dedicated to treating acute stroke by using therapeutic strategies that include intravascular thrombolysis.

R.M. Quencer, M.D.

Problems and Pitfalls of 3-D TOF Magnetic Resonance Angiography of the Intracranial Circulation
Wilcock DJ, Jaspan T, Worthington BS (Univ Hosp, Nottingham, England)
Clin Radiol 50:526–532, 1995   9–5

Introduction.—The 3-dimensional time of flight (TOF) technique of MR angiography is being used increasingly to evaluate the intracranial circulation. The problems encountered with this method were reviewed in 5 patients with cerebral aneurysms who also underwent conventional angiography.

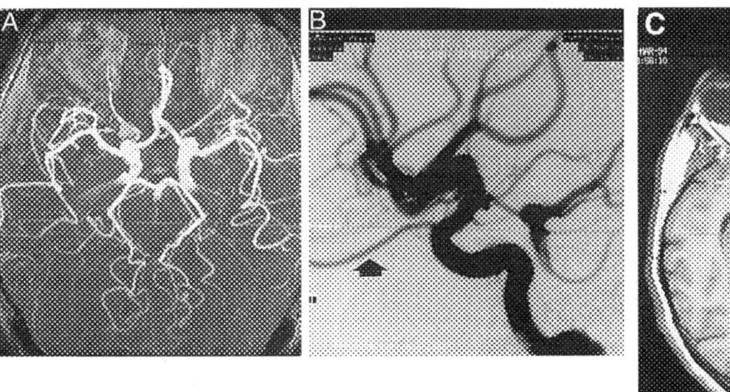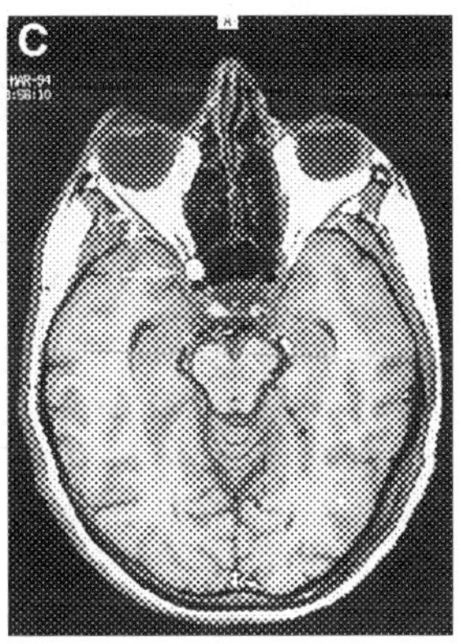

FIGURE 1.—**A**, magnetic resonance angiograph of a 33-year-old woman appears to demonstrate a 6-mm aneurysm arising from the right ophthalmic artery (*arrow*). **B**, however, digital subtraction angiography did not visualize the aneurysm (*arrow* indicates the ophthalmic artery). Repeat MRI was performed. **C**, T1-weighted spin-echo image demonstrated a high-signal intensity structure (*arrow*) within the right optic nerve canal. (Courtesy of Wilcock DJ, Jaspan T, Worthington BS: Problems and pitfalls of 3-D TOF magnetic resonance angiography of the intracranial circulation. *Clin Radiol* 50:526–532, 1995.)

Case Report.—Woman, 33, developed right-sided retro-orbital pain. Axial T2-weighted spin-echo MR images were negative, but MR angiography was thought to demonstrate a 6-mm aneurysm arising from the right ophthalmic artery (Fig 1, A). Embolization was planned, but preliminary digital subtraction angiography failed to identify the aneurysm (Fig 1, B). A repeat MR study employing T1-weighted spin-echo and fat-suppressed T1-weighted spin-echo sequences demonstrated a high-intensity structure within the right optic nerve canal (Fig 1, C). Post-processed MR angiographic images showed a cleavage plane between the high-signal lesion and artery, suggesting a thrombosed varix or, less likely, arteriovenous malformation.

Observations.—When 3-dimensional TOF MR angiography is performed, there is a risk that other phenomena, including acute thrombosis and high-signal structures, will be incorporated into the Maximal Intensity Projection (MIP) reconstruction and thereby be mistaken for vascular abnormalities. A sizeable hematoma may impede the interpretation of MIP reconstructions. There also is a risk that vascular structures will not be recognized because of a loss of signal from saturation effects or dephasing secondary to slow or complex blood flow. Slow flow in a large aneurysm may cause saturation effects that will be increased if the structure under study is near the margin of the imaging volume. In addition, local artifacts created by aneurysm clips or coils may suppress signal from vascular structures.

Suggestions.—The most reliable interpretation can be made by considering the MR angiographic source data and spin-echo axial images, as well as the MIP reconstructions. Phase contrast angiography may help distinguish subacute thrombus from blood flow.

▶ Although MR angiography has added to the diagnostic capabilities of conventional MR, caution is required in the interpretation of intracranial vascular lesions. As this article nicely summarized, saturation effects can partially or totally obscure certain abnormalities such as large aneurysms in which slow flow is present. In these situations the blood is repeatedly stimulated by radiofrequency pulsations so that full relaxation does not occur; the effect is to lower the signal from the blood within the aneurysm. On the other hand, the presence of a focal high signal (see Fig 1) when near a vessel can simulate an aneurysm or vascular malformation. It remains crucial, therefore, to evaluate each source image (i.e., those individual thin slices that in the composite are used to construct the MIP image).

R.M. Quencer, M.D.

Cervical Disk Prolapse

Houser OW, Onofrio BM, Miller GM, et al (Mayo Clinic, Rochester, Minn)
Mayo Clin Proc 70:939–945, 1995   9–6

Objective.—Several studies of imaging in cervical disk disease have compared CT myelography with MRI or described the changing MRI scanning techniques. In contrast, relatively few studies have correlated the results of these imaging techniques with the surgical and pathologic findings. The CT myelography and surgical findings of patients with prolapsed cervical disk were correlated and the clinical relevance of specific CT myelographic features defined in a retrospective study.

Patients.—The study sample was composed of 734 patients with suspected degenerative cervical disk disease who underwent CT myelography over a 4-year period. Two hundred ninety-seven patients (197 men and 100 women), most of whom were in their fifties or sixties, were found to have an extruded disk. The results of MRI in 28 patients and CT in 14 were evaluated as well.

Findings.—The surgical reports of the 297 patients with an extruded disk revealed cervical radiculopathy in 280 and myelopathy in 17. Of the patients, 87% had at least 1 prolapsed disk, and 13% had a prolapsed disk with a bony spur. More than 90% of the extruded cervical disks were identified by CT myelography. The CT myelographic and surgical findings were consistent with each other in 260 cases of radiculopathy and all 17 cases of myelopathy. However, CT myelography was unable to differentiate between an osteophytic cartilaginous cap and a disk and failed to identify the source of cervical radiculopathy in 102 patients. Magnetic resonance and CT imaging did not seem to be as sensitive as CT myelography in detecting prolapsed disks, although the number of MRI studies performed was too small for a proper comparison.

Conclusion.—The imaging of cervical disk prolapse poses a challenging problem with sometimes nonspecific results. The most sensitive imaging study in this situation seems to be CT myelography, although it is not always specific. Further advances in MRI for this purpose may be forthcoming, but they will require pathologic confirmation.

▶ This article analyzed a large number of cervical CT myelograms (34), which were performed in 1 institution over 3 years. Although the studies were done during the years when MR techniques were evolving (1986–1989), the imaging preferences of the referring clinicians for CT myelograms at that institution were clear. The perspective on how to image a patient with a cervical radiculopathy or a myelopathy has, however, changed. Under both clinical situations, MRI is now the first and very commonly the only imaging study required. Because a myelopathy can be caused by lesions intrinsic or extrinsic to the spinal cord, MRI is the preferred examination. Even for a cervical radiculopathy or radiculomyelopathy, MRI is the procedure of choice because now high-resolution and thin sections (e.g., in 3-dimensional data acquisition) are possible. Only in those instances where the history is complex (e.g., previous surgery or instrumentation) could justification be given to performing a CT myelogram, but even in those cases CT myelogram would usually follow an MRI study.

R.M. Quencer, M.D.

Brain Metastases: Comparison of Gadodiamide Injection-Enhanced MR Imaging at Standard and High Dose, Contrast-Enhanced CT and Non-Contrast-Enhanced MR Imaging
Åkeson P, Larsson E-M, Kristoffersen DT, et al (Univ Hosp, Lund, Sweden; Nycomed AB, Stockholm; Nycomed Imaging AS, Oslo, Norway)
Acta Radiol 36:300–306, 1995   9–7

Background.—The diagnostic sensitivity of imaging techniques used for the evaluation of patients with brain metastases is crucial, because metastasis number has a profound effect on treatment and prognosis. The abilities of contrast-enhanced MRI using standard and high-dose Gadodiamide injection were compared with that of contrast-enhanced CT imaging in the detection of multiple brain metastases.

Methods.—Sixteen adult patients with at least 2 brain metastases found during contrast-enhanced CT studies composed the study group. All patients were examined by CT no more than 1 week before MR examination. All patients had a T2-weighted spin-echo MR examination, then a T1-weighted spin-echo examination before contrast injection, then again after Gadodiamide injection of 0.1 mmol/kg of body weight, and again after additional contrast injection for a cumulative dose of 0.3 mmol of Gadodiamide/kg. The time between injection initiation and scanning was 5 minutes. An open analysis and a blinded analysis of these images were performed.

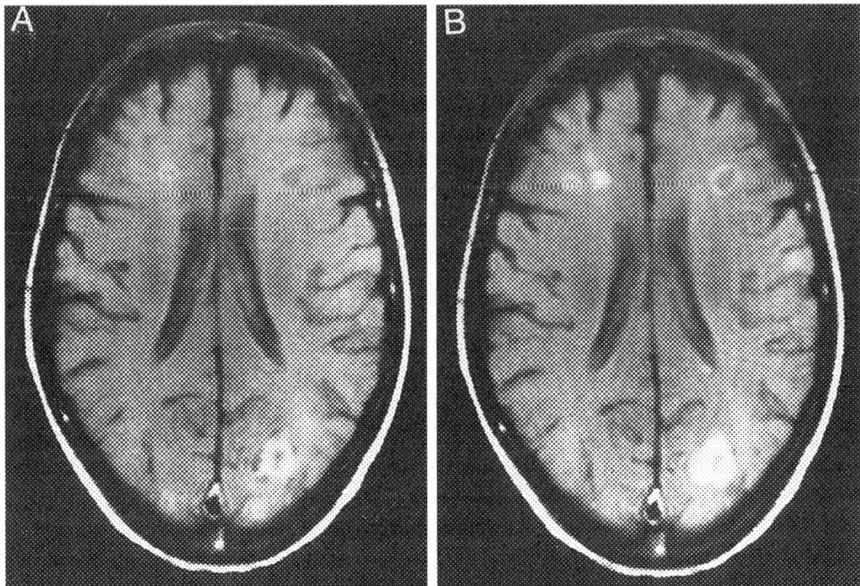

FIGURE 1.—**A,** standard-dose contrast-enhanced spin-echo MRI: 3 metastases found—2 certain, 1 probable, right-sided parasagittal lesion. **B,** high-dose contrast-enhanced spin-echo MRI: 8 metastases found—7 certain, 1 probable, small left-sided frontal lesion. (Courtesy of Åkeson P, Larsson E-M, Kristoffersen DT, et al: Brain metastases: Comparison of Gadodiamide injection-enhanced MR imaging at standard and high dose, contrast-enhanced CT and noncontrast-enhanced MR imaging. *Acta Radiol* 36:300–306, 1995.)

Results.—There were no adverse events attributed to the contrast media. High-dose contrast-enhanced MRI detected significantly more metastases, detected smaller metastases, and had more diagnostic certainty than any other technique (Fig 2). Both blinded investigators judged the high-dose contrast-enhanced MR images superior to all others.

Conclusion.—High-dose contrast-enhancing MRI is significantly more sensitive and has increased diagnostic certainty compared with standard-dose contrast-enhanced MRI or CT imaging. Spin-echo MRI with a high-dose Gadodiamide injection is an effective method to imrove the detection of small brain metastases.

▶ The issue raised by this and other previously published articles involves the most efficacious and clinically useful way of evaluating the brain for possible metastasis. Although, for example, Figure 2 does demonstrate that a higher dose of gadolinium is capable of showing more lesions and with a greater degree of confidence, the critical question, unanswered by this paper, is not only how this may help in patient management but, more important, what is the comparative clinical outcome in those patients who are determined to have an increased number of metastasis as detected by high-dose injection. That is, can it be shown that this technique sufficiently influences treatment protocols that improve patient outcome? In the absence of such proof, one must question the added expense of high-dose contrast in MRI. Also, note should be made of the fact that magnetization transfer contrast in conjunction with routine doses of Gd improves detection rates of many intracerebral lesions, including metastasis.

R.M. Quencer, M.D.

MR Findings in Adult-Onset Adrenoleukodystrophy
Kumar AJ, Köhler W, Kruse B, et al (Johns Hopkins Med Insts, Baltimore, Md; Moabit Hosp, Berlin; Kennedy Krieger Inst, Baltimore, Md)
AJNR 16:1227–1237, 1995   9–8

Background.—Adrenoleukodystrophy (ALD) is an X-linked disorder associated with increased very low–chain saturated fatty acids in the brain and adrenal gland, red blood cells, and plasma attributed to defective peroxisomal fatty acid oxidation. The phenotypic expression of ALD varies widely, ranging from the most severe childhood cerebral form to the milder adult forms. The adult neurologic variant affects approximately 30% of men and 15% to 20% of women heterozygotes. The most common form is adrenomyeloneuropathy (AMN), which involves mainly the spinal cord and peripheral nerves with mild to absent inflammatory response in cerebral white matter. This study examined the MRI findings of the brain and spinal cord in adult-onset ALD.

Methods.—Magnetic resonance imaging of the brain was performed in 164 adult patients aged 19 to 74 with clinically and biochemically proved ALD. In 30 patients, MRI of the spine was also performed.

Findings.—The brain MRI findings were abnormal in 46% of male AMN and in 20% of female heterozygotes. The brain abnormalities consisted of varying degrees of demyelination of the cerebral white matter in 46 patients, corpus callosum in 25, corticospinal tracts in 46, visual tracts in 31, and auditory tracts in 18. Diffuse spinal cord atrophy, mainly in the thoracic regions, was evident on MRI in 18 of 20 men and 8 of 10 women. There were no focal T2-weighted abnormalities in the spinal cord.

Correlation of the MRI findings with clinical features allowed tentative subdivision of adult-onset ALD into 4 subtypes that appeared to differ with respect to prognosis and possibly pathogenesis. Sixty-five male patients had "pure" AMN with normal brain MRI findings and disease confined to the spinal cord and peripheral nerves. Another 16 male AMN patients had adrenoleukomyeloneuropathy type 1 (ALMN 1) with brain MRI abnormality confined to the long-fiber tract systems, mainly bilateral involvement of the corticospinal tract. In this group, the more than 25-year interval between onset of neurologic symptoms and tract degeneration represented a "dying back" mechanism of these long tracts, possibly due to a defective axonal protein transport secondary to metabolic alterations of the perikarya. Thirty-two male AMN patients had ALMN 2 with diffuse lobar cerebral involvement (Figs 1 and 3). The most common pattern was a bilateral parieto-occipital involvement extending across the splenium of the corpus callosum in combination with bilateral pyramidal

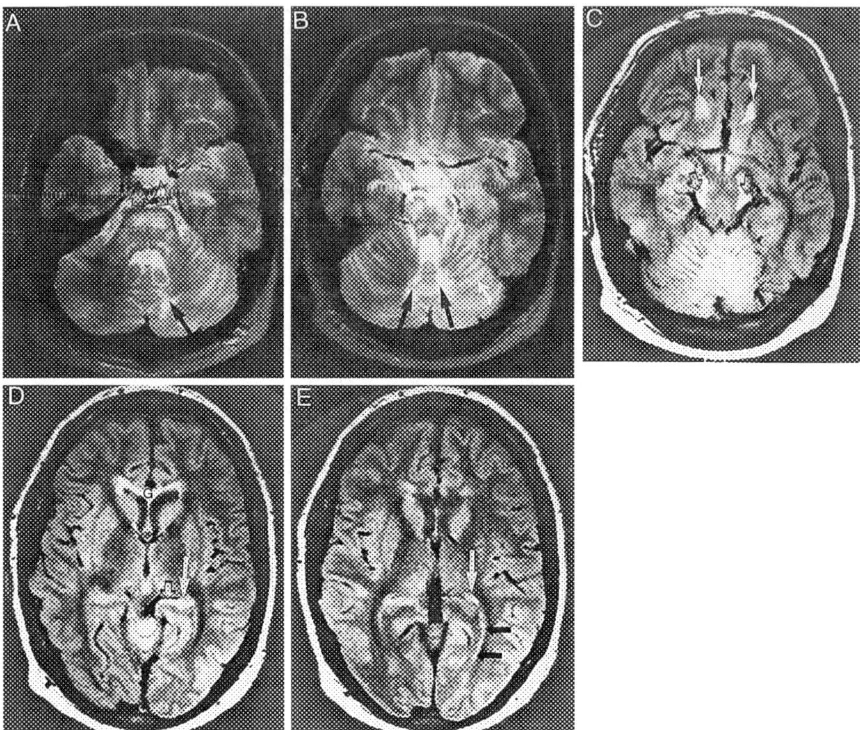

FIGURE 1.—Adrenoleukomyeloneuropathy type 2. Adrenomyeloneuropathy with severe white matter tract demyelination with early cerebral and cerebellar white matter involvement with cerebellar atrophy. A 29-year-old patient at age 22 sought medical advice for gait disturbance and was diagnosed with multiple sclerosis. Patient's clinical symptoms were difficulty with speech, memory loss, and weakness of lower extremities with sensory level at T6 level, including autonomic dysfunction. A and B, MR T2-weighted images of the brain reveal demyelination of pyramidal tracts in the pons (*open arrows* in A) and in cerebral peduncles (*white arrows* in B). *Black arrows* in A and B point to white matter demyelination, and *white arrowheads* point to cerebellar atrophy. C–E, proton density–weighted images of the brain at successive levels. Auditory tract demyelination of brachium of the inferior colliculus (*open arrows* in C and D) as it joins the demyelinated medial geniculate body (*large arrow* in D) is beautifully depicted. Visual pathway demyelination involving lateral geniculate body (*arrow*) and optic radiations (*black arrows*) is shown in E. Lobar white matter demyelination. In addition to specific tract demyelination, focal frontal lobe white matter demyelination (*white arrows* in C), and cerebellar white matter demyelination (*black arrows* in A and B) are observed. Genu of the corpus callosum (*G* in D) shows demyelination. Cerebellum shows diffuse atrophy (*white arrowheads* in A and B). (AJ Kumar, W Kohler, B Kruse, et al: MR findings in adult-onset adrenoleukodystrophy. *AJNR* 16:1227–1237, 1995, Copyright by American Society of Neuroradiology.)

tract involvement in the brain stem and internal capsule. Six patients had adult cerebral ALD with severe lobar white matter demyelination or severe brain atrophy and severe and rapidly progressive course.

Conclusion.—The clinical course in adult phenotypes of ALD differs significantly. The evaluation of the brain with MRI allows differentiation of adult ALD phenotypes for prognostic considerations and allows patient selection for experimental dietary therapy and bone marrow therapy, which can be effective if given in the early stage of the disease.

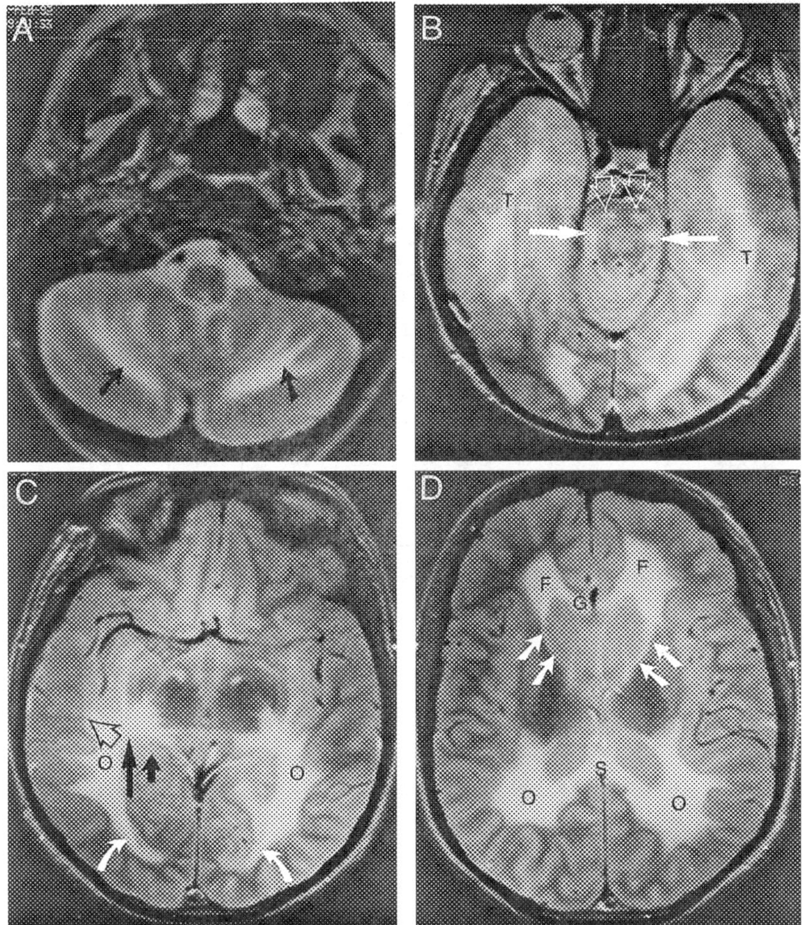

FIGURE 3.—Adrenomyeloneuropathy with severe lobar white matter demyelination and including white matter tract demyelination (adrenoleukomyeloneuropathy type 2); MR axial T2-weighted images of the brain. Extensive lobar white matter demyelination. Large areas of demyelination of the frontal lobe white matter (*F* in D), occipital white matter (*O* in C and D), temporal lobe white matter (*T* in B), and cerebellar white matter (*arrows* in A) are shown. Pyramidal tract demyelination. Frontopontine fibers in internal capsule (*arrows* in D) and corticospinal tracts in pons (*open arrows* in B) show demyelination. Auditory tract demyelination is evidenced by abnormal hyperintensity involving the lateral lemnisci in the pons (*white arrows* in B), the region of medial geniculate body (*small black arrow* in C), and acoustic radiations (*open arrow* in C). Visual tract demyelination involving the region of lateral geniculate body (*large black arrow* in C) and optic radiations (*curved white arrows* in C) are shown. Genu (*G*) and splenium (*S*) of the corpus callosum show evidence of demyelination (D). (AJ Kumar, W Kohler, B Kruse, et al: MR findings in adult-onset adrenoleukodystrophy. *AJNR* 16:1227–1237, 1995, Copyright by American Society of Neuroradiology.)

▶ This article thoroughly described the clinical and MRI findings of a large number of adult patients (164) with ALD (a disease commonly thought of as occurring only in children) and its variant AMN. Of additional interest is the fact that nearly one third of this adult population was female. In the spinal cord, atrophy is seen in conjunction with the clinical features of progressive paraparesis, sensory disturbances, and bowel and bladder dysfunction. Although the authors maintained that there were no focal T2 abnormalities in the cord, this is surprising given the fact that the major pathologic finding is loss of myelin predominately in the lateral columns. Of the 4 types of ALD, the patients in the group (type 1) in which there is no cerebral white matter involvement but only spinal cord atrophy would pose the greatest problem in arriving at a proper diagnosis.

R.M. Quencer, M.D.

Progressive Multifocal Leukoencephalopathy: Unusual MR Findings

Ng S, Tse VCK, Rubinstein J, et al (Stanford Univ, Calif; Palo Alto Veterans Affairs Med Ctr, Calif)
J Comput Assist Tomogr 19:302–305, 1995

9–9

Background.—Progressive multifocal leukoencephalopathy (PML) is a rapidly progressive demyelinating disorder caused by a papovavirus. Bleeding is rare, and cerebral atrophy is noted only in patients who also have HIV encephalitis. Typically, lesions of PML do not enhance, but contrast enhancement has been demonstrated using T1-weighted spin-echo magnetization transfer (MT) imaging with gadolinium–diethylenetriamine pentaacetic acid.

Case Report.—Man, 50, had become forgetful and mildly ataxic 4 years after having tested positive for HIV and receiving treatment. Deficits in attention and processing were evident, but there were no neurologic abnormalities and the CSF was normal. Axial T2-weighted MR images revealed poorly defined regions of increased signal in the white matter of both temporal, parietal, and occipital lobes, the right frontal lobe, and the right cerebellum (Fig 1). Cortical atrophy was visible in the left occipital lobe; on T1-weighted images, high signal was visible in the cortex and subcortical white matter (Fig 2). There was enhancement bilaterally in the parietal and occipital lobes, as well as in the right frontal lobe. Biopsy specimens of the right frontal lobe showed typical changes of PML, including abnormal oligodendroglia, reactive astrocytes, and lipid-laden macrophages, and also evidence of previous hemorrhage. There were no signs of HIV encephalitis. The patient continued to deteriorate cognitively and became disoriented, apraxic, agitated, and incontinent.

FIGURE 1.—**A,** first echo (TR = 2,200 msec; TE = 30 msec) of the T2-weighted scan shows the left occipital lobe lesion. Abnormal high-signal intensity is seen in the left occipital subcortical white matter. In addition, a thin rim of low-signal intensity is seen between the cortex and this white matter abnormality. **B,** second echo (TR = 2,200 msec; TE = 80 msec) of the T2-weighted scan shows the same occipital abnormality and lower signal intensity of the thin rim separating the cortex from the underlying white matter. This decrease in signal on the second echo suggests a magnetic susceptibility effect that can be seen in hemosiderin deposition in the brain. **C and D,** first (TR = 2,200 msec; TE = 30 msec) and second (TR 2,200 msec; TE = 80 msec) echo scans of the high parietal region show abnormal high-signal intensity in
(Continued)

FIGURE 1 (cont.)

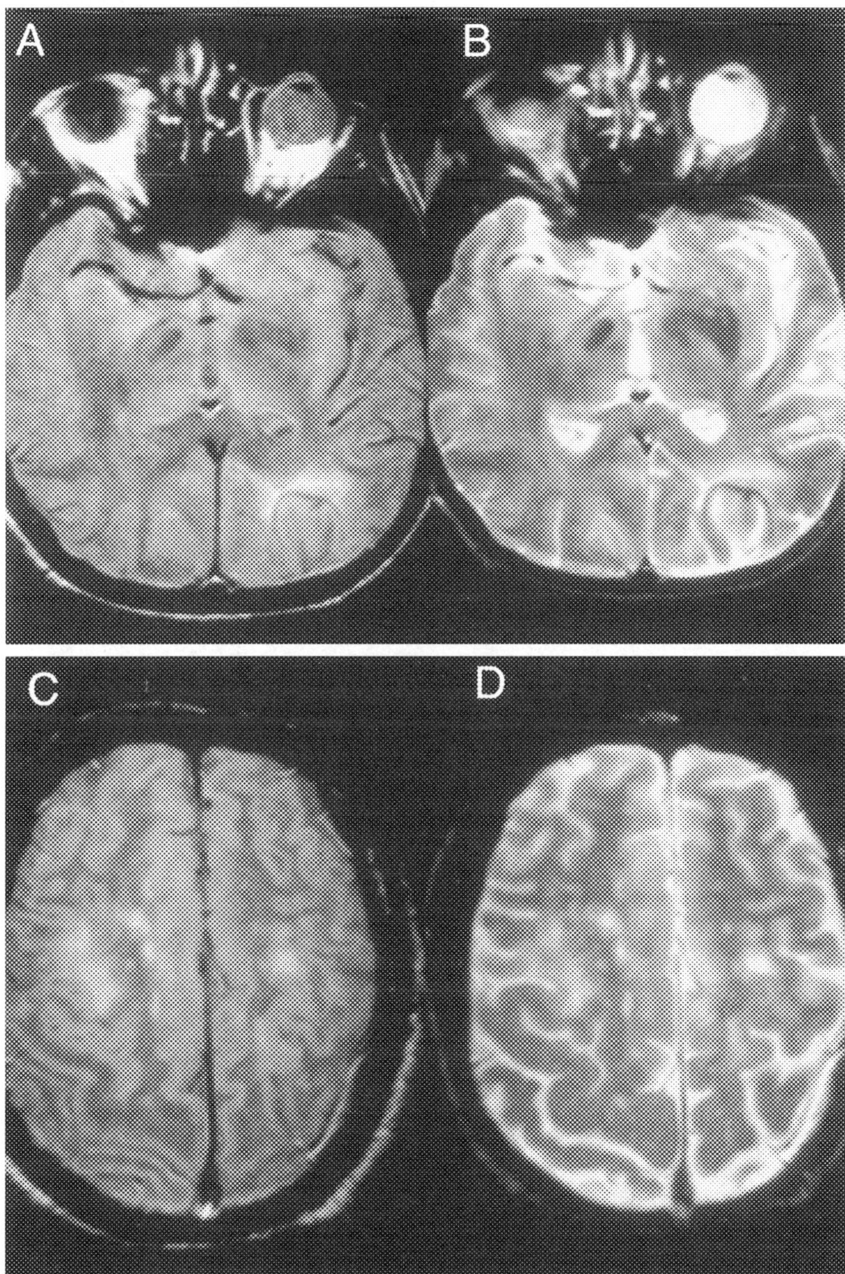

the subcortical region in both parietal lobes, somewhat greater on the right. The abnormal high-signal intensity areas are scattered, patchy, not yet confluent, but clearly restricted to the white matter. (Courtesy of Ng S, Tse VCK, Rubinstein J, et al: Progressive multifocal leukoencephalopathy: Unusual MR findings. *J Comput Assist Tomogr* 19:302–305, 1995.)

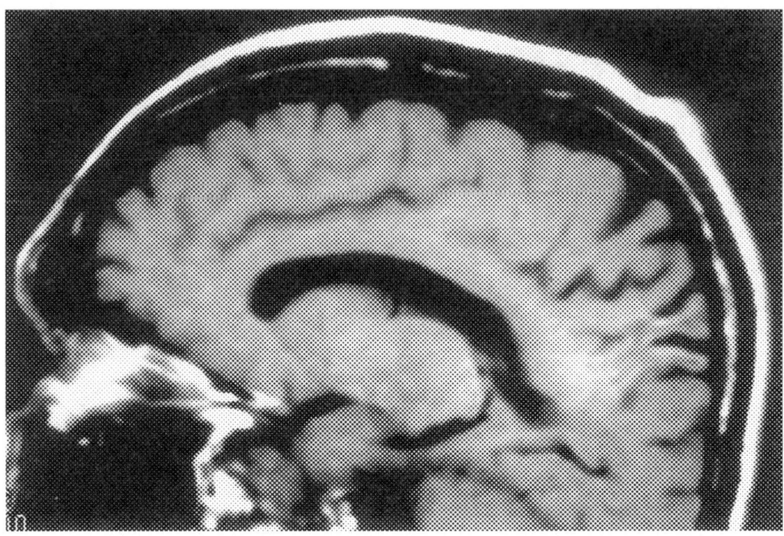

FIGURE 2.—Sagittal T1-weighted scan (TR = 800 msec; TE = 16 msec) shows increased signal intensity on a noncontrast scan in the left occipital white matter and also in the overlying cortical gray matter, which is atrophic (i.e., the cortex is thinned). *Abbreviations: TR*, recovery time; *TE*, echo time. (Courtesy of Ng S, Tse VCK, Rubinstein J, et al: Progressive multifocal leukoencephalopathy: Unusual MR findings. *J Comput Assist Tomogr* 19:302–305, 1995.)

Conclusion.—Patients with suspected PML should undergo MRI using the MT technique to determine the extent of disease and to identify lesions for biopsy.

▶ A common teaching is that PML rarely shows enhancement on postcontrast MRI. This article described and illustrated that with the MR technique MT (which suppresses the signal from macromolecules but not from enhancing lesions), localization of abnormalities suitable for biopsy can be identified. This is critical when one is deciding where the site of a biopsy should be. What we say enhances or does not enhance must be predicated on the MR parameters that are used. Similarly, if gradient echo imaging (T2) were used, small areas of hemorrhage that otherwise are not visible on routine T2-weighted spin-echo imaging might be seen more frequently.

R.M. Quencer, M.D.

Radiologic-Pathologic Correlation: Cerebral Toxoplasmosis and Lymphoma in AIDS

Chang L, Cornford ME, Chiang FL, et al (Univ of California, Los Angeles)
AJNR 16:1653–1663, 1995   9–10

Objective.—Distinguishing between cerebral toxoplasmosis and lymphoma in patients with AIDS can be difficult. Both lesions are commonly multifocal; they can also occur simultaneously. Preliminary studies suggest that MR spectroscopy may be helpful in making the differentiation. The radiologic findings of a patient with AIDS and cerebral toxoplasmosis were reported.

Case Report.—Man, 37, with HIV seropositivity but no previous AIDS-defining illness was admitted with progressive left-sided weakness and sensory loss, fever, and slow speech and comprehension with decreased attention. The patient had a large right parietooccipital periventricular lesion detected on CT. Further examination with MRI showed that the periphery of the mass was hypointense to gray matter, with a thick, irregular wall and extensive edema around the lesion. The central region was isointense, with some slightly hypointense regions and additional hypointense nodules along the frontal horns of the lateral ventricles. Gadolinium contrast revealed a nodular and irregular ring enhancement pattern in the periphery of the mass, as well as enhancement of the additional small nodules (Fig 1, B–C). Localized proton MR spectroscopy showed marked increased levels of lactate and lipid, along with decreased levels of *N*-acetyl compounds, total creatine, and *myo*-inositol, with relative preservation of the choline peak. These findings were consistent with both toxoplasmosis and lymphoma.

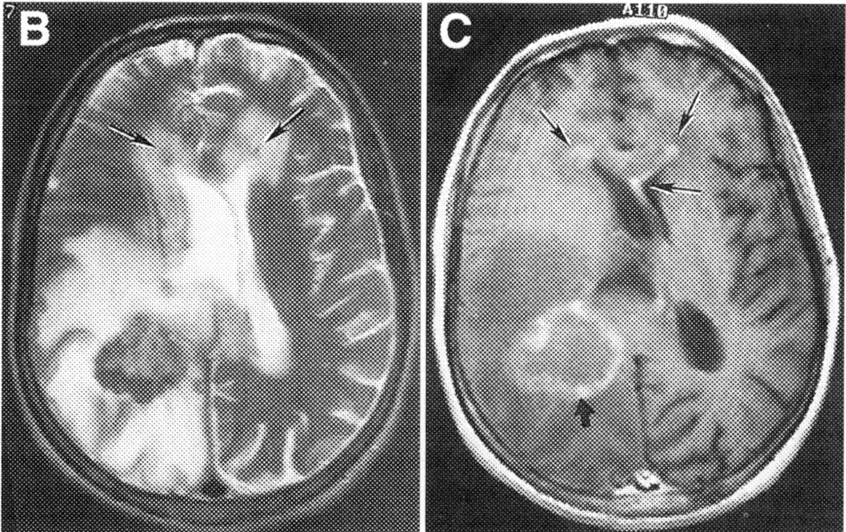

FIGURE 1.—**B**, axial T2-weighted MR image (TR = 3,000 msec; TE = 102 msec) shows hypointense small nodules along the borders of the frontal horns of the lateral ventricles (*arrows*) and confluent increased T2-weighted signal in a periventricular pattern. **C**, postgadolinium axial image (TR = 600 msec; TE = 10 msec) shows a nodular and irregular ring enhancement pattern (*short arrow*) in the periphery of the right parietooccipital periventricular mass. The additional small nodules along the borders of the frontal horns of the lateral ventricles and the septum pellucidum also are enhanced (*arrows with white shadows*). *Abbreviations:* TR, repetition time; *TE*, echo time. (L Chang, ME Cornford, FL Chiang, et al: Radiologic-pathologic correlation: Cerebral toxoplasmosis and lymphoma in AIDS. *AJNR* 16:1653–1663, 1995, Copyright by American Society of Neuroradiology.)

Although his mental status improved briefly with empiric anti-toxoplasmosis medication and dexamethasone, seizures and obtundation soon developed. He died in hospice 2 months after hospital discharge, having declined a brain biopsy. Postmortem specimens from the medial edge of the right parieto-occipital lesion showed peripheral multifocal areas of atypical lymphocytic infiltration around blood vessels. There were many mitotic figures and abundant macrophages around the angiocentric lymphocytes. Intermixed with these macrophages were basophilic cysts containing multiple ovoid organisms, which stained positive for Giemsa and immunohistochemically for *Toxoplasma* antigen. The staining pattern of the atypical angiocentric lymphocytes was consistent with B-cell lymphoma. Staining for Epstein-Barr virus latent membrane protein was apparent in many neoplastic lymphocytes. The perihippocampal region and the right frontal white matter showed focal microglial nodules, multinucleated giant cells with small hyperchromatic nuclei and eosinophilic cytoplasm characteristic of HIV giant cells, and white matter astrogliosis and edema characteristic of AIDS leukoencephaly.

Discussion.—Toxoplasmosis and lymphoma can be difficult to distinguish in patients with AIDS. Toxoplasmosis can lead to vessel adventitial proliferation and perivascular lymphocytic infiltration, thus mimicking angiocentric lymphoma. Immunohistochemical studies will reveal markers for B cells to identify lymphoma. The finding of central necrotic tissue is also consistent with high-grade B-cell lymphoma. On MR spectroscopy of toxoplasmosis lesions, lactate and lipid levels will be markedly elevated, but other normal brain metabolites will be absent. Lymphoproliferative lesions, on the other hand, are characterized by a mild to moderate increase in lactate and lipid levels, preservation of some normal metabolites, and a marked elevation in choline levels.

▶ The case described and illustrated here points out the frequent dilemma encountered in trying to decide which 1 of the 2 most common intracerebral mass-producing lesions (toxoplasmosis or lymphoma) is present in a patient with AIDS. There are clues on MRI that favor lymphoma such as a single lesion, hypointensity on T2-weighted images, intraventricular spread, and periventricular location; however, none of these findings is uniformly reliable. The study that can be useful in the differential diagnosis of lesions as shown in Figure 1 is thallium single-photon emission CT (SPECT) imaging; with this an inflammatory process such as toxoplasmosis will not show activity, but a neoplastic process such as lymphoma will. Of course, with superimposed pathologic changes this examination is not helpful, but such an occurrence is rare. Thallium SPECT is recommended in the early workup of these patients and would seem to be more efficacious than MR spectroscopy.

R.M. Quencer, M.D.

10 Infectious Diseases of the Nervous System

AIDS Dementia Complex and HIV-1 Brain Infection: Clinical-Virological Correlations
Brew BJ, Rosenblum M, Cronin K, et al (St Vincent's Hosp, Sydney, Australia; Mem Sloan-Kettering Cancer Ctr, New York; Univ of Minnesota, Minneapolis)
Ann Neurol 38:563–570, 1995   10–1

Background.—One of the most clinically important CNS disorders associated with HIV-1 infection is subcortical dementia, characterized by distinct cognitive, motor, and behavioral abnormalities. This disorder is known by several names, including AIDS dementia complex (ADC). Though its prevalence and laboratory correlates have been well defined, its pathogenesis continues to be unclear, especially in relation to brain HIV-1 infection.

Methods.—Immunohistochemical methods were used to map the HIV-1 p24 core protein in the brains of 55 patients with AIDS at autopsy. In 40 of these patients, who had had antemortem neurologic assessment of ADC, the relationship between the severities of the viral infection and clinical dysfunction was analyzed.

Findings.—Viral antigen was found in macrophages, cells with morphologic and immunohistochemical characteristics of microglia, and multinucleated cells. The antigen-positive cell distribution preferentially involved certain deep brain structures, particularly the globus pallidus, other basal ganglia nuclei, and the central white matter. Overall there was a strong correlation between the presence and frequency of infected cells and the histologic findings of multinucleated-cell encephalitis. Infected cells were also generally associated with clinical ADC stage. Commonly, however, infection was more limited than expected from the severity of patients' clinical condition. Detectable antigen was found in only 61% of patients with at least ADC stage 1. Of these, only about 30% of brain sections were antigen positive.

Conclusion.—Previous findings of a subcortical dominance to the distribution of the infection were confirmed in this study. Also, cells of monocyte/macrophage lineage were the primary, if not only, cell type productively infected. The most important new finding is that of a clinical-virologic dissociation in which the clinical deficit is more severe than the amount of demonstrable productive brain infection. Thus, moderate to severe ADC may occur with relatively little evidence of productive brain infection, and mild to moderate ADC may occur when there is no detectable brain infection.

▶ Among the observations in this study, 2 seem to stand out. First, patients with AIDS dementia complex, particularly in its earliest stages, may not have large amounts of virus demonstrated in their brain. Therefore, the investigators suggested that there is an amplification of the effects of the virus by the elaboration of toxic factors (e.g., cytokines). Second, the study confirmed the previously reported observation that the highest viral burden is in deep nuclear structure, especially the basal ganglia. This localization may be responsible for the many clinical parallels between AIDS dementia complex and parkinsonism. Among the latter are the psychomotor slowing, hypomimetic facies, poor balance, and extreme sensitivity to dopamine receptor blockade.

J.R. Berger, M.D.

Syphilis and Neurosyphilis in a Human Immunodeficiency Virus Type-1 Seropositive Population: Evidence for Frequent Serologic Relapse After Therapy

Malone JL, Wallace MR, Hendrick BB, et al (Naval Med Ctr, San Diego, Calif; Naval Hosp, Portsmouth, Va)
Am J Med 99:55–63, 1995   10–2

Introduction.—Disagreement exists about how syphilis should be managed in an HIV-infected patient. Some suggest that syphilis has a more rapid and aggressive course when HIV infection is also present and that standard antisyphilitic treatment regimens may be inadequate. Others have found no difference in the outcomes of syphilis treatment between patients with and without HIV infection. A review of 100 HIV-infected patients with syphilis was conducted.

Methods.—The patients represented 8% of a cohort of HIV-infected patients in a tertiary care military HIV program and 12% of patients with confirmed syphilis at the study medical facility. Syphilis did not require therapy in 35 patients, who had received adequate treatment for syphilis before HIV infection. Sixty-nine patients were treated for active syphilis. The patients' records were reviewed to determine the results of serologic tests for syphilis, CD4$^+$ T-lymphocyte counts, and clinical responses to therapy.

Results.—Follow-up was available in 56 of the treated patients. Of these, 18% had serologic or clinical relapse. Seven of the 10 patients with relapse had previously been treated with high-dose IV or procaine penicillin therapy. Six of the 10 did not experience relapse until more than 1 year after they were first treated, and 5 had more than 1 relapse. Relapse was not predicted by the patients' mean CD4$^+$ T-lymphocyte count. At an average of 2 years' monitoring, risk of relapse or treatment failure was greatest for patients with reactive CSF Venereal Disease Research Laboratory (VDRL) test titers or a secondary syphilis rash.

Conclusion.—High-dose IV penicillin and other standard treatments for syphilis will temporarily lower serum VDRL titers in nearly all HIV-infected patients with syphilis. However, these treatments may fail to prevent serologic and clinical relapse in some patients, particularly those with secondary syphilis and reactive CSF VDRL titers. Patients who have syphilis with HIV coinfection need careful long-term follow-up and may require repeated courses of therapy.

▶ Perhaps one can never fully eradicate *Treponema pallidum* from the body. Studies in the early 1950s of syphilis in a rabbit model demonstrated that viable organisms could be recovered in a small percentage of animals after 30 days of high-dose penicillin therapy. The explanation for the persistence of these organisms after therapy remains uncertain, but factors such as long doubling times, occasional intracellular location of the pathogen, and its presence in the CNS and other sites relatively inaccessible to therapy may contribute. Conceivably an effective immune response coupled with a marked decline in the number of infecting pathogens is responsible for the lack of appearance of subsequent neurologic disease in treated persons.

This study by Malone et al. confirmed earlier observations about the need for follow-up of the HIV-infected person who has neurosyphilis, and syphilis in general, carefully after what has been widely regarded as "curative" therapy. The absence of an effective immunologic response to *T. pallidum* may explain the high frequency of recurrence in this population.

J.R. Berger, M.D.

Central Nervous System Tuberculosis in HIV-Infected Patients: Clinical and Radiographic Findings
Whiteman M, Espinoza L, Post MJD, et al (Univ of Miami, Fla; Palm Beach County Med Examiners' Office, Fla)
AJNR 16:1319–1327, 1995   10–3

Background.—Tuberculosis is a significant infection in patients with HIV. Central nervous system tuberculosis is clearly an important cause of cerebral infection. Prompt diagnosis may enable earlier treatment. The radiographic findings of neuroimaging performed on HIV-infected patients with proved CNS tuberculosis were reported.

Methods.—Twenty-five patients were included. The diagnosis of CNS tuberculosis was based on CSF culture in 20 patients, biopsy in 4, autopsy in 5, or combination thereof. One patient had a clinical diagnosis of CNS tuberculosis. Findings were correlated with CD4 counts and chest radiographs.

Findings.—Thirty-six percent of the patients had meningeal enhancement. Forty-four percent had enhancing parenchymal lesions. Tuberculomata were present in 6 patients and tuberculous abscesses in 5. Thirty-two percent of the patients had communicating hydrocephalus, and 36% had infarction. Fifteen of 23 chest radiographs suggested pulmonary tuberculosis. The average CD4 count was 162. Thirty-eight percent of 24 patients had a history of pulmonary tuberculosis. In 21%, no history of tuberculosis or any other opportunistic infection was documented. Seventy-nine percent of the patients died.

Conclusion.—Among patients with HIV infection, CNS tuberculosis is associated with a very high mortality. Neuroradiologists can play a critical role in treatment by suggesting the correct diagnosis based on imaging findings before the results of CSF cultures are available. Suggestive radiographic features are multiloculated abscess, cisternal enhancement, basal ganglia infarction, and communicating hydrocephalus. These are not features associated with the more commonly seen CNS lymphoma and *Toxoplasma* encephalitis.

▶ Tuberculosis of the CNS has been increasing in frequency since 1986, largely as a consequence of the increased prevalence of HIV infection. Its manifestations in the latter population appear to be different from those in nonimmunocompromised hosts. For instance, these University of Miami investigators found that 11 (44%) of 25 patients with CNS tuberculosis had enhancing parenchymal lesions, a number far higher than expected in a nonimmunosuppressed population. The features of meningeal enhancement, communicating hydrocephalus, and infarction are common to both groups. The routine application of polymerase chain reaction for *Mycobacterium tuberculosis* on CSF will greatly enhance the rapidity and accuracy of diagnosis.

J.R. Berger, M.D.

Lyme Encephalopathy: Long-Term Neuropsychological Deficits Years After Acute Neuroborreliosis
Benke T, Gasse T, Hittmair-Delazer M, et al (Univ of Innsbruck, Austria)
Acta Neurol Scand 91:353–357, 1995   10–4

Background.—Lyme disease is a tick-borne spirochete infection caused by *Borrelia burgdorferi*. Acute neuroborreliosis manifests with the triad of meningitis, cranial neuritis, and painful radiculoneuritis and may be accompanied by behavioral changes. The neuropsychological deficit in chronic Lyme encephalopathy is rarely reported.

Methods.—Long-term cognitive deficits were studied in 20 patients an average of 51.6 months after the acute phase of Lyme borreliosis. Cognitive abilities, psychomotor speed, memory, attention, mental flexibility, constructional praxis, articulatory functions, and reasoning in chronic Lyme patients were compared with those of 20 control individuals matched for age and education.

Findings.—Despite minor residual neurologic symptoms, patients with chronic Lyme disease exhibited significant neuropsychological deficit. Memory was most impaired, particularly in learning and spontaneous retrieval of word list, whereas recognition memory was relatively preserved. Memory deficit was particularly dense in half of the patients, including 6 with sole verbal memory deficit and 4 with a moderate to severe global cognitive impairment. Chronic Lyme patients also performed poorly on tests of mental flexibility, letter fluency, and articulatory agility but performed adequately on intellectual and problem-solving skills, visuospatial functions, psychomotor speed, and sustained attention. The long-term cognitive outcome was not related to several clinical variables from the acute disease stage or to the time elapsed since infection.

Conclusion.—Lyme encephalopathy may be associated with a long-lasting neuropsychological deficit predominantly from loss of learning and memory. The localization of the deficits, although restricted, suggest a relatively focal, preferentially temporal and frontal pathologic condition.

▶ Benke et al. reported cognitive abnormalities in 20 patients previously treated for neuroborreliosis when compared with age- and education-matched controls. The pattern observed is suggestive of residual frontal and temporal lobe damage. The findings, if valid, are not insignificant. Lyme disease has a worldwide distribution with endemic pockets in the United States in New York, New Jersey, Massachusetts, Connecticut, Rhode Island, Wisconsin, and Minnesota. However, the results should be interpreted cautiously because the group studied was small, highly selected (chosen from among 68 patients with diagnosed neuroborreliosis), inhomogeneous (the group included 1 patient with cerebral vasculitis, 2 patients with very long duration from symptom onset to recovery), and not fully matched to controls (e.g., there is no mention of matching by sex). Additional studies addressing this very important issue are clearly warranted. If their results are confirmed, the mechanism by which CNS infection by *B. burgdorferi* results in this pattern of neuropsychological abnormality will need to be addressed. Does the pathogen result in vascular injury to the brain (akin to meningovascular neurosyphilis)? Does it injure neurons through the local elaboration of cytokines as has been suggested in AIDS?

J.R. Berger, M.D.

The Vasculopathy of Varicella-Zoster Virus Encephalitis

Amlie-Lefond C, Kleinschmidt-DeMasters BK, Mahalingam R, et al (Univ of Colorado Health Sciences Ctr, Denver; Univ of New Mexico, Albuquerque)
Ann Neurol 37:784–790, 1995
10–5

Background.—The prevalence of varicella-zoster virus (VZV) encephalitis has increased along with AIDS and other immunosuppressive diseases. The diagnosis and treatment of VZV encephalitis are a challenge. The patterns and pathogenesis of this disorder were illustrated in 6 patients.

Patients and Findings.—Patients consisted of 5 men and 1 woman aged 29 to 69. Four patients had AIDS. Two were being treated with cyclophosphamide and corticosteroids or only corticosteroids. Varicella-zoster virus was confirmed by pathologic or virologic examination. In 5 patients, zoster occurred days to months before encephalitis, and was recurrent in 2. In 1 case, VZV encephalitis developed in the absence of a history of rash. The manifestations of encephalitis included fever, seizures, focal deficit, and mental status changes. Brain imaging showed multifocal lesions in the distribution of large and small arteries, most of which were consistent with infarction. Some of these lesions enhanced. Lesions were ischemic and hemorrhagic. Pathologic examination showed that the lesions in all patients were a combination of ischemia and demyelination. Large-vessel arteritis was associated with infarction in the distribution of large arteries. Deap-seated infarction, often with demyelination, was caused by small-artery vasculopathy. This vasculopathy was characterized by endothelial swelling and scant chronic inflammation. The smaller demyelinative lesions observed were usually characterized by Cowdry A inclusions in glia at the periphery of lesions.

Conclusion.—In immunocompromised patients, VZV encephalitis typically develops concurrent with rash or weeks to months after acute herpes zoster. It is usually accompanied by mental status changes and multifocal neurologic deficits. Radiographically the spectrum of lesions ranges from ischemic and hemorrhagic infarctions of various sizes, depending on the caliber of blood vessels involved, to small ovoid lesions with mixed ischemic and demyelinative or primarily demyelinative abnormalities. The diagnosis of VZV encephalitis should be suspected when both infarctive and demyelinative lesions are detected radiologically in immunocompromised patients with or without a history of zoster rash.

▶ Varicella-zoster virus encephalitis is a disease that occurs chiefly with immunosuppression. The greater prevalence of HIV infection has resulted in a considerably increased experience with this disorder. Amlie-Lefond et al. demonstrated in these 6 cases that both ischemic and demyelinating lesions occur and frequently coexist. The former may result from involvement of small, medium, or large cerebral vessels. The encephalitis may occur weeks or months after the rash of VZV has resolved, complicating diagnostic efforts.

J.R. Berger, M.D.

The Transient Syndrome of Headache With Neurologic Deficits and CSF Lymphocytosis

Berg MJ, Williams LS (Univ of Rochester, New York)
Neurology 45:1648–1654, 1995

10–6

Purpose.—Since 1981, there have been reports of 33 patients without previous migraine who had 3 to 12 episodes of headache along with neurologic deficits and CSF lymphocytosis. This self-limited condition is probably more common than recognized, but no diagnostic criteria have been published. Diagnostic criteria of this syndrome, called headache with neurologic deficits and CSF lymphocytosis (HaNDL), were specified.

Findings.—A review combining 7 new and the 33 previously reported patients found that 56% were female and 44% male (mean age 27). Patients had 1 to 20 episodes of a severe migrainous headache of a type not previously experienced. They also had temporary focal neurologic deficits lasting hours to 3 days. The deficits were referable to different parts of the brain and evolved progressively. Cerebrospinal fluid lymphocytosis was a distinguishing feature, accompanied by elevated CSF opening pressure and total protein levels. Other findings encountered in some patients included a preceding viral syndrome, increased intracranial pressure, elevated CSF protein level, and focal electroencephalographic abnormalities. In all 40 patients, the episodes of HaNDL ceased within 3 months.

Conclusion.—Findings suggestive of the diagnosis of HaNDL include severe headache associated with temporary neurologic deficit and CSF

TABLE 3.—Characteristics of Headache With Neurologic Deficits and
Cerebrospinal Fluid Lymphocytosis

Diagnostic criteria	
Severe headache(s)	100%
Temporary neurologic deficit(s)	100%
(each deficit resolves within 3 days)	
CSF lymphocytosis	100%
(range, 16–350 WBCs/mm³; mean, 136;	
at least 86% mononuclear cells,	
predominantly lymphocytes)	
Self-limited	100%
(range, 1–84 days; mean, 21 days)	
Single episode	27%
Greater than one episode	73%
Neurologic deficit same in each	41%
Neurologic deficit different	59%
Associated features	
Increased CSF protein (>45 mg/dL)	91%
(range, 35–247 mg/dL; mean, 100 mg/dL)	
Increased opening pressure (>18 cm CSF)	73%
(range, 10–40 cm CSF; mean, 22.7 cm CSF)	
Transient focal, nonepileptiform EEG changes	72%
Viral prodrome or fever	50%

Abbreviations: WBCs, white blood cells; *EEG*, electroencephalographic.
(Reprinted from *Neurology* volume; 45:1648–1654, 1995: by permission of Little, Brown and Company [Inc.].)

lymphocyte pleocytosis (Table 3). Repeated episodes are common but resolve within 2 months, and the condition does not progress to chronic migraine or other neurologic disease. Thus, if HaNDL is recognized, invasive diagnostic procedures and long-term drug therapy can be avoided. The cause of this benign syndrome is unknown; it may be related to a single virus or may represent an idiosyncratic response to a variety of viral agents.

▶ This interesting article by Berg and Williams contributed a number of cases of the benign syndrome of headaches with CSF lymphocytosis to the world's literature. Rather than being a single disorder, it is quite likely that this entity represents a spectrum of disorders. There is a real possibility that most, if not all, are simply the consequence of a self-limited viral meningitis that was unrecognized. Candidate viruses would include Herpes simplex virus type 1 or 2, enteroviruses, and adenoviruses. A drug-induced meningitis, as seen with nonsteroidal anti-inflammatory agents, may also explain some cases. A description of seasonal variations and the application of polymerase chain reaction technology would be of great interest.

J.R. Berger, M.D.

11 Metabolic and Genetic Disorders

Mutations in the Gene for X-Linked Adrenoleukodystrophy in Patients With Different Clinical Phenotypes
Braun A, Ambach H, Kammerer S, et al (Univ of Munich; Technical Univ of Munich; Univ of Graz, Germany; et al)
Am J Hum Genet 56:854–861, 1995

Background.—X-linked adrenoleukodystrophy (X-ALD) is the most common of the inherited peroxisomal disorders. As many as 1 in 15,000 white males are affected by the disease, which produces severe, progressive demyelination of the white matter, as well as adrenocortical insufficiency. Peroxisomal β-oxidation of unbranched saturated very long–chain fatty acids is impaired in most tissues. A disease-related gene encoding a peroxisomal membrane transporter protein recently was described.

Objective and Methods.—With the techniques of reverse-transcription polymerase chain reaction analysis and DNA sequencing, the entire protein-coding sequence of the ALD protein was analyzed in 5 patients having varying phenotypical forms of X-ALD and in their female relatives.

Findings.—All 5 patients had mutations in the X-ALD gene. Three patients had the cerebral childhood form of ALD (CALD). They became ill when aged 6 or 7 years, and had severe, rapidly progressive CNS signs in addition to ocular and adrenal abnormalities. The 5' part of the gene contained a 38–base pair (bp) deletion, producing a frameshift mutation; a 3-bp deletion, resulting in deletion of an amino acid in the ATP-binding domain of the ALD protein; and a missense mutation. The patient with adrenomyeloneuropathy had 2 point mutations, a nonsense mutation in codon 212 and a mutation at codon 178. The remaining patient, who had the Addison disease–only phenotype, had a single point mutation, a missense mutation leading to an arginine-to-histidine substitution at a highly conserved site.

Implications.—A critical role for mutations in this gene in the development of X-ALD was supported. That current biochemical methods of detecting carriers are unreliable makes systematic screening for mutations a logical approach to prenatal diagnosis and genetic counseling.

▶ The ALD gene was recently cloned[1]; it encodes for a peroxisomal adenosine triphosphate–binding cassette (ABC) transporter.[2] Prenatal genetic diagnosis is now possible.[3] All families thus far tested have mutations in this gene.[4] Now the genotype-phenotypic correlations are possible, as described in this paper and elsewhere. The various mutations do not predict the possible phenotypes: ALD, adrenomyeloneuropathy, Addison disease only, or asymptomatic. This will rekindle the discussions about modifier genes that further influence the expression of ALD gene mutations.[5] The final conclusion of this paper is important and should change our practice pattern: Carriers are missed in very long–chain fatty acid assays, and genetic diagnosis should soon replace this test. It's a new world for ALD!

D.A. Stumpf, M.D., Ph.D.

References

1. Mosser J, Douar AM, Sarde CO, et al: Putative X-linked adrenoleukodystrophy gene shares unexpected homology with ABC transporters. *Nature* 361:726–730, 1993.
2. Mosser J, Lutz Y, Stoeckel ME, et al: The gene responsible for adrenoleukodystrophy encodes a peroxisomal membrane protein. *Hum Mol Genet* 3:265–271, 1994.
3. Matsumoto T, Kondoh T, Masuzaki H, et al: A point mutation at ATP-binding region of the ALD gene in a family with X-linked adrenoleukodystrophy. *Jpn J Hum Genet* 39:345–351, 1994.
4. Ligtenberg MJ, Kemp S, Sarde CO, et al: Spectrum of mutations in the gene encoding the adrenoleukodystrophy protein. *Am J Hum Genet* 56:44–50, 1995.
5. Maestri NE, Beaty TH: Predictions of a 2-locus model for disease heterogeneity: Application to adrenoleukodystrophy. *Am J Med Genet* 44:576-582, 1992.

Clinical Symptoms of Adult Metachromatic Leukodystrophy and Arylsulfatase A Pseudodeficiency

Hageman ATM, Gabreëls FJM, de Jong JGN, et al (Univ Hosp Nijmegen, The Netherlands)
Arch Neurol 52:408–413, 1995

11–2

Introduction.—Metachromatic leukodystrophy (MLD), an autosomal recessive lysosomal disorder, is manifested as demyelination of the white matter in the CNS and the peripheral nerves, and it is caused by a deficiency of arylsulfatase A (ASA). The deficiency of this enzyme results in neural accumulation of sulfatides. Twenty-five adult patients with ASA deficiency were studied.

Methods.—Twenty-five patients, older than 16, with very low ASA activity in the leukocytes were evaluated. The presence or absence of stored sulfatides in the sural nerve or brain, elevated sulfatide levels in urinary sediment, or both was established. Morphologic changes were assessed using electromyography (EMG), CT, MRI, or peripheral nerve biopsy. Analysis of DNA was performed in all patients.

Results.—Thirteen patients in whom elevated sulfatide accumulation was found, were given a diagnosis of MLD. Twelve others had a pseudodeficiency (PD) mutation, in which ASA deficiency was not associated with organic accumulation of sulfatides. Four patients with adult MLD initially had abnormalities, 4 had ataxia, 2 had polyneuropathy, 2 had dementia, and 1 had paraparesis. These patients had a second symptom develop an average of 3.7 years after onset of MLD, and a third symptom developed 2 years later. Electromyography revealed reduced nerve conduction velocities. Neuropathic examination of nerve biopsy material revealed a clear reduction in myelin sheath thickness and accumulation of metachromatic material. Areas of hypodensity in the white matter were seen on CT. Magnetic resonance imaging showed diffuse periventricular white matter demyelination. Analysis of DNA confirmed homozygosity for the PD allele in the other 12 patients. Diagnoses in this group of patients included multiple sclerosis in 1, Parkinson's disease in 1, Huntington's disease in 1, and ischemic optic neuropathy in 1. They had normal findings on EMG, CT, MRI, CSF analysis, and urinalysis. Sural nerve biopsy specimens showed normal tissue in 1 patient and accumulated metachromatic material in the other patients tested.

Discussion.—In contrast with late-infantile MLD in which initial symptoms are predominantly motor, both mental/behavioral symptoms and ataxia predominate in the early stage of adult MLD, which then progresses slowly and with great variability. Electromyography, CT, MRI, and urinalysis all can contribute to the diagnosis of MLD. A diagnosis of PD can be excluded only with DNA analysis. Determinations of ASA activity alone could not differentiate between MLD and PD. Patients with PD did not demonstrate a characteristic clinical syndrome.

▶ This article drove home the message that we cannot stop at ASA assay in diagnosing MLD. Half the patients in this series carried the MLD diagnosis based on ASA assays but had a common European allele not associated with pathologic accumulations of sulfatide. This PD group lacks a consistent clinical phenotype, indicating that the deficiency is an irrelevant finding (a "red herring"). The diagnostic enzyme assay does not accurately reflect the situation with the natural substrate in tissue. Thus, ASA "deficiency" should be followed with specific DNA diagnosis. As DNA diagnosis becomes more readily available, we will likely bypass ASA assays altogether and avoid this dilemma!

D.A. Stumpf, M.D., Ph.D.

Cognitive Function and Academic Performance in Children With Neurofibromatosis Type 1

North K, Joy P, Yuille D, et al (Children's Hosp, Sydney, Australia)
Dev Med Child Neurol 37:427–436, 1995

11–3

Objectives.—The frequency of intellectual impairment and learning disability due to neurofibromatosis 1 (NF1) alone was determined; the profile of learning disability specific to NF1 was characterized; the effects of clinical severity, age, sex, socioeconomic status, macrocephaly, family history of NF1, and family history of learning disability were determined; and the implications of these variables for the assessment and management of learning disability in 51 children aged 8 to 16 years with NF1 were examined.

Methods.—The evaluation included assessment of intellectual ability using the revised Wechsler Intelligence Scale for Children; language using the revised Clinical Evaluation of Language Fundamentals; motor development using the Beery developmental test of visual-motor integration; academic achievement on reading, spelling, and mathematics; and behavior using the Child Behavioral Checklist.

Findings.—Forty children completed the full assessment protocol. The prevalence of intellectual disability due to NF1 alone was 4.8%. The distribution of full scale intelligence quotient (IQ) scores was bimodal, suggesting 2 populations of patients with NF1: 1 with and another without a degree of cognitive impairment (Fig 1). Overall there was a left shift

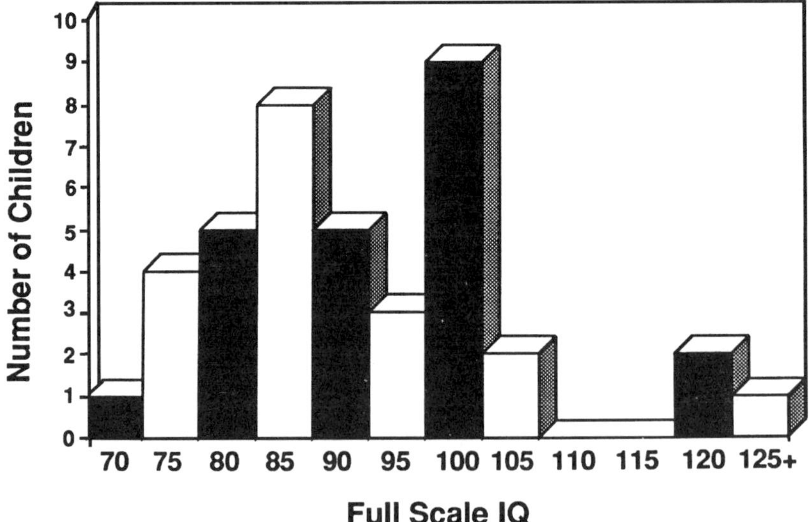

FIGURE 1.—Distribution of full-scale IQ scores for study population (N = 40). Note bimodal distribution with peaks at 85 and 100. *Abbreviation: IQ,* intelligence quotient. (Courtesy of North K, Joy P, Yuille D, et al: Cognitive function and academic performance in children with neurofibromatosis type 1. *Dev Med Child Neurol* 37:427–436, 1995.)

TABLE 3.—Mean Scores in Tests of Intellectual, Language, and Motor Function

	Mean	*(SD)*	*Range*
Verbal IQ	92.6	(13.4)	67–124
Performance IQ	95.4	(12.9)	67–133
Full-scale IQ	93.3	(12.6)	74–131
Expressive language score	90.8	(18.3)	54–130
Receptive language score	91.4	(13.6)	63–120
Total language score	90.3	(16.2)	55–121
PPVT-R (measure of receptive vocabulary)	92.7	(16.0)	56–139
Visual motor integration	92.4	(10.4)	71–119

Abbreviations: SD, standard deviation; *IQ*, intelligence quotient; *PPVT-R*, Peabody Picture Vocabulary test, Revised. (Courtesy of North K, Joy P, Yuille D, et al: Cognitive function and academic performance in children with neurofibromatosis type 1. *Dev Med Child Neurol* 37:427–436, 1995.)

in performance in tests of development and learning (Table 3). However, a distinct profile of learning disability could not be identified. Contrary to previous reports, there was no support for a profile of predominantly visuospatial deficits. One-fourth of the children had articulation errors, but there was no discrepancy between verbal and performance IQ, and the deficits in function varied widely. Twenty-six children had impaired performance on at least 1 test of academic achievement. The occurrence of cognitive deficits was not associated with clinical severity of disease or other clinical variables. Reports of parents indicated that the children had attentional problems and difficulties with social interaction.

Implications.—Children with NF1 are at high risk for learning disability, but no specific profile of learning disability has been identified in these children. Individual test scores on formal tests of intellectual, language, and motor function rarely fall below 2 standard deviations from the mean, suggesting that the use of this cutoff point to define impaired performance would underestimate the incidence of learning disabilities in this population. A developmental evaluation of children with NF1 should include performance across a range of subtests, a qualitative assessment of the child's approach to problem solving, and more detailed neuropsychological assessment.

▶ von Recklinghausen's syndrome (NF1), caused by mutations in the neurofibromin gene, has an incidence of 1 in 3,000. Neurofibromin is a GTPase-activating protein (GAP), likely involved in *ras* signal transduction. Studies of tumors from NF1 patients suggest a tumor suppressor role.[1] But neurofibromin also modulates trophic factors important in neuroembryology.[2] Cognitive changes, often seen in NF1, likely result from abnormal embryogenesis of the brain. This paper confirmed the overall shift in IQ, the frequent occurrence of specific learning problems, but also the lack of a stereotyped pattern.

D.A. Stumpf, M.D., Ph.D.

References

1. Yan N, Ricca C, Fletcher J, et al: Farnesyltransferase inhibitors block the neurofibromatosis type I (NF1) malignant phenotype. *Cancer Res* 55:3569–3575, 1995.
2. Vogel KS, Brannan CI, Jenkins NA, et al: Loss of neurofibromin results in neurotrophin-independent survival of embryonic sensory and sympathetic neurons. *Cell* 82:733–742, 1995.

Presymptomatic DNA and MRI Diagnosis of Neurofibromatosis 2 With Mild Clinical Course in an Extended Pedigree

Sainio M, Strachan T, Blomstedt G, et al (Univ of Helsinki; Natl Public Health Inst, Helsinki; Univ of Newcastle-upon-Tyne, England)
Neurology 45:1314–1322, 1995   11–4

Introduction.—Neurofibromatosis 2 (NF2) is a dominantly inherited condition that characteristically manifests with bilateral schwannomas of the vestibular branch of the eighth cranial nerve. Patients may also have other tumors of neural tissue including peripheral schwannomas, meningiomas, gliomas, and ependymomas. Gardner described a mild type of NF2 with a relatively late onset, slow-growing vestibular tumors, and few other neoplasms.

Objective.—A large Finnish pedigree having benign NF2 of the Gardner type was examined in a study of intrafamilial clinical homogeneity. Blood samples were obtained for DNA analysis from 49 of 63 living family members. Twenty-two individuals were thoroughly evaluated clinically, and 21 had gadolinium-enhanced MRI of the head and spine.

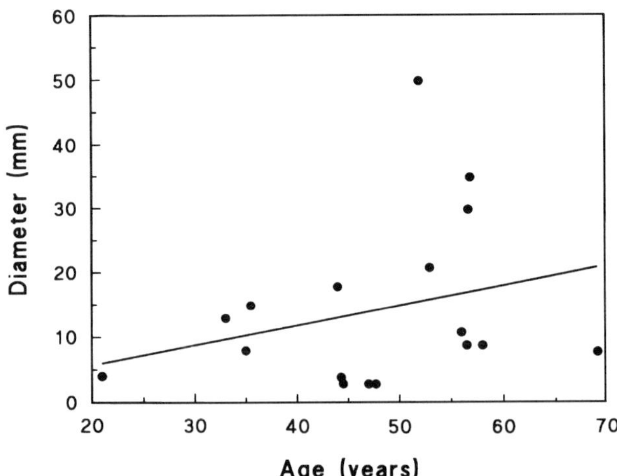

FIGURE 3.—Age of patient and diameter of vestibular schwannoma ($r = 0.280$; $P =$ not significant). (Reprinted from *Neurology* volume; 45:1314–1322, 1995; by permission of Little, Brown and Company [Inc.].)

Findings.—Linkage analyses employing 4 DNA markers flanking the *NF2* locus identified carriers of the *NF2* mutation with a high degree of certainty. Eight members of the pedigree had symptomatic NF2. Two others who were asymptomatic were identified by MRI, and 1 obligate carrier was identified from his position in the pedigree. Generations 2 to 4 included 17 persons with NF2, 16 of whom were identified as carrying the *NF2* haplotype in linkage analysis. Only 10 had clinically apparent disease. The disorder was for the most part limited to vestibular schwannomas. All 8 histologically confirmed tumors were schwannomas. Patient age did not correlate significantly with tumor size (Fig 3). Hearing deteriorated at ages 40 to 50. No patient died of the disease. Eight tumors in 6 patients were operated on, but hearing preservation was feasible in only a single instance.

Conclusion.—It now is possible to identify presymptomatic vestibular schwannomas by MRI in those carrying the *NF2* mutation, but no effective means has been found to prevent deafness.

▶ As a "nonexpert" in the field, NIH provided me an opportunity to chair their 1988 Consensus Conference on NF. Since then, an explosion of information has changed the field. Tumor suppressor genes are now implicated not only in NF1 (encoding neurofibromin) and NF2 (merlin) but also in retinoblastoma, Li-Fraumeni syndrome, familial breast and ovarian cancer, multiple endocrine neoplasia type I, tuberous sclerosis, and von Hippel-Lindau disease.[1] Furthermore, mutations exist and appear relevant in *spontaneous* tumors such as neurofibromas and pheochromocytomas (*NF1* gene) and meningiomas and schwannomas (*NF2* gene). Tumor studies in NF patients support the "2-hit" hypothesis in which 1 allele is constitutionally inactivated while the other allele is subsequently inactivated (second hit) at the somatic level.[2] Also, NF1 and NF2 are among the expanding group of neurologic disorders with "imprinting" in which gene methylation influences the parent most likely to transmit the disorder.[3] New phenotypes have now been identified, and we appreciate a role of the genes in embryogenesis. Although the multitude of mutations still makes molecular diagnosis difficult, we are looking at a new landscape since the Consensus Conference.

D.A. Stumpf, M.D., Ph.D.

References

1. Muller H, Scott RJ: Tumorsuppressorgen-Mutationen in der Keimbahn: ihre Bedeutung bei familiaren und sporadischen Tumorkrankheiten. *Schweiz Med Wochenschr* 125:1445–1454, 1995.
2. Colman SD, Williams CA, Wallace MR: Benign neurofibromas in type I neurofibromatosis (NF1) show somatic deletions of the NF1 gene. *Nat Genet* 11:90–92, 1995.
3. Chatkupt S, Antonowicz M, Johnson WG: Parents do matter: Genomic imprinting and parental sex effects in neurological disorders. *J Neurol Sci* 130:1–10, 1995.

A Clinical and Molecular Genetic Study of Dentatorubropallidoluysian Atrophy in Four European Families

Warner TT, Williams LDS, Walker RWH, et al (Inst of Neurology, London; St Bartholomew's Hosp, London; Guy's Hosp, London; et al)
Ann Neurol 37:452–459, 1995

11–5

Background.—Dentatorubropallidoluysian atrophy (DRPLA) is a rare neurodegenerative disorder with autosomal dominant inheritance, characterized by movement disorder, epilepsy, cerebellar ataxia, and cognitive impairment. It appears to be most common in Japan, where it is associated with an expanded CAG repeat on chromosome 12p. Four European families with hereditary DRPLA were described.

Study Design.—Four families, 3 British and 1 Maltese, and 55 patients with sporadic cases with symptoms compatible with DRPLA underwent DNA analysis and were compared with 50 healthy unrelated controls.

Findings.—None of the sporadic cases had mutations in the 12p region. All affected members of the 4 families had expanded *DRPLA* alleles. Affected individuals had 58 to 74 repeats, whereas control chromosomes had 2 to 26 repeats. There was some evidence of anticipation. Age of onset was inversely correlated with size of repeat. Clinical features were diverse even within 1 affected family.

Conclusion.—Dentatorubropallidoluysian atrophy is probably more common in the non-Japanese population than has previously been thought. It appears to have the same molecular genetic basis in European families as in Japanese families. It should be considered as a diagnosis in patients with a dominantly inherited neurodegenerative disorder, combining movement disorder, ataxia, epilepsy, psychosis, and dementia. This diagnosis can be confirmed by genomic DNA analysis.

▶ Repeat mutations of CAG-trinucleotide are associated with anticipation. The expansion of the repeat may occur in either coding (*SCA1*) or noncoding (myotonic dystrophy) regions of the gene. Greater expansion in 1 parent[1] explains the clinical observation of earlier onset when the father has Huntington's disease or the mother has myotonic dystrophy. Phenotypic variation also correlates with degree of repeat expansion.[2] We have yet to uncover the common mechanistic theme leading from these novel mutations to neurodegeneration. Given the diverse nature of the clinical syndromes, we can expect impairment of a fundamental process. Translation may be impaired.[3] Recently trinucleotide repeat-binding proteins (*TRIP1* and *TRIP2*), which may alter the function of these genes, were identified in the brain.[4] Abnormally expanded CAG-encoded polyglutamine stretches in the protein are also seen in diseased-patient brain, and these may participate in the disease process.[5] Hopefully further insights will lead to effective therapeutic strategies.

D.A. Stumpf, M.D., Ph.D.

References

1. Ranen NG, Stine OC, Abbott MH, et al: Anticipation and instability of IT-15 (CAG)n repeats in parent-offspring pairs with Huntington disease. *Am J Hum Genet* 57:593–602, 1995.
2. Ikeuchi T, Onodera O, Oyake M, et al: Dentatorubral-pallidoluysian atrophy (DRPLA): Close correlation of CAG repeat expansions with the wide spectrum of clinical presentations and prominent anticipation. *Semin Cell Biol* 6:37–44, 1995.
3. Feng Y, Zhang F, Lokey LK, et al: Translational suppression by trinucleotide repeat expansion at FMR1. *Science* 268:731–734, 1995.
4. Yano-Yanagisawa H, Li Y, Wang H, et al: Single-stranded DNA binding proteins isolated from mouse brain recognize specific trinucleotide repeat sequences in vitro. *Nucleic Acids Res* 23:2654–2660, 1995.
5. Yazawa I, Nukina N, Hashida H, et al: Abnormal gene product identified in hereditary dentatorubral-pallidoluysian atrophy (DRPLA) brain. *Nat Genet* 10:99–103, 1995.

Copper Deficiency Secondary to a Copper Transport Defect: A New Copper Metabolic Disturbance

Buchman AL, Keen CL, Vinters HV, et al (Baylor College of Medicine, Houston; Univ of California, Los Angeles; Univ of California, Davis; et al)
Metabolism 43:1462–1469, 1994   11–6

Background.—A unique copper deficiency, likely caused by insufficient hepatic processing, was reported in a 21-year-old man.

Case Report.—Man, 21, initially had incoordination at age 13 years that progressed to ataxia. He also had headaches and an acute temporary hearing loss. Brain MRI revealed an area of increased signal in the deep white matter of each cerebral hemisphere (Fig 1). An electroencephalogram was abnormal, but a brain biopsy specimen showed no significant abnormality. Results of a sural nerve biopsy, performed after the patient could no longer walk or sit upright, showed loss of myelination and Schwann cell hyperplasia. He had retinal degeneration, and by age 19 was nearly blind.

He had had cyclic vomiting and occasional urinary incontinence since he weas 10 years old. A diagnosis of pseudo-obstruction was clinically made. A serum copper level, performed before total parenteral nutrition (TPN) was begun for malnutrition, was decreased. Additional copper was added to the TPN solution when the copper level did not increase with supportive therapy. Plasma ceruloplasmin oxidase activity was low (19.6 IU/L).

The patient had testicular failure, cardiomyopathy, and severe osteoporosis. Normal hepatic copper levels were found during 1 liver biopsy, but a second liver biopsy revealed excessive copper deposition. He became febrile, and Coombs-positive hemolytic anemia developed. He had a cardiac arrest, and he died 1 week later.

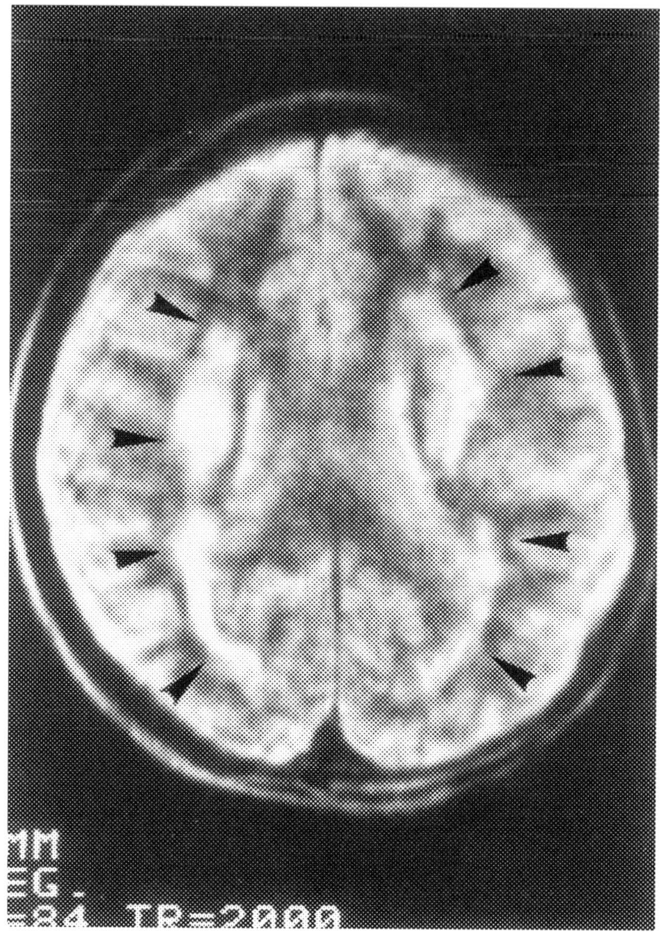

FIGURE 1.—T2-weighted brain MR image showing increased signal density in the deep white matter of each hemisphere (*arrows*). (Courtesy of Buchman AL, Keen CL, Vinters HV, et al: Copper deficiency secondary to a copper transport defect: A new copper metabolic disturbance. *Metabolism* 43:1462–1469, 1994.)

Discussion.—Because the patient had no Kayser-Fleischer rings at the first liver biopsy, had peripheral neuropathy, and his positron-emission tomography scan showed normal glucose metabolism in the basal ganglia, it was concluded that this patient did not have Wilson's disease. Several of his symptoms are attributed to his copper deficiency, however. He was considered copper deficient on the basis of defective ceruloplasmin transport and was unable to utilize intravenously infused copper.

▶ Molecular genetics brought clarity concerning copper disorders, and many disorders are now discernible. The Wilson disease gene affects the copper-transporting P-type adenosinetriphosphatase gene,[1] and many mutations are identified.[2] Menkes' tricopoliodystrophy involves a highly homologous X-chromosome copper-transporting P-type adenosinetriphosphatase gene,[3] and its clinical features also point to the dramatic import of copper in neuroembryology. An allelic mutation of the Menkes' gene produces occipital horn syndrome.[4] Primary ceruloplasmin deficiency causes hemosiderosis, dementia, ataxia, and extrapyramidal symptoms.[5] This leaves another group (including those described here) with copper deficiency. These patients are heterogeneous, suggesting that there are several additional mutations.

D.A. Stumpf, M.D., Ph.D.

References

1. Tanzi RE, Petrukhin K, Chernov I, et al: The Wilson disease gene is a copper transporting ATPase with homology to the Menkes disease gene. *Nat Genet* 5:344–350, 1993.
2. Thomas GR, Roberts EA, Walshe JM, et al: Haplotypes and mutations in Wilson disease. *Am J Hum Genet* 56:1315–1319, 1995.
3. Das S, Levinson B, Vulpe C, et al: Similar splicing mutations of the Menkes/mottled copper-transporting ATPase gene in occipital horn syndrome and the blotchy mouse. *Am J Hum Genet* 56:570–576, 1995.
4. Kaler SG, Gallo LK, Proud VK, et al: Occipital horn syndrome and a mild Menkes phenotype associated with splice site mutations at the MNK locus. *Nat Genet* 8:195–202, 1994.
5. Harris ZL, Takahashi Y, Miyajima H, et al: Aceruloplasminemia: Molecular characterization of this disorder of iron metabolism. *Proc Natl Acad Sci USA* 92:2539–2543, 1995.

12 Neuro-oncology

Neurologic Manifestations of Intravascular Lymphomatosis
Chapin JE, Davis LE, Kornfeld M, et al (Univ of New Mexico, Albuquerque; Albuquerque Veterans Med Ctr, New Mexico)
Acta Neurol Scand 91:494–499, 1995   12–1

Introduction.—Intravascular lymphomatosis (IL), a rare but fatal neoplastic disorder characterized by vascular occlusions, often has neurologic involvement. Because of its protean clinical features, however, it is rarely part of the differential diagnosis of neurologic disease. Malignant cells of lymphocytic origin produce occlusions, particularly of cerebral vessels. Two new patients with neurologic manifestations of IL were added to the 64 previously reported.

> *Case Report.*—Man, 71, had had progressive paraparesis and urinary incontinence for 1 month when examination revealed mild spastic weakness with a bilateral sensory level at T4. Cerebral MRI showed areas of increased signal intensity on T2-weighted images in the basal pons. After 2 weeks the patient became confused and somnolent, with markedly impaired memory, and was found to have an elevated sedimentation rate and a CSF protein concentration of 116 mg/dL. Electroencephalography showed diffuse slowing bilaterally and triphasic waves frontally. The patient rapidly worsened cognitively and died a few days later.
>
> Autopsy of the brain showed that many small- to medium-sized vessels in the cerebral white matter, cortex, brain stem, and cerebellum were occluded by large mononuclear cells with infrequent mitotic figures. Many involved vessels were surrounded by an infiltrate of small mononuclear cells distinct from those present intravascularly (Fig 2). The intraluminal cells were stained by a murine monoclonal antibody B-cell marker, whereas rabbit polyclonal antibody against T cells stained many of the perivascular lymphocytes. Focal degeneration was evident near vessels in the deep white matter.

Clinical Aspects.—In a substantial majority of the 66 patients, the diagnosis was ascertained only at autopsy. The patients' median age at the onset of illness was 61. Males predominated in a ratio of 2:1. There

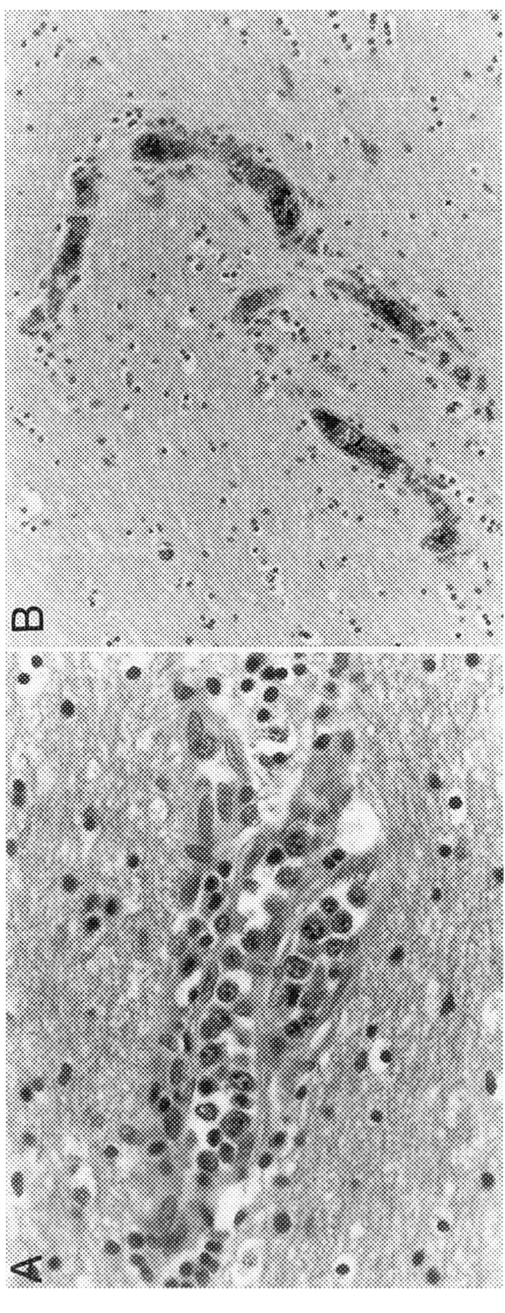

FIGURE 2.—A, frontal lobe white matter shows neoplastic mononuclear cells in lumina of small blood vessels; hematosylin-eosin, original magnification ×460. (Courtesy of Chapin JE, Davis LE, Kornfeld M, et al: Neurologic manifestations of intravascular Lymphomatosis. *Acta Neurol Scand* 91:494–499, Copyright 1995 Munksgaard International Publishers Ltd, Copenhagen, Denmark.)

TABLE 1.—Clinical Signs and Symptoms of Intravascular Lymphomatosis (N = 66)

Sign/Symptom	Initial Manifestation %	Manifestation During Clinical Course, %
Encephalopathy	37	82
Focal signs		
Hemiparesis	19	39
Myelopathy	20	34
Aphasia	5	9
Transient neurologic deficits	5	19
Headache	14	22
Seizures	5	25
Fever	5	31
Skin lesions	3	8

(Courtesy of Chapin JE, Davis LE, Kornfeld M, et al: Neurologic manifestations of intravascular lymphomatosis. *Acta Neurol Scand* 91:494–499, Copyright 1995 Munksgaard International Publishers Ltd, Copenhagen, Denmark.)

were no pathognomonic findings at the initial examination, but encephalopathy was the most common initial feature (Table 1). Most patients had a subacute course. More than one fourth were febrile. It was rare to find malignant cells in the CSF, peripheral blood, or bone marrow. Neuroimaging frequently showed changes consistent with cerebral infarction.

Pathologic Findings.—Brain biopsies were consistently diagnostic, and examination of skin lesions sometimes permitted a diagnosis of IL. A number of patients had malignant cells in the adrenal gland or lymphatic tissue. Typically autopsy revealed intravascular malignant cells in many organs, particularly the brain and adrenal tissue. It was rare for the cells to extend into the adjacent parenchyma.

Course.—Most treatments have proved ineffective in the long term. The median survival after the onset of symptoms is only months. High-dose corticosteroid treatment may have a favorable effect on encephalopathy, but focal deficits are usually unaffected. Spontaneous remissions have been recorded but are rare.

▶ Intravascular lymphomatosis usually makes its presence known by causing neurologic signs. As Table 1 shows, encephalopathy, multifocal motor and sensory abnormalities, myopathy, myelopathy, and even mononeuritis multiplex are the multifocal symptoms, and their subacute course suggests a diagnosis of CNS vasculitis.[1] However, many patients with IL have evidence of systemic illness, including fever, anemia, and an elevated erythrocyte sedimentation rate. The diagnosis is made by biopsy, but a biopsy is likely to be performed only if vascular lymphoma is considered in the differential diagnosis. Contrary to the conclusions of this paper, if the diagnosis can be established and combination chemotherapy is started, long-term remission can be achieved in some patients.[2] Because this potentially treatable systemic illness usually begins with neurologic symptoms, the neurologist has the responsibility to establish the diagnosis quickly to begin chemotherapy in a timely fashion.

J.D. Posner, M.D.

References

1. Roux S, Grossin M, de Bandt M, et al: *J Neurol Neurosurg Psychiatry* 58:363–366, 1995.
2. DeGiuseppe JA, Nelson WG, Seifter EJ, et al: *J Clin Oncol* 12:2573–2579, 1994.

Angiotropic Large Cell Lymphoma With Mononeuritis Multiplex Mimicking Systemic Vasculitis
Roux S, Grossin M, De Bandt M, et al (Bichat Hosp, Paris)
J Neurol Neurosurg Psychiatry 58:363–366, 1995   12–2

Introduction.—The angiotropic large-cell lymphoma (ALCL), also termed malignant angioendotheliomatosis, consists of proliferating tumor cells within small blood vessels, manifested chiefly in the CNS and skin. Angiotropic large-cell lymphoma was reviewed using a case report.

Case Report.—Man, 77, had lost weight and been febrile for 2 months. He had a history of hypertension. Widespread inflammatory and infiltrated skin lesions had developed 1 month earlier, regressing within 7 to 10 days. One lesion closely resembled livedo reticularis. Inflammatory arthralgia and myalgia also developed, followed by asymmetrical sensorimotor neuropathy in the legs that first involved the popliteal nerves and then became progressively worse. Testicular pain resolved within a few days. The lactate dehydrogenase level was elevated, and an axonal neuropathy was demonstrated in the legs. The CSF was normal, as were abdominothoracic CT and medullary MR studies. A skin biopsy specimen demonstrated leukocytoclastic vasculitis. Muscle and bone marrow biopsy specimens were normal, as was a myelogram. Flaccid paraplegia had developed 4 months after his initial symptoms. Urinary retention and anal incontinence also were noted. Reflexes in the legs disappeared. The patient became hypotensive and markedly hyponatremic, and he also had massive edema develop. Central hypothyroidism was documented. Abdominal ultrasonography showed splenic nodules. Corticosteroids and cyclophosphamide were given, but the patient became bedridden. He died 6 months after the onset of symptoms.

The splenic parenchyma was disrupted by atypical pleomorphic cells resembling large lymphoid cells. A B-cell lymphoma seemed likely, but the immunohistologic findings were inconclusive. Many small vessels in the kidneys, liver, bladder, lungs, and muscle tissue were filled with neoplastic cells, which occasionally occluded them. Proliferating cells were prominent in the perineural capillaries of peripheral nerves. The hypophysis was markedly involuted.

Discussion.—Nearly two thirds of patients with ALCL have neurologic abnormalities, which often include multifocal, progressive cerebrovascular events, subacute encephalopathy, and spinal cord and nerve root problems. Occlusion of small vessels by lymphomatous cells may lead to ischemic tissue damage. The condition usually is rapidly fatal, but combination chemotherapy reportedly has produced some clinical remissions.

▶ A number of recent reports have described patients with intravascular lymphomatosis who initially are seen with a fluctuating neurologic disorder involving brain, spinal cord, or peripheral nerves. The pathophysiology is occlusion of vessels by B-cell lymphoma. The symptoms range from progressive dementia to mononeuritis multiplex. Chapin et al.[1] reviewed 64 reported cases with neurologic involvement and reported 2 patients of their own. The diagnosis is rarely made before death. However, if the diagnosis can be made, usually by biopsy, anticancer therapy may ameliorate symptoms. Harris et al.[2] reported amelioration of neurologic symptoms by plasmapheresis. Corticosteroids, chemotherapy, and radiation therapy have also been reported to be beneficial in some instances.

J.D. Posner, M.D.

References

1. Chapin JE, et al: Neurologic manifestations of intravascular lymphomatosis. *Acta Neurol Scand* 91:494–499, 1995.
2. Harris CP, Sigman JD, Joekle KA: Intravascular malignant lymphomatosis: Amelioration of neurological symptoms with plasmapheresis. *Ann Neurol* 35:357–359, 1994.

Central Nervous System Metastases in Patients With Ovarian Carcinoma: A Report of 23 Cases and a Literature Review
Cormio G, Maneo A, Parma G, et al (Univ degli Studi di Milano, Italy; Ospedale S Gerardo, Monza, Italy)
Ann Oncol 6:571–574, 1995   12–3

Introduction.—Central nervous system involvement in patients with ovarian carcinoma is rare and carries a very poor prognosis. However, with early diagnosis and aggressive multimodality treatment, it may be possible to achieve significant palliation and even a few complete remissions. The experience of 23 patients with CNS metastases from ovarian carcinoma was reported.

Patients.—The patients were referred to 1 cancer center over a 12-year period. Patients' median age was 59, and the CNS metastases were documented a median of 35 months after the diagnosis of ovarian cancer. In 17 cases, the diagnosis of CNS metastases was made on clinical and radiographic grounds. Motor weakness, headache, seizure, dizziness, visual disturbances, confusion, and paresthesia were common symptoms of brain metastases. The diagnosis was made by CT in 22 patients. The negative CT scan was in a patient with meningeal carcinomatosis; all the rest had parenchymal lesions, 18 cerebral and 4 cerebellar. Fifty-nine percent of patients had multiple sites of metastases involving the brain. Eight patients had metastases detected at extraperitoneal sites at the same time, whereas the CNS was the only detectable disease site in 9 patients.

Outcomes.—Patients' median survival after diagnosis of cerebral metastases was 5 months. Median survival was 3 months for 4 untreated patients, 5.5 months for 14 patients treated by radiotherapy, and 17 months for 5 patients treated by resection of solitary metastases followed by radiotherapy. Survival was significantly affected by the number of CNS lesions, the absence of other metastatic sites, and the type of treatment.

Conclusion.—Central nervous system metastases in patients with ovarian carcinoma carries a poor prognosis. In selected patients, prompt diagnosis and multimodal treatment may produce clinically significant palliation and improve overall survival. Any patient with ovarian cancer who has neurologic symptoms should undergo CT or MRI scanning of the brain.

▶ The CNS is a rare site for ovarian cancer metastasis. Nevertheless, as this article illustrated, more than 100 patients with brain or other CNS metastases from ovarian cancer have been reported. In about one third of these patients, the CNS is the only site of relapse. In patients with single (or sometimes 2) metastatic lesions in the brain and absent or minimal systemic disease, surgical extirpation of the brain metastasis is probably the treatment of choice. Whether this should be followed by whole brain radiation or not is still an unresolved issue. Patients with multiple brain metastases or widespread systemic disease should be treated with radiation or chemotherapy. Because tumor growth has broken down the blood-brain barrier, as indicated by gadolinium enhancement on MRI, tumor cells previously sequestered behind the blood-brain barrier are now accessible to systemic chemotherapy. Systemic chemotherapy may be effective in shrinking the tumor and may even allow tumor control in the absence of radiation. Systemic chemotherapy may also control leptomeningeal metastases.

J.D. Posner, M.D.

Neuroimaging and Cerebrospinal Fluid Cytology in the Diagnosis of Leptomeningeal Metastasis
Freilich RJ, Krol G, DeAngelis LM (Memorial Sloan-Kettering Cancer Ctr, New York)
Ann Neurol 38:51–57, 1995   12–4

Introduction.—Definitive diagnosis of leptomeningeal metastasis (LM) can be a challenging clinical problem. It is usually based on the detection of malignant cells in the CSF. However, several lumbar punctures may be required. Computed tomography and MRI scans have demonstrated abnormalities in patients with LM. The clinical utility of neuroimaging in the diagnosis of LM was assessed retrospectively.

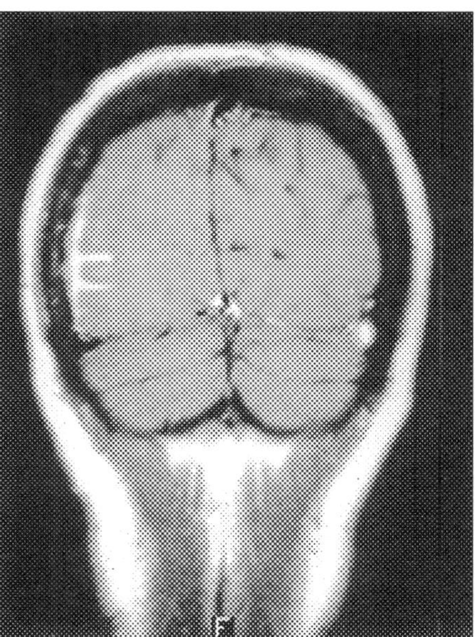

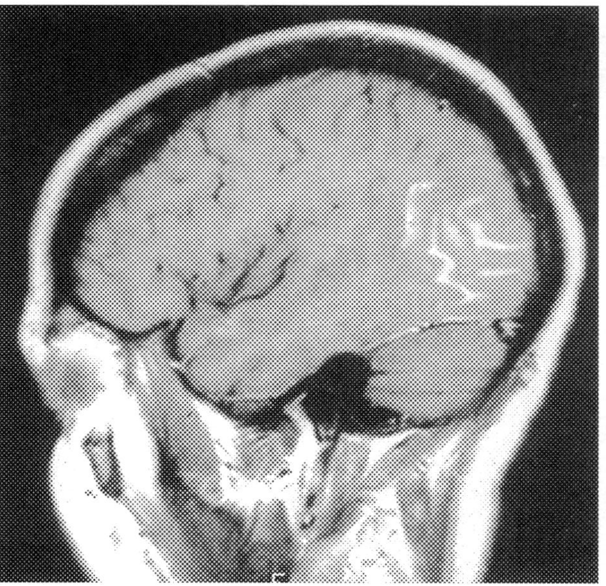

FIGURE 1.—Sagittal (*left*) and coronal (*right*) gadolinium-enhanced brain MR images of a patient with lymphoma demonstrating leptomeningeal enhancement. Lumbar CSF cytologic results were negative on 5 occasions, but cytologic results of ventricular fluid obtained through an intraventricular reservoir were positive. (Reprinted from *Annals of Neurology* volume; 38:51–57, 1995; by permission of Little, Brown and Company [Inc.].)

Methods.—The records of 137 patients undergoing evaluation for possible LM over an 18-month period were reviewed. The tumors were classified as hematologic or solid. The neuroimaging results were classified as positive, suggestive, or negative for LM. The results of CSF cytologic analysis were reviewed.

Results.—Of the 137 patients, 79 had solid tumors and 58 had hematologic tumors. Diagnostic procedures included CSF cytology in 115, neuroimaging in 128, and both evaluations in 106. Of those who underwent neuroimaging, the findings were positive in 40, suggestive in 30, and negative in 58. The CSF cytologic findings were positive in 65% of the patients with positive neuroimaging findings, 63% of those with suggestive findings, and 25% of those with negative neuroimaging findings. Leptomeningeal metastasis was ultimately diagnosed in 98% of the patients with positive neuroimaging findings, 73% of those with suggestive findings, and 21% of those with negative findings. Abnormal neuroimaging findings were detected in 44 of the 49 patients with solid tumors and 17 of the 28 patients with hematologic tumors (Fig 1).

Discussion.—Neuroimaging has clinical utility for the confirmation of clinically suspected LM and for the exclusion of other causes of neurologic signs and symptoms. Cytologic analysis of CSF also can be used to confirm the diagnosis or exclude other causes of symptoms. The 2 evaluations produce complementary information adding to the diagnostic process. Neuroimaging may allow earlier diagnosis. However, diagnosis of LM cannot be based solely on abnormal neuroimaging findings but must be placed within the clinical context. Patients with cancer who have clear clinical signs and symptoms of LM and consistent neuroimaging findings should be treated even in the absence of a positive cytologic result.

▶ Malignant cells in the CSF establish the diagnosis of LM with virtually 100% specificity. Sensitivity, however, is poor; in some series a single CSF examination yields malignant cells in only 50% of patients subsequently proved to have LM. Repetitive CSF examinations increase the yield but are invasive and time consuming. Freilich et al. indicated that neuroimaging using gadolinium-enhanced MRI scans of the head and spine to look for meningeal, subependymal, dural, or cranial nerve enhancement strongly indicates the presence of LM even when malignant cells are not found on CSF cytologic examination. Superficial cerebral lesions or communicating hydrocephalus also suggest the diagnosis. These neuroimaging findings are present in more than half of the patients with LM and thus assist CSF examination in establishing the diagnosis in a timely fashion. In the correct clinical context, leptomeningeal enhancement of the brain or spinal cord on MRI scanning eliminates the need for lumbar puncture and allows one to proceed immediately to therapy. Remember, however, that spinal root enhancement can be caused by other diseases, including inflammatory, immune, and degenerative disorders.[1]

J.D. Posner, M.D.

Reference

1. Georgy BA, Snow RD, Hesselink JR: MR imaging of spinal nerve roots: Techniques, enhancement patterns, and imaging findings. *AJR* 166:173–179, 1996.

Clinical Case Seminar: Lymphocytic Hypophysitis: Clinicopathological Findings
Thodou E, Asa SL, Kontogeorgos G, et al (Univ of Toronto)
J Clin Endocrinol Metab 80:2302–2311, 1995   12–5

Objective.—The rare pituitary inflammatory lesion lymphocytic hypophysitis may have a clinically acute outcome and sometimes leads to severe complications or death. Histologic examination is the only way to make the definite diagnosis. Sixteen cases of lymphocytic adenohypophysitis—the largest series reported to date—were described.

Patients.—Patients consisted of 14 women (mean age 31) and 2 men (mean age 42). Initial symptoms of 71% of the women occurred during pregnancy. An expanding pituitary sellar mass was noted in 56%, anterior pituitary hypofunction in 63%, and diabetes insipidus in 19%. In 19% of patients, progressive undiagnosed hypopituitarism led to death. Thirty-eight percent of the patients had hyperprolactinemia, and 1 had elevated growth hormone levels leading to insulin-like growth factor 1 excess.

A pituitary mass mimicking adenoma was seen on MRI in 83% of patients, and an associated autoimmune thyroiditis was seen in 25% (Fig 1). Morphologic and immunohistochemical studies revealed a polyclonal lymphoplasmacytic infiltrate with occasional neutrophils, eosinophils, and macrophages. Focal or diffuse adenohypophysial destruction of varying severity with associated fibrosis occurred as a result of the inflammatory process. In at least 1 patient with diabetes insipidus, the inflammatory infiltrate involved the neurohypophysis.

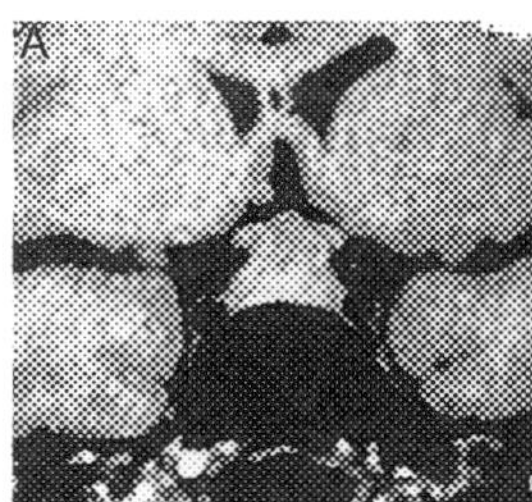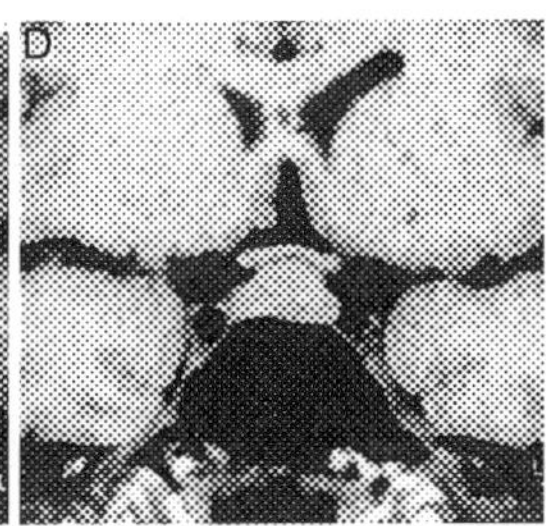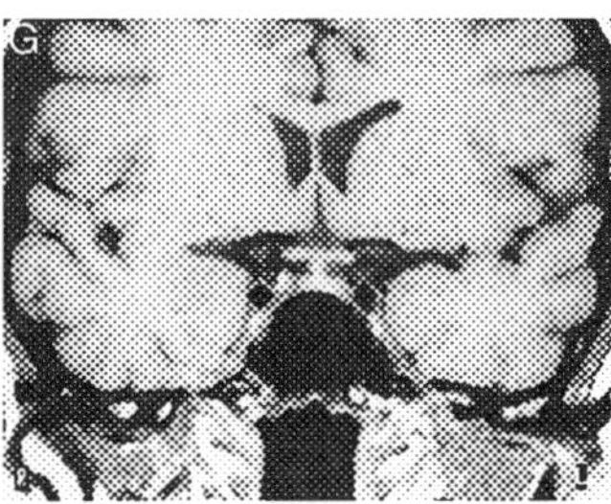

FIGURE 1.—Coronal views of the appearance of the pituitary gland in lymphocytic hypophysitis. Serial MR scans show size progression, lack of response to treatment, and resolution. A, preoperatively there is a large intrasellar mass, with significant change in the MR image of the sellar mass. D, 3 months later, with the patient off therapy, the sellar mass persists. G, 30 months after therapy was discontinued, the sellar mass has involuted, and the patient is asymptomatic. (E. Thodou, SL Asa, G Kontogeorgos, et al: Clinical case seminar: Lymphocytic hypophysitis: Clinicopathological findings: 80[8]:2302–2311, 1995; Copyright The Endocrine Society.)

Conclusion.—The clinicopathologic features of lymphocytic hypophysitis were described. This diagnosis should be considered in women whose pituitary gland enlarges during the peripartum period and in patients with pituitary hormone deficiency or excess (or both) and a coexisting autoimmune disorder. Lymphocytic hypophysitis should probably also be considered in patients with rapidly growing pituitary masses and compressive symptoms, with or without pituitary hormone dysfunction. For many patients, it may be possible to avoid aggressive pituitary surgery by being treated conservatively on the basis of clinical suspicion.

▶ Symptomatic, noninfectious, inflammatory disease of the pituitary is rare. Hypophysitis generally affects women during pregnancy or the postpartum period and usually manifests with a combination of an expanding pituitary mass and pituitary failure. Pathologically, the enlarged pituitary shows either plasma cell and lymphocytic infiltrates with multifocal or diffuse pituitary destruction (lymphocytic hypophysitis) or giant-cell granulomas (granulomatous hypophysitis).[1] The serum of some patients contains antipituitary or antinuclear antibodies, suggesting an autoimmune disorder. The MRI findings of global and symmetrical mass effect, diffuse enhancement and thickening of the pituitary stalk, and enlargement and absence of the normal hyperintense signal of the neurohypophysis, when combined with the rapid clinical course and early thyroid failure, should lead one to suspect an inflammatory rather than a neoplastic pituitary disorder. Conservative treatment with corticosteroids may obviate the need for surgery. If a surgical approach is taken, biopsy and frozen section diagnosis should be undertaken before the pituitary gland is removed.[2]

J.D. Posner, M.D.

References

1. Scanarini M, d'Avella D, Rotilio A, et al: Giant-cell granulomatous hypophysitis: A distinct clinicopathological entity. *J Neurosurg* 71:681–688, 1989.
2. Sautner D, et al: Hypophysitis in surgical and autoptical specimens. *Acta Neuropathol* 90:637, 1995.

13 Neurotoxicology

The Poisoned Patient With Altered Consciousness: Controversies in the Use of a 'Coma Cocktail'
Hoffman RS, Goldfrank LR (New York Univ; Bellevue Hosp Ctr, New York; New York City Poison Control Ctr/Bureau of Labs; et al)
JAMA 274:562–569, 1995   13–1

Introduction.—Nearly 2 million Americans are reportedly exposed to drugs and toxins each year. When a potentially poisoned patient with altered consciousness is treated, the focus is on the first 5 minutes of management. The overall results of management are excellent, but the use of a so-called coma cocktail consisting of hypertonic dextrose, thiamine, and naloxone remains controversial.

Objective.—A MEDLINE search was made for English language publications in the years 1966 through 1994 that deal with use of a coma cocktail. Analysis of diagnostic usefulness and efficacy were limited to large trials, but smaller trials and case reports were reviewed to identify adverse effects.

Consensus Findings.—Some physicians believe that routine use of a 50% dextrose solution is warranted because as many as 1 in 12 patients with altered mental status may be hypoglycemic. There is a risk of hyperkalemia from glucose loading. The literature review supports the empirical use of both hypertonic dextrose and thiamine for patients whose consciousness is altered. Rapid reagent strips may be used, but they may fail to detect clinical hypoglycemia that does not correspond to "numerical" hypoglycemia. Thiamine is used to treat Wernicke's encephalopathy (a rare cause of altered mental status) and to prevent administered carbohydrate from precipitating encephalopathy when nutritional stores are limited. The use of naloxone should be limited to patients with clinically evident opioid intoxication. Flumazenil is used to reverse sedation that results from treatment and also in the rare case of benzodiazepine overdose.

▶ In patients with potential CNS intoxication, the "coma cocktail" is used to facilitate early diagnosis or provide emergent treatment in cases where therapeutic delay may be detrimental. Risk-benefit ratios differ for the various components of the "cocktail," depending on the underlying cause (e.g., hypoglycemia vs. benzodiazepine overdose) and physical setting (e.g., prehospital vs. emergency department). As indicated in this article, conditions where treatment delays are intolerable, such as hypoglycemia or thiamine deficiency, are best served by the immediate IV administration of hypertonic dextrose and thiamine. In patients with potential opiate or benzodiazepine intoxications, mortality usually results from respiratory depression and consequent anoxia or aspiration. In these cases, airway management is the immediate concern. Once this is achieved, the prehospital use of naloxone to reverse opiate toxicity and flumazenil to treat benzodiazepine toxicity becomes of dubious value.

A.R. Berger, M.D.

Peripheral Neurologic Abnormalities Among Roofing Workers: Sentinel Case and Clinical Screening
Herbert R, Harris-Abbott D, Gerr F, et al (Mount Sinai School of Medicine, New York; Emory Univ, Atlanta, Ga)
Arch Environ Health 50:349–354, 1995   13–2

Background.—The effects of exposure to organic solvents used in a new "1-ply," or "single-ply," roofing system have not been adequately studied. Substances used in these systems that could cause neurotoxicity include toluene, xylene, heptane, *n*-hexane, trichloroethylene, methylethyl ketone, and methyl-isobutyl ketone. Peripheral neuropathy, discovered in a roofer working with 1-ply roof systems, prompted screening of other roofers for neurologic abnormalities.

> *Case Report.*—Man, 52, complained of balance problems, lightheadedness, headache, irritability, and fatigue, with the symptoms intensifying over the preceding 1.5 years. He had worked as a roofer for 16 years and had used 1-ply roofing systems for the last 4 years. He reported symmetrical paresthesias in both his feet and hands, which was confirmed in the physical examination. Laboratory findings were normal. One year later, electrophysiologic testing revealed severe symmetric sensory-motor axonal polyneuropathy, which confirmed the physical examination findings of a stocking-glove loss of temperature and vibration sensation, particularly in the lower extremities.

Methods.—Forty roofers underwent an occupational health screening examination, which included the collection of data regarding demographics, occupational exposures, medical history, and current symptoms; a physical and neurologic examination; laboratory evaluation; and vibrotactile thresholds determinations.

Results.—The most common symptoms related to solvent exposure were light-headedness, headache, and irritability. There were no neurologic abnormalities except for a diminished perception of sharp touch or vibration in the extremities, particularly the lower extremities. There were abnormal vibrotactile thresholds noted in the nondominant index finger of 9% of the patients, in the nondominant great toe of 36%, and in the dominant great toe of 42%.

Conclusion.—There was a highly significantly increased frequency of lower extremity sensory impairment among the roofers who underwent screening, indicating that peripheral neuropathy may be a previously undiscovered health hazard for roofers. Formal epidemiologic study of roofing-related peripheral nerve dysfunction is warranted.

▶ Quantitative sensory testing (QST) is a reproducible, noninvasive method of determining vibration and thermal thresholds and is used increasingly to screen for neurotoxic peripheral neuropathies. Because QST abnormalities reflect dysfunction anywhere along the somatosensory pathway (not just peripheral nerve), its value as a screen for subclinical nerve disease is enhanced when patients with alternative explanations for sensory dysfunction are excluded (e.g., radiculopathies, nontoxic nerve disease, myelopathies, cortical lesions). In addition, QST abnormalities need to be interpreted in context of the clinical history, examination, and (occasionally) neuroimaging to increase the likelihood that threshold abnormalities reflect peripheral nerve disease. Ideally QST testing should be combined with quantitative electrophysiology to confirm peripheral nerve dysfunction. There may be times, however, when QST thresholds but not nerve conduction studies are abnormal. Such instances can occur when sensory dysfunction is limited to the sensory end-organ, without the more proximal axon being involved.

A.R. Berger, M.D.

White Matter Changes Caused by Chronic Solvent Abuse
Yamanouchi N, Okada S-I, Kodama K, et al (Chiba Univ, Japan; Natl Psychiatric Inst of Shimofusa, Chiba, Japan; Kisarazu Hosp, Japan)
AJNR 16:1643–1649, 1995   13–3

Introduction.—Chronic abuse of organic solvents causes toxic encephalopathy. Atrophy and changes in the white matter of the CNS of these patients have been shown in MRI studies. A group of abusers in Japan were studied using MRI examinations to further characterize CNS changes associated with organic solvent abuse.

Methods.—Fifteen men and 5 women who had abused organic solvents for at least 1 year were examined for neurologic and MRI abnormalities. Magnetic resonance images were obtained at 1.5 tesla in 4 modes: sagittal T1-weighted imaging, axial T2-weighted and proton density–weighted imaging, axial T1-weighted imaging, and coronal T1-weighted imaging.

Results.—Patients were found to have 2 types of white matter changes: restricted and diffuse, which were shown best on proton density–weighted images. Restricted white matter changes appeared on T2-weighted images as hyperintense areas in the brain stem, middle cerebellar peduncles, and cerebellar white matter around the dentate nuclei. Patients with diffuse white matter changes had evidence of brain atrophy, including a thin corpus callosum and hippocampal atrophy. The 7 patients with restricted white matter changes had neurologic symptoms, including cerebellar ataxia, tremor, and pyramidal signs. Long-term abuse of lacquer thinner was associated with diffuse white matter changes, whereas abuse of pure toluene was associated with restricted and intermediate white matter change.

Conclusion.—Restricted white matter change in chronic solvent abusers may represent either a qualitatively different change from diffuse white matter change or an early stage of diffuse white matter change. If there is a qualitative difference, it may be related to the substance abused, with pure toluene causing neurologic symptoms associated with restricted white matter change and lacquer thinner or glues causing neurologic symptoms after diffuse white matter changes.

▶ The ability of MRI to visualize early or subtle pathologic changes has facilitated the study of regional or selective vulnerability of different regions of the brain to various neurotoxins. Selective vulnerability may reflect differences in metabolic rate, neurotransmitters, substrate utilization, or blood-brain barrier. In some cases, the clinical condition and MRI appearance reflect the dose or length of exposure to the neurotoxin. This paper questioned whether differences in MRI patterns between exposure to toluene and lacquer reflect regional vulnerability or severity and length of exposure. The few pathologic studies of brains exposed to chronic high-dose toluene did not show the cortical atrophy seen with lacquer exposure. This may reflect a cortical toxin present in lacquer. Functional and echo planar MRI studies will probably help to identify early sites of involvement before persistent structural changes have occurred.

A.R. Berger, M.D.

Manganese and Chronic Hepatic Encephalopathy

Krieger D, Krieger S, Jansen O, et al (Ruprecht-Karls Univ of Heidelberg, Germany)
Lancet 346:270–274, 1995

13–4

Background.—Both clinical and laboratory observations have suggested that an increased circulating level of manganese might lead to its accumulation in the basal ganglia in patients with end-stage liver disease. Magnetic resonance imaging has demonstrated symmetric hyperintensity of the globus pallidus, pituitary gland, and mesencephalon not only in patients with chronic liver failure but also in those receiving long-term total parenteral nutrition and workers with Mn toxicity. Chronic exposure to Mn has been related to extrapyramidal symptoms and to psychological effects resembling chronic hepatic encephalopathy.

Objective.—Cranial MRI was carried out in 10 consecutive, unselected hospitalized patients having Child's grade C hepatic cirrhosis who were

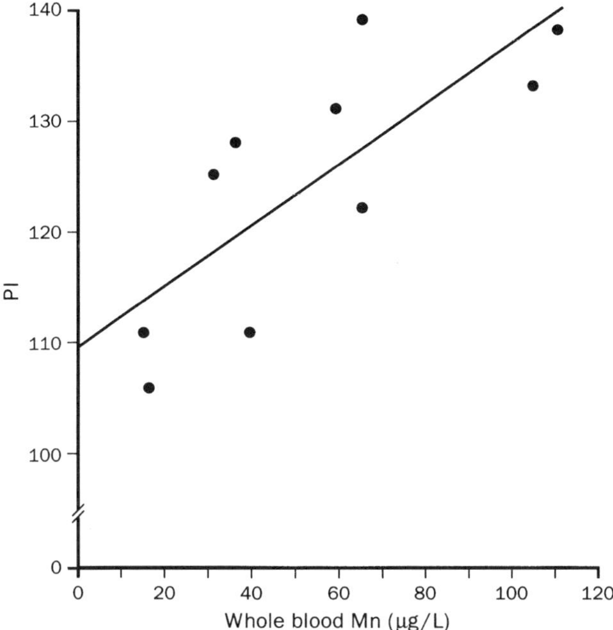

FIGURE 2.—Pallidal signal intensity and whole blood manganese levels in 10 patients with end-stage liver failure (R_s = 0.8; P = 0.0058). *Abbreviation: PI*, pallidal signal intensity. (Courtesy of Krieger D, Krieger S, Jansen O, et al: Manganese and chronic hepatic encephalopathy. *Lancet* 346:270–274, 1995.)

being considered for liver transplantation. Ten neurology inpatients with no history of liver disease served as a control group. Three of the study patients died and underwent postmortem MRI of the brain; in addition, brain tissue levels of Mn were determined.

Findings.—The median whole-blood Mn concentration was 50 µg/L in the patients with end-stage liver disease and 10 µg/L in controls. Pallidal signal intensity (PI) also was greater in the patients with liver disease. Blood Mn levels correlated significantly with pallidal signal intensity (Fig 2), but in neither group did Mn levels correlate with age. The postmortem MRI studies demonstrated uniform hyperintensity in the globus pallidus, putamen, and caudate nucleus. Concentrations of Mn were increased in the same structures and also in the substantia nigra and mesencephalic tegmentum. The same regions contained increased number of Alzheimer type II astrocytes.

Conclusion.—Manganese accumulates within the basal ganglia in patients with end-stage liver disease. It seems likely that Mn has a role in the development of chronic hepatic encephalopathy (CHE).

▶ Chronic manganese intoxication and CHE share many clinical features. This paper suggested that some clinical manifestations of CHE are caused by the toxic effects of endogenously accumulated Mn. Exogenously administered Mn tends to accumulate in the basal ganglia, substantia nigra, and subthalamic nuclei. In this study, patients with CHE had higher blood and tissue Mn levels (striatum and pallidum) than controls, possibly due to impaired biliary excretion. T1-weighted MR images of patients with CHE showed hyperintense signal in the basal ganglia, a finding the authors believed to be caused by accumulated Mn. They postulated that excessive Mn interferes with enzymatic detoxification of ammonia, thereby causing the clinical manifestations of CHE.

This paper raised an intriguing but unproven hypothesis regarding the pathogenesis of symptoms in CHE. One problem is that the pathology of CHE and Mn intoxication is different. Chronic hepatic encephalopathy is characterized by diffuse cortical necrosis and cavitation at the corticomedullary junctions and degenerative changes in the striatum, cerebellar cortex, dentate nuclei, thalamus, and red nuclei. Although occasional patients with Mn intoxication may have widespread changes, pathologic changes are limited mainly to the basal ganglia and subthalamic nuclei, and cavitation is most unusual.

A.R. Berger, M.D.

Cyclosporin A Toxicity: MRI Appearance of the Brain
Pace MT, Slovis TL, Kelly JK, et al (Harper-Grace Hosp, Detroit; Children's Hosp of Michigan, Detroit)
Pediatr Radiol 25:180–183, 1995   13–5

Introduction.—Neurotoxicity is a recognized complication of cyclosporine therapy for bone marrow and organ transplantation. Transient neurotoxic episodes that developed in 3 patients receiving cyclosporine after a bone marrow transplant were evaluated, with particular attention to MRI findings.

Clinical Features.—All patients developed an acute seizure activity 2 to 4 days after receiving IV cyclosporine and methylprednisolone. One patient also became encephalopathic with disorientation, and 2 had visual or auditory hallucinations (or both). There was no linear correlation between blood levels of cyclosporine and the neurologic symptoms. The cyclosporine dosage was reduced, and all symptoms resolved with time.

Imaging Findings.—The first patient demonstrated high T2-weighted signal changes in the parietal cortex bilaterally, and these changes were nearly resolved by 4 months (Fig 1). In the second patient, nonenhancing areas of low attenuation were seen in the occipital cortex bilaterally with extension into the periatrial white matter on CT; the same areas showed high T2-weighted signal changes on MRI. In the third patient, both CT and MRI showed abnormal attenuation and signal changes in both hippocampal and uncal regions without evidence of enhancement. Follow-up CT scans showed eventual resolutions of the lesions, although bilateral temporal lobe atrophy with resultant temporal horn dilatation became evident.

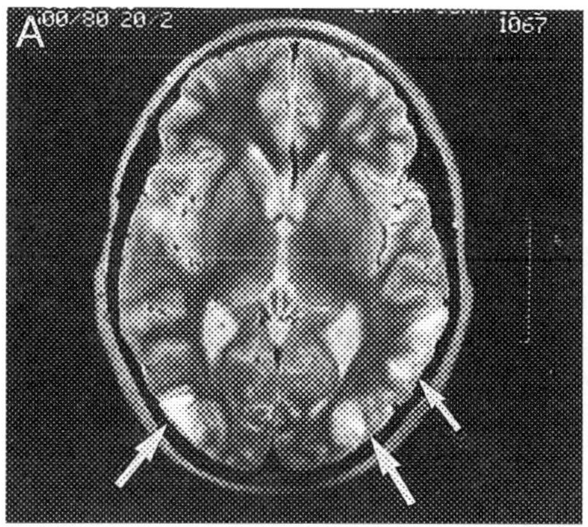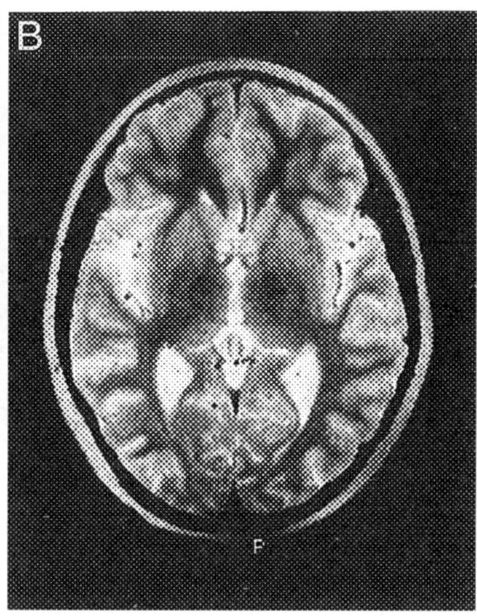

FIGURE 1.—First patient. **A**, high-signal changes are seen on this T2-weighted MR image in the parietal cortex bilaterally (*arrows*). **B**, 4 months later, the signal abnormalities have resolved. (*Pediatr Radiol*; Cyclosporin A toxicity: MRI appearance of the brain; Pace MT, Slovis TL, Kelly JK, et al; vol 25; p 181; Fig 1; 1995; Copyright notice of Springer-Verlag.)

Implications.—Patients on cyclosporine therapy should be monitored for neurotoxicity regardless of cyclosporine blood levels. Both MRI and CT demonstrate symmetric, nonenhancing cortical or white matter changes (or both), and these abnormalities usually resolve with a reduction or discontinuation of cyclosporine.

▶ Cyclosporine has become an important immunosuppressive agent. It has a wide spectrum of neurotoxicity; about 10% of patients receiving cyclosporine develop severe headaches, seizures, visual disturbances, and encephalopathy. This paper (and others similar to it) reported reversible MRI abnormalities consisting of high-intensity T2-weighted signal changes in occipital and posterior parietal cortical and subcortical areas. Both the clinical syndrome and MRI findings are reminiscent of hypertensive encephalopathy. Some studies have reported systemic hypertension to be an invariable accompaniment to cyclosporine neurotoxicity, suggesting a pathogenetic role. It is unclear what role the usual administration of IV corticosteroids plays in the pathogenesis of both the neurotoxicity and the hypertension. Although MRI changes seem fairly prevalent in patients with clinical neurotoxicity, the relationship between clinical symptoms and radiographic localization is poor. With both a reduction of cyclosporine dose and systemic blood pressure, MRI and clinical symptoms tend to resolve.

A.R. Berger, M.D.

Pattern of Neurobehavioral Deficits Associated With Interferon Alfa Therapy for Leukemia

Pavol MA, Meyers CA, Rexer JL, et al (Univ of Texas MD Anderson Cancer Ctr, Houston)
Neurology 45:947–950, 1995

13–6

Objective.—Interferon causes a wide range of neurologic side effects when used to treat cancer, and these often prove to be the dose-limiting factor. This study took a close look at the cognitive and emotional status of patients with chronic myelogenous leukemia who were treated with interferon-alfa (IFN-α).

Patients and Treatment.—Fifteen men and 10 women aged 24 to 70 participated in the study. Patients tended to be well educated, and many were professionals. The mean time since leukemia had been diagnosed was 33 months, and patients had received IFN-α for 26 months on average. Treatment was given subcutaneously, usually on a daily basis, in an average weekly dose of 5.1 × 10⁷ IU. Sixteen leukemic patients not given IFN-α served as a control group.

Findings.—An unexpectedly large number of interferon-treated patients had scores in the impairment range on tests of verbal memory, delayed visual memory, verbal fluency, visual sequencing, and motor dexterity. Both verbal memory and graphomotor performance on the Digit Symbol test correlated with the time since diagnosis. About half the study patients had increased Minnesota Multiphasic Personality Inventory scores for hypochondriasis, depression, and hysteria, but scores did not correlate with the time since diagnosis.

Conclusion.—These findings suggest frontal-subcortical dysfunction in many leukemic patients who are treated with IFN-α.

▶ Interferon-alfa is becoming an important agent in treating the different lymphoid malignancies and leukemia. As with many of the newer cancer treatments, neurologic side effects are either dose limiting or an important source of comorbidity. This paper illustrated the subtle cognitive deficits that may result from IFN-α treatment. Although these side effects are not dose limiting, they may substantially interfere with the patient's cognitive function and, if not identified as a toxic effect, may be misdiagnosed as a component of the underlying malignancy. Increasingly, the pathophysiologic mechanisms underlying toxic adverse effects are being identified and specific protective agents that increase the tolerable dose and duration of treatment are being employed.

A.R. Berger, M.D.

14 Sleep Disorders

Manifestations and Consequences of Obstructive Sleep Apnoea
Peter JH, Koehler U, Grote L, et al (Klinikum der Philipps-Univ, Marburg, Germany)
Eur Respir J 8:1572–1583, 1995   14–1

Background.—The last 15 years have seen major advances in the technology used for diagnosis of patients with suspected sleep-related breathing disorders (SRBDs). The past emphasis on obstructive sleep apnea (OSA) syndrome is no longer sufficient to deal with consequences of SRBD, which include cardiovascular effects and "human error" caused by hypersomnolence. The characteristics and consequences of SRBDs were reviewed as part of a discussion of the current state of research into OSA.

Manifestations and Consequences.—Some of the diagnostic advances in SRBD include serial monitoring devices that permit detailed study of the interactions of SRBD with cardiovascular function and the autonomic nervous system, as well as its impact on various physiologic procedures while the patient is awake. Major advances have been made in surgical treatment, and the availability of various modes of nasal ventilation permits all forms of SRBD to be treated. Early diagnosis and treatment can prevent the acute and long-term consequences of OSA.

Hypersomnia is the main symptom in about one third of patients with SRBD. In this situation, upper airway obstruction during sleep induces CNS activation, which the patient usually fails to notice (Fig 1). This form of arousal results in increased muscle tone, heart rate, blood pressure, and ventilation. In severe OSA, arousal caused by upper airway obstruction may be a major cause of hypertension. The amount of rapid-eye movement (REM) and of stage 3 and 4 non-REM sleep decreases as the apnea index increases (Fig 2). Hypersomnolence, fragmented sleep, and sleep deprivation combine to interfere with breathing control and with hypercapnia and hypoxic ventilatory responsiveness. Accidents resulting from hypersomnolence and human error are a major problem. Obstructive sleep apnea has also been linked to cardiac arrhythmias, though this seems confined to the more severe cases. The link between OSA, snoring, and arterial hypertension has also received major attention in recent years.

Future of Sleep-Related Breathing Disorder Research.—The resources are available to treat patients with severe OSA. Further attention to conditions associated with the milder forms of OSA is needed, especially to

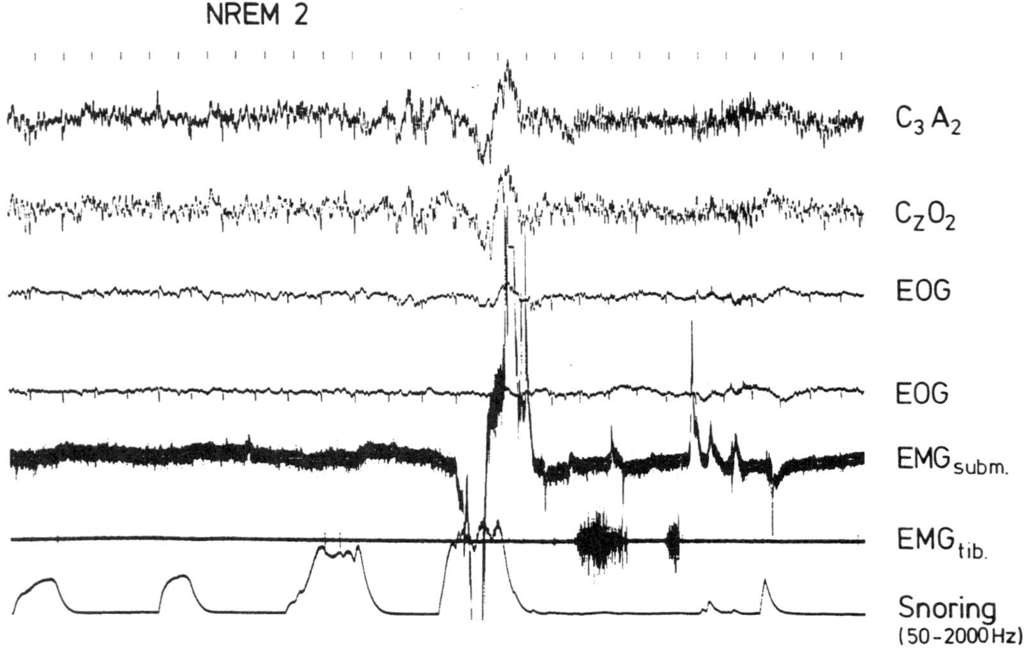

FIGURE 1.—Arousal caused by snoring during stage 2 non–rapid eye movement sleep. The figure shows 2 electroencephalographic leads (C_3-A_2; C_2-O_2), 2 electro-oculogram leads, submental and tibial electromyographic activity and integrated snoring activity. *Abbreviations: NREM*, non–rapid eye movement; *EOG*, electro-oculogram; *EMG_{subm}*, submental electromyographic; *EMG_{tib}*, tibial electromyographic. (Courtesy of Peter JH, Koehler U, Grote L, at al: Manifestations and consequences of obstructive sleep apnoea. *Eur Respir J* 8:1572–1583, 1995.)

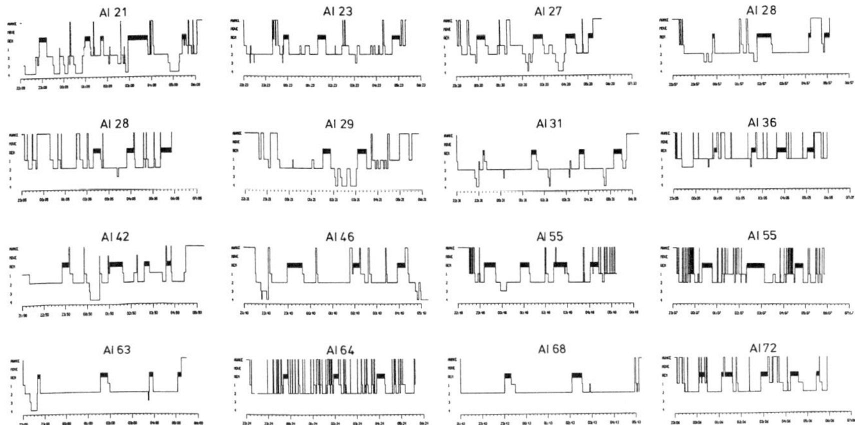

FIGURE 2.—Hypnograms from 16 randomly selected patients with obstructive sleep apnea arranged according to the corresponding AI, starting from *top left*. Although there is considerable interindividual variability, the amount of stage 3 and 4 non-REM sleep and REM sleep decreases with increasing AI. *Abbreviations: AI*, apnea index; *REM*, rapid eye movement. (From Peter JH, Koehler U, Grote L, at al: Manifestations and consequences of obstructive sleep apnoea. *Eur Respir J* 8:1572–1583, 1995. Courtesy of Penzel T: Zur Pathophysiologie der Interaktion von Schlaf, Atmung und Kreislauf-Konzepte der kardiorespiratorischen Polysomnographic [in preparation].)

the cardiac arrhythmias, arterial hypertension, and hypersomnolence associated with SRBDs. These conditions also raise some important economic issues, including the costs of accidents resulting from hypersomnolence. The authors called for a European program of early detection, treatment, and prevention of SRBDs in an attempt to reduce the incidence of human error accidents and to reduce the associated cardiovascular morbidity and mortality.

▶ The authors shared with us their large experience in dealing with SRBDs. Evidence they cited continues to mount that SRBDs contribute to morbidity and mortality of affected individuals in many established ways. The current trend suggests that as our understanding of these disorders increases, we will further appreciate the huge toll that SRBDs take on industrial society. Readers should be mindful that prevalence rates for these SRBDs are substantially higher in selected subgroups of patients with hypertension and neurologic disorders. Because excellent treatments are available for most patients with SRBD, recognition and early diagnosis are especially important.

B. Nolan, M.D.

Pharyngeal Narrowing/Occlusion During Central Sleep Apnea

Badr MS, Toiber F, Skatrud JB, et al (William S Middleton Mem Veterans Hosp, Madison, Wis; John Rankin Lab of Preventive Medicine, Madison, Wis; Univ of Wisconsin, Madison)
J Appl Physiol 78:1806–1815, 1995   14–2

Introduction.—Experimental studies have shown that negative intraluminal pressure can cause pharyngeal obstruction. However, the extent to which this observation applies to spontaneous pharyngeal obstruction during sleep in humans is unclear. The hypothesis that subatmospheric intraluminal pressure is not required for the development of pharyngeal occlusion during non–rapid eye movement (non-REM) sleep in humans was tested.

Methods.—Six patients with sleep apnea or hypopnea (SAH) and 6 normal controls were studied during non-REM sleep. Fiber-optic nasopharyngoscopy was used to assess the subjects' pharyngeal patency during spontaneous central apnea in 4 subjects and during nasal mechanical ventilation to induce hypocapnic central apnea in 10 patients.

Results.—The patients with central sleep apnea syndrome had a total of 160 spontaneously occurring central apneas; of these, 146 were associated with complete pharyngeal occlusion. The pharynx narrowed gradually and progressively during induced hypocapnic central apnea (Fig 2). The narrowing was more pronounced at the velopharynx than the oropharynx and in patients with SAH than in controls. Of 44 episodes of apnea in the patients with SAH, 31 were associated with complete pharyngeal occlusion compared with 3 of 25 episodes in controls. When the patients started trying to inhale again, narrowing or occlusion persisted until electroencephalographic signs of arousal were observed.

Conclusion.—Central apnea is associated with a reduced cross-sectional area of the pharynx in the absence of inspiratory effort. Induced hypocapnic central apnea produces velopharyngeal narrowing even in normal subjects. In patients with SAH, spontaneous or induced apnea is associated with complete pharyngeal occlusion. Thus, pharyngeal occlusion can occur in the absence of subatmospheric intraluminal pressure. The pharyngeal narrowing or occlusion that occurs during central apnea may result from either passive collapse or active constriction.

▶ The authors carefully measured mechanical responses of the upper airway to passively induced hypocapnea, followed by central apnea. Despite daunting technical considerations addressed in the full text of the original article, the conclusions appear noteworthy. Persons with predominantly central sleep apnea experienced significant associated obstructive components. Fortunately, nasal continuous positive airway pressure is often effective in subjects with central sleep apnea, as well as in those with obstructive

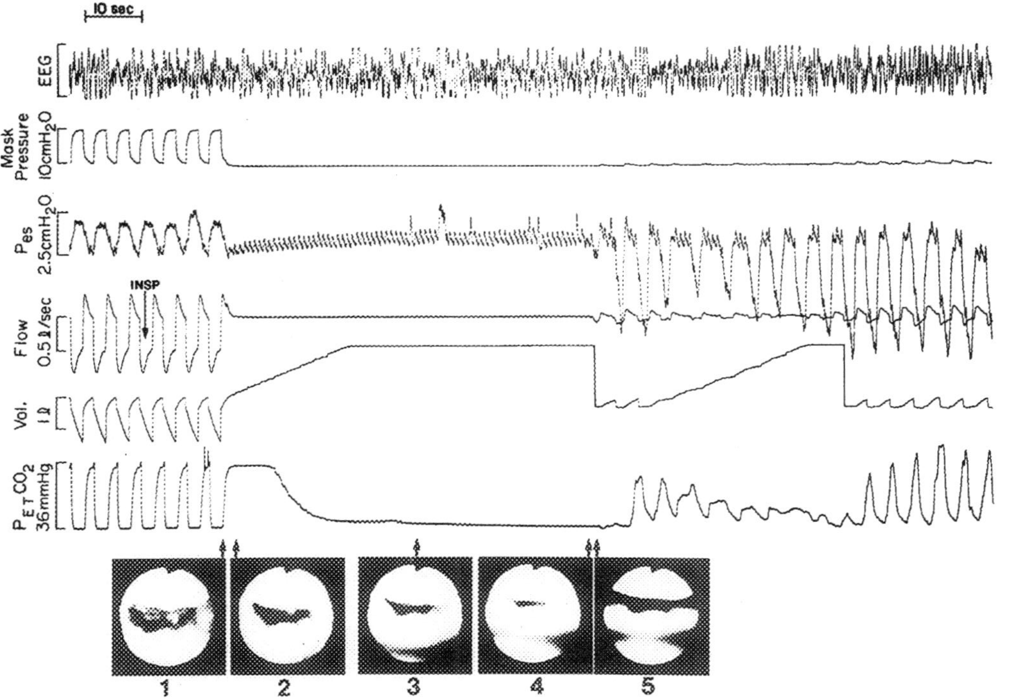

FIGURE 2.—Velopharyngeal narrowing during induced hypocapnic central apnea (28 sec) in normal subject. Note gradual narrowing from control (*image 1*) to end of central apnea (*image 4*), to almost complete occlusion. Also note persistent narrowing, augmented P_{es}, and flow rates during recovery period. *Abbreviations:* P_{es}, esophageal pressure; $P_{ET}CO_2$, end-tidal carbon dioxide pressure; *EEG*, electroencephalogram; *INSP*, inspiration. (Courtesy of Badr MS, Toiber F, Skatrud JB, et al: Pharyngeal narrowing/occlusion during central sleep apnea. *J Appl Physiol* 78:1806–1815, 1995.)

sleep apnea. This study helped to further our understanding of the mechanics and relationships of central and obstructive sleep apnea.

B. Nolan, M.D.

Fluctuations in Autonomic Nervous Activity During Sleep Displayed by Power Spectrum Analysis of Heart Rate Variability

Baharav A, Kotagal S, Gibbons V, et al (Saint Louis Univ, Mo; Tel Aviv Univ, Israel)

Neurology 45:1183–1187, 1995

14–3

Background.—Beat-to-beat heart rate variability has 2 main components: a low-frequency (LF) component between 0.02 and 0.15 Hz, representing vasomotor and baroreceptor activity (which are under both sympathetic and parasympathetic control) and a high-frequency (HF) component higher than 0.2 Hz (which is under parasympathetic control). A noninvasive power spectrum analysis was performed on healthy sleeping children to investigate autonomic cardiovascular control during the stages of sleep.

Methods.—Ten children with normal sleep patterns were chosen from a chart review of children who had undergone all-night polysomnographic studies. The time intervals analyzed were the beginning of the night awake stage, non–rapid-eye movement (non-REM) sleep stages I and II, light sleep, non-REM sleep stages III and IV, slow-wave sleep, and REM sleep. Both the HF and LF ranges were examined on 256-sec traces of heart rate and respiration.

Findings.—There was a decrease in LF during sleep, with minimal values during non-REM sleep and elevated levels during REM sleep. High frequency inceased with the onset of sleep, was maximal during slow-wave sleep, and had a pattern that was the inverse of LF. The LF/HF ratio (Fig 2) had changes during sleep that paralleled the changes in LF.

Conclusion.—The sympathetic component that characterizes wakefulness decreases during non-REM sleep is at its lowest during slow-wave sleep and approaches awake levels during REM sleep in healthy children. During slow-wave sleep, the autonomic balance is shifted toward the parasympathetic component. This noninvasive approach of continuous measurement of autonomic cardiorespiratory control used in this study permits simple, on-line monitoring of autonomic activity during all sleep stages. The results obtained with this noninvasive method are in agreement with those obtained with more invasive techniques.

▶ Numerous physiologic changes in function of the nervous system occur in association with changes from wake to non-REM sleep to REM sleep. This study reported the use of power spectrum analysis of beat-to-beat variability in heart rate during waking and sleep states as 1 means of measuring such changes in function. Although they were not asymptomatic normal children, subjects reportedly had normal sleep recordings as part of an evaluation for

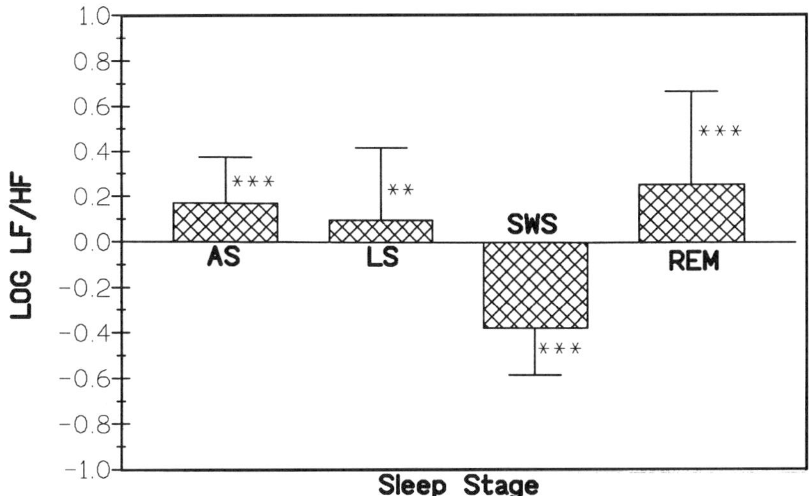

FIGURE 2.—Autonomic balance during sleep. The balance points toward *HF* during *SWS*, with significant differences between this stage and *AS, LS,* and *REM*. The *error bars* show standard deviation. ***P* < 0.001; ****P* < 0.0001 on 2-tailed *t* test. *Abbreviations: AS,* awake at the beginning of the night; *LS,* light sleep; *SWS,* slow-wave sleep; *REM,* rapid eye movement; *LF,* low frequency; *HF,* high frequency. (Reprinted from *Neurology* volume; 45:1183–1187, 1995; by permission of Little, Brown and Company [Inc.].)

such disorders as excessive sleepiness and cleft palate. The technique described has the advantage of being noninvasive but utilized epochs of 256 sec or more than 4 minutes for the power spectrum measures. Such techniques may facilitate the identification and understanding of state-dependent autonomic changes in normal individuals and in disease.

B. Nolan, M.D.

A Questionnaire Study of 138 Patients With Restless Legs Syndrome: The 'Night-Walkers' Survey

Walters AS, Hickey K, Maltzman J, et al (UMDNJ-Robert Wood Johnson Med School, New Brunswick, NJ; Rutgers Univ, New Brunswick, NJ; Dept of Veterans Affairs Med Ctr, Lyons, NJ; et al)
Neurology 46:92–95, 1996
14–4

Introduction.—Restless legs syndrome (RLS) can be diagnosed by clinical criteria and a neurologic examination. Diagnosis is strengthened by the finding of a clinically significant periodic limb movement in sleep (PLMS) index of more than 5 (number per hour of sleep). Although RLS is considered a condition of middle to older age, reports have documented its onset in childhood and adolescence. Additional information on the age of onset, symptoms, and course of RLS was obtained by interviewing a group of patients by telephone.

Methods.—A standardized questionnaire was administered to 107 patients who were members of the RLS Foundation support group and 33 patients in the authors' own practice. All met the 4 minimal criteria for diagnosis of RLS: needing to move the legs because of discomfort, pacing the floor or practicing other methods to relieve discomfort, feeling more discomfort at rest, and experiencing worsening of symptoms at night. All the patients from the authors' practice had undergone neurologic examination and met the PLMS index requirement.

Results.—Age of onset varied widely but was most common between 11 and 30 (86 of 138 patients). More females (96) than males (42) were affected. Incorrect diagnosis or failure to make a diagnosis occurred often, especially in patients who were young at the onset of symptoms. A psychological diagnosis was common at all ages, and children with severe symptoms were at times diagnosed with attention deficit hyperactivity disorder. "Growing pains" was offered as a diagnosis in many younger patients. Symptoms of RLS tended to progress in frequency and severity. The 33 patients from the authors' practice responded to various combinations of opiods, L-dopa, dopamine agonists, or benzodiazepines.

Conclusion.—This large-scale survey of patients with RLS indicated that onset of the condition is often in childhood and can be severe at this time. Misdiagnosis is common, especially among younger patients, but adults were misdiagnosed as well. About half of the patients had first-degree relatives affected with RLS. Diabetic peripheral neuropathy or lumbosacral neuropathy was known to have triggered RLS in 5 cases.

▶ I was much surprised to learn that 30% of adults with RLS dated the onset of symptoms to childhood. It is never diagnosed at that age, in part because it is not considered a disease of childhood and also because it is often considered psychogenic at all ages. Children who sought medical attention were diagnosed as having attention deficit hyperactivity syndrome or growing pains. Those of us who see children will need to be alert to the possibility of RLS as a cause of "hyperactivity".

G.M. Fenichel, M.D.

15 Neuro-otology

Meniere's Disease: Etiologic Considerations
Parker W (Cleveland Clinic Found, Ohio)
Arch Otolaryngol Head Neck Surg 121:377–382, 1995   15–1

Objective.—Data from 85 cases of Meniere's disease were reviewed to assess the possibility that a common vascular mechanism underlies both idiopathic Meniere's disease and migraine. Twenty-nine patients (34%) also had migraine.

Observations.—Migraine was more prevalent in these patients than in the general population. More women than men had Meniere's disease alone and combined Meniere's disease and migraine. The age at onset was similar in the 2 groups of patients. In most patients having both diagnoses, both disorders were present at the time when Meniere's disease was diagnosed. Individual episodes of each disorder did not always occur together at the time of manifestation. Occasionally Meniere's symptoms were associated with a migraine episode without headache. Treatment with methysergide maleate or prednisone sometimes lessened the Meniere's symptoms.

Implications.—Further studies of this type should clarify the relationship between Meniere's disease and migraine in patients who seemingly have both disorders; in those with active Meniere's disease and a personal or family history of migraine; and in patients with Meniere's disease and mild, paroxysmal neurologic symptoms that might represent migraine equivalent.

▶ Migraine is a common and unrecognized cause of vertigo spells. Patients with migraine-induced vertigo are frequently misdiagnosed with Meniere's disease or with vestibular hydrops when there is no fluctuation in hearing. This is especially true in patients with migraine aura without headache. Patients with both migraine and Meniere's disease can be very challenging with regard to diagnosis and management. These patients usually require evaluation during or immediately after a spell of vertigo to determine whether there is associated hearing loss, which is more consistent with Meniere's disease. Several articles have shown an increased incidence of migraine in patients with Meniere's disease. Because these are 2 common disorders, it is still not clear whether there is a causal link. Migraine-induced vertigo should be treated the same way as migraine headaches.

R.J. Tusa, M.D., Ph.D.

Persistent Direction-Changing Positional Nystagmus: Another Variant of Benign Positional Nystagmus?

Baloh RW, Yue Q, Jacobson KM, et al (Univ of California, Los Angeles)
Neurology 45:1297–1301, 1995   15–2

Background.—An occasional brain lesion such as a posterior fossa tumor may manifest with positional vertigo, making it important to distinguish between peripheral and central positional vertigo. Benign peripheral positional vertigo (BPPV) generally is associated with paroxysmal positional nystagmus that lasts less than 1 minute, has a latency, and fatigues on repeated positioning. In contrast, central positional nystagmus has no latency, often lasts for as long as the position is maintained, and does not fatigue. Three patients with positional vertigo who had positional nystagmus of benign peripheral origin were reported.

Case Reports.—Three patients with positional vertigo had positional nystagmus of the type usually attributed to a central lesion. The nystagmus changed direction in each lateral position, consistently beating away from the ground. In 2 patients positional nystagmus had developed after being treated for typical benign

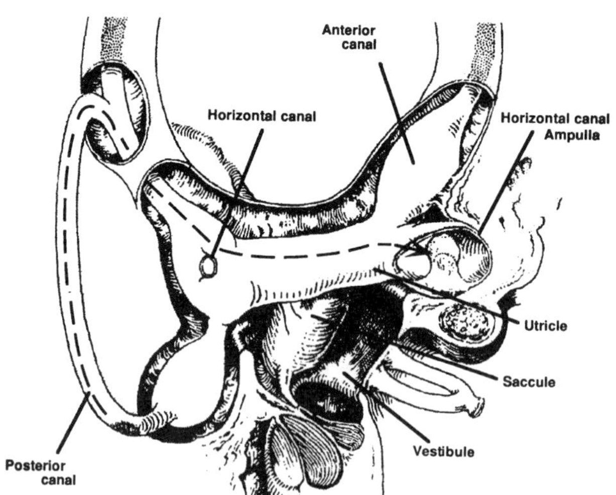

FIGURE 2.—Schematic drawing of the inner ear showing how the debris could move from the posterior semicircular canal and attach to the cupula of the horizontal semicircular canal (*dashed line* and *arrow*). (Reprinted from *Neurology* volume; 45:1297–1301, 1995; by permission of Little, Brown and Company [Inc.].)

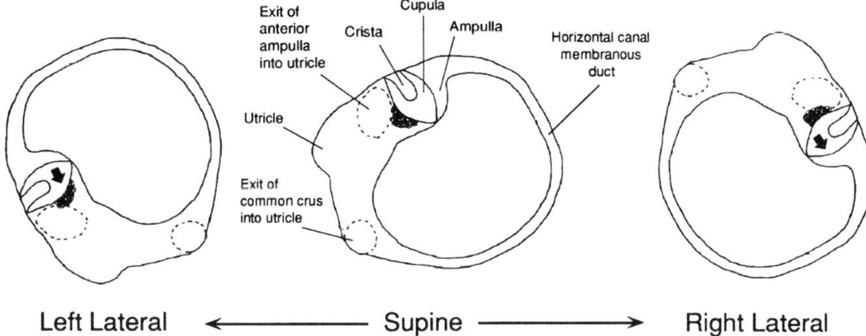

FIGURE 3.—Schematic drawing illustrating how a mass attached to the cupula of the right horizontal semicircular canal can produce apogeotropic direction-changing positional nystagmus. The shape of the horizontal canal is taken from drawings of a semicircular membranous canal dissected from a fetus by Curthoys and Oman (see original article for complete reference information). The position of the utricle and ampulla relative to the head was derived from CTs of normal human temporal bones with cuts through the horizontal semicircular canals. *Arrows* indicate the direction of cupula deviation. (Reprinted from *Neurology* volume; 45:1297–1301, 1995; by permission of Little, Brown and Company [Inc.].)

positional vertigo by the positioning maneuver used to remove debris from the posterior semicircular canal (SCC).

Clinical Findings.—Each patient initially described brief vertigo when turning in bed, bending down and straightening up, and extending the head back to look upward. Subsequently vertigo was induced by turning to either side when the patient was lying down, and it lasted for 1 minute or so after sitting up. Vertigo no longer occurred on bending down and straightening up or when the head was extended backward. Nystagmus lasted as long as the position was held, and its fast phase beat away from the ground. Vestibular function testing gave normal results.

Interpretation.—It seems likely that the static direction-changing positional nystagmus in these patients developed when debris from the posterior SCC became attached to the cupula of the horizontal canal (Fig 2). When patients turned over onto the abnormal side, the mass atop the cupula would cause it to deviate away from the utricle, inhibiting the ampullary nerve of the horizontal canal and nystagmus away from the undermost area of the ear (Fig 3). The condition in 1 patient remitted after she performed rapid side-to-side positional changes, presumably because the debris was dislodged from the cupula.

▶ Benign paroxysmal positional vertigo is the most common cause of vertigo from a peripheral abnormality. It is caused by debris (usually calcium carbonate material from the utricle) in 1 of the SCCs. Most commonly, the debris is free floating (canalithiasis) in the posterior SCC, which induces vertigo and transient upbeat/torsional nystagmus during the Hallpike-Dix maneuver. Occasionally the debris may be located in the anterior SCC, which would induce a transient downbeat/torsional nystagmus, or horizontal SCC, which would induce geotropic (beats toward the earth) nystagmus. Rarely the debris is attached to the cupula of 1 of the SCCs (cupulolithiasis), which causes sustained nystagmus and vertigo during performance of the Hallpike-Dix maneuver. For the posterior and anterior SCCs, the direction of nystagmus for cupulolithiasis is the same as canalithiasis. For the horizontal SCC, the direction of nystagmus for cupulolithiasis is in the opposite direction (ageotropic) as canalithiasis. Baloh et al. provided clear descriptions and mechanisms of the different types of BPPV. This is a particularly important paper because most cases of persistent ageotropic nystagmus have previously been attributed to either cerebellar or vestibular nuclear lesions. It is important to recognize the various types of BPPV, because all types should respond to specific types of physical therapy that relocate the debris back to the utricle. One cautionary note: Horizontal canal BPPV should not be confused with the sustained geotropic or ageotropic nystagmus occasionally seen in patients many months after labyrinthitis or vestibular neuritis. In these cases, the patient does not complain of vertigo when performing the Hallpike-Dix or roll maneuver.

R.J. Tusa, M.D., Ph.D.

Post-Prandial Hypotension in the Elderly

Aronow WS (Hebrew Hosp Home, Bronx, NY)
J R Soc Med 88:499–501, 1995

15–3

Background and Findings.—Postprandial declines in systolic blood pressure may predispose elderly persons to symptomatic hypotension and syncope or falls. However, the relationship of a marked drop in postprandial systolic blood pressure and the long-term incidence of falls, syncope, new coronary events, new stroke, and total mortality is still unclear. This relationship and management of postprandial hypotension were discussed using a recent large-scale study by Aronow and Ahn.[1] In their investigation, mean maximal decrease in postprandial systolic blood pressure was found to be 24 mm Hg in elderly nursing home residents with a recent history of syncope and 14 mm Hg in those without such a history. The mean maximal reduction in postprandial systolic pressure was 21 mm Hg in elderly residents with a recent history of falls and 13 mm Hg in those without such a history. Elderly residents treated with angiotensin-converting enzyme (ACE) inhibitors, calcium channel blockers, diuretics, nitrates, and psychotropic drugs had a significantly greater mean maximal reduction in postprandial systolic blood pressure than residents not treated with these drugs. Elderly residents with and without β-blocker treatment had similar mean maximal reductions in postprandial systolic pressure.

Pathologic Mechanisms.—Several changes that occur with aging can result in hypotension if preload is reduced. Left ventricular stiffness increases, left ventricular compliance declines, and left ventricular wall thickness increases. Also, left ventricular diastolic filling is reduced, and left ventricular relaxation is impaired. Age-associated rises in systolic pressure also hinder left ventricular filling. The reduction in baroreflex sensitivity related to aging and systemic hypertension results in impaired baroreflex-mediated increases in total systemic vascular resistance and in an inability to increase heart rate. Thus, elderly patients with systemic hypertension have more seriously impaired baroreflex sensitivity and are more likely to have postprandial hypotension. Oral glucose and insulin administration also damage baroreflex mechanisms, particularly in those with autonomic nervous system dysfunction. Some researchers have suggested that postprandial hypotension in elderly patients may partly be the result of failed sympathetic nervous system stimulation in response to insulin.

Management.—Ethyl alcohol predisposes susceptible patients to postprandial hypotension and should be avoided. Also, such patients should eat less readily digestible carbohydrates that reduce the increase in glucose level and the release of insulin. A significantly greater drop in postprandial systolic blood pressure has been associated with drugs such as ACE inhibitors, calcium channel blockers, digoxin, diuretics, nitrates, and psychotropic drugs. Greater numbers of these drugs result in greater declines in postprandial systolic blood pressure. Patients with postprandial hypotension must stop taking inessential drugs.

Conclusion.—The hemodynamic, biochemical, and hormonal responses that occur after a meal contribute to postprandial hypotension in elderly persons. Postprandial declines in systolic blood pressure can result in symptomatic hypotension and syncope or falls. Perfusion impairment in different vascular beds may produce symptoms. Research is under way to determine whether a marked decline in postprandial blood pressure is correlated with an increased incidence of falls, syncope, new coronary events, new stroke, and total mortality in the long term.

Reference

1. Aronow WS, Ahn C: Postprandial hypotension in 499 elderly persons in a long-term health care facility. *J Am Geriatr Soc* 42:930–932, 1994.

► This is an excellent, short review article on the occurrence of transient orthostatic hypotension ($\geq$ 20 mm Hg decrease in systolic pressure) in the elderly after meals. Key issues were discussed, including the unexpected high prevalence (as high as 36% in debilitated nursing home residents), risk factors (ACE inhibitors, calcium channel blockers, diuretics, nitrates, and psychotropic drugs), pathophysiology, and, most important, management. Surprisingly, β-blockers do not appear to be a problem. Current studies are under way to determine to what extent postprandial hypotension correlates with increased falls, syncope, myocardial infarctions, and cerebrovascular accidents. Because postprandial hypotension may be avoided with a change in diet and medication, we need to maintain a high degree of vigilance in ruling out this problem in our elderly patients.

R.J. Tusa, M.D., Ph.D.

Aphysiologic Performance on Dynamic Posturography

Cevette MJ, Puetz B, Marion MS, et al (Mayo Clinic Scottsdale, Ariz)
Otolaryngol Head Neck Surg 112:676–688, 1995   15–4

Background.—The evaluation of patients with disturbances in balance and inconsistencies between reported problem and performance in diagnostic tests often lacks quantitative data to demonstrate these differences. Traditional tests that examine the vestibular ocular reflex evaluate only the horizontal canal and superior vestibular nerve and may be insensitive to disorders of the otolith organs, posterior and superior semicircular canals, inferior vestibular nerves, and extravestibular causes of imbalance. Computerized dynamic posturography (CDP), a test that isolates contributions from the vestibular, visual, and somatosensory systems in patients with dizziness or imbalance, was evaluated.

Principles.—The sensory organization (SO) of CDP evaluates the amount of anteroposterior sway under varying degrees of sensory conflict with a computer-controlled, menu-driven, movable platform and visual surround. Under 6 different conditions in the SO portion of CDP (Fig 1), patients who perform relatively better on the more difficult conditions of sensory conflict than on easier ones demonstrate an aphysiologic pattern, suggesting a functional component to their on-feet balance problems.

Methods.—The performance on 6 20-sec sensory subtests of 22 patients with aphysiologic performance of on-feet balance was compared with that of 22 age-matched patients with vestibular deficits based on clinical examination and 22 age-matched patients with normal patterns (Table 1). Patients with aphysiologic CDP pattern demonstrated unusual symptoms of imbalance, gait disturbance, or vertigo, but findings on physical examination failed to correlate the patients' symptoms with any organic disease.

Results.—Patients in the aphysiologic group performed significantly better than patients in the vestibular dysfunction group on the most difficult subtests of CDP, conditions 5 and 6 in which both vision and somatosensory function were compromised. Moreover, the aphysiologic group performed significantly poorer on the easiest subtests of CDP, conditions 1 to 4. In addition, patients in the aphysiologic group tended to show greater intertrial variability compared with patients with either normal pattern or vestibular system dysfunction. A statistical model using stepwise linear discriminant analysis correctly classified 95.5% of the patients to their respective groups.

Implications.—Computerized dynamic posturography offers a quantitative analysis of a patient's balance under various sensory conditions. The data may be clinically useful in the evaluation of patients whose history and diagnostic test results provide conflicting information regarding dizziness, vertigo, or imbalance.

▶ Dynamic posturography has been used in the clinic to evaluate patients with balance problems in only the last 5 years. The diagnostic value of this test is still being evaluated. One clear value is the ability to objectively

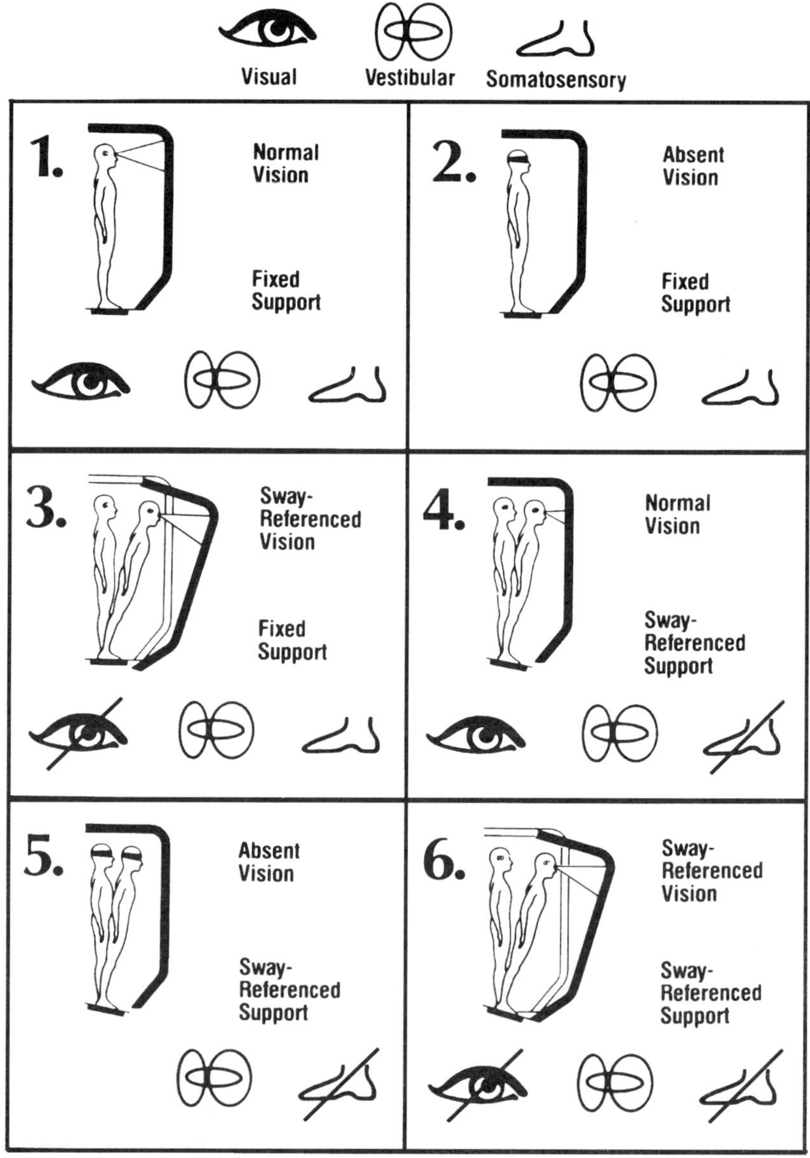

FIGURE 1.—Sensory organization protocol showing 6 sensory subtests. (Courtesy of Cevette MJ, Puetz B, Marion MS, et al: Aphysiologic performance on dynamic posturography. *Otolaryngol Head Neck Surg* 112:676–688, 1995.)

demonstrate a functional component to a balance disorder, which this article summarized extremely well. One item not discussed by this article is the possibility of missing a superimposed organic defect masked by significant functional overlay. One additional caution is the concept of a "vestibular

TABLE 1.—Patient Characteristics

Characteristics	Normal	Vestibular	Aphysiologic
Mean age (yr)	53	52	52
Age range (yr)	29–69	22–69	21–67
Sex			
Male (%)	9 (41)	8 (36)	7 (32)
Female (%)	13 (59)	14 (64)	15 (68)
Disorder (no. of patients)	No vestibular or neurologic disorder (22)	Bilateral vestibular loss (7), uncompensated unilateral vestibular loss (4), vestibulotoxicity (2), gunshot wound to left temporal bone (1), hydrocephalus (1), large acoustic neuroma (1), multiple sclerosis (1), primary cerebellar degenerative disease (1), cerebellar vascular disorder (1), postlabyrinthectomy (1), acute vertigo (2)	Possible malingering (2), somatoform disorder [conversion (2), somatization (1), NOS (10)], anxiety disorder [posttraumatic stress (2), panic disorder (1)], depressive disorder [dysthymic (1), NOS (3)]

Abbreviation: NOS, not otherwise specified.
(Courtesy of Cevette MJ, Puetz B, Marion MS, et al: Aphysiologic performance on dynamic posturography. *Otolaryngol Head Neck Surg* 112:676–688, 1995.)

pattern" seen during CDP. Although this article used this term regarding patients with increased sway or fall during sensory tests 5 and 6, this pattern is not diagnostic of a vestibular disorder. Sensory tests 5 and 6 are inherently more difficult, and patients with postural instability from nonvestibular causes also may have difficulty with these tests.

R.J. Tusa, M.D., Ph.D.

16 Neuro-ophthalmology

Leber's "Plus": Neurological Abnormalities in Patients With Leber's Hereditary Optic Neuropathy
Nikoskelainen EK, Marttila RJ, Huoponen K, et al (Univ of Turku, Finland; Emory Univ, Atlanta, Ga)
J Neurol Neurosurg Psychiatry 59:160–164, 1995   16–1

Background.—Leber's hereditary optic neuropathy (LHON) appears to be a systemic disorder with manifestations in organs other than the optic nerves. The frequency and type of neurologic dysfunctions in patients with this disorder were investigated.

Patients and Findings.—Thirty-eight men and 8 women were examined. The patients were divided into 3 groups based on mitochondrial DNA analysis: patients with the 11778 mutation, patients with the 3460 mutation, and patients with neither primary mutation. Overall, 59% had neurologic abnormalities. However, this did not differ significantly in the 3 groups. The most common finding was movement disorders. Nine patients had constant postural tremor, 1 had chronic motor tic disorder, and 1 had parkinsonism with dystonia. Peripheral neuropathy with no other apparent cause was noted in 4 patients. Two patients had a multiple sclerosis (MS)–like syndrome and MR changes in the periventricular white matter. Seven patients, 5 with the 3460 mutation, had thoracic kyphosis. The 3460 mutation was related to brain-stem involvement in 1 patient.

Conclusion.—The association of neuropathy with LHON is still uncertain. Various movement disorders, MS-like disease, and vertebral column deformities may be associated pathogenetically with LHON.

▶ The extent of neurologic involvement in LHON has been evolving. The "plus" syndromes now include an MS-like syndrome, brain-stem syndromes with ophthalmoplegia, and dystonias.

In the present report of 46 patients (38 men and 8 women), 27 patients (59%) had other neurologic abnormalities. The most common abnormality (14 patients) was a postural and action tremor of the hands. The usual tremor was identical to essential tremor. Further studies may suggest a more specific connection of tremor with LHON.

N.J. Schatz, M.D.

Noninvasive Investigation of Pericarotid Syndrome: Role of MR Angiography in the Diagnosis of Internal Carotid Dissection
Auer D, Karnath H-O, Nägele T, et al (Univ of Tübingen, Germany)
Headache 35:163–168, 1995

16–2

Background.—Magnetic resonance imaging and MR angiography (MRA) were used to diagnose pericarotid syndrome in a patient and to differentiate it from Raeder's syndrome. These noninvasive modalities proved useful in establishing the diagnosis and preclude the use of intra-arterial angiography for diagnosis.

> *Case Report.*—Male, 52, with facial pain, ptosis, and miosis underwent carotid Doppler sonography, which showed no abnormalities. Enhanced CT of the skull and orbits was normal. Magnetic resonance imaging revealed a hyperintense ring around the left internal carotid artery on T1- and T2-weighted images. Narrowing of the remaining lumen was also noted and was confirmed by a subsequent MRA. A second MRA examination of the bifurcation level demonstrated the extent of the dissection down to 1 cm above the carotid bifurcation. The patient's pain resolved after treatment with warfarin for 3 months. A follow-up MRI and MRA revealed that the hematoma had disappeared.

Discussion.—Magnetic resonance imaging and MRA are accurate, noninvasive methods that are useful in distinguishing between pericarotid syndrome and Raeder's syndrome.

▶ Magnetic resonance angiography is of localizing value in the evaluation of Horner's syndromes with acute onset of facial pain. The carotid artery in the neck, base of the skull, and cavernous sinus can be well visualized. Carotid dissections are visualized and differentiated from cavernous sinus causes and Tolosa-Hunt syndrome, without intra-arterial angiography.

N.J. Schatz, M.D.

17 Neurorehabilitation

Incidence and Consequences of Falls Due to Stroke: A Systematic Inquiry
Forster A, Young J (Saint Luke's Hosp, Bradford, England)
BMJ 311:83–86, 1995   17–1

Objective.—Falling is the most common type of accident experienced by elderly persons at home, and they are a significant threat to their health and continued independence. The specific case of falls in stroke victims was studied in a series of 108 patients aged 60 and older who lived at home after a stroke but had some degree of residual disability.

Observations.—Whereas only about one fifth of patients had fallen in the year before their stroke, nearly half fell at least once while hospitalized, and nearly three fourths fell in the 6 months after discharge. Thirty-one of the latter patients had not fallen previously. A majority of falls occurred during the day as patients undertook basic activities such as walking and transferring. Most patients who fell required help in getting up. Only 4 patients had a fracture, and only 1 was hospitalized as a direct result of falling. Soft-tissue injuries were, however, frequent.

TABLE 6.—Category Analysis of Nottingham Health Profile for Fallers and Nonfallers and General Health Questionnaire Completed by Main Carer 6 Months After Discharge From Hospital*†

Index	Non-fallers (0 or 1 falls)	Fallers ($\geq$2 falls)	χ^2	P value
Nottingham health profile:				
No of patients	50	47		
Score				
0–29	36 (72)	22 (47)	6·4	0·01
$\geq$30 (depressed mood)	14 (28)	25 (53)		
General health questionnaire†:				
No of carers	33	30		
Score:				
0–4	27 (82)	14 (47)	8·5	0·003
$\geq$5	6 (18)	16 (53)		

Note: Figures are numbers (percentages) of those able to answer questions.
 * Eleven patients (7 nonfallers and 4 fallers) had comprehension difficulties and were therefore unable to complete the profile.
 † Eleven carers (3 of nonfallers and 8 of fallers) were unable to complete the questionnaire.
 (Courtesy of Forster A, Young J: Incidence and consequences of falls due to stroke: A systematic inquiry. *BMJ* 311:83–86, 1995.)

"

Correlates.—Fifty-one of the 108 patients were classified as "fallers" because they had fallen at least twice. Fallers had significantly poorer balance at the time of hospital discharge, and they remained more disabled 6 months later than the nonfallers. There was no significant difference in comorbid conditions. Fallers were less active socially when evaluated 6 months after discharge, and more of them reported being depressed. Health profiles are contrasted in Table 6. On logistic regression analysis, only falling while hospitalized was a significant predictor of falling at home; the odds ratio was 2.0.

Conclusion.—Elderly individuals who have a stroke are at risk of falling at home. Both falling itself and the fear of falling must be addressed.

▶ This systematic natural history study of falls in older people who have been hospitalized for stroke and discharged to their homes recorded a surprisingly high incidence of falls; a full 73% fell at least once during the 6 months after discharge. The predictors of falls were degree of disability (Barthel's score), problems with balance in the hospital, and a history of falling either before the stroke or while in the hospital. Although the incidence of serious complications was low, their falls frightened and upset many patients. These observations indicate that training stroke patients how to avoid falls and how to get up after a fall should be part of their rehabilitation.

J.P. Blass, M.D., Ph.D.

Peripheral Neuropathy: A True Risk Factor for Falls
Richardson JK, Hurvitz EA (Univ of Michigan Med Ctr, Ann Arbor)
J Gerontol 50A:M211–M215, 1995   17–2

Introduction.—Recently several studies have linked peripheral nerve dysfunction in the elderly with postural instability and falls. Given the potentially high association between peripheral neuropathy (PN) and other diseases and impairments, the hypothesis that PN is not a risk factor for falls but simply a marker for a comorbidity (e.g., CNS dysfunction) that is the true cause of falls in the elderly was examined.

Methods.—Twenty patients with electromyographically documented axonal PN affecting the lower extremities were matched by age and sex with 20 individuals with normal lower extremity nerve conduction responses. Mean age was 67 for both groups. All participants underwent a focused history and physical examination designed to identify factors other than PN that might cause falls. All participants were asked about history of falls or postural instability over the previous year.

Findings.—Eleven (55%) patients with PN reported a fall within the previous year compared with only 2 (10%) control persons (odds ratio = 17; 95% confidence interval [CI] = 2.5, >100). In addition, 7 PN patients reported repetitive stumbles or a sense of unsteadiness within the previous year, but none of the control individuals did (odds ratio = 13, 95% CI = 1.5, >100). The total number of risk factors associated with falls did not

TABLE 4.—Physical Findings Within Peripheral Neuropathy Group

	Fallers	Nonfallers	*p*-value
Vibratory sense			
Toe	23.6	25.1	n.s.
Ankle	13.8 sec	9.4 sec	< .05
Finger	8.5	5.0	< .05
Unipedal stance			
(10 subjects)	3.1 sec	9.1 sec	< .05

(Courtesy of *Journal of Gerontology*; 50:M211–M215, 1995; Copyright The Gerontological Society of America.)

differ significantly between the PN and control groups. The PN group took a significantly greater number of medications associated with falls, but the usage pattern among those who did and did not fall within the PN group suggested that the medications did not play a primary role in the falls. Compared with controls, PN patients had significantly decreased unipedal stance time, more frequent abnormal Romberg testing results, areflexia at the ankle, decreased proprioception at the great toe, and decreased vibratory sensation at the toe, ankle, and finger. Among the PN group, those who reported falling in the previous year demonstrated significantly worse vibratory sensation at the ankle and finger and markedly decreased unipedal stance time than those who did not fall (Table 4).

Conclusion.—Peripheral neuropathy in the elderly is associated with an increased risk for falling, independent of other risk factors that might be expected to accompany PN, such as coincident CNS dysfunction, foot abnormality, or use of drugs associated with falls. A markedly impaired vibratory sense and a substantially diminished ability to maintain unipedal stance may identify patients with PN at particularly high risk for falls.

▶ The authors, among others, previously reported an association between PN and falls. Although this association is intuitively reasonable, the authors showed a praiseworthy willingness to test a null hypothesis. The present study tested the hypothesis that the association between PN and falls is artifactual because PN is a marker for neurologic comorbidity. In fact, their study disproved the null hypothesis and accorded with their original, intuitively attractive interpretation: Problems in motor control and in sensing the position of one's limbs make falling more likely.

J.P. Blass, M.D., Ph.D.

Pulmonary Function and Posture in Traumatic Quadriplegia

Ali J, Qi W (Univ of Toronto)
J Trauma 39:334–337, 1995   17–3

Background.—Lung volume and arterial oxygenation are influenced by body position in uninjured individuals; however, whether this same relationship exists in patients with spinal cord injury has not been determined.

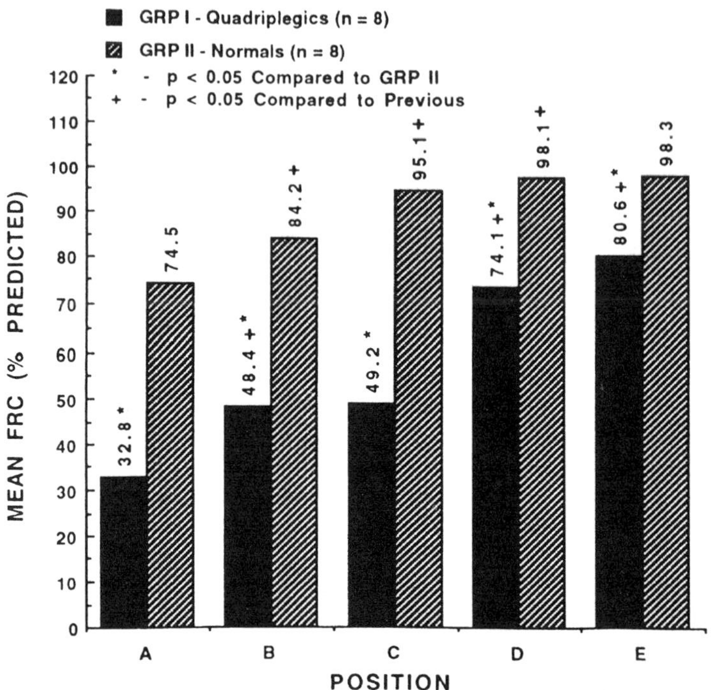

POSITION LEGEND: A = 20° Head Down; B = Horizontal; C = 35° Head Up; D = 60° Head Up; E = 90° Head Up.

FIGURE 1.—Functional residual capacity results. Functional residual capacity increased from the head-down position to the 90-degree head-up position in both groups. However, there were no changes in functional residual capacity between the horizontal position and 35-degree head-up position in quadriplegics. *Abbreviations: FRC*, functional residual capacity; *GRP*, group. (Courtesy of Ali J, Qi W: Pulmonary function and posture in traumatic quadriplegia. *J Trauma* 39[2]:334–337, 1995.)

The extent and pattern of alterations in oxygenation and lung volumes were evaluated in quadriplegic patients while they were in different body positions, and findings were compared with those noted in uninjured individuals. An understanding of the association between pulmonary function and posture may help optimize the respiratory care for spinal cord–injured patients.

Patients and Methods.—Sixteen men, aged 18 to 32, were enrolled in the study. Eight had sustained traumatic quadriplegia (C6–C7) at least 12 months before study enrollment (group 1). The remaining 8 participants were healthy volunteers who served as controls (group 2). Functional residual capacity (FRC), forced vital capacity (FVC), and arterial blood gases were measured while participants breathed room air in 5 different body positions: 20 degrees head down, horizontal, 35 degrees head up, 60 degrees head up, and 90 degrees head up. Within- and between-group findings were compared.

Results.—In group 1 patients, FRC was lower in all positions measured. A similar directional change in FRC with posture was noted, however, in both groups. Forced residual capacity was found to be highest between the 35-degree head-up and the 60-degree head-up positions among group 1 patients. Unlike group 2 controls, FVC decreased from the 35-degree head-up position to the 60-degree head-up position in group 1 patients. No significant changes in partial pressure of oxygen (PO_2) with position were observed in the controls. In contrast, PO_2 improved from the head down to the horizontal and 60-degree head-up positions in group 1 patients (Figs 1–3).

Conclusion.—Patterns of change in FRC, FVC, and arterial PO_2 with changes in posture differ between uninjured individuals and patients with traumatic quadriplegia. These differences should be considered when the best course of respiratory care for traumatic quadriplegic patients is de-

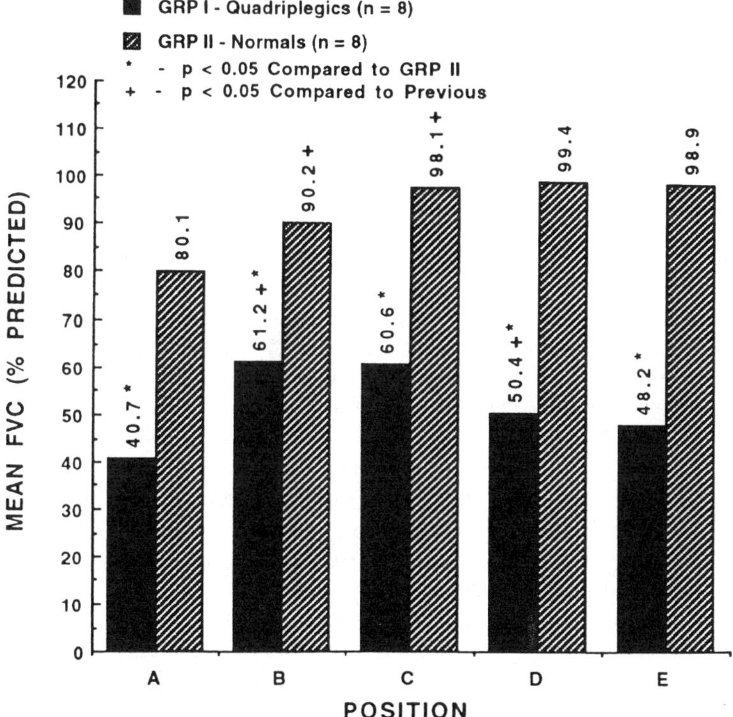

FIGURE 2.—Forced vital capacity results. Forced vital capacity was lower in all positions in quadriplegics. However, in contrast to normal, the highest forced vital capacity results in quadriplegics were in the horizontal and 35-degree head-up positions. Forced vital capacity decreased in the quadriplegic group between the 35-degree head-up position and the 60-degree head-up position. *Abbreviations: FVC,* forced vital capacity; *GRP,* group. (Courtesy of Ali J, Qi W: Pulmonary function and posture in traumatic quadriplegia. *J Trauma* 39[2]:334–337, 1995.)

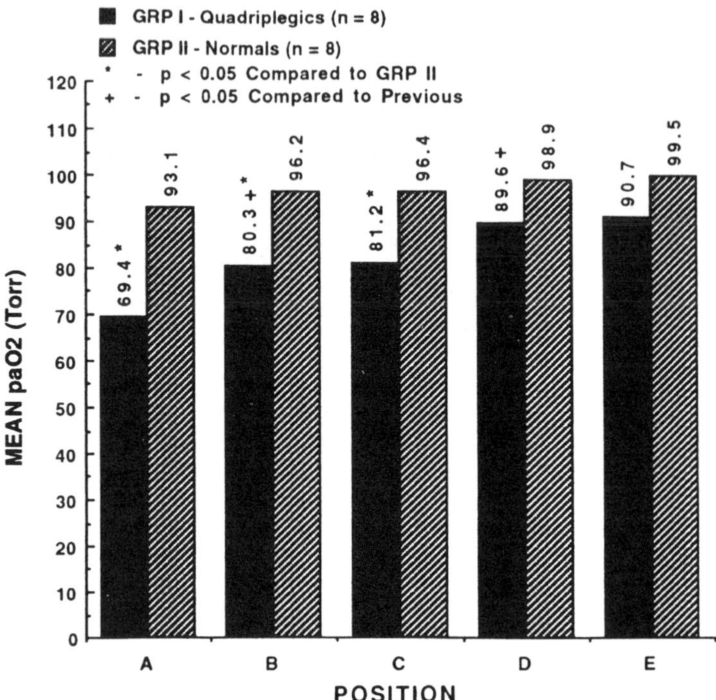

FIGURE 3.—Results of paO$_2$. In both groups the PaO$_2$ progressively increased from the head-down position to the 90-degree head-up position. However, the quadriplegic group maintained lower paO$_2$ in all positions. *Abbreviations: paO$_2$*, arterial partial pressure of oxygen; *GRP*, group. (Courtesy of Ali J, Qi W: Pulmonary function and posture in traumatic quadriplegia. *J Trauma* 39[2]:334–337, 1995.)

termined. The present findings indicate that in quadriplegic patients, the best position for respiratory physiotherapy, such as deep breathing and coughing, is between the horizontal and the 35-degree head-up position. Conversely, maximum oxygenation and patency of alveoli at rest are best achieved in the 60- to 90-degree head-up positions in these patients.

▶ This careful study provided documentation that the best position for pulmonary physiotherapy in quadriplegic patients is relatively flat, whereas the best oxygenation is achieved when the patients are more upright (between 60 and 90 degrees). Although the results are not surprising, it is gratifying that this commonly used approach is buttressed by careful physiologic measurements. It is a gratifying instance of clinical science bearing out clinical lore.

J.T. Blass, M.D., Ph.D.

Effects of Transcutaneous Electrical Nerve Stimulation (TENS) on Spasticity in Patients With Hemiplegia
Potisk KP, Gregorič M, Vodovnik L, et al (Univ of Ljubljana, Slovenia)
Scand J Rehabil Med 27:169–174, 1995   17–4

Background.—In patients with spastic muscle hypertonia and clonus, electrical stimulation of the nerves and muscles can help to suppress abnormally increased tonic and phasic stretch reflex activity. One study has found that transcutaneous electrical nerve stimulation (TENS) applied to the sural nerve produces lasting changes in sensory function and in the excitability of the soleus muscle, though some other studies have failed to confirm these results. The effects of TENS applied to the sural nerve on stretch reflex activity in the leg muscles of patients with chronic spastic hemiplegia were studied.

Methods.—The study included 20 patients with hemiplegia after stroke at least 3 months previously. All received standard cutaneous stimulation with TENS at an impulse frequency of 100 Hz, applied via stimulation electrodes applied over the sural nerve. An electrohydraulic measuring brace was used to assess leg tonus. As the biomechanical parameters were measured, surface electrodes made simultaneous recordings of electromyographic (EMG) stretch reflex activity of the tibialis anterior and triceps surae muscles. Spasticity measurements were made immediately after 20 minutes of TENS and repeated at intervals for up to 60 minutes.

Results.—Immediately after TENS, 90% of patients had significant reductions in resistive torque at all frequencies of passive ankle joint movement (Fig 1). The average reduction was 12%, with a range of 3% to 39%. In 75% of patients, resistive torque decreased along with a decrease

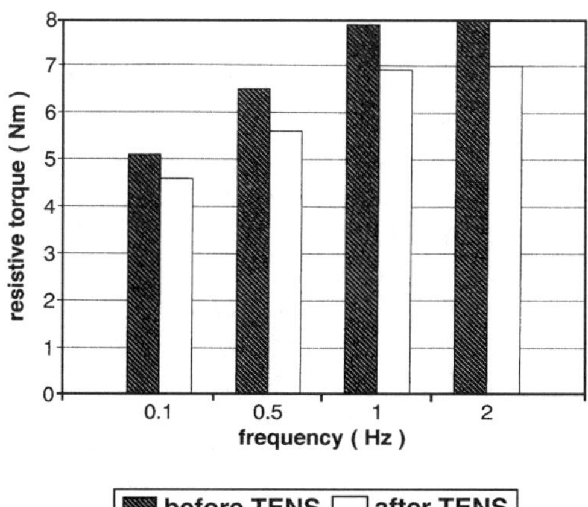

FIGURE 1.—Mean values of resistive torque at different frequencies of passive ankle joint movements (0.1, 0.5, 1, and 2 Hz) obtained before TENS and immediately after TENS in 20 patients with hemiplegia or hemiparesis. *Abbreviation: TENS,* transcutaneous electrical nerve stimulation. (Courtesy of Potisk KP, Gregorič M, Vodovnik L, et al: Effects of transcutaneous electrical nerve stimulation (TENS) on spasticity in patients with hemiplegia. *Scand J Rehabil Med* 27:169–174, 1995.)

in reflex EMG activity. The reductions in resistive torque were still present 15, 30, and 45 minutes after TENS application, though not at 60 minutes.

Conclusion.—In patients with poststroke hemiplegia, application of TENS to the sural nerve appears to produce immediate and short-term inhibition of abnormally enhanced stretch reflex activity in the spastic muscles. The neurophysiologic mechanisms underlying the beneficial effects of afferent electrical stimulation remain to be determined but could involve activation of the opiate analgetic system. A single TENS treatment has no significant prolonged effects that could be useful for therapeutic purposes.

▶ This study from Slovenia documented by objective measurements that TENS appears to reduce spasticity in hemiplegic patients. The lack of a sham-stimulated control makes it hard to specify that the effect was specific, particularly because the authors argued that the effect seen may be caused by increased level of endorphins, and an increased level of endorphins is a well-known response to placebos. Nevertheless, whatever the mechanisms, TENS is a simple, almost noninterventive procedure, applicable within the home given the proper equipment, which might help to reduce the complications and discomfort associated with spasticity. Clearly further studies, including studies of clinical relevance, are needed.

J.P. Blass, M.D.

Investigation of the Neurogenic Bladder
Fowler CJ (Natl Hosp for Neurology and Neurosurgery, London)
J Neurol Neurosurg Psychiatry 60:6–13, 1996   17–5

Introduction.—Cystometry, uroflowmetry, ultrasound scanning of the urinary tract, and neurophysiologic investigations of the sphincters and pelvic floor are used to evaluate patients with a neurogenic bladder. This article summarizes the history of the development of urodynamics and neurophysiologic investigations were summarized and the principles underlying the various methods of examination discussed. An algorithm for the management of patients with neurogenic bladder disorders was also presented.

Cystometry.—The technique of cystometry, the recording of the pressure-volume relation of the bladder, can be understood by observing the preparatory stages of cystometric recordings when the patient is asked to cough (Fig 1). Intravesical and intra-abdominal pressures are measured by passing a fine catheter through the urethra into the bladder and another into the rectum. Measurement of detrusor pressure, both during filling and while the patient attempts to micturate, provides important information. The most common finding in neurogenic bladder is an abrupt rise in detrusor pressure, usually accompanied by urinary urgency (Fig 2). This "detrusor hyperreflexia" may result from a disorder of the detrusor muscle.

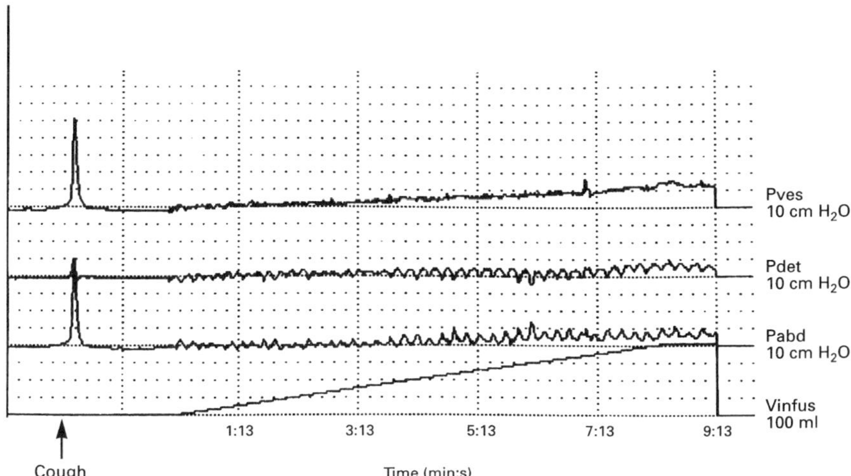

FIGURE 1.—Filling cystometry in a healthy subject. Respiratory movements were not recorded with the intravesical pressure measurements but instead were recorded with the rectal pressure line; therefore these appear as an artefact due to subtraction on Pdet. In the early part of the trace, the subject was asked to cough; the subtraction of Pabd from Pves was complete, so no rise in Pdet is recorded. Pdet = Pves = Pabd. *Abbreviations: Pves*, intravesical pressure; *Pdet*, detrusor pressure; *Pabd*, intra-abdominal pressure measured by the rectal line; *Vinfus*, infusion at 50 mL/min. (Courtesy of Fowler CJ: Investigation of the neurogenic bladder. *J Neurol Neurosurg Psychiatry* 60:6–13, 1996.)

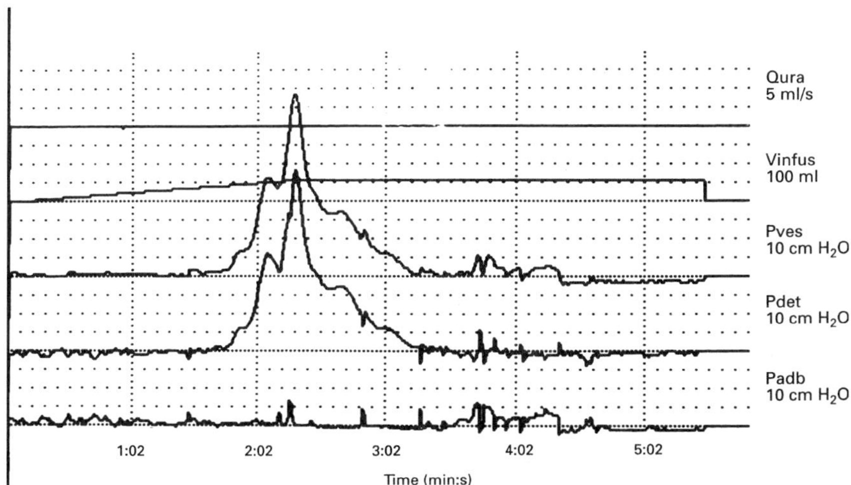

FIGURE 2.—Detrusor hyperreflexia in a woman with multiple sclerosis. After filling to 100 mL (*Vinfus*), there was a detrusor contraction, which resulted in a pressure rise of 90 cm H₂O. *Abbreviations: Qura*, rate of urine flow; *Vinfus*, infusion at 50 mL/min; *Pves*, intravesical pressure; *Pdet*, detrusor pressure; *Padb*, intra-abdominal pressure. (Courtesy of Fowler CJ: Investigation of the neurogenic bladder. *J Neurol Neurosurg Psychiatry* 60:6–13, 1996.)

Uroflowmetry.—Measurement of urinary flow rate is a noninvasive investigation performed when the patient has a full bladder. The patient voids into a receptacle with a spinning wheel in its base, and a graphical output of flow rate is produced. Combined with ultrasound scanning of postmicturition residual volume, outflow obstruction can be detected and the management of patients with neurogenic bladder planned.

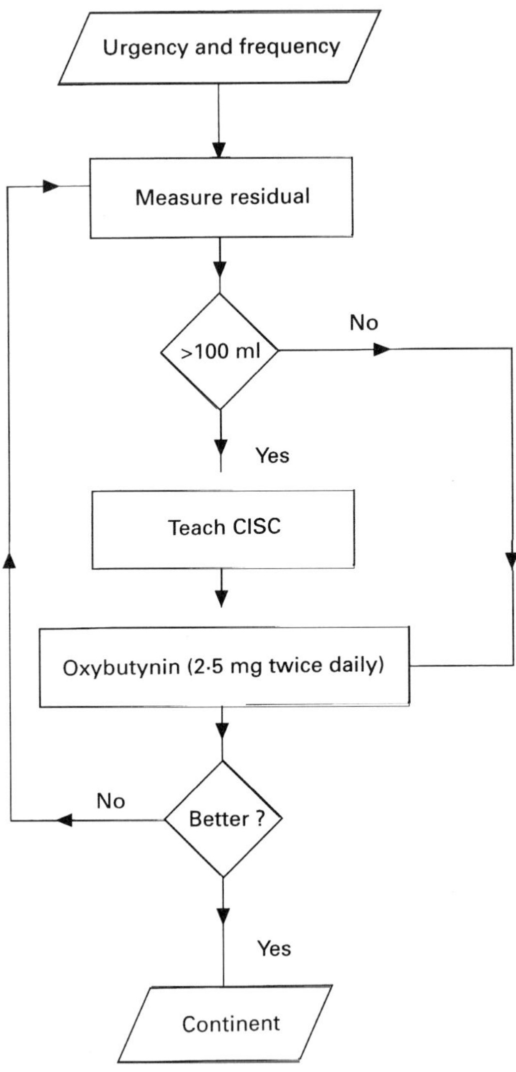

FIGURE 6.—Algorithm for management of patients with neurogenic bladder disorders. If this algorithm is followed, both aspects of bladder dysfunction (incomplete emptying and hyperreflexia) are treated. (Courtesy of Fowler CJ: Investigation of the neurogenic bladder. *J Neurol Neurosurg Psychiatry* 60:6–13, 1996.)

Neurophysiologic Investigations.—Several clinical neurophysiologic techniques that initially appeared promising have not proved to be useful investigations. Changes of denervation and chronic reinnervation in patients with cauda equina lesions or suspected multiple system atrophy can be detected, however, by electromyography (EMG) of the striated muscle of the pelvic floor. Urethral sphincter EMG is also useful in identifying a number of conditions and in ruling out others.

Conclusion.—Neurologists have met with difficulty when investigating the neurogenic bladder. Presenting symptoms may be few, the bladder cannot be examined clinically, and there are many bladder diseases of unknown cause. Patients sent by urologists to neurologists should have spinal cord disease excluded. In older patients, a high index of suspicion for multiple system atrophy is recommended. The algorithm in Figure 6 considers treatment options.

▶ Uroneurology is a new subspecialty discipline of neurology. It has advanced the understanding of the basic pathophysiology of urinary sphincter disturbance and of sexual dysfunction. The underlying concepts are relatively straightforward, and diagnosis depends on the results of relatively simple investigations. This review by Fowler set out clearly the use of these tests.

W.G. Bradley, D.M., F.R.C.P.

18 Other Neurologic Disorders

Stiff-Person Syndrome With Anti-Glutamic Acid Decarboxylase Autoantibodies: Complete Remission of Symptoms After Intrathecal Baclofen Administration

Seitz RJ, Blank B, Kiwit JCW, et al (Heinrich-Heine-Univ, Düsseldorf, Germany)

J Neurol 242:618–622, 1995

18–1

Background.—Stiff-person syndrome (SPS) is an uncommon disorder of the CNS. The condition generally progresses gradually and is known to cause stiffness of the axial and proximal muscles and startle reactions with sudden spasms. Administration of γ-aminobutyric acid (GABA) agonists has been found to result in symptom improvement in patients with SPS and anti-glutamic acid decarboxylase (GAD) autoantibodies. When given orally, however, these agents must be administered at high doses to suppress muscular hyperactivity, leading to various adverse effects, such as drowsiness and vertigo. Intrathecal administration is reportedly more efficient than oral delivery and is associated with fewer side effects. A patient with severe SPS whose stiffness was resolved with intrathecal administration of baclofen, a $GABA_B$ agonist, is described.

Case Report.—Woman, 61, received a diagnosis of severe immobilizing SPS, confirmed by electrophysiological findings, demonstration of autoantibodies against GAD in serum and CSF, and the presence of the typical clinical symptoms. The patient also had been given a diagnosis of IDDM when she was 40.

Stiffness of the legs, abdomen, back, and neck was noted, and the patient was unable to walk or sit. Startle reactions with suddenly increasing muscle stiffness caused by unanticipated acoustic, visual, or tactile stimuli also were reported.

Treatment with IV insulin, isosorbide dinitrate, nifedipine, omeprazole, heparin, pethidine, buprenorphine, metamizole, and diclofenac all failed to relieve the patient's symptoms. Symptomatic therapy with continuous intrathecal baclofen, administered at a daily dosage of 260 μg by subcutaneous pump, was subsequently initiated. The patient experienced a rapid clinical recovery and was able to walk with crutches. After 12 months, the patient had improved further. Her gait pattern also had normalized, and only 1 crutch was needed. At 24 months, her condition was stabilized, and her gait pattern was normal without crutches.

To prove that intrathecal baclofen was still effective, the patient was hospitalized and therapy interrupted. Her SPS-related symptoms returned within 18 hours of treatment termination, and she was once again unable to walk. Typical spontaneous muscle activity also was observed in surface electromyographic recordings of the trunk and leg muscles. Reinitiation of intrathecal baclofen at 260 μg daily led to complete recovery within 48 hours.

Conclusion.—Early treatment with intrathecal baclofen can effectively abolish symptoms in patients with SPS and anti-GAD autoantibodies without the systemic side effects associated with oral administration of this agent. Additional studies are needed to determine whether patients with paraneoplastic SPS and idiopathic SPS without anti-GAD autoantibodies would similarly benefit from intrathecal baclofen therapy.

▶ The SPS may be idiopathic or paraneoplastic, and may be associated with or without autoantibodies to GAD. The condition is uncommon and frequently difficult to diagnose. Oral therapy with baclofen or diazepam is usually of limited benefit. These 2 reports of 4 patients indicate that intrathecal baclofen is more effective than oral medication. The degree of benefit can vary from patient to patient, but can be very gratifying in some cases. Long infusion of baclofen by intrathecal pump will probably become the treatment of choice for this interesting condition.

W.G. Bradley, D.M., F.R.C.P.

Intrathecal Baclofen Therapy in Stiff-Man Syndrome: A Double-Blind, Placebo-Controlled Trial
Silbert PL, Matsumoto JY, McManis PG, et al (Mayo Clinic and Mayo Found, Rochester, Minn)
Neurology 45:1893–1897, 1995   18–2

Background.—Stiff-man syndrome (SMS) is an uncommon disease, the cause of which has not yet been determined. The condition is characterized by involuntary stiffness of axial and lower-extremity muscles, accompanied by painful muscle spasms. In some patients with SMS, reduced levels of CSF γ-aminobutyric acid (GABA) have been documented. Baclofen, a GABA agonist, therefore may offer appropriate therapy, although oral administration of this agent is associated with inadequate CSF penetration and patient response frequently is insufficient. Intrathecal baclofen (ITB), however, results in CSF levels up to 50 times greater using only $\frac{1}{100}$th of the oral dose, thus avoiding the high systemic levels noted with oral administration. The clinical efficacy of ITB was evaluated in a double-blind, placebo-controlled trial.

Patients and Methods.—Three patients with SMS refractory to current treatment regimens were enrolled in the study. Symptoms had been present for either 10 years, 6 years, or 4 years. Patients were assigned to receive 50 μg of ITB or placebo on sequential days and were asked to document improvement or deterioration in symptoms before, 90 minutes after, and 3.5 hours after injections. Electrophysiologic evaluations were performed approximately 90 minutes before and 90 minutes after each intrathecal injection. Clinical assessments of muscle tone and stiffness, done before and approximately 2.5 hours after the injection using the Ashworth score, also were completed.

Results.—Although subjective improvement was noted by only 1 patient after ITB treatment, improvements in reflex electromyographic (EMG) activity were observed in all 3 patients after the ITB injection. After stimulation of the medial plantar nerve, the mean reduction in total EMG activity from all muscles was 72% and 18% with ITB and placebo. A significantly extended mean latency to onset of the response also was noted for all muscles after ITB. The Ashworth score decreased from 3 to 2 in 2 patients and from 4 to 3 in the third patient after ITB, whereas no changes in scores were noted after placebo.

Conclusion.—Patients with SMS may benefit from treatment with ITB, as demonstrated by the significant postinjection electrophysiologic improvements observed in this study. The overall patient response did not, however, always correspond with this improvement. Long-term clinical efficacy of ITB remains to be established.

▶ Stiff-person syndrome may be idiopathic or paraneoplastic and may be associated with or without autoantibodies to GAD. The condition is uncommon and frequently difficult to diagnose. Oral therapy with baclofen or diazepam is usually of limited benefit. These 2 reports of 4 patients indicate that intrathecal baclofen is more effective than oral medication. The degree of benefit can vary from patient to patient but can be very gratifying in some cases. Long infusion of baclofen by intrathecal pump will probably become the treatment of choice for this interesting condition.

W.G. Bradley, D.M., F.R.C.P.

Peripheral Neuropathy With Necrotizing Vasculitis in Rheumatoid Arthritis: A Clinicopathologic and Prognostic Study of Thirty-Two Patients
Puéchal X, Said G, Hilliquin P, et al (Univ René Descartes, Paris; Univ Paris XI)
Arthritis Rheum 38:1618–1629, 1995   18–3

Introduction.—Peripheral neuropathy in patients with rheumatoid arthritis appears to be related to the presence of necrotizing vasculitis.

Thirty-two patients with sensory or sensorimotor neuropathy and documented necrotizing vasculitis in nerve or muscle biopsy specimens were examined for clinical and pathologic features and factors associated with survival.

Methods.—Eligible patients had pathologic features of classic polyarteritis nodosa and were free of any other systemic disease or malignancy. The 23 women and 9 men who entered the study had a mean age of 59 at diagnosis of vasculitis and a mean duration of arthritis of 16 years. A single examiner interpreted all of the neuromuscular biopsy specimens. Morphologic analysis included light and electron microscopy studies and teased fiber preparation. Survival was assessed by life-table analysis, and Cox proportional hazards models were used to determine the prognostic values of clinical, biological, and pathologic findings.

Results.—Common clinical features were a low-grade fever (40%), weight loss (40%), and cutaneous lesions (38%). The 32 patients had 35 episodes of peripheral neuropathy. Mononeuritis was present in 14% of patients, mononeuritis multiplex in 51%, and distal symmetric sensory or sensorimotor neuropathy in 34%. Epineural or perineural vasculitis (or both) was associated with axonal degeneration of an average of 77.7% of the nerve fibers. Corticosteroid therapy was given to 75% of patients for a mean of 8 years.

During follow-up (mean 7.2 years) 53% experienced a full, prolonged remission of the vasculitis; 25% had a relapse. Fourteen patients (44%) died of systemic vasculitis, or infectious complications, or both during the study. Survival rates after a diagnosis of vasculitis were 64% at 3 years, 57% at 5 years, and 45% at 10 years. In decreasing order of importance, factors correlated with mortality were clinical cutaneous vasculitis, neuropathy affecting 3 or 4 limbs, and a depressed complement C4 level at the time of diagnosis. The administration of high-dose corticosteroids or immunosuppressive agents at the time of diagnosis did not affect survival. Although extent of neuropathy had a significant prognostic impact, motor involvement did not.

Conclusion.—Necrotizing vasculitis accounts for the different patterns of noncompressive neuropathies in rheumatoid arthritis. The best predictors of mortality in patients with systemic rheumatoid vasculitis are clinical features at diagnosis, primarily cutaneous involvement, extent of neuropathy, and depressed C4 levels.

▶ Peripheral nerve damage occurs in a number of different forms in rheumatoid arthritis, including polyneuropathy due to local compression related to the arthritis, multiple mononeuropathies, a mild distal sensory neuropathy, and a sensorimotor polyneuropathy. This is an excellent report of 32 patients studied clinically and pathologically. It has previously been suggested that patients with a rapidly progressive symmetric sensorimotor neuropathy and those treated with corticosteroids have a worse prognosis. This study allowed a greater insight into prognostic factors. A caveat is that the treatment regime was not standardized, and hence more studies are needed to define the best therapy. For patients with a worse prognosis, combined high-dose prednisone and oral cyclophosphamide therapy is probably the treatment of choice.

W.G. Bradley, D.M., F.R.C.P.

Lupus Transverse Myelopathy: Better Outcome With Early Recognition and Aggressive High-Dose Intravenous Corticosteroid Pulse Treatment

Harisdangkul V, Doorenbos D, Subramony SH (Univ of Mississippi Med Ctr, Jackson)
J Neurol 242:326–331, 1995   18–4

Background.—Although uncommon, transverse myelopathy (TM) can be associated with systemic lupus erythematosus (SLE). In such patients, this syndrome tends to be severe, with a poor prognosis. Intravenous methylprednisolone and cyclophosphamide pulse treatment may yield better outcomes. Seven patients with TM associated with SLE were retrospectively identified at 1 center. Diagnostic and clinical features, treatment, and outcomes were reported.

Methods.—The 7 patients were treated between 1975 and 1990. All patients were female aged 16 to 52. Four had not been previously diagnosed as having SLE. Antinuclear antibody testing results were positive in all 6 patients. A spinal syndrome progressing to TM with cervical or thoracic levels was documented in all patients. Neurologic and neuroradiographic studies confirmed the diagnosis of TM. Outcomes were poor when the diagnosis and treatment were delayed. Four women died, and 1 was confined to a wheelchair. The 2 patients who retained their ability to walk without assistance were treated with high-dose IV pulse corticosteroid within 1 week of TM onset.

Conclusion.—Patients with TM associated with SLE have a poor prognosis if diagnosis and aggressive treatment are delayed. In this series, the 2 patients treated with IV methylprednisolone within 1 week of TM onset had better outcomes.

▶ Transverse myelopathy occurring as a consequence of SLE, although rare, is associated with a high morbidity and mortality. As illustrated in this study, in which only 2 of their 7 patients had an established diagnosis of SLE before developing TM, a high index of suspicion must be maintained for the diagnosis because it may occur as the heralding manifestation of SLE. Although this study was small, a compelling argument for early aggressive treatment with high-dose, IV corticosteroid pulse therapy was made. The appropriate duration of this high-dose corticosteroid therapy remained uncertain, but relapse of the TM after discontinuation of conventional doses of prednisone once ambulatory ability had returned suggests that many months, if not years, of immunosuppressive is warranted.

J.R. Berger, M.D.

Natural Course of Cervical Spine Lesions in Rheumatoid Arthritis

Oda T, Fujiwara K, Yonenobu K, et al (Osaka Univ, Suita, Japan; Hoshigaoka Koseinenkin Hosp, Hirakata, Japan; Kansai Rosai Hosp, Amagasaki, Japan)
Spine 20:1128–1135, 1995   18–5

Objective.—Widely varying proportions of patients with rheumatoid arthritis are reported to have cervical spine involvement. The course of cervical spine lesions was examined by longitudinal radiographic review in 49 patients with a diagnosis of classic or definite rheumatoid disease and at least a 5-year follow-up. Dynamic cervical radiographs were obtained for an average of nearly 8 years. Forty-seven patients were followed for longer than 10 years.

Methods.—Criteria for cervical subluxation included an anterior atlantodental interval (ADI) of 3 mm or more on a lateral flexion radiograph, a Ranawat vertical subluxation measurement of less than 13 mm, and a distance of 3 mm or more between the posterior borders of adjacent vertebrae (Fig 1).

Findings.—Sixteen patients initially had anterior atlantoaxial subluxation (AAS) alone, and 8 had vertical subluxation (VS). By the time of final follow-up, all but 11 patients exhibited subluxation. Nineteen patients had

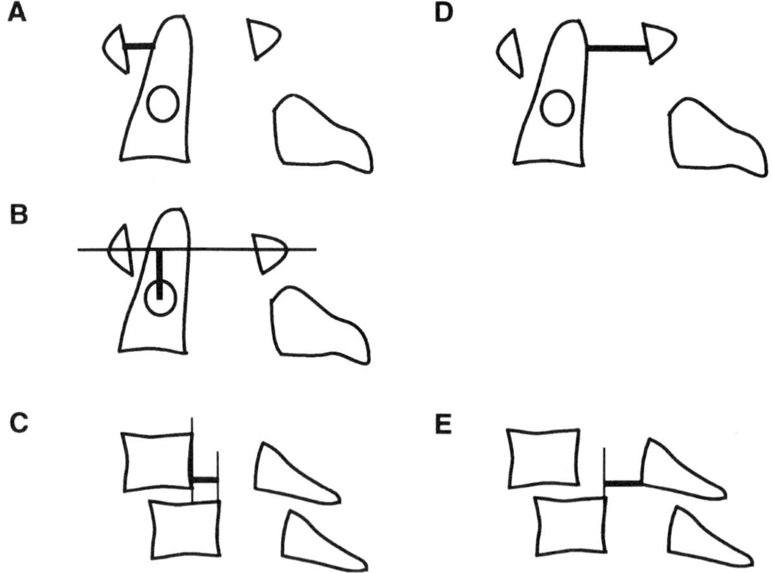

FIGURE 1.—Measurements of cervical lateral radiographs. **A,** anterior ADI for the diagnosis of anterior AAS. **B,** measuring method of Ranawat et al. (see original article for complete reference information) for the diagnosis of vertical subluxation of the axis. **C,** measurement for the diagnosis of subaxial subluxation. **D,** posterior ADI as an indirect indication of the space available for the spinal cord at the anterior AAS. **E,** sagittal canal diameter as an indirect indication of the space available for the spinal cord at the subaxial subluxation. *Abbreviations: ADI,* atlantodental interval; *AAS,* atlantoaxial subluxation. (Courtesy of Oda T, Fujiwara K, Yonenobu K, et al: Natural course of cervical spine lesions in rheumatoid arthritis. *Spine* 20:1128–1135, 1995.)

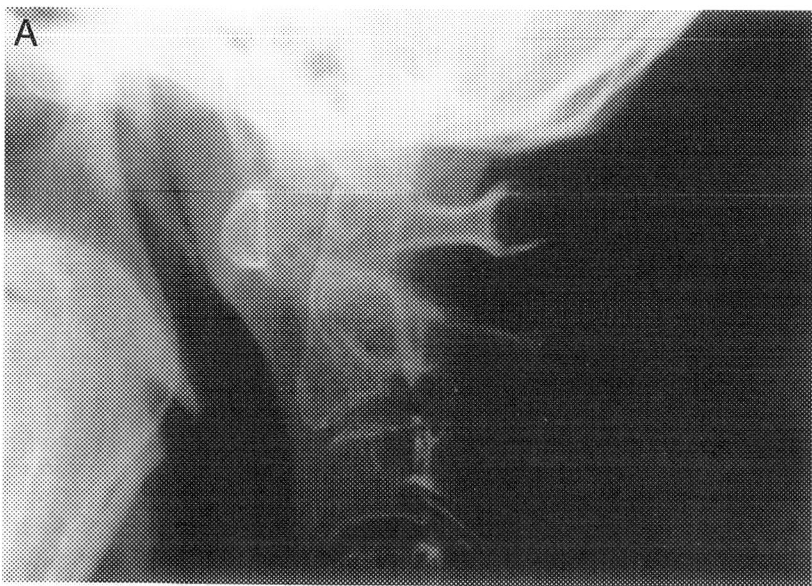

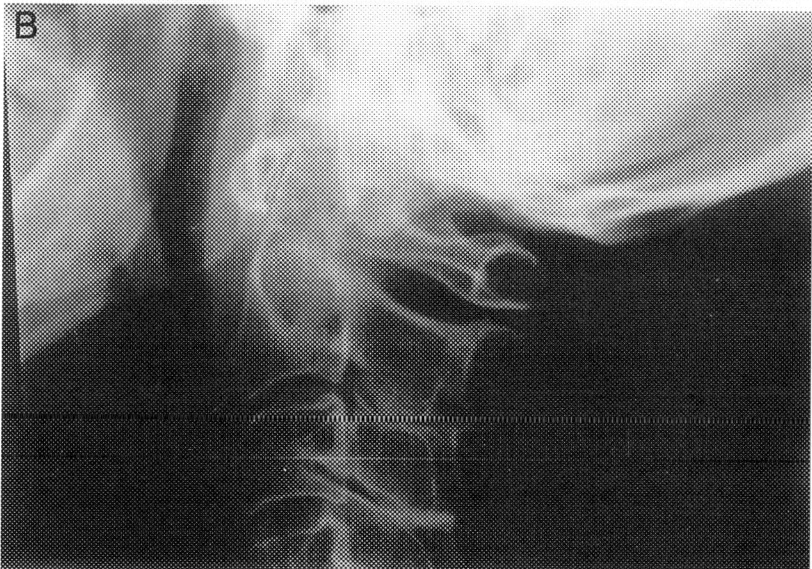

FIGURE 3.—Anterior atlantoaxial subluxation. **A,** flexion (atlantodental interval = 10 mm). **B,** extension (atlantodental interval = 1.5 mm). Subluxation was reduced. (Courtesy of Oda T, Fujiwara K, Yonenobu K, et al: Natural course of cervical spine lesions in rheumatoid arthritis. *Spine* 20:1128–1135, 1995.)

AAS alone at this time, and 19 had VS. A common initial finding in patients in whom AAS developed was erosive change at the posterior surface of the odontoid process. In all cases AAS was reducible by extending the neck (Fig 3). Anterior atlantodental subluxation that was initially reducible often became irreducible when VS developed. Seven patients had subaxial subluxation (SS) initially, and in 4 others it developed during follow-up. Neurologic deficits developed in only 3 patients, 2 of them secondary to AAS and 1 from SS.

Conclusion.—In patients with rheumatoid disease of the cervical spine, involvement progresses from reducible AAS to irreducible subluxation with a vertical component. The most caudal area of fusion should be followed closely in postoperative patients so that new subluxation may be detected at an early stage.

▶ Rheumatoid arthritis undoubtedly causes degenerative cervical spine changes. The most dramatic is the atlantoaxial dislocation that can be clinically demonstrated by the somewhat horrifying "clunk sign," elicited when the flexed head is moved backward and forward by the examiner. Although radiologically demonstrated disease is frequent in cross-sectional studies of a population of patients with rheumatoid arthritis, the progress of the disorder and its relationship to the development of neurologic signs remain undetermined. This longitudinal study nicely demonstrated the progression of cervical spine degeneration of quite dramatic type. Interestingly, it appears that cervical myelopathy developed in only 3 patients (6%) during an average of 8 years' follow-up. Sudden death from medullary compression is a risk in patients with atlantoaxial subluxation, but this study confirmed that spinal cord damage in severe rheumatoid arthritis is relatively rare. Patients should, however, be strongly advised about the need for high headrests in motor vehicles.

W.G. Bradley, D.M., F.R.C.P.

Therapeutic Considerations in Patients With Refractory Neurosarcoidosis
Agbogu BN, Stern BJ, Sewell C, et al (Sinai Hosp of Baltimore, Md; Johns Hopkins Hosp, Baltimore, Md)
Arch Neurol 52:875–879, 1995   18–6

Background.—Patients with the multisystem granulomatous disorder sarcoidosis have enhanced cellular immune processes at the sites involved with the disease. About 5% of affected patients have neurosarcoidosis (NS), and about one third of patients with NS will have refractory disease. Morbidity and mortality are high in refractory NS, which may involve mass lesions of the CNS, hydrocephalus, or diffuse encephalopathy or vasculopathy. Treatment to control the symptoms of refractory NS may require long-term, high-dose corticosteroids. Cyclosporine or other immunosuppressive agents may be used, but there have been no critical evaluations of these alternative forms of therapy. The clinical course of patients with refractory NS receiving alternative treatment was reviewed.

Patients.—The review included 14 women and 12 men (mean age 44) with refractory NS. Common clinical manifestations of NS included cra-

TABLE 2.—Percentage Frequency of Clinical Manifestations
of Neurosarcoidosis

Clinical Manifestation	Approximate Overall Frequency, %	Refractory Neurosarcoidosis (n = 26)
Cranial neuropathy	50–75	54
Facial palsy	25–50	12
Aseptic meningitis	10–20	31
Hydrocephalus	10	38
Parenchymal disease		
Endocrinopathy	10–15	54
Mass lesion	5–10	50
Encephalopathy/vasculopathy	5–10	42
Seizures	5–10	39
Neuropathy	5–10	46
Myopathy	10	46

(From Agbogu BN, Stern BJ, Sewell C, et al: Therapeutic considerations in patients with refractory neurosarcoidosis. *Arch Neurol* 532:875–879, 1995. Courtesy of Stern BJ, Schonfeld A: Neurosarcoidosis, in Arieff AI, Griggs RC [eds]: *Metabolic Brain Dysfunction in Systemic Disorders*. Boston, Little, Brown, 1992, pp 289–312.)

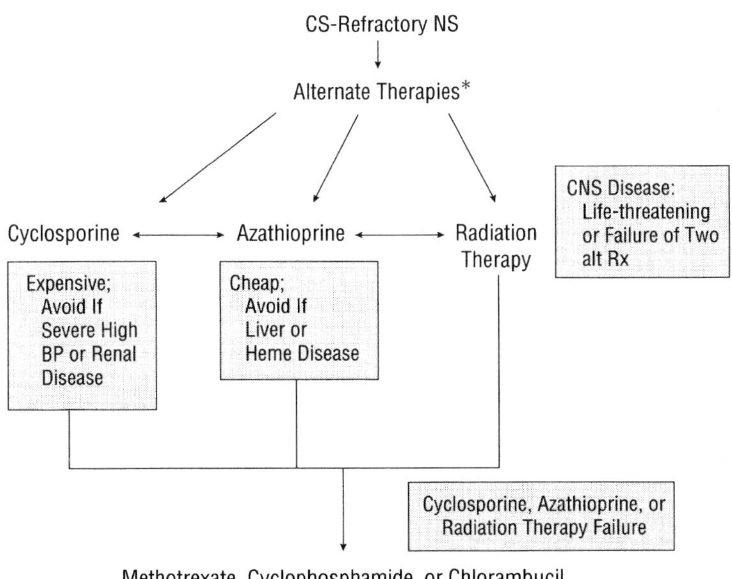

FIGURE 3.—Algorithm for the use of alternate treatment for refractory neurosarcoidosis. *Asterisk* means excluding surgery. *Abbreviations: CS,* corticosteroid; *NS,* neurosarcoidosis; *BP,* blood pressure; *alt Rx,* alternative treatments; *Heme,* hematologic; *Pulm,* pulmonary. (Courtesy of Agbogu BN, Stern BJ, Sewell C, et al: Therapeutic considerations in patients with refractory neurosarcoidosis. *Arch Neurol* 52:875–879, 1995.)

nial neuropathy, endocrinopathy, and mass lesions (Table 2). All patients received alternate treatments in addition to corticosteroids, including azathioprine, cyclosporine, cyclophosphamide, chlorambucil, methotrexate, and radiation therapy. Mean follow-up was 81 months.

Outcomes.—In 38% of patients, prednisone dosage was tapered to 10 to 20 mg/day without a worsening effect on symptoms. Alternative medications were associated with an improvement in condition for 23% of patients and with stabilization in 35%. One of 3 patients receiving radiotherapy seemed to benefit. Fifteen percent of patients failed to respond to alternative treatment; these 4 patients eventually died of worsening symptoms or infection. Although the alternative treatments had some adverse effects, these resolved when the treatment was discontinued.

Conclusion.—Some patients with refractory NS will benefit from alternative forms of therapy in addition to corticosteroids. An algorithm for the use of such treatments is presented (Fig 3). Alternative treatments should be chosen according to their potential adverse effects and the extent of the patient's systemic disease; it is best to select a treatment with adverse effects that spare organs that are already inflamed. Some patients' conditions will continue to deteriorate despite the use of alternative therapies.

▶ Having recently confronted a large number of patients with refractory NS (this disorder seems to be far more prevalent in Kentucky than it was in South Florida), I found this article by Agbogu et al. to be quite helpful. They described the ability to treat some patients with low-dose corticosteroids using alternative (chiefly cytotoxic) therapies as an adjunct, described deterioration and death that occurred in 15% despite the best therapeutic efforts, and highlighted the importance of the side effect profile in choosing an adjunctive therapy. What is needed now is a prospective study of the various treatment options and some fresh approaches to this often vexing disease.

J.R. Berger, M.D.

Spinal Dural Arteriovenous Fistula: The Pathology of Venous Hypertensive Myelopathy

Hurst RW, Kenyon LC, Lavi E, et al (Univ of Pennsylvania, Philadelphia)
Neurology 45:1309–1313, 1995   18–7

Background.—Spinal dural arteriovenous fistula (SDAVF) is the most common vascular anomaly that affects the spinal cord. They cause slow, progressive development of sensory and motor deficits, which can be accompanied by bowel, bladder, and sexual dysfunction. These deficits are believed to be caused by venous hypertension within the veins of the spinal cord, resulting in subacute necrotic myelopathy. A patient with SDAVF who underwent spinal cord biopsy was described. The findings in this case support increased venous pressure as a mechanism of neurologic dysfunction in SDAVF.

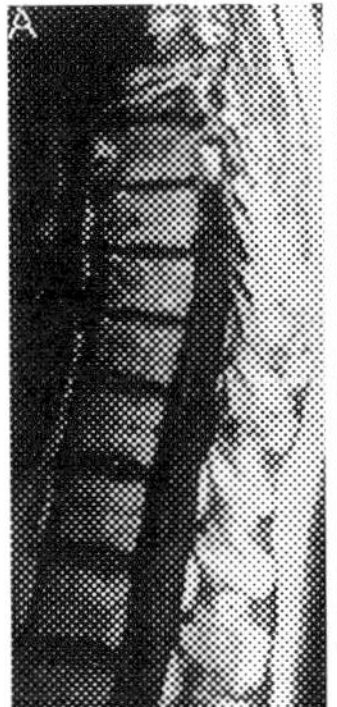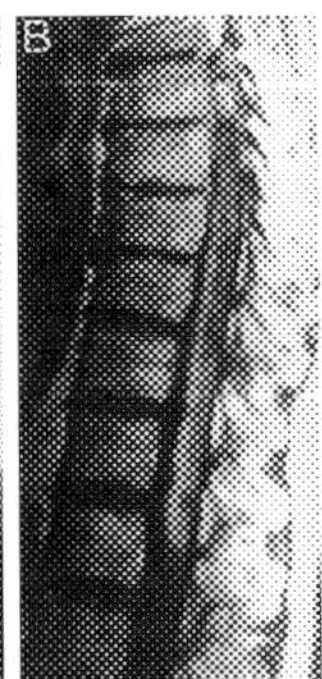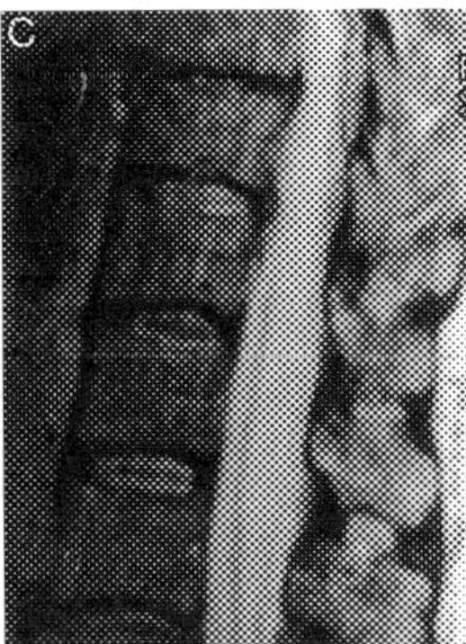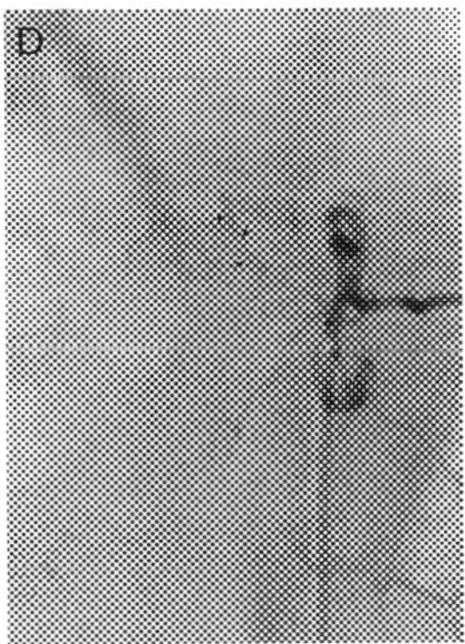

FIGURE 1.—Sagittal unenhanced (**A**) and enhanced (**B**) T1-weighted (TR = 500 msec; TE = 15 msec) MRI demonstrates enlarged spinal cord with diffuse heterogeneous enhancement. Sagittal T2-weighted (TR = 4,000 msec; TE = 87 msec) image (**C**) with increased intramedullary cord signal. Anteroposterior angiographic injection of left T12 intercostal artery (**D**) shows early filling of pial vein of the spinal cord (*arrows*). *Open arrow* is at the catheter tip. (Reprinted from *Neurology* volume; 43:1309–1313, 1195; by permission of Little, Brown and Company [Inc.].)

Case Report.—Woman, 77, had progressive bilateral leg weakness of 22 months' duration. There was no history of trauma or family history of neurologic disease. There were no other neurologic or constitutional symptoms. All laboratory test results were normal, but MRI of the spinal cord revealed diffuse enlargement of the cord below the midthoracic (Fig 1). Spinal cord biopsy revealed a midline posterior spinal vein that was dilated and tortuous. Biopsy specimen from the T5 level revealed white matter with hypocelullarity and small vessels with thickened hyalinized walls. There was myelin and axonal loss. These findings suggested an ischemic myelopathy secondary to a vasculopathy. Spinal angiography demonstrated AV shunting into an enlarged pial vein of the spinal cord, indicating an SDAVF (see Fig 1, D). The lesion was embolized, and more than 1 year later, the patient had no further progression of neurologic deficits.

Conclusion.—These findings support the mechanism of venous hypertension as a cause of cord dysfunction and progressive neurologic deficit in SDAVF. Because this condition is progressive, aggressive evaluation of subacute myelopathy, including spinal angiography, to ensure early diagnosis should result in a greater chance of neurologic recovery for patients with this common spinal vascular malformation.

▶ The syndrome of Foix and Alajouanine, subacute necrotizing myelopathy, and its interrelationship with a venous angioma of the spinal cord and with an underlying carcinoma (frequently lung) has caused great confusion in the literature. Reports of SDAVFs have been appearing for several years with the suggestion that they might be responsible for a progressive myelopathy. These fistulas may be fed by radicular vessels on any nerve root and even by more remote vessels. For instance, in 1 case that I have seen, the fistula was supplied by a vesicular (bladder) artery. For a period I had considerable skepticism about whether such fistulas truly caused a myelopathy. They are presumably present from birth, though the symptoms may first appear late in life, as in the case of the 72-year-old patient described in this report. However, I have eventually become convinced that in many cases the DAVF is truly responsible for producing venous hypertension and, hence, impaired capillary perfusion, leading to hypoxic/ischemic damage to the spinal cord. The pathologic finding in such a disorder, as well illustrated by this case, is hyalinized arterialized veins. These appearances are very similar to the autopsy reports in the literature of the Foix and Alajouanine syndrome. I would still like to see some anatomical correlation between the level of the fistula and the level of the myelopathy, and for complete confidence I would like to see that closure of the fistula produces stabilization or even improvement, as in the present case. Magnetic resonance imaging seems about as good as myelography for demonstrating the tortuous dilated spinal veins, and MR angiography or venography may demonstrate the fistula or at least provide sufficient evidence of the location to allow efficient performance of selective spinal angiography.

W.G. Bradley, D.M., F.R.C.P.

Superficial Siderosis of the Central Nervous System

Fearnley JM, Stevens JM, Rudge P (Natl Hosp for Neurology and Neurosurgery, London)
Brain 118:1051–1066, 1995

18–8

Objective.—Superficial siderosis of the CNS is an uncommon condition, with only 87 cases reported worldwide. A review of reported cases with sufficient clinical details was conducted to characterize this distinct syndrome.

Findings.—Of the 87 cases reported to date, adequate clinical details were available for review in 67 patients. Sensorineural deafness was present in 95%, cerebellar ataxia in 88%, and pyramidal signs in 76%. Additional characteristics included dementia in 24%, bladder disturbances in 24%, anosmia in at least 17%, anisocoria in at least 10%, and sensory signs in 13%. Extraocular motor palsies, neck pain or backache, bilateral sciatica, and lower motor neuron signs, although less frequently observed, were present in 5% to 10% of the patients.

Males were affected to a greater frequency than females, with a ratio of 3:1 noted. Age of onset ranged from 14 to 77, and age at death ranged from 29 to 78. After deaths resulting from underlying conditions or surgery were excluded, syndrome duration until death ranged from 1 to 38 years.

Approximately 27% of the patients became bedridden because of cerebellar ataxia, myelopathic syndrome, or both 1 to 37 years after the first symptoms. Symptomatic subarachnoid hemorrhage was noted in 37%, and the CSF was hemorrhagic or xanthochromic in 75%.

Conclusion.—Superficial siderosis is now believed to be caused by chronic subarachnoid hemorrhage. A source of bleeding has been documented in 54% of patients, caused by dural abnormalities in 47%, a vascular tumor in 35%, or a vascular irregularity in 18%. It also is argued that the remaining cases have resulted from chronic hemorrhage and that evidence for a nonhemorrhagic form of superficial siderosis is nonexistent. An incidental diagnosis by MRI or at death was made in an additional 14 patients free from symptoms of superficial siderosis during life, supporting a possible presymptomatic phase. This phase was estimated in 22 patients in whom the syndrome developed, and it ranged from 4 months to 30 years (average 15 years). The most effective therapy for superficial siderosis is surgical ablation of the bleeding source.

▶ Superficial hemosiderosis of the CNS is potentially more easily diagnosable than previously with the advent of MRI. The clinical features of the syndrome can be quite diverse and reminiscent of a system degeneration, with cerebellar ataxia, sensorineural deafness, pyramidal signs, and dementia. Although the condition is responsible for only a small proportion of patients who have such clinical features, this potentially treatable disorder must always be kept in mind.

W.G. Bradley, D.M., F.R.C.P.

NEUROSURGERY

ROBERT H. WILKINS, M.D.

Electronic Publishing

ROBERT H. WILKINS, M.D., AND JEFFREY K. WILKINS, M.S.E.E., M.B.A., PH.D.

The senior author of this article (RHW) is sitting at his desk at home, having just returned from the medical center library, and is enjoying reading the book that he brought home with him. He has always liked books and has bought and kept many of those of special importance to him. They and several series of bound journals line the shelves that surround him in his personal home library. Yet as he looks across the desk to his computer, he wonders how much longer medical information will continue to be transmitted in book and journal form. With the dawning of the age of electronic publishing, the established methods of printing and binding material for sale and distribution may become little more than a curiosity for aficionados in the future.

As background, it is helpful to review the origin and development of electronic networks. In 1945, Vannevar Bush[1] pointed the way with his seminal article, "As We May Think." Bush was director of the Office of Scientific Research and Development and coordinated the activities of some 6,000 leading American scientists in the application of science to warfare during World War II. In his article he pointed out the need for better scientific interchange during the peace ahead. Bush envisioned ways of collecting, storing, retrieving, and manipulating data that predicted the computer techniques used today. Some of his thoughts follow:

> Consider a future device for individual use, which is a sort of mechanized private file and library. It needs a name, and, to coin one at random, "memex" will do. A memex is a device in which an individual stores all his books, records, and communications, and which is mechanized so that it may be consulted with exceeding speed and flexibility. It is an enlarged intimate supplement to his memory.
>
> It consists of a desk, and while it can presumably be operated from a distance, it is primarily the piece of furniture at which he works. On the top are slanting translucent screens, on which material can be projected for convenient reading. There is a keyboard, and sets of buttons and levers... .
>
> It affords an immediate step...to associative indexing, the basic idea of which is a provision whereby any item may be caused at will to select immediately and automatically another... . The process of tying two items together is the important thing.
>
> When the user is building a trail, he names it, inserts the name in his code book, and taps it out on his keyboard. Before him are the two items to be joined... . The user taps a single key, and the items are permanently joined... . Thereafter, at any time, when one of these items is in view, the other can be instantly recalled merely by taping a button below the corresponding code space. Moreover, when numerous items have been thus joined together to form a

> trail, they can be reviewed in turn, rapidly or slowly.... It is exactly as though the physical items had been gathered together from widely separated sources and bound together to form a new book. It is more than this, for any item can be joined into numerous trails....
>
> Wholly new forms of encyclopedias will appear, ready-made with a mesh of associative trails running through them.... The patent attorney has on call the millions of issued patents, with familiar trails to every point of his client's interest. The physician, puzzled by a patient's reactions, strikes the trail established in studying an earlier similar case, and runs rapidly through analogous case histories, with side references to the classics for the pertinent anatomy and histology.... *

Little did the early pioneers of the present Internet realize that they were building an infrastructure that would ultimately bring the concept of the memex to fruition. More than 2 decades after Vannevar Bush's article appeared in the *Atlantic Monthly,* the Advanced Research Projects Agency (ARPA) of the U.S. Department of Defense funded the development of a computer network based on packet switching.[2, 3] The initial intent of the network was to connect a small number of computers made by different companies, which used different operating systems and were too far apart to connect with electrical wires. Work began on software for the new ARPANET in January 1969. By the fall the network's 4 Interface Message Processors (at the University of California, Los Angeles; the Stanford Research Institute; the University of California, Santa Barbara; and the University of Utah, Salt Lake City) were successfully exchanging packets of information with each other.[3] This project laid the groundwork for the subsequent Internet.

Since its origin, the Internet has grown to a worldwide network connecting more than 40 million users to each other and to a dizzying array of information. The methods by which users have accessed the Internet have also evolved rapidly. The first program to send e-mail across the Internet was developed in 1972. Internet-wide bulletin boards, called USENET newsgroups, were established in 1979.

Without question, the service that has most contributed to the popularization of the Internet is the World Wide Web (WWW). The WWW implements many ideas originally introduced by Vannevar Bush. The WWW was proposed by Tim Berners-Lee in March 1989, as an Internet-based hypertext system to serve the needs of the high-energy physics community. The growth of the WWW was further accelerated with the release of Mosaic in February 1993. Developed by the National Center for Supercomputing Applications (NCSA), at the University of Illinois, Champaign-Urbana, Mosaic provides a web browser with a graphic user interface. With graphic user interface web browsers, still images, video images,

---

*Courtesy of Bush V: As we may think. *Atlantic Monthly* 176:101–108, July 1945.

sound, and text all can be delivered seamlessly through the Internet. This friendly interface has enabled a large number of nontechnical users to access the Internet.

Another important recent development is the creation of directory and search services that allow users to quickly find information of interest on the Internet. Novice and experienced users alike will find web directories (e.g., Yahoo, http://www.yahoo.com) and search services (e.g., AltaVista, http://altavista.digital.com and Reference.COM, http://www.reference.com) extremely useful research tools.

How big will the Internet ultimately be? Some experts forecast 1 billion users by the year 2000.[4] Regardless of the accuracy of such claims, it is clear that the Internet is having a profound impact on the way we live and work. This is particularly true for the academic physician. A review of the history of on-line medical information services provides a glimpse of the changes that the Internet will likely bring.

Concerning computerized access to published medical information, especially journal articles and books, in 1964 the National Library of Medicine had the foresight to introduce the MEDLARS (Medical Literature Analysis and Retrieval System) method of accessing published medical information, and this was brought on-line in 1966 as MEDLINE. Subsequently a variety of database producers, vendors, or suppliers and telecommunications networks began to take part in the electronic transmission of information, including medical information. By 1976 there were just more than 300 on-line databases, 28 of which were in the life sciences. By 1983 there were more than 1,600 on-line databases covering topics from accounting to wines, available through 225 vendors. By 1990 there were more than 7,600 computer-readable databases.

Computer techniques have allowed both librarians and library users to get better control over the ever-increasing volume of printed medical information. Yet the time consumed by manuscript preparation, peer review, and publication has remained essentially the same. The time from an author's submission of a manuscript to its appearance in print frequently consumes 6 to 18 months for a journal and longer for a textbook. Because of such delays, authors may be concerned that their work might not be accorded the appropriate priority or that it will be out of date by the time it is published. For years, both authors and journal and book editors have been looking for methods to speed up the review and publication process while also reducing the costs of publication and distribution. One method under development at present in many scientific fields, including neurosurgery, is electronic publication.[5, 6] By 1995 there were nearly 700 electronic journals and newsletters, including 142 peer-reviewed electronic journals.[6]

The majority of neurosurgical material currently available on the Internet consists of nonscientific information such as socioeconomic topics, listings of meetings and courses, information about neurosurgical organizations, and bulletin boards. But now there is also an interest in publishing peer-reviewed scientific information as well. Several aspects still must be finalized, such as matters of copyright, advertising, and subscription, but the movement is under way. For example, in 1996, the *Journal of Neurosurgery* inaugurated a new on-line journal. *Neurosurgical Focus.*

If electronic journal publishing takes hold, if review publications switch to an electronic format, and if textbooks convert to a CD-ROM or similar computer format, printed journals and books actually may be on the way out. The senior author is going to save his, though, not only because they can comfort him in his old age but also because they may increase in value as collectors' oddities in an age that is increasingly more suitable for those like the junior author (JKW), an electrical engineer.

References

1. Bush V: As we may think. *Atlantic Monthly* 176:101–108, July 1945.
2. Computer Science and Telecommunications Board, National Research Council: *Realizing the Information Future. The Internet and Beyond.* Washington, DC, National Academy Press, 1994, p 237.
3. Dern DP: *The Internet Guide for New Users.* New York, McGraw-Hill, 1994, pp 8, 9.
4. Negroponte N: *Being Digital.* New York, Alfred A Knopf, 1995, pp 181–182.
5. Anonymous: Electronic science journals. Paperless papers. *Economist* 337:78–79, Dec 16, 1995.
6. Hayes JR: The Internet's first victim? *Forbes* 156:200–201, Dec 18, 1995.

Chance Discovery in Neurosurgery

Robert H. Wilkins, M.D.

As with other branches of medicine and with science in general, neurosurgery has developed gradually, mainly by the planned efforts of many people. On occasion, however, a significant discovery has been made by accident or unique opportunity, usually by an individual who has encountered an unexpected circumstance and has had the wit to recognize its potential value. "Pasteur reiterated, time and time again, 'In the field of experimentation, chance favors only the prepared mind.'"[1]

Beveridge[2] states that there are 3 different types of discovery in which chance is a vital factor. The first of these is intuition from the random juxtaposition of ideas, that is, "the sudden linking of apparently unconnected ideas or pieces of information in the mind to form a new meaningful relationship."[2] Beveridge[2] terms the second type a eureka intuition: "The scientist observes some rather common event and suddenly perceives the analogy between it and some aspect of the problem he has been puzzling over: this triggers off a flash of illumination in a mind already loaded with a mass of relevant information." The third type of chance discovery is serendipity.[3]

The word serendipity was coined by Horace Walpole, the fourth Earl of Oxford, and used in a letter to Horace Mann, the English resident in Florence, on January 28, 1754. To quote Walpole, "I once read a silly fairy tale, called *The Three Princes of Serendip*: as their highnesses travelled, they were always making discoveries, by accidents and sagacity, of things which they were not in quest of... ."[4] Walpole emphasized that serendipity means accidental sagacity, stating that "*no* discovery of a thing you *are* looking for, comes under this description... ."[4]

Beveridge[2] states that "in *serendipity* the scientist encounters an unusual event or a curious coincidence of two not unusual events, or an unexpected experimental result. There is no question here of clinching already half-formed ideas, or seeing suggestive analogies, because the observed event is itself the discovery, or a strong clue to it; it comes as a surprise and it may be met with doubt or even incredulity."

In relation to the development of neurosurgery, there have been at least 9 examples of discovery by chance or through an opportunity afforded by a unique circumstance.

Pierre Paul Broca (1824–1880)

Paul Broca was a man of many talents.[5] Among his various interests was physical anthropology, a field he helped establish. He was especially involved with craniology and craniocerebral topography. In regard to craniometry, Broca invented various measuring devices, including a craniograph, various goniometers, a stereograph, a craniostat, optic and acoustic sounds, and a cranioscope. His pioneering studies of trepanation resulted in a number of his more than 500 articles and monographs. Broca was instrumental in founding the Société d'Anthropologie and the *Revue d'Anthropologie*. Early in 1861 there were debates at the meetings of this newly formed society concerning the localization of function within the human brain. Broca, who was Secretary of the society, became interested in the topic and joined in the debate.[6]

On April 11, 1861, a patient was admitted to the hospital on Broca's surgical service because of a diffuse lower extremity cellulitis. Of interest was the fact that 21 years earlier the patient had lost the ability to speak except for 1 syllable, and starting 10 years later he had gradually developed a right hemiparesis. This man died 6 days after admission, and at a meeting of the Société d'Anthropologie the following day, Broca described the findings present at autopsy: softening and cavitation in the left frontal lobe.

On October 27, 1961, an 84-year-old man was hospitalized under Broca's care because of a fracture of the neck of the femur. In April 1860, he had suddenly become unconscious, and although he had partially recovered, he was unable to speak except for 5 words. This patient died 12 days after admission, and cavitation was found in the posterior third of the left inferior frontal gyrus and, to a lesser extent, the adjacent middle frontal gyrus.

With the publication of his 2 case reports, Broca became 1 of the champions of the idea of discrete localization of function within the brain. This concept of cerebral localization was vital to the subsequent development of neurosurgery. Of interest is the fact that in 1871 Broca performed the first craniotomy based on cerebral localization when he drained an intracranial abscess of a patient who had developed dysphasia and right-sided weakness a month after a head injury.[7]

Roberts Bartholow (1831–1904)

Roberts Bartholow,[8] professor of Materia Medica and Therapeutics and of Clinical Medicine in the Medical College of Ohio, also made a significant contribution to cerebral localization with his 1874 report of the first instance of electrical stimulation of the human brain.[9, 10] Bartholow knew about the studies of Gustav Fritsch and Eduard Hitzig and of David Ferrier, who had studied electrical stimulation of the cerebrum of animals. However, he[8] noted that "the researches recently made in animals on the functions of the brain, although of great importance, need to be complemented by similar investigations, or by corresponding pathological alterations, in the human brain."

A 30-year-old mentally retarded woman, Mary Rafferty, was admitted to the Good Samaritan Hospital in Cincinnati under Bartholow's care in January 1874. As an infant she had fallen into a fire and her scalp had been badly burned. Thirteen months before her hospitalization a small rodent ulcer of the scalp had appeared. This had gradually enlarged into an open, nearly circular ulcer extending laterally to a point 3½ to 4 inches above each external auditory meatus, anteriorly to a point 4 inches from the nasion, and posteriorly to within 2¼ inches of the inion. The skull was missing over a space 2 inches in diameter, and the excavation secreted a great quantity of pus.

Bartholow decided to make use of this circumstance to stimulate Mary's brain with galvanic and faradic current. "As portions of brain-substance have been lost by injury or by the surgeon's knife, and as the brain has been deeply penetrated by incisions made for the escape of pus, it was supposed that fine needles could be introduced without material injury to the cerebral matter. The needles being insulated to near their points, it was believed that diffusion of the current could be as restricted as in the experiments of Fritsch and Hitzig and Ferrier."[8] Bartholow conducted a series of experiments to test the sensibility of the dura mater and brain, to test faradic reaction of the surface of the dura, and to test faradic reaction of the posterior lobes. He produced muscular contractions and unpleasant tingling on the side opposite the stimulation, but during the third experiment the electrical stimulation produced a focal seizure with generalization. On a subsequent day, when Bartholow had planned to test galvanic stimulation, Mary had a seizure and the testing was not performed. Her condition worsened, with another seizure the next day, and she died subsequently. At autopsy there was a thick layer of pus over the left hemisphere and thrombosis of the superior sagittal sinus was verified.

Bartholow was criticized severely at home and abroad, especially in regard to the ethical aspects of his experimentation.[9,10] "In 1879, Bartholow accepted the chair of materia medica at Jefferson Medical College and spent the rest of his career at Philadelphia. Notwithstanding the comments of his censors, thought at the time to be damaging to his reputation, Bartholow was elected to membership in many medical and scientific societies, as well as being a founder of the American Neurological Association. He was a noted and prolific medical writer, and while at Philadelphia published his major works."[10]

William Gibson Spiller (1863–1940)

During the early development of modern neurosurgery, it was common for a neurologist to diagnose a disease and direct a surgeon in its surgical treatment. In fact, some new operations were devised by neurologists. For example, in 1898 William G. Spiller proposed that tic douloureux be treated by cutting the sensory root of the trigeminal nerve. After appropriate animal experimentation in dogs (done in association with Charles H. Frazier, Professor of Clinical Surgery at the University of Pennsylvania) to show that nerve regeneration would not occur, Spiller, who was Assistant Clinical Professor of Nervous Diseases at the University of Pennsylvania, persuaded Frazier to perform the procedure in 1901.[6]

In September 1904, Spiller, who by then was Professor of Neuropathology and Associate Professor of Neurology in the University of Pennsylvania, had under his care a 23-year-old man with a loss of the normal ability to perceive the sensations of pain and temperature in the lower extremities but with relative preservation of the ability to appreciate touch. The patient died in January 1905 and at autopsy was found to have small bilateral tuberculomas in the anterolateral portions of the spinal cord; on the right the lesion was at the extreme lower end of the thoracic cord and on the left it was ½ to 1 inch higher. Gowers interpreted these findings as

"...the best evidence that has as yet been offered for the location of the fibers for temperature and pain within the tracts of Gowers."[11]

In March 1909, a 47-year-old man was admitted to Spiller's service at the Philadelphia General Hospital with a 2-month history of pain in the lower extremities and pelvis.[6] By August this had progressed to painful paraparesis. In November the patient was found at operation to have a malignant tumor involving the lower part of the spinal cord. By January 1910 the patient suffered greatly from pain in the lower limbs. As noted previously, Spiller already had first-hand knowledge about the pain pathways within the spinal cord. He enlisted Edward Martin, John Rhea Barton Professor of Surgery in the University of Pennsylvania, to divide each anterolateral column of the spinal cord through a T6–T8 laminectomy on January 19, 1911.[12] This first cordotomy provided the patient significant pain relief and initiated the subsequent widespread use of this procedure and its later percutaneous variant.

Walter Edward Dandy (1886–1946)

Pneumoventriculography[13] and pneumoencephalography[14] were important neuroradiologic diagnostic tests performed frequently during the half century between 1925 and 1975.[6] These were initiated by Walter Dandy, an innovative and truly preeminent neurosurgeon while he was still a resident.[15–17]

To quote Dandy[13]:

> Since the X-rays penetrate normal brain tissues, blood, cerebrospinal fluid and non-calcified tumor tissue almost equally, any changes in the brain produced by altered proportions of these components will not materially alter the röntgenogram....For some time I have considered the possibility of filling the cerebral ventricles with a medium that will produce a shadow in the radiogram....The various solutions and suspensions used in pyelography...were injected into the ventricles of dogs, but always with fatal results, owing to the injurious effects on the brain.

On January 3, 1917, Dandy saw a patient with a suspected intestinal perforation.[15] A preoperative roentgenogram of the chest was made to exclude miliary tuberculosis, and Dandy noticed air under the patient's diaphragm, a radiologic sign that had been useful since that time for the diagnosis of intestinal perforation. At operation, Dandy confirmed the presence of intraperitoneal air, as well as the typhoid ulcer through which it had escaped.[15] Based on this experience, as well as Halsted's observations about the striking roentgenographic appearances of intestinal gases and Dandy's recognition of various other radiographic properties of air, Dandy began using air to outline the ventricular system. By the time he had completed his first report, Dandy[13] had injected air into the cerebral ventricles at least 20 times. Thus, the chance observation of air under the diaphragm stimulated a prepared mind to institute 2 important neuroradiologic techniques.

Jean Athanase Sicard (1872–1929) and Jacques Forestier (1890–1978)

In 1921 Jean Sicard, a French clinician, and his pupil Jacques Forestier reported their use of an iodized poppyseed oil, lipiodol, as a pain-relieving medication.[18] Lipiodol was known to be radiopaque, but this property had been regarded as a curiosity.[6] Sicard and Forestier[18, 19] found that if they injected the lipiodol into the epidural space for treatment of lumbar hyperesthesia, lumbar arthritis, or lumboischialgia, they could also visualize the epidural space radiographically. It was then just a short step for them to inject lipiodol into the spinal subarachnoid space, and positive contrast myelography was born.[20]

Subsequently lipiodol was used widely for myelography, but it was associated with meningeal irritation, and its viscosity made it difficult to remove. It was eventually replaced by another oily iodinated organic liquid with the trade name Pantopaque[6] and subsequently by water-soluble agents. However, even though lipiodol did not remain the agent of choice for myelography, Sicard and Forestier recognized the potential value of its radiographic properties and turned a marginally useful approach to treatment into a method of diagnosis that is still used today.

W. Gayle Crutchfield (1900–1972) and Claude C. Coleman (1879–1953)

In 1932, Gayle Crutchfield was a house officer in the Neuro-Surgical Department of the Medical College of Virginia. A 22-year-old woman was hospitalized on June 27, 1932 within 1 hour of an automobile accident. She was found to have Erb's paralysis of the right arm, with loss of sensation over the distribution of the second and third cervical nerves. In addition to a C2–C3 fracture-dislocation, she had a compound comminuted fracture of the mandible that prevented the use of halter traction. At the suggestion of his chief, Claude Coleman, Crutchfield[21] inserted Edmonton extension tongs into the patient's skull for cervical traction. Later he[22] perfected the Crutchfield tongs that came into widespread use until being supplanted in more recent years by Gardner-Wells tongs and then by the halo device. Skeletal traction has been a significant advancement in the treatment of cervical spinal injuries,[23] and it was begun by Crutchfield and Coleman because of a coincidental mandibular fracture.

Antonio Caetano de Abreu Freire Egas Moniz (1874–1955)

The Portuguese neurologist Egas Moniz led an unusually varied and productive life. He created and directed a political party; he was a political prisoner at 1 point in his career, and at another he was almost assassinated. During World War I he was Ambassador to Spain and later was Minister of Foreign Affairs. He was president of the Portuguese delegation to the Paris Peace Conference in 1918. In 1951 he was asked to be President of Portugal but refused.

Egas Moniz was also active in other nonmedical fields. "He wrote an operetta, taught mathematics, fought a duel, became a gourmet, and still found time to write on the history of playing cards and to publish a biography of Pope John XXI."[6]

> Even more outstanding were the medical achievements of Egas Moniz. After distinguishing himself as a student at the University of Coimbra, he studied neurology at La Salpêtrière with Raymond, Pierre Marie and Dejerine, and at L'Hôpital de la Pitié with Babinski. Egas Moniz became a professor of medicine at the age of 28, the first occupant of the chair of neurology at the University of Lisbon, and the author of over 300 medical publications.[6]

Partly in collaboration with the neurosurgeon Pedro Manuel de Almeida Lima, he developed 2 major techniques: cerebral angiography and prefrontal leucotomy. The latter work brought Egas Moniz a Nobel Prize for Physiology or Medicine in 1949.

After trials of cerebral angiography in dogs and human cadavers, Egas Moniz tried the technique in 9 patients and reported the results in 1927. His experience grew, and in 1931 he published a book describing his first 180 arteriograms. Then in 1935, at age 61, he had an exhibit on the subject at the Second International Neurological Congress in London. At that time frontal lobe function was of great interest.

> Because of the advances in neurosurgery between 1910 and 1935, patients with lesions in the frontal lobes began to survive for longer periods of time. The careful clinical analysis of these patients, combined with more sophisticated animal experiments, resulted in the gradual elucidation of the functions of the frontal lobes. The entire problem was of such fundamental importance that many of the world's foremost neurologists, neurophysiologists, and neurosurgeons became involved.[6]

At the 1935 Congress an all-day symposium on frontal lobe function was scheduled, and Egas Moniz attended.

> Most of the presentations were by clinical neurologists, reporting changes in patients after damage to their frontal lobes. Participating in the symposium were some of Europe's leading neurologist....The American neurologist Richard Brickner and the neurosurgeon Wilder Penfield described patients studied for several years following extensive destruction of their frontal lobes. There was also an experimental report by Carlyle Jacobsen and John Fulton from Yale on the effect of removing a large part of the frontal lobes of chimpanzees.[24]

Although Egas Moniz had probably been thinking about the possibility of psychosurgery for several years, this presentation by Jacobsen and Fulton stimulated him to action. As recalled by Fulton[25]:

> Both Jacobsen and I were alarmed when Moniz raised the question of whether a similar operation might not relieve anxiety states in man. Being something of a neurosurgeon myself, the idea of a bilateral frontal ablation, which is difficult enough in the chimpanzee, seemed a particularly hazardous procedure in the human subject. But Professor Moniz...had other ideas and with Lima developed the leucotomy by which the major frontal projections could be interrupted through two superiorly placed burr holes.

Egas Moniz returned to Lisbon in August 1935 and immediately assembled a team that included the neurosurgeon Almeida Lima, a neurologically oriented clinician, and 2 psychiatrists.

> Three months later he and Lima carried out their first lobotomy by injecting alcohol in the white matter of the frontal lobes. This technique was used in three additional patients before the two investigators moved to the use of a "leucotome" to sever volumes of white matter about 1 cm in diameter; several such lesions were placed in each frontal lobe. In June of 1936 Egas Moniz published his now classic paper describing the results of these surgical procedures in the first 20 patients: 7 were felt to be greatly benefited, another 7 were helped and the psychiatric status of the remaining 6 was unchanged.[26]

Psychosurgery rapidly came into widespread use in many countries. In the United States this form of treatment was pioneered at George Washington University by Walter J. Freeman, a neurologist, and James W. Watts, a neurosurgeon. Throughout the world, various surgical procedures were introduced to achieve the same goal, modification of mood and behavior in patients with certain forms of psychiatric illness. Eventually psychosurgery waned because of the development of effective psychoactive medications and because of public opposition to surgery having the potential of interfering with personal freedom by altering the individual's mind and personality.

Few psychiatric patients are treated surgically at the present time, and psychosurgery is largely obsolete. Yet from a historical perspective it is interesting to recall the spark that lit the fire in Egas Moniz at the International Congress in London in 1935.

Irving S. Cooper (1922–1985)

In 1951, Irving Cooper accidentally discovered a technique that has found widespread usefulness in its later, modified forms. Before that time, the tremor and rigidity of Parkinson's disease had been treated by a number of different surgical procedures, none very effective.[27] On October 9,

1951, during a craniotomy for a proposed section of the cerebral peduncle of a 39-year-old man incapacitated by postencephalitic parkinsonism with tremor and rigidity, Cooper[27, 28] accidentally tore the anterior choroidal artery and had to occlude it.

The following is Cooper's account of his surgical accident and his use of the information gained to develop a better surgical approach to Parkinson's disease:

> During the operation, before I had a chance to cut the crucial motor fibers, a small artery at the base of the brain…bled profusely. Tiny silver clips were placed on each open end of the artery to stop it from hemorrhaging… . I decided not to proceed any further with the operation….
>
> The patient, who might have suffered serious complications as a result of the torn artery, awoke promptly from the effects of the anesthetic. There was no tremor or rigidity in the left arm and leg, which had been so seriously afflicted….By the time the results had persisted for several months, I decided that I had serendipitously found a clue that could lead to the surgical relief of tremor and rigidity without paralyzing the patient….
>
> I decided to carry the evidence to Dr. Fred Mettler, professor of anatomy at Columbia University, located diametrically across the island of Manhattan from the New York University Bellevue Medical Center where I had elected to start my clinical, research, and teaching career that very same year, an unknown, embryonic brain surgeon. Mettler was already a famed neuroanatomist, whose principal interest had been the study of involuntary movements in experimental animals….
>
> He suggested that I perform the same operation on some large chimpanzees in his own laboratory, so that I could examine the anatomic effects upon the brain produced by the closure of the anterior choroidal artery. One of the chimps, Rosebud, weighed in at close to one hundred fifty pounds. It took longer to corner her, and for capable anesthetists from the Columbia Medical Center to anesthetize her, than to carry out the operation. Rosebud was subsequently sacrificed, and Professor Mettler's meticulous examination of her brain demonstrated that certain of the…basal ganglia…were affected irreversibly by the operation.*

Cooper practiced the operation in cadavers but needed additional patients to prove its value in patients with parkinsonism. He then saw in consultation a patient named Raymond Walker at the Central Islip State Hospital, a New York State psychiatric center located on Long Island. Mr. Walker had had viral encephalitis in 1936 and had been left with a severe postencephalitic parkinsonian syndrome. After a suicide attempt when he

---

*From *The Vital Probe. My Life as a Brain Surgeon* by IS Cooper, M.D. Copyright © 1981 by IS Cooper. Reprinted by permission of WW Norton & Company, Inc.

was 31 years old, he was placed in the psychiatric hospital and ended up on a back ward, which he shared with 29 other patients whose conditions were considered hopeless. The superintendent of the hospital, Dr. O'Neill, was reluctant to give Cooper permission to proceed with his experimental procedure but finally agreed when Walker's sister, his closest living relative, was located and granted permission.

> Raymond lay there, expressionless, his gaze seemingly fixed on the cciling twenty feet overhead. The only sign of life was the constant violent shaking of his arms and legs, which in turn shook the metal frame hospital bed so violently that it was impossible for me to talk across him to Dr. Francis O'Neill....It was the beat of persistent, merciless oscillation of the entire body of this silent young man whose cadaverous appearance made him look almost twice his chronological age of thirty-five. His uncontrollably trembling muscles, paradoxically, were so stiff and rigid that he could not move them voluntarily. In constant motion, he could not choose to move himself....
>
> On February 27, 1952, Raymond Walker was wheeled into the small, freshly scrubbed, old-fashioned white-tiled operating room of Building A in Central Islip State Hospital....Quickly, I performed the steps I had practiced so many times on bodies in the morgue; upon still, silent teachers from whom I had learned so much....The target, the anterior choroidal artery....was too tiny to bear the weight of the silver clips. Quickly, I sizzled and coagulated it with an electric current. Satisfying myself that the vessel had been clotted, I divided it with a scissors....*
>
> With my assistant, Dr. Aldo Morello..., I sat by Raymond's side in the tiny recovery room adjacent to the operating theater. Shortly, Raymond was awake. He became restless and started to move about....He had not been paralyzed. Thank God.
>
> Almost instantaneously, the stretcher on which he lay could be heard to squeak and groan. The squeaks were repetitive,...and within an hour violent. However, the tremors were present only on the left side of the body.
>
> "Raymond, raise your right arm."
>
> Briskly, without any sign of stiffness, Raymond lifted his right arm in the air....His hand aloft, Raymond snapped the thumb and forefinger of his right hand... . I turned to Dr. Morello who was at my side....We embraced each other. We pulled up chairs and sat by the patient's side without speaking. We could not express to each other the unique joy we experienced....There was nothing that could be said that would surpass the expression or the significance of Raymond's fingers snapping.*

---

*From *The Vital Probe. My Life as a Brain Surgeon* by IS Cooper, M.D. Copyright ® 1981 by IS Cooper. Reprinted by permission of WW Norton & Company, Inc.

Raymond's immediate postoperative course was complicated by the development of an epidural hematoma, which was evacuated that night. Cooper and Morello spent the next 3 days and nights at the hospital.

> Raymond demonstrated physical improvement beyond anything we had hoped for....On the third day after surgery, he fed himself with his right hand....On the fifth day he stood by himself and walked out of the recovery room....
>
> About fifty feet down the corridor was a Coca-Cola vending machine. Raymond walked to the machine and stood there gazing at it. He turned and walked back, approaching one of the nurses who stood watching with us. In a whisper, barely audible, he asked her for a nickel. Granted the gift, he turned and went back to the Coke machine, placed the nickel in the slot, and reached down with his new right hand to grasp the Coke bottle as it emerged. He placed the head of the bottle into the machine and snapped off the cap.
>
> Raymond lifted the bottle to eye level and gazed at it for a few seconds, then carefully carried it to his mouth. Tilting his head back, he drank the contents of the bottle without stopping. He placed the bottle in the box alongside the Coke machine, turned and walked back to the recovery room, dragging his still rigid left side, but allowing his loose right arm to swing joyfully at his side....
>
> On March 25, 1952, the same operation was carried out on the right side of Raymond's brain, so that his left arm and leg might be relieved. This time the anterior choroidal artery was larger. Two silver clips were placed on it and squeezed tightly in order to occlude the vessel. There was no joy in Central Islip this time in that tiny recovery cubicle....This time the result was failure.*

Cooper was perplexed initially but then reasoned that the silver clips might not have occluded the artery, a circumstance that was verified by a postoperative arteriogram. On April 11, 1952, Cooper operated again, squeezing the existing clips more tightly and coagulating and dividing the artery.

> Raymond's postoperative course was marked by the fact that tremor and rigidity were relieved in the left arm and leg....Expression returned to his previously frozen features....On June 21, 1952, Raymond walked out of Central Islip State Hospital to seek a new life. Within a few weeks he had sought and found a job.

As Cooper and others gained experience with his new operation, it became apparent that the results were not consistent, largely because of

*From *The Vital Probe. My Life as a Brain Surgeon* by IS Cooper, M.D. Copyright ® 1981 by IS Cooper. Reprinted by permission of WW Norton & Company, Inc.

individual variations in the areas of the brain supplied by the anterior choroidal artery. Cooper thought that the preferred target for destruction was the medial globus pallidus, and he devised another way of achieving this with a procedure he called a chemopallidectomy. This was done by a freehand technique initially; a catheter was passed through a temporal craniectomy so that its tip entered the medial globus pallidus. Procaine was injected, and if the desired effect was achieved, alcohol was then injected to create a permanent lesion. The catheter was left in place for 7 to 10 days so that subsequent injections could be given if necessary.[27]

Additional changes and refinements in the surgical treatment of Parkinson's disease were introduced by Cooper and many others, including the adaptation of stereotactic techniques to improve accuracy, the development of other methods of lesion production, and the preferential use of targets in the thalamus rather than the globus pallidus. Surgery for Parkinson's disease and other movement disorders is now much safer, with a more predictable outcome than was the case with Cooper's early procedures. Yet, as Redfern[29] has concluded, "Although anterior choroidal artery ligation was soon superseded, demonstration of relief of tremor without hemiparesis nonetheless represented a significant milestone in the evolution of the surgery of movement disorders and encouraged continued search for safer methods of reaching targets in the basal ganglia."

Sten Håkanson (Contemporary)

Lars Leksell, the innovative neurosurgeon who spent the majority of his career in Stockholm, introduced stereotactic radiosurgery in 1951 when he was Head of the Department of Neurosurgery at the University of Lund.[30–32] He[32] designed a stereotactic arc frame and used it to focus radiation on an intracranial target:

> The principle of the instrument, with the target in the centre of a semicircular arc, made it easily adaptable for cross-firing of the target with narrow beams of radiation. The first attempt...with ionizing radiation was made...with X-rays....It was tempting to try to reduce the hazards of open surgery and by the administration of a single heavy dose of radiation it appeared possible to destroy any deep brain structure, without risk of bleeding or infection.
>
> Ten years later considerable progress had been made, due in considerable measure to the contribution of the physicists Kurt Liden and Börje Larsson....The heavy particle beam was an excellent knife blade but the syncho-cyclotron was too clumsy. A similar technique was developed for a linear accelerator. The next step was to get to a practical, precise and simple tool which could be handled by the surgeon himself.
>
> The first stereotactic Gamma Unit, using Cobalt 60..., was installed at the Sophiahemmet Hospital in 1968... . The results were promising and a second Gamma Unit, with more generally suitable spherical fields of radiation, was constructed and installed at the Karolinska Hospital in Stockholm in 1974.

Leksell[33] first used stereotactic radiosurgery to treat trigeminal neuralgia on April 20, 1953 using the gasserian ganglion as the target. The patient's pain gradually subsided over 5 months and did not return over the next 18 years. To better visualize the location of the gasserian ganglion radiographically, Sten Håkanson,[34–36] working in Leksell's Department of Neurosurgery at the Karolinska Sjukhuset, developed the technique of injecting a water-soluble contrast medium, metrizamide, into the trigeminal cistern. As a more permanent marker, tantalum powder was tried. Then Håkanson[36] encountered an unexpected occurrence:

> During the development of a stereotactic technique for gamma irradiation of the trigeminal ganglion and root in the treatment of trigeminal neuralgia, glycerol was used as a vehicle to introduce tantalum dust into the trigeminal cistern....The tantalum dust was used to mark permanently the trigeminal cistern for the precise, stereotactic localization of the trigeminal ganglion and root. Quite unexpectedly it was observed that the intracisternal injection of glycerol alone rendered the patient completely free from the paroxysmal pain without producing any significant sensory loss.

The technique of percutaneously injecting a liquid through the foramen ovale to destroy part of the gasserian ganglion and trigeminal sensory root dates back to the first use of alcohol for this purpose by Wilfred Harris[37] in 1910. Among the various agents used was phenol in glycerine by Antony Jefferson,[38] as reported in 1963. However, it was because of the unexpected observation by Håkanson that the currently used procedure of percutaneous retrogasserian glycerol rhizotomy was initiated.

Conclusion

Chance occurrences and serendipity have been part of many scientific advancements, including in areas of importance to neurosurgeons. To quote Rossman[3]:

> The importance of chance in medical discoveries is seldom realized, and is often neglected in treatises on the scientific method....Serendipity occurs in small discoveries as well as in revolutionary ones. However, its prerequisites of astute observation, curiosity, insight, opportunism, and receptivity are the same in both instances....The scientist ought to realize that "chance favors only those who know how to court her"....It is therefore not insulting to the integrity of a discoverer to admit that his discovery was accidental, for serendipity does not depend entirely on chance....It involves both the phenomenon to be observed and the appreciative, intelligent observer. Chance merely provides the most suitable circumstances, but it must be recognized opportunely and turned to advantage.

References

1. Dubos RJ: *Louis Pasteur, Free Lance of Science.* Boston, Little Brown, 1950, p 101.
2. Beveridge WIB: *Seeds of Discovery.* New York, WW Norton, 1980, pp 18–20.
3. Rossman RE: The history and significance of serendipity in medical discovery. *Trans Stud Coll Physicians Phila* 33:104–120, 1965.
4. Remer TG: Serendipity and the Three Princes, from the *Peregrinaggio* of 1557. Norman, Okla, University of Oklahoma Press, 1965, pp 6, 15.
5. Schiller F: *Paul Broca. Founder of French Anthropology, Explorer of the Brain.* New York, Oxford University Press, 1992.
6. Wilkins RH: *Neurosurgical Classics.* New York, Johnson Reprint, 1965, pp 61–68, 242–256, 257–263, 264–276, 418–427, 442–448, 477–483.
7. Stone JL: Paul Broca and the first craniotomy based on cerebral localization. *J Neurosurg* 75:154–159, 1991.
8. Bartholow R: Experimental investigations into the functions of the human brain. *Am J Med Sci* 67:305–313, 1874.
9. Holmes GL: Roberts Bartholow. In search of anatomic localization. *NY State J Med* 82:238–241, 1982.
10. Morgan JP: The first reported case of electrical stimulation of the human brain. *J Hist Med* 37:51–64, 1982.
11. Spiller WG: The location within the spinal cord of the fibers for temperature and pain sensations. *J Nerv Ment Dis* 32:318–320, 1905.
12. Spiller WG, Martin E: The treatment of persistent pain of organic origin in the lower part of the body by division of the anterolateral column of the spinal cord. *JAMA* 58:1489–1490, 1912.
13. Dandy WE: Ventriculography following the injection of air into the cerebral ventricles. *Ann Surg* 68:5–11, 1918.
14. Dandy WE: Röntgenography of the brain after the injection of air into the spinal canal. *Ann Surg* 70:397–403, 1919.
15. Campbell E: Walter E. Dandy—surgeon, 1886–1946. *J Neurosurg* 8:249–262, 1951.
16. Fox WL: *Dandy of Johns Hopkins.* Baltimore, Md, Williams & Wilkins, 1984.
17. Pinkus RL: Innovation in neurosurgery: Walter Dandy in his day. *Neurosurgery* 14:623–631, 1984.
18. Sicard JA, Forestier J: Méthode radiographique d'exploration de la cavité épidurale par le lipiodol. *Rev Neurol* 37:1264–1266, 1921.
19. Sicard [JA], Forestier [J]: Méthode générale d'exploration radiologique par l'huile iodée (lipiodol). *Bull Soc Med Hop Paris* 46:463–468, 1922.
20. Sicard JA, Forestier J: *The Use of Lipiodol in Diagnosis and Treatment. A Clinical and Radiological Survey.* New York, Oxford University Press, 1932.
21. Crutchfield WG: Skeletal traction for dislocation of the cervical spine. Report of a case. *South Surg* 2:156–159, 1933.
22. Crutchfield WG: Redesigned Crutchfield skull tongs. Technical note describing the combined "squeeze" and "hook" principle. *J Neurosurg* 25:656–657, 1966.
23. Loeser JD: History of skeletal traction in the treatment of cervical spine injuries. *J Neurosurg* 33:54–59, 1970.
24. Valenstein ES: *Great and Desperate Cures. The Rise and Decline of Psychosurgery and Other Radical Treatments for Mental Illness.* New York, Basic Books, 1986, pp 77–78.
25. Fulton JF: *The Frontal Lobes and Human Behaviour.* Springfield, Ill, Charles C Thomas, 1952, pp 6, 7.
26. Ballantine HT Jr: Historical overview of psychosurgery and its problematic. *Acta Neurochir (Wien)* 44 (suppl):125–128, 1988.
27. Cooper IS: *The Neurosurgical Alleviation of Parkinsonism.* Springfield, Ill, Charles C Thomas, 1956, pp 7–17, 25–44.
28. Cooper IS: *The Vital Probe. My Life as a Brain Surgeon.* New York, WW Norton, 1981, pp 25–43.

29. Redfern RM: History of stereotactic surgery for Parkinson's disease. *Br J Neurosurg* 3:271–304, 1989.
30. Leksell L: The stereotaxic method and radiosurgery of the brain. *Acta Chir Scand* 102:316–319, 1951.
31. Leksell L: *Stereotaxis and Radiosurgery. An Operative System.* Springfield, Ill, Charles C Thomas, 1971.
32. Leksell L: Stereotactic radiosurgery. *J Neurol Neurosurg Psychiatry* 46:797–803, 1983.
33. Leksell L: Stereotaxic radiosurgery in trigeminal neuralgia. *Acta Chir Scand* 137:311–314, 1971.
34. Håkanson S, Leksell L: Stereotactic gamma radiation in trigeminal neuralgia (abstract). *Excerpta Med Int Congr Series* 418:57, 1977.
35. Håkanson S: Transoval trigeminal cisternography. *Surg Neurol* 10:137–144, 1978.
36. Håkanson S: Trigeminal neuralgia treated by the injection of glycerol into the trigeminal cistern. *Neurosurgery* 9:638–646, 1981.
37. Harris W: Alcohol injection of the Gasserian ganglion for trigeminal neuralgia. *Lancet* 1:218–221, 1912.
38. Jefferson A: Trigeminal root and ganglion injections using phenol in glycerine for the relief of trigeminal neuralgia. *J Neurol Neurosurg Psychiatry* 26:345–352, 1963.

The History of Minimally Invasive Neurosurgery

ROBERT H. WILKINS, M.D.

Definitions

The term "minimally invasive neurosurgery" has been used often in recent years. Two collections of papers with this title were published as supplements to *Acta Neurochirurgica* in 1992[1] and 1994[2]. A book entitled *Minimally Invasive Techniques in Neurosurgery* appeared in 1995[3]. The journal *Neurochirurgia*, which had been in existence since 1958, changed its name to *Minimally Invasive Neurosurgery* with Volume 37 in 1994. Also of interest is the fact that the Sixth International Congress of Neurological Surgery, which was held in São Paulo in 1977, used the following title for its proceedings: "Neurological Surgery with Emphasis on Noninvasive Methods of Diagnosis and Treatment."

What is meant by "minimally invasive neurosurgery?" Does it mean the introduction and development of techniques that significantly reduce neurosurgical operative exposure? Does it mean the reduction of operative risk? Does it mean both? And is this really a recent phenomenon?

The journal *Minimally Invasive Neurosurgery* states on its cover that it is the international journal for microsurgery, keyhole surgery, endoscopy, stereotactic guided surgery, endovascular surgery, radiosurgery, and technological developments. This list represents the key components of minimally invasive neurosurgery as viewed by the editors of that journal.

As stated by Perneczky et al.,[4] "The term 'minimally invasive' is now being used in a wide variety of disciplines of medicine and often in a very different sense in each discipline. As far as surgery is concerned, we may use the term only if we realise that every surgical manipulation involves traumatisation of the patient. This applies in particular to neurosurgery, for nothing can be more traumatic for a human being than touching his brain, even if this is performed by means of a small needle as in biopsy. Hence, the prinicpal aim in neurosurgery has always been to minimise surgical traumatisation while increasing the therapeutic effect."

Said another way by Bauer and Hellwig,[5] "Minimally Invasive Neurosurgery is neither a new discipline nor another type of neurosurgery—we have not given birth to a new child."

If minimally invasive neurosurgery is defined as surgery of the nervous system done from the surface of the body, its inclusive components are somewhat different from those listed on the cover of the journal bearing that name. It also includes procedures with a long history and procedures that have become obsolete.

Microneurosurgery is a term that ordinarily implies the use of an operating microscope, microinstruments, and microtechnique to perform an operation at some depth on some aspect of the nervous system through an appropriate opening through the skin and other covering tissues. This type of surgery usually can be done through smaller access corridors than procedures performed without the magnification and added illumination of the operating microscope, but it is still more invasive than a percutaneous procedure or 1 done through a burr hole. Likewise, stereotactic guided surgery is more accurate than surgery performed without such guidance, but if it involves a craniotomy exposure, it is not necessarily less invasive. Therefore, I will not include microneurosurgery or "open" stereotactic guided surgery in the following discussion. Also, I will not include peripheral nerve surgery performed by an open operative exposure of the involved nerve or nerves even though such procedures (e.g., a standard carpal tunnel release) may not be very invasive. Similarly, I will not include procedures such as the insertion of medication pumps or stimulators because, even though the tubing or electrodes are placed percutaneously or stereotactically, dissection is required for insertion and attachment of the pump or receptor unit. The topics to be discussed will include only therapeutic procedures; minimally invasive neurodiagnostic procedures will not be considered. In addition, other topics that will not be dealt with here include procedures usually done by other specialists such as peripheral nerve blocks (by anesthesiologists), some of questionable value such as percutaneous spinal facet denervation (medial branch neurotomy), and some not widely performed such as stereotactic C1 central myelotomy or stereotactic pontine spinothalamic tractotomy.

In the following material, no claim is made regarding absolute priority about the introduction of the various minimally invasive neurosurgical procedures. Some uncertainty always exists about who was the first to describe an approach to treatment.[6] As an example, although the intrasellar injection of alcohol for pain relief in patients with cancer has frequently been dated back to the work of Moricca in 1974, Carbonin[7] in a "Letter to the Editor" of the *Journal of Neurosurgery* supplied 12 references to such treatment in Italy published between 1957 and 1965.

Procedures Introduced Before the Twentieth Century

Trepanation

Trepanation has been carried out in many parts of the world since its inception in the Neolithic period.[8–13] However, although trepanation has involved opening only the scalp and skull, the bony openings made in ancient times with a stone instrument or metal tumi were sometimes relatively large, and until the introduction of aseptic technique, the threat of infection was significant. Beginning as early as the sixteenth century, surgeons trepanned patients to evacuate intracranial collections of pus or blood.[14–16]

The modern counterpart of trepanation is the burr hole or twist drill hole. These relatively small openings can be used to drain intracranial fluid collections or provide access to deeper lesions by freehand, stereotactic, or endoscopic techniques.

Cervical Traction

According to Schneider,[17] Glisson et al.[18] in 1650 introduced halter traction for overcoming deformities of the spine due to rickets. More than 2 centuries later, Lewis A. Sayre[19] used such a sling in his overhead suspension technique for reducing spinal deformity. Then in 1932, 1 of the most important contributions to the nonoperative treatment of cervical dislocations resulted from an unusual set of circumstances. W. Gayle Crutchfield[20] had under his care a young woman who had sustained a complete fracture-dislocation of C2 on C3 in an automobile accident but who also had a compound comminuted fracture of the mandible that prevented the use of halter traction. At the suggestion of his chief, Claude C. Coleman, he modified an instrument used for femur traction, Edmonton extension tongs, and used this for craniocervical traction, thus introducing skeletal traction for the reduction and stabilization of cervical spinal deformities. Subsequently Crutchfield developed his own cranial tongs that were widely used until being superseded more recently by other types of tongs[17, 21] and by the halo device.[22, 23] Of historical interest is the fact that Kenneth G. McKenzie[24] of Toronto independently introduced skeletal traction for treating severe cervical spinal injuries using ice tongs, which he reported in 1935.

Procedures Introduced During the Twentieth Century

Percutaneous Treatments

TRIGEMINAL NEURALGIA

Injection.—In about 1900 the manufacture of appropriate needles permitted physicians to begin treating trigeminal neuralgia by injecting a destructive liquid such as ethyl alcohol into the vicinity of the external opening of the foramen ovale, the foramen rotundum, or the infraorbital foramen to destroy a peripheral division or branch of the trigeminal nerve.[25] With experience, physicians realized that peripheral nerve blocks provide only temporary relief from the pain of trigeminal neuralgia. The injection of a destructive liquid directly into the gasserian ganglion was then proposed as a means of providing a more permanent effect. Beginning in 1907, a few surgeons did so after performing a surgical approach to the foramen ovale.[25]

> According to Stookey and Ransohoff,[30] The first suggestion of the possibility of injecting alcohol directly into the ganglion without a surgical incision was made by Harris (1909) [26].... Harris's first gasserian ganglion injection with alcohol in an actual case of trigeminal neuralgia was carried out in November 1910 [27], producing complete anaesthesia and pain relief, which lasted until the patient's death twenty-seven years later.... Four months after Harris's report appeared, Härtel (1912) [28] described a method of injecting the ganglion with procaine, which he employed in Bier's clinic in Berlin, so that facial operations might be done without a general anaesthetic.... Subsequently, in a very complete study, Härtel (1914) [29] detailed the...technique for alcohol injection of the gasserian ganglion. The procedure was done entirely outside the oral cavity, the skin being pierced anterior to the coronoid process.

In addition to Harris and Härtel, Taptas was another pioneer in the injection of alcohol via the foramen ovale into Meckel's cave.[31] His first publication on this subject was in 1911.[32]

Glycerol has been used for percutaneous injection into the trigeminal cistern since 1975. The first use of this agent for this purpose by Sten Håkanson represents 1 of the classic examples of chance discovery in neurosurgery.[33] Lars Leksell[34] had first used stereotactic radiosurgery to treat tic douloureux in 1953 using the gasserian ganglion as the target.

"In order to better visualize the location of the gasserian ganglion radiographically, Sten Håkanson, working in Leksell's Department of Neurosurgery at the Karolinska Sjukhuset, developed the technique of injecting a water-soluble contrast medium, metrizamide, into the trigeminal cistern... . As a more permanent marker, tantalum powder was tried. Then Håkanson encountered an unexpected occurrence"[33]

To quote Håkanson,[35] "During the development of a stereotactic technique for gamma irradiation of the trigeminal ganglion and root in the treatment of trigeminal neuralgia, glycerol was used as a vehicle to introduce tantalum dust into the trigeminal cistern... . The tantalum dust was used to mark permanently the trigeminal cistern for the precise, stereotactic localization of the trigeminal ganglion and root. Quite unexpectedly it was observed that the intracisternal injection of glycerol alone rendered the patient completely free from the paroxysmal pain without producing any significant sensory loss."

Jefferson[36] had previously used glycerine as a vehicle for injecting phenol into the trigeminal root and ganglion. However, it was Håkanson who discovered that glycerine alone could provide relief of trigeminal neuralgia, and it is he who merits the credit for the introduction of percutaneous retrogasserian glycerol rhizotomy.

Electrocoagulation.—Electrocoagulation of peripheral aspects of the trigeminal nerve was tried soon after peripheral injections were begun. For example, Réthi[37] reported such treatment in 1913. As with alcohol injections, attention later shifted to the gasserian ganglion as the target for electrocoagulation.

According to Stookey and Ransohoff,[30] "Kirschner (1931 [38] and 1933 [39]) suggested electrocoagulation of the gasserian ganglion. A needle, insulated except at its tip, was inserted through the foramen ovale with the aid of a special frame attached to the head."

Penman[40] gave credit to Bauer,[41] as well as to Kirschner,[42] citing references by each author in 1932. He also pointed out that despite the use of the elaborate needle-aiming apparatus, the needle failed to enter the foramen ovale on the first attempt in 10% of Kirschner's cases. Although many patients were treated by electrocoagulation of the gasserian ganglion over the next decade, the procedure gradually fell out of favor until it was resurrected in 1965 by Sweet,[31] who took advantage of advances in electronics and pharmacology to design a procedure that includes electrode localization by electrophysiologic stimulation, intermittent patient sedation with a short-acting IV drug, and controlled lesion production.

In 1938, Sjöqvist[43] introduced an operation for trigeminal neuralgia that involved open sectioning of the descending tract of the trigeminal nerve in the brain stem. In 1967, Crue et al.[44] reported a patient in whom they had performed this procedure percutaneously using a stereotactic approach to create a radiofrequency lesion in the trigeminal tract. However, although it has been tried by Hitchcock[45] and Tsukamoto[46] and others,[47] percutaneous stereotactic trigeminal tractotomy has not caught on as a treatment for trigeminal neuralgia.

Compression.—In 1953, Shelden et al.[48] began to compress the posterior root of the trigeminal nerve after its surgical exposure in the hope that such mild trauma might provide pain relief without significant sensory impairment. However, because of the relatively high rate of pain recurrence, such procedures lost their appeal. In 1978, Mullan and Lichtor[49] revived compression of the gasserian ganglion but introduced a simpler percutaneous technique using a Fogarty-type balloon for this purpose. Their method has since become an accepted low-risk form of surgical treatment of trigeminal.[50]

HEMIFACIAL SPASM.—In a fashion analogous to the introduction of certain surgical treatments of trigeminal neuralgia, hemifacial spasm at 1 time was treated by procedures directed at dividing or otherwise injuring the peripheral branches or the main trunk of the facial nerve.[51] The percutaneous versions of these techniques included injections of alcohol or phenol, radiofrequency thermocoagulation, or compression with a needle; the main target was the facial nerve trunk at the stylomastoid foramen. The dissatisfaction with these approaches to treatment related to the replacement of the abnormal muscle contractions by subtotal or complete facial muscle paralysis, followed by eventual return of hemifacial spasm as the nerve recovered and the weakness resolved. In recent years, type A botulinum exotoxin has been injected in small doses into various facial muscles to reduce their contractions; this has been effective in relieving the hemifacial spasm without producing major weakness, with the beneficial effects usually lasting 3 to 4 months.

GLOSSOPHARYNGEAL NEURALGIA.—Percutaneous radiofrequency glossopharyngeal rhizotomy has been used occasionally by Tew[52] and others[53, 54] in patients with secondary or primary glossopharyngeal neuralgia who are too debilitated to undergo open nerve sectioning in the posterior fossa. Despite the fact that the target of the electrode is the glossopharyngeal nerve at or external to the neural portion of the jugular foramen (and especially the inferior petrous ganglion), ipsilateral vocal cord paralysis and interference with deglutition may occur, as the result of either suboptimal needle placement or the spread of the heat produced by the radiofrequency current to the vagus nerve. On the other hand, if only the glossopharyngeal nerve is injured, the pain may not be relieved as well or as long.[55] Because of such vagaries, this treatment technique has not gained widespread acceptance.

INTERVERTEBRAL DISK DISEASE

Epidural Steroid Injection.—Sicard was an early champion of the treatment of back and leg pain by the epidural injection of medication.[33] In 1901 he[56] published an account of the epidural injection of cocaine. In 1930 Evans[57] published his experience of treating 40 patients with sciatica using epidural injections of normal saline or a procaine solution; more than 60% of the patients obtained relief. After his analysis of this experience, Evans[57] concluded that "relief from sciatic pain is in no way dependent on the nature of the solution introduced.... A mechanical stretching of the nerve roots that go to form the sciatic nerve appears to be the important factor...."

In the 1950s, reports of epidural steroid injection for the treatment of back and leg pain began appearing in the European literature, and these were then followed in the 1960s and subsequently by reports from the United States and elsewhere.[58-62] It has become a widely and frequently used form of treatment, and yet its efficacy is still in doubt.

For example, after a systematic review of randomized clinical trials of epidural steroid injections for low-back pain and sciatica, Koes et al.[63] concluded that "there are flaws in the design of most studies. The best studies showed inconsistent results of epidural steroid injections. The efficacy of epidural steroid injections has not yet been established. The benefits of epidural steroid injections, if any, seem to be of short duration only."

Similarly, Spaccarelli[62] concluded after a review of 9 controlled studies that "at *long-term* follow-up, no difference may be noted between the group that received epidural corticosteroid injections and the control group. This can be explained by the fact that long-term prognosis of a nonsurgically treated herniated disk is improvement in most patients.... [However,] a therapeutic effect seems to occur in patients with lower-extremity radicular pain syndromes at intermediate-term follow-up (2 weeks to 3 months)."

Intradiscal Enzyme Injection.—Because the intervertebral disk is composed of different types of cartilage, the idea arose that perhaps disk herniation or protrusion could be treated by the percutaneous injection of an enzyme that could digest the nucleus pulposus differentially. Although collagenase was tested,[64] chymopapain was the enzyme chosen for this purpose.

"Chymopapain is a proteolytic enzyme first isolated in 1941....Following extensive animal investigations, Smith...commenced his study of the effects of chymopapain on the human disc in 1963, and recorded his first series of patients in 1964 [65–67]. He termed the process of treatment of lumbar intervertebral disc disease with chymopapin 'chemonucleolysis.'"

In the United States, the performance of chemonucleolysis has had peaks and valleys. For a time, the Food and Drug Administration (FDA) did not approve the use of chymopapain for chemonucleolysis, and some patients went to Canada for this treatment. Approval from the FDA was granted in

1982, and there was an immediate widespread interest in such treatment. The American Association of Neurological Surgeons and the American Academy of Orthopaedic Surgeons jointly organized a series of training courses, and over a short period more than 6,000 orthopedic and neurologic surgeons were instructed in chemonucleolysis.[69] However, interest in this form of treatment waned as microdiscectomy and other treatment techniques were developed.

Percutaneous Discectomy.—After the percutaneous approaches to intervertebral disks had been developed for biopsy and for chymopapain injection, there was a natural evolution to the use of such approaches for mechanical discectomy. Starting in 1973, several surgeons began performing radiographically monitored lumbar discectomy through a percutaneously inserted cannula.[70–72] Over time the instrumentation has been modified, and a wider variety of techniques have been employed, including endoscopy and laser tissue removal, such that percutaneous discectomy is a well-recognized option for the treatment of certain types of lumbar disk disease.[73–75] Currently percutaneous endoscopic approaches are being developed not only for discectomy in the thoracic and lumbar areas but also for vertebrectomy, anterior fusion, and anterior instrumentation.[76–79]

RHIZOTOMY AND CORDOTOMY.—As an open operation, posterior rhizotomy of spinal nerve roots to treat pain was introduced independently in 1889 by Bennett in London and Abbe in New York.[80] Spiller and Martin devised and first performed open cordotomy for pain in 1911; unaware of this, Foerster and Tietze sectioned the anterolateral spinal tracts for tabetic pain in 1912.[80] Cordotomy and, to a lesser extent, rhizotomy became standard neurosurgical procedures for many decades.

Then in the 1960s and 1970s percutaneous versions of these procedures were developed. In 1963, Mullan et al.[81] introduced percutaneous cordotomy using a strontium-90 needle, which destroyed the ipsilateral anterolateral aspects of the spinal cord by radiation. By 1965, Mullan et al.[82] had begun to make unipolar anodal electrolytic lesions, and Rosomoff et al.[83] had begun making radiofrequency lesions. Percutaneous radiofrequency cordotomy is still performed, more than 30 years after its introduction. Percutaneous rhizotomy, as introduced by Uematsu et al.[84] in 1974, is also still used occasionally not only for the relief of pain but also for the amelioration of spasticity.[85]

SUBARACHNOID INJECTIONS FOR PAIN OR SPASTICITY.—The subarachnoid injection of alcohol for the treatment of pain was reported by Dogliotti[86] in 1931, and the subsequent experience with the intrathecal injection of alcohol and phenol was reviewed by Rétif[87] in 1977. Although technical variations were introduced to limit the neurolytic effect of these agents, there was always a threat of paraplegia with incontinence, and that restricted their usefulness. For a time there was interest in using hypothermic or hypertonic saline solutions instead of alcohol or phenol in the hope that such solutions would be less injurious, and might relieve pain or spasticity without causing paraplegia with incontinence, thus increasing the numbers of patients who might benefit.[88-90] This hope was not realized, and the use of subarachnoid injections of neurolytic agents waned as better methods of treatment were developed.

SYMPATHECTOMY.—In the third edition of their important book *The Autonomic Nervous System: Anatomy, Physiology, and Surgical Application*, White et al.[91] described in detail the techniques available in 1952 for performing sympathectomy in various areas of the body. They included descriptions of the paravertebral injection of the thoracic and lumbar sympathetic rami and ganglia with alcohol and noted that such paravertebral injections in the thoracic area to relieve cardiac pain had been reported in 1925 by Mandl[92] using local anesthetic agents and in 1926 by Swetlow[93] using alcohol.

Starting in 1979, Wilkinson[94] developed the procedure of percutaneous upper thoracic sympathectomy using radiofrequency lesioning. He has refined this technique in 3 stages to make it a viable alternative to open or endoscopic sympathectomy techniques.

Endoscopy

Endoscopy in neurosurgery began as ventriculoscopy more than 70 years ago. Important to its origin was Walter E. Dandy.

Before he started his residency training in surgery, Walter Dandy began a series of studies at the Johns Hopkins University and Hospital in association with Kenneth Blackfan of the Department of Pediatrics. The 2 men[95-97] performed a series of animal experiments and human investigations that clarified where CSF is produced, how it circulates, where it is absorbed, and what types of hydrocephalus result from the various abnormalities that alter its production, circulation, and absorption.[80] Dandy subsequently developed the operations of choroid plexectomy, cannulation of the aqueduct of Sylvius, and third ventriculostomy to treat hydrocephalus. In 1922, Dandy[98] performed ventriculoscopy utilizing a Kelley cystoscope for inspection of the lateral ventricles in 2 patients and as an aid to choroid plexus coagulation in 1.

In 1923, Fay and Grant[99] took ventriculoscopy 1 step further. They recorded the use of intraventricular photography.

Also in 1923, Mixter[100] reported the use of ventriculoscopy (with a small urethroscope) for puncture of the floor of the third ventricle:

> On February 6, 1923, under ether anaesthesia, an opening was made through the fontanelle.... A small incision was made in the dura and a direct vision urethroscope passed into the ventricle. Under visual guidance the urethroscope was passed through the dilated foramen of Munro [sic] and the third ventricle explored. The dilated aqueduct could be easily seen, but could not be entered with the urethroscope. Under visual guidance, a flexible sound was pushed through the floor of the third ventricle and the opening was enlarged by moving the sound from side to side until it was about four mm. across. The edges of this opening immediately began to

vibrate, apparently due to the passage of a current through the opening and this continued during the short period that the opening was under observation. The urethroscope was withdrawn and the dura and scalp closed with fine silk.

The procedure of excision of the choroid plexus had a high mortality rate and was abandoned early. However, endoscopic cauterization of the choroid plexus, which had also been tried by Lespinasse[101] in 1910, was developed and used by Dandy, Putnam, Scarff, Feld, and others for 30 to 40 years, when the combination of the equivocal results of this procedure and the introduction of successful valved shunt systems led to its abandonment as well.[102]

> In 1953, Scarff developed a new endoscope....His improvements included an angled lens system permitting better lateral visualization, a movable unipolar electrode allowing more flexibility in cauterizing tissue, and an irrigating system enabling blood to be cleared from the operative field. The system maintained an adequate cerebrospinal fluid volume and pressure within the ventricles and thereby prevented collapse of the ventricular walls.... These improvements are retained in most modern day ventriculoscopes.[103]

Yet, despite such improvements, neurosurgical endoscopes were still relatively primitive. In 1960, Harold Hopkins devised a new lens system that substituted a train of glass rods in a metal tube (thus creating a series of air lenses in glass) for the older system that consisted of a series of biconvex glass lenses in a metal tube otherwise filled with air.[104] Hopkins also pioneered the congruent fiber bundle, which led to further improvements in endoscope design.[104] Such changes led to a resurgence of interest in neurosurgical endoscopy in the 1960s and 1970s.[103–105]

Even so, neurosurgical endoscopy was not used widely until relatively recently, when further technical advances made this possible. Endoscopes have been miniaturized and made flexible, and video systems, lasers, and other instruments have been developed for or adapted to endoscopy.[105–108]

Although choroid plexectomy and coagulation are no longer employed, endoscopy is now used for third ventriculostomy; the biopsy, evacuation, or resection of intraventricular tumors and cysts; and the fenestration of intraventricular septa.[1–3, 102–108] The scope of neurosurgical endoscopy has been expanded remarkably in recent years to include a wide variety of procedures such as the biopsy and evacuation of extraventricular intracranial cysts; the resection of membranes and drainage of chronic subdural hematomas; the drainage of brain abscesses; the evacuation of intracerebral hematomas; the resection of angiographically occult vascular malformations; the resection of sellar and suprasellar tumors and cysts; the inspection of the cerebellopontine angle; the inspection of the spinal subarachnoid space; the endocavitary treatment of septated syringomyelia;

the removal of intervertebral disk material; the resection of spinal lesions; the biopsy or drainage of intraspinal cysts; the repair of anterior, lateral, or intrasacral meningoceles; the performance of spinal fusion and instrumentation procedures; and the decompression of the median nerve at the wrist and hand.

Psychosurgery

In the nineteenth century, as evidence of localization of function within the nervous system was accumulating, it became apparent that the anterior aspects of the frontal lobes had some relationship with mental functions and personality. Although a few physicians tried to use this information for therapeutic benefit, psychosurgery did not really begin until 1935.[80, 109-118]

In that year the prominent Portuguese neurologist Antonio Caetano de Abreu Freire Egas Moniz attended the Second International Neurological Congress in London to present an exhibit of his pioneering investigations of cerebral angiography. There he heard the presentation of the work of John Fulton and Carlyle Jacobsen concerning primate frontal lobe function; on his return to Lisbon in August, Egas Moniz organized a team to determine whether the creation of lesions in the frontal lobes would have a beneficial effect for certain psychiatric illnesses. Three months later, the neurosurgical member of the team, Pedro Manuel de Almeida Lima, injected alcohol into the white matter of the frontal lobes of a psychiatric patient, thereby initiating the subsequent widespread use of psychosurgery in various areas around the world. Numerous procedures were developed to produce frontal lobe lesions. Several of them can be thought of as minimally invasive procedures that used limited routes of access such as bilateral burr holes in the frontal calvaria or a puncture wound through the roof of each orbit. Most of the procedures were performed with free-hand technique, but some used stereotactic guidance.

In 1949, at the peak of the worldwide use of psychosurgery, Egas Moniz was awarded the Nobel Prize in Physiology and Medicine. This form of neurosurgery declined thereafter as effective antipsychotic medications were developed and as public opposition to psychosurgery rose.[117]

Other Minimally Invasive Treatments of Trigeminal Neuralgia (Other than Percutaneous Treatments)

RADIOSURGERY.—The innovative neurosurgeon Lars Leksell[119, 120] introduced stereotactic radiosurgery in 1951. In 1953 he[34] began to use radiation focused on the gasserian ganglion to treat trigeminal neuralgia, and by 1983 he[121] had treated 63 patients with this condition. More recently, investigators from several centers have used the Leksell Gamma Knife to treat trigeminal neuralgia but have used the trigeminal sensory root (between the pons and Meckel's cave) as the target. Kondziolka et al.[122] report encouraging results, but the length of follow-up is still relatively short. More time will be required for the assessment of pain recurrence and delayed complications related to the long-term effects of γ-radiation.

ENDOSCOPY.—With the advances in the technological aspects of endoscopy in recent years, there has been a preliminary interest in performing partial sectioning of the main sensory root[123] and in possibly performing microvascular decompression of the trigeminal nerve[124] endoscopically. Whether this less invasive approach to sectioning or decompressing the trigeminal nerve and perhaps other cranial nerves will develop into a worthwhile and widely used form of treatment remains to be seen.

Minimally Invasive Treatments of Other Types of Pain (Other Than Percutaneous Treatments)

HYPOPHYSECTOMY.—For a period starting in 1952, transcranial hypophysectomy was used in an attempt to control the growth of hormonally responsive tumors such as carcinoma of the breast and carcinoma of the prostate.[125] It was discovered that hypophysectomy might ameliorate pain caused by metastatic carcinoma (especially metastatic to bone), as well as other conditions. And as time passed, various radiologically monitored transnasal transsphenoidal probe techniques were developed in an attempt to simplify hypophysectomy and reduce its risks. Among the methods tried were brachytherapy using implanted radioisotopes such as radon, yttrium-90, gold-198, or phosphorus-32,[126, 127] cryosurgery,[128, 129] radiofrequency lesioning,[130, 131] and alcohol injection.[7, 132, 133] Traditional radiotherapy proved inadequate, but beginning in 1954, beams of high-energy particles such as protons were used for hypophysectomy.[134] These techniques of performing hypophysectomy for pain relief have become outmoded as other, more effective, pain management techniques have been developed.

STEREOTACTIC ABLATIVE PROCEDURES.—As stereotactic techniques were developed to permit neurosurgeons to make lesions accurately within the brain, certain areas became targets for the alleviation of pain and suffering. Targets were chosen within pain pathways and also within the limbic system.[135–138]

Spiegel and Wycis, pioneers in the initiation and development of stereotactic neurosurgery, began in 1947 to make precise lesions in the mesencephalon for the relief of pain.[139–141] With subsequent modifications, this procedure is still used today. Stereotactic thalamotomy has also been employed since 1947,[139–144] but there has been much more controversy about the choice of target within the thalamus.[135–138, 144] The posteromedial hypothalamus,[145, 146] the cingulum,[147, 148] and other areas of the brain[149] also have been targeted, but overall the results have been somewhat disappointing. To quote Young,[138] "Stereotactic ablative lesions may provide pain relief in about two-thirds of patients with somatic pain, but early recurrences are frequent and loss of normal sensory function and disabling dysesthesias are fairly frequent occurrences. Ablative lesions for treatment of central pain due to deafferentation are effective in less than 50% of patients."

ENDOSCOPIC THORACIC SYMPATHECTOMY.—Although it is often employed for hyperhidrosis and other nonpainful conditions, endoscopic thoracic sympathectomy is also used to treat pain. In particular, upper thoracic sympathectomy has been used for painful disorders of an upper extremity such as causalgia or reflex sympathetic dystrophy and for pain of cardiac origin. As already noted, there has been a resurgence of interest in endoscopy in recent years. It is good to remember, however, that in the early 1940s Houghes, Goetz, and Marr and Kux independently reported the endoscopic approach for operations on the sympathetic chain in the chest, and in 1954 Kux[150] published a book based on an experience with 1,104 patents![151]

Reservoir and Shunt Insertions

Access to the ventricular system has been and continues to be important to surgeons not only for diagnosis but also for therapy. To avoid the need for serial ventricular punctures, several surgeons such as McKenzie,[152] Ommaya,[153] and Rickham[154] have introduced implantable reservoirs with attached ventricular catheters that can be inserted to provide repetitive ventricular access via simple puncture of the scalp.

In contrast to the relatively simple and straightforward development and introduction of ventricular reservoirs, the development and introduction of shunts for the treatment of hydrocephalus have had a long and fascinating history, with many ingenious approaches taken but with only a few surviving the test of time.[155–163] Furthermore, the search for better shunt systems continues on at present.

From the beginning of successful ventriculoatrial, ventriculoperitoneal, and ventriculopleural shunting, the ventricular end has been inserted through a burr hole or twist drill hole. Also, for these shunts, as well as the lumboperitoneal shunt, the subcutaneous catheter was tunneled from 1 skin incision to another using a temporarily inserted guide tube. More recently techniques have been developed to insert peritoneal, lumbar, pleural, and atrial catheters through needles or peel-away sheath systems, thus simplifying current shunting procedures for hydrocephalus and making them truly minimally invasive operations.[164–166] The same holds true for procedures to shunt other intracranial fluid collections such as arachnoid cysts or chronic subdural hematomas.

A related issue is the antenatal shunting of hydrocephalus discovered in utero. When ultrasonography became sufficiently advanced to permit the diagnosis of hydrocephalus before birth, interest developed in the possibility of treating it in utero to provide ventricular decompression until a standard shunting technique could be performed at birth. The first technique used in human patients was serial ultrasonically guided percutaneous cephalocenteses, as reported by Birnholz and Frigoletto[167] in 1981. Soon thereafter, valved and unvalved tubes were used for ventriculoamniotic shunting.[168, 169] The initial enthusiasm for such treatment rapidly waned when it became apparent that fetal shunting improved survival somewhat without improving functional outcome.[170, 171]

Stereotactic Neurosurgery

During the nineteenth century 2 concepts evolved that were important to the development of neurosurgery. The first was the idea that certain areas of the brain are especially important for certain brain functions—the concept of cerebral localization. The second was the idea that the surface of the brain has a predictable relationship with the overlying calvaria and that specific brain areas can be located by the use of external calvarial landmarks—the concept of craniocerebral topography.[172] However, when individuals attempted to use such external landmarks to guide them to specific areas within the brain, they[173] discovered that there is significant variability in the relationships between skull landmarks and brain structures. The early instruments used for surface localization, such as the kephalograph of Harting (1861), the encephalometer of Zernov (1889), and the cerebral topograph of Rossolima (1907), were not based on truly cartesian (3-dimensional) coordinates.[174, 175] This deficiency was overcome by Robert Henry Clarke, who laid the real foundation for stereotactic neurosurgery in his initial experimental work with Victor Horsley regarding the structure and functions of the cerebellum of animals.

According to Schurr and Merrington,[176] "It was Clarke's inspiration to apply geometry to the study of the brain. He realized that there was no constant relationship between the skull and the structures within the cranium, and that the only way to find out where to place an instrument in a given internal part was to build a map on which everything could be related to three zero planes."

Clarke's original stereotaxic instrument was constructed in 1905 and was first used by Horsley and Clarke in 1906. Their initial reports appeared in 1906[177] and 1908.[178]

> Instructions for developing an atlas and section of the brain of the cat and monkey were published by Clarke and Henderson in 1911..., 1914...and in 1920... . Clarke, who realized the limitations of his original rectilinear system, later developed an equatorial system which enabled the electrode to be introduced anywhere over the skull and at any inclination... . In addition to producing a cerebral stereotaxic apparatus, Clarke invented a similar instrument for use on the spinal cord... . The cerebral stereotaxic instrument was patented by Clarke in 1914... .
>
> Aubrey Mussen..., a graduate from McGill Medical School in Montreal, worked with Horsley and Clarke in London in 1905, 1906 and 1908... . Based upon the original Clarke instrument, Mussen designed his own stereotaxic apparatus for use in humans. It was built in London [in] 1918 and a stereotaxic atlas followed 4 years later... . Mussen, who was a neuroanatomist and neurophysiologist, never managed to convince any neurosurgeon to use it [179, 180]... .
>
> In 1925 Dr. Ernest Spiegel, who at that time lived in Vienna, made inquiries about having a...Clarke's apparatus constructed... .

> Because of Clarke's death the plan was never realized. Twenty-two years later Spiegel et al….became the first to apply Clarke's idea for human stereotaxis….[181]

Spiegel Wycis[182, 183] constructed the first of a series of devices (stereo-encephalotomes) with which in 1947 they began to perform stereotactic brain operations in patients with various conditions such as psychiatric disorders, intractable pain, movement disorders, and epilepsy. They added accuracy to such surgery by using structures within the brain as reference points for their method of stereotaxis.

> In 1947, as the world was recovering from a devastating war…, Ernest Spiegel, a neurologist in Philadelphia, expressed grave concerns over the then current surgical technique of frontal lobotomy which was used to control disturbance of emotion and behavior. The initial impetus to construct a stereotactic frame was Spiegel's concern over the crudeness of frontal lobotomy suggested that therapeutic lesions could be made in the medial dorsal thalamic nucleic interrupting the projection of the fibers to the frontal lobe, accomplishing the same clinical effect without the serious side effects often associated with open frontal lobotomy. Collaborating with Henry Wycis, the neurosurgeon, they conceived and built the first stereotactic instrument for humans….instead of using landmarks on the skull for localization of intracranial structures, Spiegel et al. [139] used intracranial structures around the third ventricle…, which were visualized after introduction of air into the ventricular system. Spiegel…classified stereotactic frames into three general types… . Type I is a cuboidal or rectangular frame… . Type II was constructed on the principle of a semicircular arc and the Leksell…and Riechert-Mundinger…instruments are examples. Type III is an instrument fixed in or above the trephine opening to guide a probe into the brain and early examples of these are Spiegel (1953)…, Cooper (1955)…, Austin and Lee (1958)…and Rand (1961)… .[184]

Stereotactic techniques were used for several purposes initially[184–189] but especially for producing accurate focal ablations for the treatment of movement disorders, the main 1 of which was Parkinson's disease.[33, 190, 191] With the introduction of effective pharmacologic agents for movement disorders, the need for stereotactic surgery diminished significantly in the 1960s. However, as CT came into use in the 1970s and MRI in the 1980s, and as the problems of long-term medical treatment of Parkinson's disease became apparent, such as secondary levodopa resistance, there was a resurgence of interest in the stereotactic surgical treatment of movement disorders.

In fact, the adaptation of computer technology to neuroradiology has not only revolutionized neuroradiologic diagnosis but has also permitted the use of the computerized data from such diagnostic studies to improve the accuracy of modern stereotactic cranial and spinal surgery,[192] including procedures done in minimally invasive fashion such as ventricular endoscopy, tumor biopsy, cyst or abscess drainage, ablative functional neurosurgery, and the injection or insertion of drugs, radioisotope solutions, solid brachytherapy radiation sources, neural grafts, or genes.[174, 187, 193, 194] Such stereotactic procedures now involve interaction of the surgeon with the computer, as well as with the patient, and with the stereotactic equipment. At present, interactive stereotactic neurosurgery is usually performed using 1 of the large variety of frames that have been introduced since 1947.[189] Frameless techniques are being developed,[195–198] however, and these have the potential of rendering stereotactic frames obsolete before the year 2000. Furthermore, robotic technology could play an increasingly important role in stereotactic neurosurgery by that time.[199–201]

Radiosurgery

A natural extension of the idea of stereotactic neurosurgery was the idea of focusing radiation on a target within the brain so that a small area of tissue can be destroyed without the necessity of a cranial opening. As mentioned earlier, Lars Leksell, a pioneer in stereotactic neurosurgery, used stereotactic radiosurgery to treat tic douloureux in 1953.

Leksell "visited Wycis in Philadelphia in 1947 and then developed the Leksell instrument [202], which is a type II stereotactic instrument based on a semicircular arc... . He reported his results in 1949... ."[184]

Lars Leksell was an innovative man with a lifelong interest in engineering.[203] In 1971, Leksell[120] commented on the origination of radiosurgery:

> The first attempts to supplant instruments with stereotaxically directed narrow beams of ionizing radiation were made in 1951 [119]... . The development of this method was begun in 1948... . From the beginning the localization of the target has been based on the pneumoencephalographic visualization of ventricular reference points... . Initially, relatively low energy x-rays were used, but even then the use of high energy gamma rays appeared an attractive possibility... . Extensive studies in goats, using the proton beam of the 185 MeV synchrocyclotron in Uppsala, and clinical tests in a small group of patients with Parkinsonism gave valuable information concerning the anatomy of the radiolesions and the doses of radiation required... . The use of heavy particles in cerebral surgery was also studied by Kjellberg and Lawrence and their co-workers [204, 205]. However, although the synchrocyclotron is a valuable research tool, it has proved too complicated for general neurosurgical application. The final choice of gamma rays rather than high energy x-rays from a linear accelerator was determined on technical grounds and on the need for a practical and reliable clinical method. The present ^{60}Co Gamma Unit was specially designed to be included in this stereotaxic system... . The first operations on man were performed in February, 1968.

Since its inception, radiosurgery with Leksell's Gamma Knife has become a method of treatment used around the world for a variety of conditions.[206–208] In addition, radiosurgery using a linear accelerator or a source of heavy particles is also widely employed.[206–208]

Endovascular Neurosurgery (Therapeutic or Interventional Neuroradiology)

The vascular system is an obvious route of access to the CNS. For many years, medications have been given through the arterial system, and venous blood has been sampled for diagnostic purposes.

In 1927, Myerson et al.[209] described percutaneous methods for obtaining blood from the internal jugular vein and the internal carotid artery. They[209] noted that:

> ...while a method of injecting therapeutic solutions into the internal carotid artery so that these substances might reach the brain directly was being worked on, the technic broadened out into a new method of studying the metabolism of the brain. It seemed theoretically correct that if one could study the blood directly before it reached the brain, and then could study it directly as it came from the brain, without admixture with venous blood from other parts of the body, something might be learned of what takes place within the brain.

These 1927 puncture techniques are of interest from an historical point of view in light of the fact that cerebral arteriography was first described by Moniz in 1927.[80] Furthermore, the seminal studies of human cerebral circulation and cerebral metabolism by Kety and Schmidt, using the internal jugular vein puncture technique of Myerson et al., did not appear until 1945[210] and 1946.[211]

In 1958, Woodhall et al.[212] began to treat brain tumors by the intracarotid injection of chemotherapeutic agents. However, for such localized cerebral perfusion they exposed and cannulated the carotid arteries and internal jugular veins in the neck rather than accessing these structures percutaneously.

Therapeutic ligation of the common or internal carotid artery in the neck has a long history.[213–215] To quote Johnson,[213]

> The first adequate description in medical literature of a ligation of the common carotid artery was by John Abernethy...who in 1798 ligated the common carotid for the treatment of hemorrhage in a patient who had been gored in the neck by an ox... . Several years later, in 1805, the first ligation for carotid aneurysm in the neck was performed by Sir Astley Cooper...but proved unsuccessful... . In 1808 Cooper performed the operation successfully in a similar case... . In 1809..., Travers performed his carotid ligation for pulsating exophthalmos.

According to Hamby,[215] "Warren was probably the first American surgeon to ligate the common carotid artery for a carotid-cavernous fistula, around 1837. Maury was reported by Harkness and by Dandy to have been the first to ligate the internal carotid artery for this disease, although the vessel had been ligated for other reasons as early as 1847 by Wood of New York."

Carotid ligation was a commonly used treatment for certain intracranial aneurysms and for carotid-cavernous fistulas in the 1950s and 1960s. For the latter condition, intracranial ligation of the internal carotid and ophthalmic arteries was often added to extracranial ligation of the internal carotid artery, but even such trapping did not produce obliteration of the fistula in some cases.

In 1930, "in discussing a paper by Noland and Taylor before the Southern Surgical Association [216], Dr. Barney Brooks, of Nashville, reported a unique method by which he attempted to obliterate a carotid-cavernous fistula [217]. He opened the internal carotid artery in the neck between clamps and packed a long, thin, strip of muscle into the artery. The incision in the artery then was closed and the clamps were removed."[215] It was thought that the bloodstream forced the muscle into the fistula, effectively plugging it.

Variations on this theme were used subsequently by a number of surgeons. Embolization of muscle was often used in association with open arterial ligation in the treatment of carotid-cavernous fistulas.

Although the use of vascular occlusion to treat certain neurologic conditions has a long history, endovascular neurosurgery is a relatively recent development.[218] Endovascular embolization and occlusion techniques have advanced from open arteriotomy, through percutaneous methods, to superselective catheterization. Materials used for embolization have evolved and improved, and balloon catheters have been developed, first with nondetachable balloons and later with detachable balloons.

Such advancements have also occurred simultaneously in other areas of radiology and medicine. Interventional cardiology has grown rapidly from its modest beginnings in the diagnostic cardiac catheterization laboratory to its present important position in the treatment of various conditions affecting the heart. The specialty of vascular and interventional radiology has developed, and by 1990 there were approximately 100 fellowship training programs in North America.[219] The Society of Cardiovascular and Interventional Radiology was founded, and since 1990 it has published the *Journal of Vascular and Interventional Radiology.*

Starting in 1959, Luessenhop and Spence[220] and then Luessenhop et al.[221] began to occlude intracranial arteriovenous malformations (AVMs) with artificial emboli which were introduced through a plastic tube inserted into a surgically created stump of the external carotid artery. Initially they used hand-molded spheres of methylmethacrylate containing a fragment of steel or tantalum that was visible radiographically. Subsequently they used molded spheres of Marlex plastic and, later, molded silicone spheres containing a steel ball. Luessenhop et al.[221] noted that "multiple lengths of silk suture can be sewn through each sphere to project from the surface about 1 mm. to encourage thrombosis over a wider area in the malformation."

Such emboli were carried preferentially to the AVM by its increased blood flow, which diminished as the malformation was progressively occluded. Because of this and other factors, the emboli at times ended up in vessels other than those of the AVM. In an effort to gain more control over the fate of artificial emboli, Luessenhop and Velasquez[222] developed a catheter that could be led into the intracranial circulation by an artificial embolus or by an inflatable balloon at its tip, a technique that they described in 1964.

In Japan, Sano et al.[223] experimented with a liquid plastic (dimethyl-polysiloxane) for endovascular embolization. They[223] first tested this agent in the superior mesenteric artery of dogs and then used it to treat 2 patients with AVMs as reported in 1966.

In the United States, 2 magnetically controlled intravascular catheter systems were introduced in 1968.[224, 225] And in 1970, Taren and Gabrielsen[226] reported the radiofrequency thrombosis of 2 extracranial AVMs with a transvascular magnetic catheter. However, magnet catheter systems did not prove to be sufficiently effective for widespread use, and other techniques took their place.

By 1963, Fogarty et al.[227] had already developed a balloon catheter for the extraction of arterial emboli and thrombi. In 1969, Prolo and Hanbery[228] used a Fogarty catheter to occlude the internal carotid artery at the site of a carotid-cavernous fistula. Also in 1969, Kessler and Wholey[229] inflated a latex balloon on a polyvinyl catheter in the proximal 1 to 2 cm of the internal carotid artery to treat an intracranial aneurysm on that artery; the balloon was deflated and withdrawn after being left for 48 hours, and the aneurysm could not be visualized angiographically then or 3 months later. Kerber[230] subsequently developed a balloon catheter with a calibrated leak suitable for superselective angiography and occlusive catheter therapy.

However, the development of endovascular neurosurgery really had its origin in the work of Fyodor Serbinenko at the Burdenko Institute in Moscow. He has been called the father of endovascular neurosurgery.[231]

> After countless hours of research and development, Serbinenko settled on the use of polyethylene catheters and latex balloons for his endovascular operations. To prevent balloon deflation, he inflated his balloons with a hardening agent; liquid silicone was his initial choice. Serbinenko and his colleague, Filatov, further refined their techniques by describing the use of a second "helper balloon," which made this a more navigable balloon catheter system.
>
> Starting in 1971, Serbinenko began turning out a number of papers in Russian detailing his years of research... . His landmark publication, "Balloon Catheterization and Occlusion of Major Cerebral Vessels" caught the neurosurgical world by surprise, stirring great interest [232].[231]

In that paper, Serbinenko mentioned that he had started his selective angiographic studies in 1963.[231] Between 1969 and 1972 he had performed temporary diagnostic balloon occlusion of 13 different major cerebral arteries in 304 cases with 2 complications; each of the 2 patients died as a result of an unexplained thrombosis of the middle cerebral artery.

Serbinenko[232] noted that "the use of a balloon provided with a lumen permits: 1, Selective angiography of a vessel located either distal or proximal to the occluded section...; 2, injection of a fluid-hardening plastics into an aneurysm; 3, Injection of radiopaque materials for tumor staining...; 4, supplying chemotherapeutic agents to a tumor."

He reported the permanent therapeutic occlusion of major cerebral vessels in 162 instances, starting in 1970, to treat a variety of conditions including aneurysms (10 operations) and arteriovenous malformations (79 operations). Concerning carotid-cavernous fistulas, various parts of the cavernous segment of the internal carotid artery were occluded in 38 operations, and in another 30 the fistulas were occluded for reconstruction of the cavernous part of the internal carotid artery. Serbinenko[232] also gave 2 examples of balloon occlusion of intracranial aneurysms, 1 at the tip of the basilar artery and the other arising from the supraclinoid portion of the internal carotid artery.

Serbinenko's paper in the *Journal of Neurosurgery* had a major effect. "Neurosurgeons around the world quickly took notice of his work. Students and admirers flocked to Moscow to watch Serbinenko work...." However, aspects of Serbinenko's work such as the construction of the balloon catheters were kept secret, which initially cast doubt on the accuracy and validity of his work and delayed the widespread use of his intravascular techniques.

For various reasons, endovascular neurosurgery flourished in the Soviet Union.[231] Victor Shcheglov at the Kiev Neurosurgical Institute quickly gained experience in treating a variety of vascular lesions, and in 1975 Zozulia and Shcheglov reported their initial series of endovascular operations for intracranial aneurysms.[231] In 1984, Zubkov et al.[233] of the Polenov Neurosurgical Institute in Leningrad published pioneering work on intracranial endovascular angioplasty for cerebral vasospasm.

Outside of the Soviet Union, endovascular neurosurgery was developed and refined at many medical centers. In 1978, Debrun et al.[234] in Paris reported their work on detachable balloon and calibrated-leak balloon techniques in the treatment of vascular lesions. At the end of 1974, Debrun,[235] without knowing Serbinenko's technique, had independently devised a detachable balloon technique and published the initial experimental and clinical results.

Since those early beginnings, numerous advancements have occurred worldwide in the field of interventional neuroradiology.[236, 237] The technology and equipment for angiography have changed significantly in the past 20 years. A variety of catheters have been developed for angiography, embolization, vascular occlusion, angioplasty, and thrombolysis. Numerous agents have been used for embolization, including particles, liquid agents, and coils. And intravascular stents and snares are under development.

Indications for endovascular neurosurgery have expanded beyond the embolization of vascular tumors and intracranial AVMs; the occlusion of parent arteries, arteriovenous fistulas, and aneurysms; the physical dilation of spastic intracranial arteries; and the selective injection of chemotherapeutic agents. For example, endovascular approaches are being used to dilate stenotic areas of the carotid and vertebral arteries and to lyse intra-arterial and IV thrombi.[238, 239] Certain carotid-cavernous fistulas and dural arteriovenous fistulas are now treated by venous endovascular techniques,[240-243] as are certain vein of Galen malformations.[244-246] And since the initial reports concerning the embolization of spinal AVMs starting in 1968,[247, 248] certain vascular spinal lesions have been treated by endovascular embolization.[249, 250]

Conclusion

The concept of minimally invasive neurosurgery is currently receiving much attention. But it is not a new idea, and the roots of its components extend back in time. In a way, a review of its history confirms Ecclesiastes 1:9: "There is nothing new under the sun."

References

1. Bauer BL, Hellwig D (eds): Minimally invasive neurosurgery I. *Acta Neurochir (Wien)* Suppl 54, 1992.
2. Bauer BL, Hellwig D (eds): Minimally invasive neurosurgery II. *Acta Neurochir (Wien)* Suppl 61, 1994.
3. Cohen AR, Haines SJ (eds): *Minimally Invasive Techniques in Neurosurgery.* Baltimore, Williams & Wilkins, 1995.
4. Perneczky A, Cohen A, George B, et al: Editorial. *Minim Invas Neurosurg* 37:1, 1994.
5. Bauer BL, Hellwig D: Preface, in Bauer BL, Hellwig D (eds): Minimally invasive neurosurgery II. *Acta Neurochir (Wien)* Suppl 61, 1994.
6. Palmer ED: Who was first? *JAMA* 239:1609–1610, 1978.
7. Carbonin G: Hypophysectomy and pain relief in cancer. Letter to the editor. *J Neurosurg* 48:666, 1978.
8. Henschen F (Thomas S, transl): *The Human Skull. A Cultural History.* London, Thames and Hudson, 1966, pp 85–102.
9. O'Connor DC, Walker AE: Prologue, in Walker AE (ed): *A History of Neurological Surgery.* Baltimore, Md, Williams & Wilkins, 1951, pp 1–22.
10. Rifkinson-Mann S: Cranial surgery in ancient Peru. *Neurosurgery* 23:411–416, 1988.
11. Stone JL, Miles ML: Skull trepanation among the early Indians of Canada and the United States. *Neurosurgery* 26:1015–1020, 1990.
12. Velasco-Suarez M, Martinez JB, Oliveros RG, et al: Archaeological origins of cranial surgery: Trephination in Mexico. *Neurosurgery* 31:313–319, 1992.
13. Walker AE: Primitive trepanation: the beginning of medical history. *Trans Stud Coll Physicians Phila* 26:99–102, 1958.
14. Stern WE: Surgery of the craniocerebral infections, in Walker AE (ed): *A History of Neurological Surgery.* Baltimore, Md, Williams & Wilkins, 1951, pp 180–212.
15. Walker AE: Surgery of craniocerebral trauma, in Walker AE (ed): *A History of Neurological Surgery.* Baltimore, Md, Williams & Wilkins, 1951, pp 216–247.

16. Wilkins RH: Treatment of craniocerebral infection and other common neurosurgical operations at the time of Lister and Macewen, in Greenblatt SH, Dagi TF, Epsteins MH (eds): *A History of Neurosurgery.* Park Ridge, Ill, American Association of Neurological Surgeons (in press).
17. Schneider RC: Cervical traction, with evaluation of methods, and treatment of complications. *Int Abstr Surg* 104:521–530, 1957.
18. Glisson F, Bate G, Regemorter A: *De Rachitide Sive Morbo Puerili, Qui Vulgo The Rickets Dicitur.* London, Roberti Beaumont, 1650.
19. Sayre LA: *Spinal Disease and Spinal Curvature. Their Treatment by Suspension and the Use of the Plaster of Paris Bandage.* London, Smith, Elder, & Co, 1877.
20. Crutchfield WG: Skeletal traction for dislocation of the cervical spine. Report of a case. *South Surg* 2:156–159, 1933.
21. Loeser JD: History of skeletal traction in the treatment of cervical spine injuries. *J Neurosurg* 33:54–59, 1970.
22. Perry J, Nickel VL: Total cervical-spine fusion for neck paralysis. *J Bone Joint Surg (Am)* 41A:37–60, 1959.
23. Nickel VL, Perry J, Garrett A, et al: The halo. A spinal skeletal traction fixation device. *J Bone Joint Surg (Am)* 50A:1400–1409, 1968.
24. McKenzie KG: Fracture, dislocation, and fracture-dislocation of the spine. *Can Med Assoc J* 32:263–269, 1935.
25. Wilkins RH: Historical perspectives. in Rovit RL, Murali R, Jannetta PJ (eds): *Trigeminal Neuralgia.* Baltimore, Md, Williams & Wilkins, 1990, pp 1–25.
26. Harris W: The alcohol injection treatment for neuralgia and spasm. *Lancet* 1:1310–1313, 1909.
27. Harris W: Alcohol injection of the gasserian ganglion for trigeminal neuralgia. *Lancet* 1:218–221, 1912.
28. Härtel F: Die Leitungsanästhesie und Injektionsbehandlung des Ganglion Gasseri und der Trigeminusstämme. *Arch Klin Chir* 100:193–292, 1912.
29. Härtel F: Ueber die intracranielle Injectionsbehandlung der Trigeminusneuralgie. *Med Klin* 10:582–584, 1914.
30. Stookey B, Ransohoff J: *Trigeminal Neuralgia: Its History and Treatment.* Springfield, Ill, Charles C Thomas, 1959, pp 149, 165.
31. Sweet WH: The history of the development of treatment for trigeminal neuralgia. *Clin Neurosurg* 32:294–318, 1985.
32. Taptas N: Les injection d'alcool dans le ganglion de Gasser a travers le trou ovale. *Presse Med* 19:798–799, 1911.
33. Wilkins RH: Chance discovery in neurosurgery, in Bradley WG, Wilkins RH (eds): 1997 Year Book of Neurology and Neurosurgery, p xxx, St Louis, Mosby, 1997.
34. Leksell L: Stereotaxic radiosurgery in trigeminal neuralgia. *Acta Chir Scand* 137:311–314, 1971.
35. Håkanson S: Trigeminal neuralgia treated by the injection of glycerol into the trigeminal cistern. *Neurosurgery* 9:638–646, 1981.
36. Jefferson A: Trigeminal root and ganglion injections using phenol in glycerine for the relief of trigeminal neuralgia. *J Neurol Neurosurg Psychiatry* 26:345–352, 1963.
37. Réthi A; Die elektrolytische Behandlung der Trigeminusneuralgien. *Munch Med Wochenschr* 60:295–296, 1913.
38. Kirschner M: Zur Elektrochirurgie. *Arch Klin Chir* 167:761–768, 1931.
39. Kirschner: Die Punktionstechnik und die Electrokoagulation des Ganglion Gasseri. Über "gezielte" Operationen. *Arch Klin Chir* 176:581–620, 1933.
40. Penman J: Trigeminal neuralgia, in Vinken PJ, Bruyn GW (eds): *Handbook of Clinical Neurology,* vol 5: *Headaches and Cranial Neuralgias.* Amsterdam, North-Holland, 1968, pp 296–322.
41. Bauer KH: Beiträge zur Hirn- and Schädelchirurgie. *Zentralbl Chir* 59:819–821, 1932.
42. Kirschner: Zur Electrokoagulation des Ganglion Gasseri. *Zentralbl Chir* 59:2841–2843, 1932.

43. Sjöqvist O: Studies on pain conduction in the trigeminal nerve: A contribution to the surgical treatment of facial pain. *Acta Psychiatr Neurol* 17(suppl):1–139, 1938.
44. Crue BL, Todd EM, Carregal EJA, et al: Percutaneous trigeminal tractotomy: Case report—utilizing stereotactic radiofrequency lesion. *Bull Los Angeles Neurol Soc* 32:86–92, 1967.
45. Hitchcock E: Stereotactic trigeminal tractotomy. *Ann Clin Res* 2:131–135, 1970.
46. Hitchcock E. Tsukamoto Y: Distal and proximal sensory responses during stereotactic spinal tractotomy in man. *Ann Clin Res* 5:68–73, 1973.
47. Kanpolat Y, Caglar S, Savas A, et al: CT-guided percutaneous trigeminal tractotomy-nucleotomy. Paper presented at the 64th Annual Meeting of the American Association of Neurological Surgeons, Minneapolis, Minn, May 1, 1996.
48. Shelden CH, Pudenz RH, Freshwater DB, et al: Compression rather than decompression for trigeminal neuralgia. *J Neurosurg* 12:123–126, 1955.
49. Mullan S, Lichtor T: Percutaneous microcompression of the trigeminal ganglion for trigeminal neuralgia. *J Neurosurg* 59:1007–1012, 1983.
50. Lichtor T, Mullan JF: A 10-year follow-up review of percutaneous microcompression of the trigeminal ganglion. *J Neurosurg* 72:49–54, 1990.
51. Wilkins RH: Hemifacial spasm: A review. *Surg Neurol* 36:251–277, 1991.
52. Tew JM Jr: Percutaneous rhizotomy in the treatment of intractable facial pain (trigeminal, glossopharyngeal, and vagal nerves), in Schmidek HH, Sweet WH (eds): *Current Techniques in Operative Neurosurgery.* New York, Grune & Stratton, 1977, pp 409–426.
53. Lazorthes Y, Verdie J-C: Radiofrequency coagulation of the petrous ganglion in glossopharyngeal neuralgia. *Neurosurgery* 4:512–516, 1979.
54. Broggi G, Siefried J: Percutaneous differential radiofrequency rhizotomy of glossopharyngeal nerve in facial pain due to cancer. *Adv Pain Res Ther* 2:469–473, 1969.
55. Apfelbaum RI: Discussion of Arbit E, Krol G: Percutaneous radiofrequency neurolysis guided by computed tomography for the treatment of glossopharyngeal neuralgia. *Neurosurgery* 29:582, 1991.
56. Sicard A: Les injection médicamenteuses extra-durales par voie sacrococcygienne. *C R Soc Biol (Paris)* 53:396–398, 1901.
57. Evans W: Intrasacral epidural injection in the treatment of sciatica. *Lancet* 2:1225–1229, 1930.
58. Liévre J-A, Bloch-Michel H, Pèan G, et al: L'hydrocortisone en injection locale. *Rev Rhum Mal Osteoartic* 20:310–313, 1953.
59. Cappio M: Il trattamento idrocortisonico par via epidurale sacrale delle lombosciatalgie: osservazione su 80 casi. *Reumatismo* 9:60–70, 1957.
60. Goeber HW Jr, Jallo SJ, Gardner WJ, et al: Painful radiculopathy treated with epidural injections of procaine and hydrocortisone acetate: results in 113 patients. *Anesth Analg* 40:130–134, 1961.
61. Dilke FW, Burry HC, Grahame R: Extradural corticosteroid injection in management of lumbar nerve root compression. *BMJ* 2:635–637, 1973.
62. Spaccarelli KC: Lumbar and caudal epidural corticosteroid injections. *Mayo Clin Proc* 71:169–178, 1996.
63. Koes BW, Scholten RJPM, Mens JMA, et al: Efficacy of epidural steroid injections for low-back pain and sciatica: A systematic review of randomized clinical trials. *Pain* 63:279–288, 1995.
64. Sussman BJ, Mann M: Experimental intervertebral discolysis with collagenase. *J Neurosurg* 31:628–635, 1969.
65. Smith L, Garvin PJ, Gesler RM, et al: Enzyme dissolution of the nucleus pulposus. *Nature* 198:1311–1312, 1963.
66. Smith L: Enzyme dissolution of the nucleus pulposus in humans. *JAMA* 187:137–140, 1964.
67. Smith L, Brown JE: Treatment of lumbar intervertebral disc lesions by direct injection of chymopapain. *J Bone Joint Surg (Br)* 49B:502–519, 1967.
68. Watts C, Knighton R, Roulhac G: Chymopapain treatment of intervertebral disc disease. *J Neurosurg* 42:374–383, 1975.

69. Javid MJ, Nordby EJ: Current status of chymopapain for herniated nucleus pulposus. *Neurosurg Q* 4:92–101, 1994.
70. Kambin P, Gellman H: Percutaneous lateral discectomy of the lumbar spine: A preliminary report. *Clin Orthop* 174:127–132, 1983.
71. Hoppenfeld S: Percutaneous removal of herniated lumbar discs: 50 cases with ten year follow-up periods. *Clin Orthop* 238:92–97, 1989.
72. Hijikata S: Percutaneous nucleotomy: A new concept technique and 12 years' experience. *Clin Orthop* 238:9–23, 1989.
73. Stern MB (ed): Symposium: Percutaneous nucleotomy. *Clin Orthop* 238:1–106, 1989.
74. Choy DSJ, Case RB, Fielding W, et al: Percutaneous laser nucleolysis of lumbar disks [letter]. *N Engl J Med* 317:771–772, 1987.
75. Kambin P (ed): *Arthroscopic Microdiscectomy: Minimal Intervention in Spinal Surgery.* Baltimore, Md, Urban & Schwarzenberg, 1991.
76. McAfee PC, Regan JR, Zdeblick T, et al: The incidence of complications in endoscopic anterior thoracolumbar spinal reconstructive surgery: A prospective multicenter study comprising the first 100 consecutive cases. *Spine* 20:1624–1632, 1995.
77. Dickman CA, Mican C: Multilevel anterior thoracic discectomies and anterior interbody fusion using a microsurgical thorascopic approach. *J Neurosurg* 84:104–109, 1996.
78. Dickman CA, Rosenthal D, Karahalios DG, et al: Thoracic vertebrectomy and reconstruction using a microsurgical thoracoscopic approach. *Neurosurgery* 38:279–293, 1996.
79. Dickman CA, Mican C: Thoracoscopic approaches for the treatment of anterior thoracic spinal pathology. *BNI Q* 12(1):4–19, 1996.
80. Wilkins RH: *Neurosurgical Classics.* New York, Johnson Reprint, 1965, pp 69–118, 162–185, 264–276, 442–448, 477–483, 504–515.
81. Mullan S, Harper PV, Hekmatpanah J, et al: Percutaneous interruption of spinal-pain tracts by means of a strontium^{90} needle. *J Neurosurg* 20:931–939, 1963.
82. Mullan S, Hekmatpanah J, Dobben G, et al: Percutaneous, intramedullary cordotomy utilizing the unipolar anodal electrolytic lesion. *J Neurosurg* 22:548–553, 1965.
83. Rosomoff HL, Carroll F, Brown J, et al: Percutaneous radiofrequency cervical cordotomy: Technique. *J Neurosurg* 23:639–644, 1965.
84. Uematsu S, Udvarhelyi GB, Benson DW, et al. Percutaneous radiofrequency rhizotomy. *Surg Neurol* 2:319–325, 1974.
85. Uematsu S: Percutaneous radiofrequency rhizotomy for the treatment of paraplegic spasms, in Rengachary SS, Wilkins RH (eds): *Neurosurgical Operative Atlas.* Park Ridge, Ill, American Association of Neurological Surgeons, vol 2, pp 443–453, 1992.
86. Dogliotti AM: Traitement des syndromes douloureux de la périphérie par l'alcoolisation sub-arachnoïdienne des racines postérieures à leur émergence de la moelle épinière. *Presse Med* 39:1249–1252, 1931.
87. Rétif J: Intrathecal injection of a neurolytic solution for the relief of intractable pain. *Adv Tech Stand Neurosurg* 4:43–64, 1977.
88. Hitchcock E: Hypothermic subarachnoid irrigation for intractable pain. *Lancet* 1:1133–1135, 1967.
89. Hitchcock E: Hypothermic subarachnoid irrigation [letter]. *Lancet* 1:1330, 1967.
90. Ventafridda V, Spreafico R: Subarachnoid saline perfusion. *Adv Neurol* 4:477–484, 1974.
91. White JC, Smithwick RH, Simeone FA: *The Autonomic Nervous System: Anatomy, Physiology, and Surgical Application,* ed 3. New York, Macmillan, 1952.
92. Mandl F: Die Wirkung der paravertebralen Injektion bei "Angina pectoris." *Arch Klin Chir* 136:495–518, 1925.
93. Swetlow GA: Paraverteral alcohol block in cardiac pain. *Am Heart J* 1:393–412, 1926.
94. Wilkinson HA: Percutaneous radiofrequency upper thoracic sympathectomy. *Neurosurgery* 38:715–725, 1996.

95. Dandy WE, Blackfan KD: An experimental and clinical study of internal hydrocephalus. *JAMA* 61:2216–2217, 1913.

96. Dandy WE, Blackfan KD: Internal hydrocephalus: An experimental, clinical and pathological study. *Am J Dis Child* 8:406–482, 1914.

97. Dandy WE, Blackfan KD: Internal hydrocephalus: Second paper. *Am J Dis Child* 14:424–443, 1917.

98. Dandy WE: III. Cerebral ventriculoscopy. *Johns Hopkins Hosp Bull* 33:189, 1922.

99. Fay T, Grant FC: Ventriculoscopy and intraventricular photography in internal hydrocephalus: Report of case. *JAMA* 80:461–463, 1923.

100. Mixter WJ: Ventriculoscopy and puncture of the floor of the third ventricle. Preliminary report of a case. *Boston Med Surg J* 188:277–278, 1923.

101. Lespinasse VL: Cited by Davis L: *Neurological Surgery.* Philadelphia, Lea & Febiger, 1936, p 405.

102. Wilkins RH: History of surgery of the third ventricular region, in Apuzzo MJL: *Surgery of the Third Ventricle,* ed 2. Baltimore, Md, Williams & Wilkins (in press).

103. Gieger M, Cohen AR: The history of neuroendoscopy, in Cohen AR, Haines SJ (eds): *Minimally Invasive Techniques in Neurosurgery.* Baltimore, Md, Williams & Wilkins, 1995, pp 1–5.

104. Griffith HB: Endoneurosurgery: Endoscopic intracranial surgery. *Adv Tech Stand Neurosurg* 14:3–24, 1986.

105. Yamakawa K: Instrumentation for neuroendoscopy, in Cohen AR, Haines SJ (eds): *Minimally Invasive Techniques in Neurosurgery.* Baltimore, Md, Williams & Wilkins, 1995, pp 6–13.

106. Auer LM, Holzer P, Ascher PW, et al: Endscopic neurosurgery. *Acta Neurochir (Wien)* 90:1–14, 1988.

107. Bauer BL, Hellwig D: Minimally invasive endoscopic neurosurgery—a survey. *Acta Neurochir (Wien)* 61(suppl):1–12, 1994.

108. Zamorano L, Chavantes C, Jiang Z, et al: Stereotactic neuroendoscopy, in Cohen AR, Haines SJ (eds): *Minimally Invasive Techniques in Neurosurgery.* Baltimore, Md, Williams & Wilkins, 1995, pp 49–65.

109. Ballentine HT Jr: Historical overview of psychosurgery and its problematic. *Acta Neurochir (Wien)* 44(suppl):125–128, 1988.

110. Bridges PK, Bartlett JR: Psychosurgery: Yesterday and today. *Br J Psychiatry* 131:249–260, 1977.

111. Diering SL, Bell WO: Functional neurosurgery for psychiatric disorders: A historical perspective. *Stereotact Funct Neurosurg* 57:175–194, 1991.

112. Flor-Henry P: Psychiatric surgery—1935–1973. Evolution and current perspectives. *Can Psychiatr Assoc J* 20:157–167, 1975.

113. Jasper HH: A historical perspective. The rise and fall of prefrontal lobotomy. *Adv Neurol* 66:97–114, 1995.

114. Lichterman BL: On the history of psychosurgery in Russia. *Acta Neurochir (Wien)* 125:1–4, 1993.

115. Pressman JD: Sufficient promise: John F. Fulton and the origins of psychosurgery. *Bull Hist Med* 62:1–22, 1988.

116. Swayze VW II: Frontal leukotomy and related psychosurgical procedures in the era before antipsychotics (1935–1954): A historical overview. *Am J Psychiatry* 152:505–515, 1995.

117. Valenstein ES: *Great and Desperate Cures. The Rise and Decline of Psychosurgery and Other Radical Treatments for Mental Illness.* New York, Basic Books, 1986.

118. Walker AE: Psychosurgery: Collective review. *Int Abstr Surg* 78:1–11, 1944.

119. Leksell L: The stereotaxic method and radiosurgery of the brain. *Acta Chir Scand* 102:316–319, 1951.

120. Leksell LA: *Stereotaxis and Radiosurgery. An Operative System.* Springfield, Ill, Charles C Thomas, 1971.

121. Leksell L: Stereotactic radiosurgery. *J Neurol Neurosurg Psychiatry* 46:797–803, 1983.

122. Kondziolka DS, Lunsford LD, Flickinger JC, et al: Results from a multicenter study of trigeminal neuralgia radiosurgery. Paper presented at the 64th Annual Meeting of the American Association of Neurological Surgeons, Minneapolis, Minn, May 1, 1996.

123. Oppel F, Mulch G: Selective trigeminal root section via an endoscopic transpyramidal retrolabyrinthine approach. *Acta Neurochir (Wien)* 28(suppl):565–571, 1979.

124. Khodnevich AA, Karakhan VB: New kinds of microneuroprotectors for microsurgery and endoscopy of cerebellopontine angle neurovascular decompression. *Acta Neurochir (Wien)* 61(suppl):40–42, 1994.

125. Luft R, Olivecrona H: Experiences with hypophysectomy in man. *J Neurosurg* 10:301–316, 1953.

126. Forrest APM, Brown DAP: Pituitary-radon implant for breast cancer. *Lancet* 1:1054–1055, 1955.

127. Talairach J, Tournoux P: Appareil de stéréotaxie hypophysaire pour voie d'abord nasale. *Neurochirurgie* 1:127–131, 1955.

128. Rand RW: Stereotactic transsphenoidal cryohypophysectomy. *Bull Los Angeles Neurol Soc* 29:40–48, 1964.

129. Rand RW, Dashe AM, Paglia DE, et al: Stereotactic cryohypophysectomy. *JAMA* 189:255–259, 1964.

130. Zervas NT: Technique of radio-frequency hypophysectomy. *Confin Neurol* 26:157–160, 1965.

131. Zervas NT, Gordy PD: Radiofrequency thermal hypophysectomy: Technical note. *J Neurosurg* 30:511–514, 1969.

132. Moricca G: Chemical hypophysectomy for cancer pain. *Adv Neurol* 4:707–714, 1974.

133. Takeda F, Fujii T, Uki J, et al: Cancer pain relief and tumor regression by means of pituitary neuroadenolysis and surgical hypophysectomy. *Neurol Med Chir (Tokyo)* 23:41–49, 1983.

134. McCombs RK: Proton irradiation of the pituitary and its metabolic effects. *Radiology* 68:797–811, 1957.

135. Hassenbusch SJ: Surgical management of cancer pain. *Neurosurg Clin North Am* 6:127–134, 1995.

136. Rawlings C III, Rossitch E Jr, Nashold BS Jr: The history of neurosurgical procedures for relief of pain. *Surg Neurol* 38:454–463, 1992.

137. Sano K: Neurosurgical treatments of pain—a general survey. *Acta Neurochir (Wien)* 38 (suppl):86–96, 1987.

138. Young RF: Stereotactic methods in the management of pain, in Heilbrun MP (ed): *Stereotactic Neurosurgery.* Baltimore, Md, Williams & Wilkins, 1988, pp 149–160.

139. Spiegel EA, Wycis HT, Marks M, et al: Stereotaxic apparatus for operations on the human brain. *Science* 106:349–350, 1947.

140. Wycis HT, Soloff L, Spiegel EA: Facial pain, persisting after retrogasserian rhizotomy, relieved by mesencephalothalamotomy. *Surgery* 27:115–121, 1950.

141. Spiegel EA, Wycis HT: Mesencephalotomy in treatment of "intractable" facial pain. *Arch Neurol Psychiatry* 69:1–13, 1953.

142. Talairach J, Hecaen H, David M, et al: Recherches sur la coagulation thérapeutique des structures sous-corticales chez l'homme. *Rev Neurol* 81:4–24, 1949.

143. Hécaen H, Talairach J, David M, et al: Coagulations limitées du thalamus dans les algies du syndrome thalamique: Résultats thérapeutiques et physiologiques. *Rev Neurol* 81:917–931, 1949.

144. Pagni CA: Place of stereotactic technique in surgery for pain. *Adv Neurol* 4:699–706, 1974.

145. Fairman D: Hypothalamotomy as a new perspective for alleviation of intractable pain and regression of metastatic malignant tumors, in Fusek I, Kunc Z (eds): *Present Limits of Neurosurgery* excerpta from (Medical International Congress Series), Prague, Avicenum, 1972, pp 525–528.

146. Sano K, Sekino H, Hashimoto I, et al: Posteromedial hypothalamotomy in the treatment of intractable pain. *Confin Neurol* 37:285–290, 1975.

147. Foltz EL, White LE Jr: Pain "relief" by frontal cingulumotomy. *J Neurosurg* 19:89–100, 1962.
148. Ballantine HT Jr, Cassidy WL, Flanagan NB, et al: Stereotaxic anterior cingulotomy for neuropsychiatric illness and intractable pain. *J Neurosurg* 26:488–495, 1967.
149. Gybels JM, Sweet WH: *Neurosurgical Treatment of Persistent Pain: Physiological and Pathological Mechanisms of Human Pain.* Basel, Switzerland, Karger, 1989.
150. Kux E: *Thorakoskopische Eingriffe am Nervensystem.* Stuttgart, Germany, Georg Thieme, 1954.
151. Roedling HA, MacCarty CS, Roth GM: Encoscopic surgery of the thoracic autonomic nervous system. *Surg Clin North Am* 37:1403–1412, 1957.
152. Alexander E Jr: The McKenzie reservoir. *Surg Neurol* 31:476, 1989.
153. Ommaya AK: Subcutaneous reservoir and pump for sterile access to ventricular cerebrospinal fluid. *Lancet* 2:983–984, 1963.
154. Rickham PP: A ventriculostomy reservoir. *BMJ* 2:173, 1964.
155. Aronyk KE: The history and classification of hydrocephalus. *Neurosurg Clin North Am* 4:599–609, 1993.
156. Hirsch JF: Surgery of hydrocephalus: past, present and future. *Acta Neurochir (Wien)* 116:155–160, 1992.
157. Keen J: Casey Holter and the Spitz-Holter valve. *Eur J Pediatr Surg* 2(suppl 1):5–6, 1992.
158. McCullough DC: A history of the treatment of hydrocephalus. *Fetal Ther* 1:38–45, 1986.
159. McCullough DC: History of the treatment of hydrocephalus, in Scott RM (ed): *Hydrocephalus.* Baltimore, Md, Williams & Wilkins, 1990, pp 1–10.
160. Pudenz RH: The surgical treatment of hydrocephalus–an historical review. *Surg Neurol* 15:15–26, 1981.
161. Ring-Mrozik E, Angerpointner TA: Historical aspects of hydrocephalus. *Progr Pediatr Surg* 20:158–187, 1986.
162. Scarff JE: Treatment of hydrocephalus: An historical and critical review of methods and results. *J Neurol Neurosurg Psychiatry* 26:1–26, 1963.
163. Wallman LJ: Shunting for hydrocephalus: An oral history. *Neurosurgery* 11:308–313, 1982.
164. Raimondi AJ, Matsumoto S: A simplified technique for performing the ventriculoperitoneal shunt. Technical note. *J Neurosurg* 26:357–360, 1967.
165. Spetzler R, Wilson CB, Schulte R: Simplified percutaneous lumboperitoneal shunting. *Surg Neurol* 7:25–29, 1977.
166. Kanev PM, Park TS: The treatment of hydrocephalus. *Neurosurg Clin North Am* 4:611–619, 1993.
167. Birnholz JC, Frigoletto FD: Antenatal treatment of hydrocephalus. *N Engl J Med* 303:1021–1023, 1981.
168. Clewell WH, Johnson ML, Meier PR, et al: A surgical approach to the treatment of fetal hydrocephalus. *N Engl J Med* 306:1320–1325, 1982.
169. Frigoletto FD, Birnholz JC, Greene MF: Antenatal treatment of hydrocephalus by ventriculoamniotic shunting. *JAMA* 248:2496–2497, 1982.
170. Manning FA, Harrison MR, Rodeck C, et al: Catheter shunts for fetal hydronephrosis and hydrocephalus: Report of the International Fetal Surgery Registry. *N Engl J Med* 315:336–340, 1986.
171. Hudgins RJ, Edwards MSB: Management of hydrocephalus detected in utero, in Scott RM (ed): *Hydrocephalus,* Baltimore Md, Williams & Wilkins, 1990, pp 99–107.
172. Cushing H: Surgery of the head, in Keen WW (ed): *Surgery: Its Principles and Practice.* Philadelphia, WB Saunders, 1908, vol 3, pp 17–276 (see pp 167–173).
173. Carpenter MB, Whittier JR: Study of methods for producing experimental lesions of the central nervous system with special reference to stereotaxic technique. *J Comp Neurol* 97:73–131, 1952.
174. Iizuka J: Development of a stereotaxic endoscopy of the ventricular system. *Confin Neurol* 37:141–149, 1975.

175. Kandel EI, Schavinsky YV: Stereotaxic apparatus and operations in Russia in the 19th century. *J Neurosurg* 37:407–411, 1972.
176. Schurr PH, Merrington WR: The Horsley-Clarke stereotaxic apparatus. *Br J Surg* 65:33–36, 1978.
177. Clarke RH, Horsley V: On a method of investigating the deep ganglia and tracts of the central nervous system (cerebellum). *BMJ* 2:1799–1800, 1906.
178. Horsley V, Clarke RH: The structure and functions of the cerebellum examined by a new method. *Brain* 31:45–124, 1908.
179. Picard C, Olivier A, Bertrand G: The first human stereotaxic appparatus. The contribution of Aubrey Mussen to the field of stereotaxis. *J Neurosurg* 59:673–676, 1983.
180. Olivier A, Bertrand G, Picard C: Discovery of the first human stereotactic instrument. *Appl Neurophysiol* 46:84–91, 1983.
181. Fodstad H, Hariz M, Ljunggren B: History of Clarke's stereotactic instrument. *Stereotact Funct Neurosurg* 57:130–140, 1991.
182. Spiegel EA, Wycis HT: *Stereoencephalotomy (Thalamotomy and Related Procedures): Part I. Methods and Stereotaxic Atlas of the Human Brain.* New York, Grune & Stratton, 1952.
183. Spiegel EA, Wycis HT: *Stereoencephalotomy: Part II. Clinical and Physiological Applications.* New York, Grune & Stratton, 1962.
184. Nashold BS: The history of stereotactic neurosurgery. *Stereotact Funct Neurosurg* 62:29–40, 1994.
185. Gildenberg PL: Stereotactic surgery: Present and past, in Heilbrun MP (ed): *Stereotactic Neurosurgery.* Baltimore, Md, Williams & Wilkins, 1988, pp 1–15.
186. Gildenberg PL: The history of stereotactic neurosurgery. *Neurosurg Clin North Am* 1:765–780, 1990.
187. Iskandar BJ, Nashold BS Jr: History of functional neurosurgery. *Neurosurg Clin North Am* 6:1–25, 1995.
188. Bullard DE, Nashold BS Jr: Evolution of principles of stereotactic neurosurgery. *Neurosurg Clin North Am* 6:27–41, 1995.
189. Tasker RR: Stereotactic surgery: Principles and techniques, in Wilkins RH, Rengachary SS (eds): *Neurosurgery,* ed 2. New York, McGraw-Hill, 1996, pp 4069–4089.
190. Cooper IS: *The Neurosurgical Alleviation of Parkinsonism.* Springfield, Ill, Charles C Thomas, 1956, pp 7–17.
191. Redfern RM: History of stereotactic surgery for Parkinson's disease. *Br J Neurosurg* 3:271–304, 1989.
192. Kelly PJ, Kall BA (eds): *Computers in Stereotactic Neurosurgery.* Boston, Blackwell Scientific Publications, 1992.
193. Hitchcock E: Stereotactic neural transplantation. *Stereotact Funct Neurosurg* 62:129–133, 1994.
194. Boyer KL, Bakay RAE: The history, theory, and present status of brain transplantation. *Neurosurg Clin North Am* 6:113–125, 1995.
195. Maciunas RJ (ed): *Interactive Image-Guided Neurosurgery.* Park Ridge, Ill, American Association of Neurological Surgeons, 1993.
196. Turner DA: Frameless stereotaxy: Clinical applications and future promise, in Bradley WB, Wilkins RH (eds): *The Year Book of Neurology and Neurosurgery 1995.* St Louis, Mosby, 1995, pp xxxiii-xl.
197. Kelly PJ: Quantitative virtual reality enhances stereotactic neurosurgery. *Bull Am Coll Surg* 80.13–20, 1995.
198. Maciunas RJ (ed): Clinical frontiers of interactive image-guided neurosurgery. *Neurosurg Clin North Am* 7:171–335, 1996.
199. Kelly PJ: Robotics in neurosurgery. *Crit Rev Neurosurg* 2:54–62, 1992.
200. Lewis MA, Bekey GA: Automation and robotics in neurosurgery: Prospects and problems, in Apuzzo MLJ (ed): *Neurosurgery for the Third Millennium.* Park Ridge, Ill, American Association of Neurological Surgeons, 1992, pp 65–79.

201. Benabid AL, Hoffmann D, Munari C, et al: Surgical robotics, in Cohen AR, Haines SJ (eds): *Minimally Invasive Techniques in Neurosurgery.* Baltimore, Md, Williams & Wilkins, 1995, pp 85–97.

202. Leksell L: A stereotactic apparatus for intracerebral surgery. *Acta Chir Scand* 99:229–233, 1949.

203. Ammar A: Lars Leksell's vision—radiosurgery. *Acta Neurochir (Wien)* 62(suppl): 1–4, 1994.

204. Kjellberg RN, Koehler AM, Preston WM, et al: Intracranial lesions made by the Bragg peak of a proton beam, in Haley TJ, Snider RS (eds): *Response of the Nervous System to Ionizing Radiation.* Boston, Little, Brown, 1964, pp 36–53.

205. Lawrence JH, Tobias CA, Born JL, et al: Heavy-particle irradiation in neoplastic and neurologic disease. *J Neurosurg* 19:717–722, 1962.

206. Lunsford LD (ed): Stereotactic radiosurgery. *Neurosurg Clin North Am* 3:1–257, 1992.

207. Steiner L, Lindquist C, Steiner M: Radiosurgery. *Adv Tech Stand Neurosurg* 19:19–102, 1992.

208. Alexander E III, Loeffler JS, Lunsford LD (eds): *Stereotactic Radiosurgery.* New York, McGraw-Hill, 1993.

209. Myerson A, Halloran RD, Hirsch HL: Technic for obtaining blood from the internal jugular vein and internal carotid artery. *Arch Neurol Psychiatry* 17:807–808, 1927.

210. Kety SS, Schmidt CF: The determination of cerebral blood flow in man by the use of nitrous oxide in low concentrations. *Am J Physiol* 143:53–66, 1945.

211. Kety SS, Schmidt CF: The effects of active and passive hyperventilation on cerebral blood flow, cerebral oxygen consumption, cardiac output, and blood pressure of normal young men. *J Clin Invest* 25:107–119, 1946.

212. Woodhall B, Hall K, Mahaley S Jr, et al: Chemotherapy of brain cancer: Experimental and clinical studies in localized hypothermic cerebral perfusion. *Ann Surg* 150:640–652, 1959.

213. Johnson HC: Surgery of cerebral vascular anomalies, in Walker AE (ed): *A History of Neurological Surgery.* Baltimore, Md, Williams & Wilkins, 1951, pp 250–269.

214. Hamby WB: *Intracranial Aneurysms.* Springfield, Ill, Charles C Thomas, 1952, pp 45–55.

215. Hamby WB: *Carotid-Cavernous Fistula.* Springfield, Ill, Charles C Thomas, 1966, pp 75, 89.

216. Noland L, Taylor AS: Pulsating exophthalmos, the result of injury. *Trans South Surg Assoc* 43:171–177, 1931.

217. Brooks B: Discussion. *Trans South Surg Assoc* 43:176–177, 1931.

218. Djindjian R, Picard L, Manelfe C, et al: Développement de la neuroradiologie thérapeutique. *Neuroradiology* 16:381–384, 1978.

219. Becker GJ: Editor's page. *J Vasc Interv Radiol* 1:16, 1990.

220. Luessenhop AJ, Spence WT: Artifical embolization of cerebral arteries: Report of use in a case of arteriovenous malformation. *JAMA* 172:1153–1155, 1960.

221. Luessenhop AJ, Kachmann R Jr, Shevlin W, et al: Clinical evaluation of artificial embolization in the management of large cerebral arteriovenous malformations. *J Neurosurg* 23:400–417, 1965.

222. Luessenhop AJ, Velasquez AC: Observations on the tolerance of the intracranial arteries to catheterization. *J Neurosurg* 21:85–91, 1964.

223. Sano K, Jimbo M, Saito I, et al: Artificial embolization with liquid plastic. *Neurol Med Chir (Tokyo)* 8:198–202, 1966.

224. Alksne JF: Magnetically controlled intravascular catheter. *Surgery* 64:339–345, 1968.

225. Yodh SB, Pierce NT, Weggel RJ, et al: A new magnet system for "intravascular navigation." *Med Biol Eng* 6:143–147, 1968.

226. Taren JA, Gabrielsen TO: Radio-frequency thrombosis of vascular malformations with a transvascular magnetic catheter. *Science* 168:138–141, 1970.

227. Fogarty TJ, Cranley JJ, Krause RJ, et al: A method for extraction of arterial emboli and thrombi. *Surg Gynecol Obstet* 116:241–244, 1963.

228. Prolo DJ, Hanbery JW: Intraluminal occlusion of a carotid-cavernous sinus fistula with a balloon catheter: Technical note. *J Neurosurg* 35:237–242, 1971.
229. Kessler LA, Wholey MH: Internal carotid occlusion for treatment of intracranial aneurysms: A new percutaneous technique. *Radiology* 95:581–583, 1970.
230. Kerber C: Balloon catheter with a calibrated leak: A new system for superselective angiography and occlusive catheter therapy. *Radiology* 120:547–550, 1976.
231. Alexander LF, Ward BA: The history of endovascular therapy. *Neurosurg Clin North Am* 5:383–391, 1994.
232. Serbinenko FA: Balloon catheterization and occlusion of major cerebral vessels. *J Neurosurg* 14:125–145, 1974.
233. Zubkov YN, Nikiforov BM, Shustin VA: Balloon catheter technique for dilatation of constricted cerebral arteries after aneurysmal SAH. *Acta Neurochir (Wien)* 70:65–79, 1984.
234. Debrun G, Lacour P, Caron J-P, et al: Detachable balloon and calibrated-leak balloon techniques in the treatment of cerebral vascular lesions. *J Neurosurg* 49:635–649, 1978.
235. Debrun GM: Balloon catheter techniques in neuroradiology, in Athanasoulis CA, Pfister RC, Greene RE, et al (eds): *Interventional Radiology*. Philadelphia, WB Saunders, 1982, pp 707–730.
236. Tsai FY: Introduction to neurointerventional treatment for cerebrovascular diseases, in Rumbaugh CL, Wang A-M, Tsai FY (eds): *Cerebrovascular Disease: Imaging and Interventional Treatment Options*. New York, Igaku-Shoin, 1995, pp 423–438.
237. Maciunas RJ (ed): *Endovascular Neurological Intervention*. Park Ridge, Ill, American Association of Neurological Surgeons, 1995.
238. Ferguson RDG, Ferguson JG, Lee LI: Endovascular revascularization therapy in cerebral athero-occlusive disease: Angioplasty and stents, systemic and local thrombolysis. *Neurosurg Clin North Am* 5:511–527, 1994.
239. Alfiere K, Tsai FY: Thrombolytic treatment in the setting of an acute stroke, in Rumbaugh CL, Wang A-M, Tsai FY (eds): *Cerebrovascular Disease: Imaging and Interventional Treatment Options*. New York, Igaku-Shoin, 1995, pp 470–486.
240. Mullan S: Treatment of carotid-cavernous fistulas by cavernous sinus occlusion. *J Neurosurg* 50:131–144, 1979.
241. Manelfe C, Berenstein A: Treatment of carotid cavernous fistulas by venous approach. *J Neuroradiol* 7:13–19, 1980.
242. Halbach VV, Higashida RT, Hieshima GB, et al: Transvenous embolization of direct carotid cavernous fistulas. *AJNR* 9:741–747, 1988.
243. Halbach VV, Higashida RT, Hieshima GB, et al: Transvenous embolization of dural fistulas involving the transverse and sigmoid sinuses. *AJNR* 10:385–392, 1989.
244. Mickle JP, Quisling RG, Ryan P: Transtorcular approach to vein of Galen aneurysms. *Concepts Pediatr Neurosurg* 6:230–238, 1985.
245. Dowd CF, Halbach VV, Barnwell SL, et al: Transfemoral venous embolization of vein of Galen malformation. *AJNR* 11:643–648, 1990.
246. Casasco A, Lylyk P, Hodes JE, et al: Percutaneous transvenous catheterization and embolization of vein of Galen aneurysms. *Neurosurgery* 28:260–266, 1991.
247. Doppman JL, DiChiro G, Ommaya A: Obliteration of spinal-cord arteriovenous malformation by percutaneous embolisation. *Lancet* 1:477, 1968.
248. Newton TH, Adams JE: Angiographic demonstration and nonsurgical embolization of spinal cord angioma. *Radiology* 91:873–876, 887, 1968.
249. Djindjian R: Embolization of angiomas of the spinal cord. *Surg Neurol* 4:411–420, 1975.
250. Hodes JE, Merland JJ, Casasco A, et al: Spinal vascular malformations: Endovascular therapy. *Neurosurg Clin North Am* 5:497–509, 1994.

19 Patient Management

Postoperative Pain in Neurosurgery: A Pilot Study in Brain Surgery
De Benedittis G, Lorenzetti A, Migliore M, et al (Univ of Milano, Italy)
Neurosurgery 38:466–470, 1996   19–1

Introduction.—There is a lack of well-designed clinical epidemiologic investigations on the issue of acute pain experienced by patients who have undergone neurosurgery. The incidence, magnitude, characteristics, and duration of pain after major neurosurgical procedures of the brain in 37 patients were reported.

Methods.—Neurosurgical staff members recorded patient pain intensity on a Visual Analogue Scale at frequent time intervals up to 48 hours. Patients were given the Italian equivalent of the McGill Pain Questionnaire 6 hours after surgery. Several pain characteristics were also evaluated. The Minnesota Multiphasic Personality Inventory (MMPI) and the State Trait Anxiety Inventory were administered to all patients preoperatively to assess psychological patterns.

Results.—Twenty-two of 37 patients (59.5%) complained of postoperative pain, and 15 patients (40.5%) were pain free. In the postoperative pain group, 14 patients were female and 8 were male. Patients in the pain group (mean age 42.05) were significantly younger than those in the pain-free group (mean age 56.3). There was no significant difference in the experience of postsurgical pain regarding the surgical route used. However, the subtemporal and suboccipital routes generated the greatest incidence of postoperative pain. Pain occurred most frequently in the first 48 hours, but a significant number of patients experienced pain for longer periods. Pain was described as predominantly superficial in 86% of patients, indicating somatic rather than visceral origin and possibly involving mainly pericranial muscle and soft tissue. Most patients (86%) reported partial or absolute congruence of pain with the site of operation. Pain was most often described as "pulsating and pounding," "tensive," or "steady and continuous." Pain was reported to be moderate to severe by 63.6% of patients. The only significant difference in preoperative psychological pattern between the pain and pain-free groups was that of hypochondriasis on the MMPI. Patients in the pain-free group unexpectedly scored higher than patients in the pain group.

Conclusion.—Findings suggest that postoperative pain after brain surgery was significantly higher than that reported in the literature. This important conclusion deserves greater attention by members of the surgical team to provide a more adequate and appropriate treatment approach.

▶ Traditionally neurosurgeons have been reluctant to order narcotic pain medicine other than codeine for patients during the first few days after a craniotomy because of the worry that such medication might mask the early changes in level of consciousness or pupillary function that would otherwise signal increasing intracranial pressure or brain herniation. Common wisdom holds that a craniotomy is associated with relatively little pain and therefore does not require significant narcotic medication. De Benedittis et al. provided evidence to the contrary.

R.H. Wilkins, M.D.

20 Cranial Operative Technique

The Use of Magnetic Resonance Angiography in Stereotactic Neurosurgery
Michiels J, Bosmans H, Nuttin B, et al (Univ Hosp Gasthuisberg, Leuven, Belgium)
J Neurosurg 82:982–987, 1995   20–1

Background.—Although digital subtraction angiography for stereotactic localization provides good vascular information, it is an invasive technique that carries an associated risk of complication. Magnetic resonance angiography was investigated as an alternative method of acquiring images for neurosurgical biopsy planning, because it is less invasive and offers 3-dimensional images that can provide data about stationary and flowing tissues with 1 imaging device and frame.

Methods.—Surgical planning was conducted on a 1-tesla whole-body imaging system. Either T1- or T2-weighted images or both were acquired after administration of 0.2 mmol of gadolinium-chelate contrast/kg of body weight. Thirty-six cases were planned using this method. Five different approaches were used: the calculated cross-sections of the probe trajectory were evaluated; the safety of the trajectory was determined in a reslice, the maximum intensity projection (MIP) algorithm was used in 2 approaches, or a stereoscopic MIP image pair was calculated.

Discussion.—Magnetic resonance angiography offers several benefits for stereotactic neurosurgical planning. Compared with digital subtraction angiography, it provides better delineation of neuroanatomy and a reduced risk of complication, because it is less invasive and offers a single modality to acquire anatomy and vessel information. Reslicing provides information in only 1 image and can be used to measure distances from any point on the trajectory. Despite the advantages of MR-based planning, the process is sensitive to patient motion; patients who are noncooperative may require sedation. In addition, because both arteries and veins are visualized, differentiation among all the information acquired may be a more difficult task.

► The authors demonstrated that MR angiography is of value to the neurosurgeon who is planning a stereotactic procedure because it provides

3-dimensional information about the relationship of intracranial blood vessels to the pathologic lesion, as well as to the proposed operative approach.

R.H. Wilkins, M.D.

Functional Magnetic Resonance Imaging of Somatosensory Stimulation

Hammeke TA, Yetkin FZ, Mueller WM, et al (Med College of Wisconsin, Milwaukee)
Neurosurgery 35:677–681, 1994

20–2

Purpose.—Functional MRI (FMRI) is capable of detecting changes in regional cerebral blood flow and volume in response to tactile stimuli. The sensitivity of FMRI to activation of the somatosensory cortex by tactile stimulation was examined.

Methods.—Six right-handed patients aged 21 to 54 with chronic epilepsy who were candidates for temporal lobe lobectomy underwent echo-planar imaging with a 1.5-tesla MR scanner equipped with local gradient and radiofrequency coils. In each patient, the palm of the right hand was stimulated for 20 secs, followed by a 20-sec rest period. This cycle was repeated 3 times during the image sequence. Two 15-mm or 3 10-mm adjacent sagittal slices in the left hemisphere that included the postcentral gyrus and surrounding regions were selected and analyzed. In addition, 7 contiguous 10-mm coronal slices were obtained in 1 patient.

Results.—Temporally correlated activation in the perirolandic region could be identified in all 6 patients. Strong changes in MR signal occurred in the sensorimotor cortex, and these changes were highly correlated with the tactile stimulation cycles.

Conclusion.—Cortical activation of the primary sensory area by tactile stimulation can be imaged by FMRI.

▶ Although the clinical value of MR spectroscopy has not yet been demonstrated, the imaging aspects of MR have proved their worth without any doubt. In this paper, Hammeke et al demonstrated a new and rapidly developing area of MRI that has potential importance in defining both brain function and brain morphology.

R.H. Wilkins, M.E.

Functional Magnetic Resonance Imaging of Sensory and Motor Cortex: Comparison With Electrophysiological Localization

Puce A, Constable RT, Luby ML, et al (Veterans Affairs Med Ctr, West Haven, Conn; Yale Univ, New Haven, Conn)
J Neurosurg 83:262–270, 1995

20–3

Introduction.—Functional MRI scanning could be a valuable part of preoperative neurosurgical planning, with the potential to avoid invasive preoperative studies. Functional MRI, which exploits the paramagnetic effect of deoxyhemoglobin as an endogenous contrast agent, is noninvasive and repeatable and offers high spatial resolution. The results of functional MRI in identifying the sensory and motor cortex in normal controls and neurosurgical patients were reported.

Methods.—Functional MRI was performed in 6 neurologically normal controls and 4 patients scheduled for surgery: 3 with focal seizure disorder caused by a lesion impinging on the sensorimotor cortex and 1 with intractable posttraumatic seizures. The subjects were studied during a motor task (repetitively squeezing a sponge) and 3 sensory tasks: electrical stimulation of the median nerve, continuous brushing over the thenar region, and pulsed flow of compressed air over the palm and digits. Functional MRI scans were performed with a 1.5-tesla unit. Axial gradient-echo images were used in the controls and echo-planar imaging sequences in the patients, who also underwent electrophysiologic localization studies.

Results.—In the controls, the motor task and 2 of the sensory tasks were associated with an increased MR signal in or near the central sulcus. This corresponded to the location of the primary sensory and motor cortex. Electrical stimulation of the median nerve did not reliably activate the sensorimotor cortex in control subjects. In the patients, the activation observed on functional MRI was coextensive with the location of the sensorimotor area, as assessed by subdural recordings of somatosensory evoked potentials and electrical stimulation of the brain.

Conclusion.—Functional MRI offers a noninvasive technique for localization and functional assessment of the sensorimotor cortex. The results correspond well to those of electrophysiologic mapping in neurosurgical patients. Effective sensory tasks for use in functional MRI are identified.

▶ Accurate localization of cerebral areas that are critical to movement, sensation, and speech is important to surgeons who are planning the excision of a lesion in the vicinity. A number of investigators, including the authors of this paper, are now defining the sensitivity and specificity of various functional MRI paradigms. There is a real possibility that this noninvasive method could become widely used by neurosurgeons in preoperative planning to the benefit of their patients.

R.H. Wilkins, M.D.

Magnetic Resonance Image–Directed Stereotactic Neurosurgery: Use of Image Fusion With Computerized Tomography to Enhance Spatial Accuracy

Alexander E III, Kooy HM, van Herk M, et al (Brigham and Women's Hosp, Boston; Children's Hosp, Boston; Harvard Med School, Boston)
J Neurosurg 83:271–276, 1995 20–4

Background.—Magnetic field distortions, such as those resulting from susceptibility artifacts and peripheral magnetic field warping, can compromise geometric precision in MR stereotactic procedures. In the experien e of several physicians, systematic error occurs routinely in MR stereotactic coordinates compared with CT coordinates. In some cases, this error may jeopardize critical neural structures. An image fusion technique was developed that combines MRI and stereotactic CT for better tumor localization in the planning of stereotactic neurosurgery and radiosurgery. The technique incorporates a chamfer matching algorithm. The use of this image fusion method in 1 patient was described.

> *Case Report.*—Woman, 59, with a progressive, 2-year hearing loss caused by an acoustic neurinoma was scheduled for radiosurgery. Axial MR images with the stereotactic localizer ring in place showed that the MR tumor image was displaced posteriorly, directly into the anterolateral brain stem. On the basis of the MR stereotactic frame-defined tumor plan, all of the tumor volume was covered by 80% of the total dose. However, image fusion showed that the 0.96-cc target volume was displaced 4 mm posteriorly. Thus, only 83% of the actual tumor volume would have been covered by the dose prescribed. In addition, the radiation dose to the anterolateral pons and cerebellar peduncle would have been greater than expected.

Conclusion.—This image fusion technique combines the advantages of MRI in anatomical definition with the geometric precision of CT and eliminates most of the anatomical spatial distortion occurring on stereotactic MR images. In the patient described, MR localization alone would have resulted in irradiation of vital neural structures outside the target volume and underdose of the intended target volume.

▶ In 28 consecutive cases of radiosurgical treatment planning based on stereotactic MRI using an MR-compatible localizer frame and stereotactic CT in the same patient, the authors routinely noted 3-dimensional offsets of 3 to 5 mm of MRI compared with CT reconstructions. For biopsy of a glioma, such a difference probably would not be important. For a thalamotomy, using physiologic parameters to guide the final location of the lesioning electrode, it also might not be crucial. But for radiosurgical treatment, this type of error could alter the outcome adversely. The authors called this problem to our attention and also showed how they have dealt with it.

R.H. Wilkins, M.D.

Clinical Use of a Frameless Stereotactic Arm: Results of 325 Cases
Golfinos JG, Fitzpatrick BC, Smith LR, et al (Barrow Neurological Inst, Phoenix, Ariz; St Joseph's Hosp and Med Ctr, Phoenix, Ariz)
J Neurosurg 83:197–205, 1995 20–5

Objective.—Frameless stereotactic systems have been developed in an attempt to overcome the disadvantages of frame-based systems, especially the lack of continuous anatomical feedback. One device of this type is the viewing wand, a frameless stereotactic arm used with CT or MRI to provide image-based intraoperative navigation. A large experience with the use of the viewing wand in neurosurgical patients was reviewed, with an emphasis on its real-world accuracy.

Methods.—The viewing wand was used in 325 operations over a 2-year period. The system was abandoned because of technical problems in 15 cases; this left 144 male and 166 female patients available for analysis. Patients' ages ranged from 1 to 83. Patients were selected at the discretion of the operating surgeon; malignant cerebral glioma was the most common indication for craniotomy.

The viewing wand system used the Surgicom articulated position-sensing arm with sophisticated 3-dimensional imaging software. The position of the viewing wand tip is updated 30 times/sec and transferred to an image processor for 3-dimensional reconstruction. The operations were performed under CT guidance in 165 cases and MRI guidance in 145. The experience was analyzed to assess the viewing wand's usefulness, ease of integration into the surgical setup, reliability, and accuracy.

Results.—Use of the viewing wand required little additional effort or time in setup, provided that a trained technician was available to perform data transfer and reconstruction. Useful registration was achieved in 95% of cases. Accuracy was better with fiducial-based registration than with an anatomical landmark–surface fit method; mean error was 2.8 vs. 5.6 mm with CT and 3.0 vs. 6.2 mm with MRI. In 92% of the MRI cases and 82% of the CT cases, the surgeon judged the system's actual error in estimating probe position just after registration to be less than 2 mm. In only about 1% of the cases was this error judged to be greater than 5 mm. As the operation proceeded, the system's accuracy decreased. By the final evaluation the estimated error was less than 2 mm in only 77% of the MRI cases and 62% of the CT cases. However, by this time, the viewing wand was often abandoned because the resection seemed straightforward. The system's usefulness in various stages of the operation depended on the type of surgery being performed (Table 2).

Conclusion.—The viewing wand frameless stereotactic arm appears to be a reliable and accurate tool for neurosurgery. It is accurate enough for

TABLE 2.—Utility of the Viewing Wand in Relation to Pathologic Conditions as Judged by the Operating Surgeon in 310 Cases

Pathology	Planning Craniotomy				Defining Anatomy				Locating Lesion				Margin				Resection			
	Yes	No	NA	NR	Yes	No	NA	NR	Yes	No	NA	NR	Yes	No	NA	NR	Yes	No	NA	NR
Glioma (54)	64.8	14.8	20.4	0	75.9	24.1	0	0	75.9	22.2	1.9	0	81.5	13.0	5.6	0	75.9	16.7	7.4	0
Convexity meningioma (31)	71.0	9.7	19.4	0	71.0	9.0	0	0	67.7	29.0	3.2	0	48.4	41.9	9.7	0	45.2	41.9	12.9	0
Skull base tumor (29)*	17.2	27.6	55.2	0	65.5	27.6	6.9	0	48.3	41.4	6.9	0	65.5	27.6	3.4	3.4	70.0	24.1	3.4	3.4
Epilepsy surgery (26)†	15.4	11.5	73.1	0	92.3	0	3.8	3.8	3.8	7.7	88.5	0	3.8	3.8	92.3	0	84.6	3.8	11.5	0
Cavernous malformation (18)	77.8	16.7	5.6	0	66.7	33.3	0	0	77.8	16.7	5.6	0	27.8	50.0	22.2	0	22.2	55.6	22.2	0
AVM (15)	86.7	6.7	6.7	0	80.0	20.0	0	0	53.3	33.3	13.3	0	33.3	40.0	26.7	0	33.3	53.3	13.3	0
Acoustic schwannoma (13)	7.7	7.7	84.6	0	61.5	30.8	7.7	0	53.8	46.2	0	0	69.2	23.1	7.7	0	61.5	30.8	7.7	0
VP shunt (12)	16.7	75.0	8.3	0	100.0	0	0	0	8.3	0	91.7	0	0	0	100.0	0	0	0	100.0	0
Metastasis (6)	83.3	0	16.7	0	50.0	50.0	0	0	66.7	33.3	0	0	50.0	50.0	0	0	66.7	33.3	0	0
Other (90)	62.2	15.6	22.2	0	64.4	30.0	5.6	0	78.9	17.8	3.3	0	63.3	24.4	10.0	1.1	60.0	24.4	14.4	1.1
Miscellaneous (16)	56.3	0	43.8	0	68.8	25.0	6.25	0	87.5	0	12.5	0	62.5	6.3	31.3	0	62.5	25.0	12.5	0

Note: "Other" refers to other or unspecified primary brain tumor.
*Tumors include meningioma, chordoma, and juvenile angiofibroma.
†Surgery involved temporal lobectomy or callosotomy.
Abbreviations: NA, not applicable; *NR*, not rated; *AVM*, arteriovenous malformation; *VP*, ventriculoperitoneal.
(Courtesy of Golfinos JG, Fitzpatrick BC, Smith LR, et al: Clinical use of a frameless stereotactic arm: Results of 325 cases. *J Neurosurg* 83:197–205, 1995.)

use in applications ranging from glioma resection, to CSF shunting techniques, to resection of small subcortical masses, to temporal lobe resection. It permits a direct approach to intracranial lesions while avoiding the disadvantages of stereotactic frames.

▶ As they are being refined, various types of frameless stereotactic systems are becoming increasingly useful to neurosurgeons. What was once, just a few years ago, an idea under development has become an available technology with inherent value. The authors documented the accuracy and practical benefit of 1 frameless stereotactic system in daily use on a busy neurosurgical service.

R.H. Wilkins, M.D.

Supratentorial–Infraoccipital Approach for Posteromedial Temporal Lobe Lesions
Smith KA, Spetzler RF (St. Joseph's Hosp and Med Ctr, Phoenix, Ariz)
J Neurosurg 82:940–944, 1995   20–6

Objective.—If standard approaches are used to access lesions in the posteromedial part of the temporal lobe, some of the lateral temporal cortex will have to be removed or excessive retraction applied. A new posterior approach that precludes the need to retract or resect the temporal lobe, the supratentorial-infraoccipital approach, was reported. The supratentorial-infraoccipital approach was compared with the standard anterolateral route (Fig 2). A viewing wand navigational system was used.

Technique.—After an MR image or CT scan was obtained, general anesthesia was induced, a lumbar drain was placed, Mayfield tongs were used to stabilize the head, and the patient was turned prone. A moderate reverse-Trendelenburg position was used to avoid venous congestion. A U-shaped incision based on the upper cervical region was made to expose the occiput and, after the posterior cervical muscles were separated from their attachment to the nuchal ligament, an occipital craniotomy was done using a craniotome. Lumbar cisternal drainage was initiated before the dura was opened in an oblique manner to create triangular flaps over the sagittal and transverse sinuses. Deep dissection was done with the aid of the operating microscope. The ambient cistern was drained of CSF, permitting removal of the brain retractor. It is possible to anteriorly extend this approach as far as the uncus.

Experience.—The supratentorial-infraoccipital approach was used in 7 patients initially seen with seizures whose lesions were chiefly in the posteromedial temporal lobe. None had permanent morbidity or died. One patient required evacuation of an epidural hematoma. Two patients had persistent headache that resolved when epidural blood patches were placed. Three patients noted transient visual problems, probably related to retraction of the occipital lobe, that resolved fully within days of surgery.

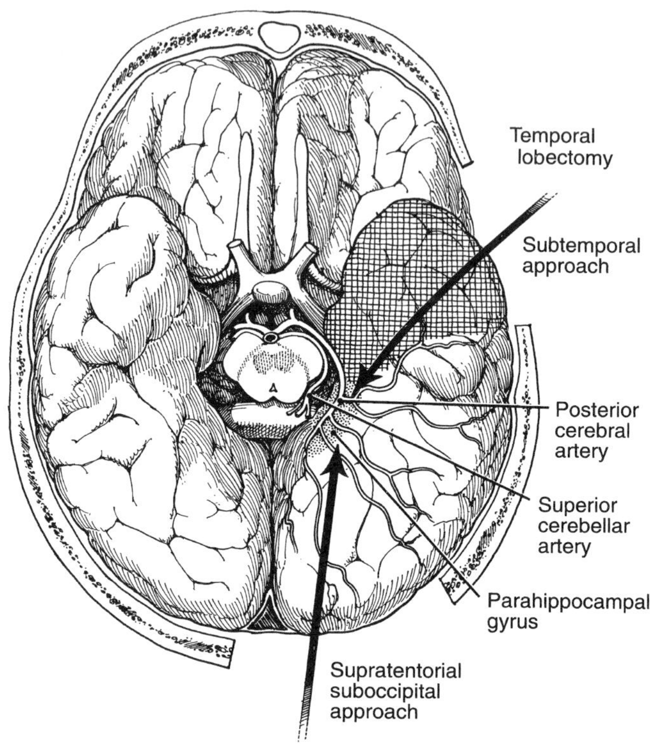

FIGURE 2.—Comparison of the supratentorial-infraoccipital approach and the standard anterolateral approach for access to the posteromedial temporal lobe. The lateral temporal lobe is markedly inferior relative to the medial temporal lobe and obscures access to medial lesions. The *cross-hatched area* depicts a standard anterolateral temporal lobe resection employed for medial exposure that may nevertheless be insufficient for complete removal of some posterior medial lesions. Note the relatively straight and slightly shorter approach from behind to posteromedial lesions without any cortical resection required for exposure. (From Smith KA, Spetzler RF: Supratentorial–infraoccipital approach for posteromedial temporal lobe lesions. *J Neurosurg* 82:940–944, 1995. Courtesy of Barrow Neurological Institute, Phoenix, Ariz.)

Six of the 7 patients remained free of seizures after an average follow-up of 15 months. The condition of 1 patient was well controlled with anticonvulsant therapy.

Conclusion.—The supratentorial-infraoccipital approach can facilitate the removal of posterior and medial temporal lobe tumors without the need to sacrifice lateral temporal cortex or transect the optic radiations.

▶ Smith and Spetzler described a posterior approach to the posteromedial temporal lobe that is somewhat similar to the supratentorial-occipital approach to the pineal region. The prone position used by the authors takes advantage of the effects of gravity to aid occipital lobe retraction.

R.H. Wilkins, M.D.

Repair of Critical Size Rat Calvarial Defects Using Extracellular Matrix Protein Gels
Sweeney TM, Opperman LA, Persing JA, et al (Univ of Virginia, Charlottesville; Yale Univ, New Haven, Conn)
J Neurosurg 83:710–715, 1995   20–7

Objective.—Although autografts are commonly used to repair bone defects, fresh autografts are not always available, and allogenic bone grafts present risks of nonunion, fatigue fracture, rejection, and infection. Extracellular matrix protein gels have been used to repair bone defects and have been shown to enhance osteogenic differentiation and angiogenesis in vitro. Efficacy studies of healing were conducted in the rat model to evaluate in vivo effects. The degree of bone repair in rat calvarial critical size defects (CSDs) treated with methylcellulose, type I collagen, reconstituted basement membrane, or laminin was compared.

Methods.—An 8-mm circular CSD was created in 36 retired male Sprague-Dawley rats. Six animals in group 1 received no treatment; 6 animals in group 2 were implanted with 50 µL of 3% methylcellulose; 6 animals in each of groups 3, 4, and 5 were implanted with 100 µL gels of type I collagen, reconstituted basement membrane, or laminin; 3 animals in group 6 were implanted with 150 µL and 3 animals in group 7 with 100 µL of type I collagen gel. Rats underwent CT scans at 12 weeks to evaluate healing. Groups 1 to 6 animals were killed at 12 weeks, and group 7 animals were killed at 20 weeks. Calvarial defects were sectioned and analyzed histologically for degree of healing.

Results.—Significant repair was noted in rats treated with reconstituted basement membrane, laminin, and type I collagen. At 87%, repair in group 3 type I collagen treated animals was significantly greater than for groups 1, 2, 4, and 5 and for the control animals. Group 7 animals at 20 weeks showed 92.5% healing. Type I collagen–implanted animals showed most of their healing (71%) in the first 6 weeks after treatment. Increasing gel volumes to 150 µL accelerated healing. Healing in control animals averaged only 7%. Histologic examination showed formation of new immature bone in the defects that were morphologically similar to cranial sutures, particularly in the animals treated with type I collagen.

Conclusion.—Extracellular protein gels may be acceptable alternatives for osteogenic repair of large bone defects when autograft material is not available.

▶ The authors showed that in rats, type I collagen gel stimulates bony healing of calvarial defects. This promising approach to cranioplasty should be tested in primates.

R.H. Wilkins, M.D.

Prefabricated Prostheses for the Reconstruction of Skull Defects

Eufinger H, Wehmöller M, Harders A, et al (Ruhr-Univ, Bochum, Germany; Univ Hosp Knappschaftskrankenhaus, Bochum, Germany)
Int J Oral Maxillofac Surg 24:104–110, 1995

20–8

Background.—The use of intraoperatively modeled prostheses in cranioplasties may not produce harmonic contours with long-term stability. Preoperative modeling would permit more sophisticated planning of the contour and better preparation of the implant material if a precise enough model of the defect site was available. The use of preoperative modeling in cranial defect reconstruction was discussed.

Methods and Outcomes.—To date, 4 patients with postoperative cranial defects have undergone reconstruction with individual prefabricated prostheses. Computer-aided design and manufacturing (CAD/CAM) techniques based on helical CT data were used for the prefabrication of prostheses. An individual computer-based 3-dimensional model of the bony defect was generated after acquisition, transfer, and assessment of the CT data. An individual and "idealized" prosthesis-geometry was derived from this freeform surface geometry, and it was fabricated by a numerically controlled milling machine using modern industrial CAD/CAM systems and design software. The margins of this prosthesis-geometry were defined using the borders of the defect and the surface, with consideration of the unaffected neighboring contours. In all patients, the resulting skull contours were harmonic and smooth. With the perioperative administration of antibiotics, wound healing was uneventful.

Conclusion.—Although experience, to date, is limited, reconstructing cranial bone defects with individual prostheses based on CAD/CAM–manipulated CT data has proved superior to conventional methods of cranioplasty in the current series. This new method should be applied in other fields of maxillofacial surgery as well.

▶ The larger the cranial defect, the harder it is to achieve an excellent cosmetic result by current methods of cranioplasty. The ideal cranioplasty plate has not yet been created. Two major areas need further work: the plate material and its shaping. Despite many centuries of experience, the perfect material has not been developed, and this development may be far in the future. In contrast, it seems that the problem of shaping the cranioplasty plate to provide an ideal cosmetic result should be solved in the near future by techniques similar to those reported here.

R.H. Wilkins, M.D.

21 Spinal Operative Technique

Microsurgical Anterior Cervical Foraminotomy for Radiculopathy: A New Approach to Cervical Disc Herniation
Jho H-D (Univ of Pittsburgh, Pa)
J Neurosurg 84:155–160, 1996   21–1

Background.—Cervical disk disorders causing radiculopathy have traditionally been treated through an anterior or posterior approach. A new microsurgical method was designed to achieve direct nerve root decompression through the anterior approach while preserving the functioning motion segment, as does the posterior approach.

Methods and Findings.—This method of microsurgical anterior foraminotomy is similar to that of Verbiest or Hakuba yet differs in its preservation of the intervertebral disk and in its simplicity. Unlike the Verbiest technique, it does not directly transpose the vertebral artery. Unlike the Hakuba technique, the disk in the intervertebral disk space is not removed. The nerve root is decompressed from its origin in the spinal cord to the point at which it passes behind the vertebral artery laterally. Because most of the disk in the intervertebral space is not disturbed, a functioning motion disk segment remains intact (Fig 1). More than 30 patients with a cervical radiculopathy were treated by this technique. Most patients showed good resolution of radicular, posterior neck, and interscapular pain. In addition, their postoperative range of motion in the neck was not restricted. Most of these operations were done on an outpatient basis.

Conclusion.—The microsurgical anterior cervical foraminotomy for radiculopathy accomplishes a direct resection of the compressive lesion (i.e., the soft disk fragment, spondylotic spur, or both). Though long-term follow-up data are not yet available, the short-term results are encouraging. Biomechanical laboratory studies will be needed to measure the actual changes occurring in cervical spine stability.

▶ Dr. Jho developed an anterior approach to the cervical intervertebral foramen for nerve root decompression. The offending spur or disk herniation is removed without the necessity for a full discectomy or a fusion. I believe that this will become a widely used procedure because of its advantages.

R.H. Wilkins, M.D.

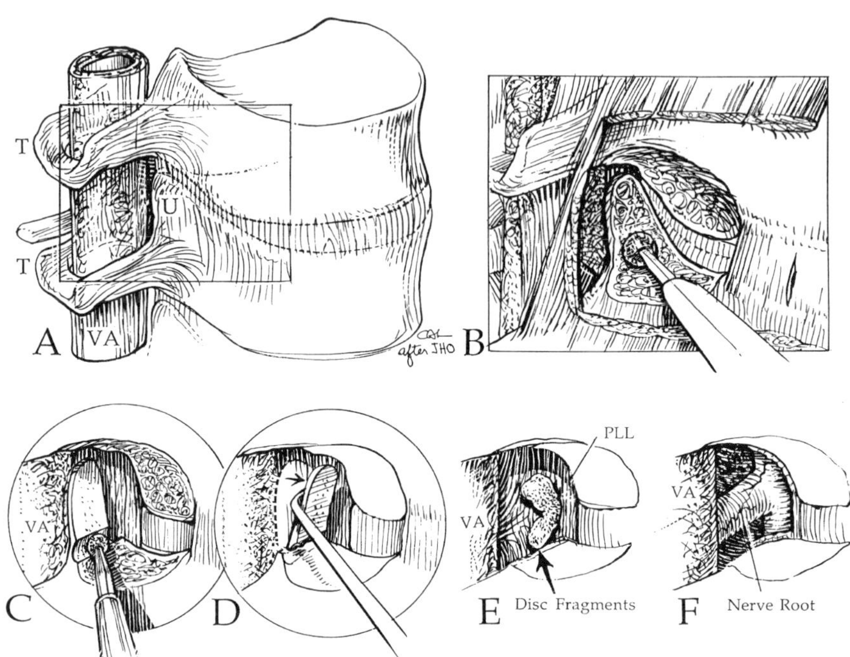

FIGURE 1.—Schematic drawings displaying microsurgical anterior foraminotomy. **A,** overview of cervical structures seen in the anterior approach. The surgical exposure is approximated in the box and enlarged in subsequent illustrations. **B,** the medial portion of the longus colli muscle is excised to expose the uncovertebral joint and the medial portion of the upper and lower transverse processes. **C,** under an operating microscope, the uncovertebral joint is drilled up to the posterior longitudinal ligament. **D,** a piece of the thin cortical bone (*small arrow*) of the uncinate process covering the vertebral artery is fractured and removed. The vertebral artery cen be identified by its pulsation. **E,** the compressed nerve root is distended forward by bone decompression. A tail of the herniated disk fragment may be visible through a tear in the posterior longitudinal ligament (*large arrow*). **F,** the posterior longitudinal ligament is removed to confirm decompression of the nerve root. The nerve root is then visible from its origin in the spinal cord to its exit behind the vertebral artery. Removal of the posterior longitudinal ligament may not be necessary if it has no defect. *Abbreviations: PLL,* posterior longitudinal ligament; *T,* transerve process; *VA,* vertebral artery; *U,* uncinate process. (Courtesy of Jho H-D: Microsurgical anterior cervical foraminotomy for radiculopathy: A new approach to cervical disc herniation. *J Neurosurg* 84:155–160, 1996.)

The Transfacet Pedicle-Sparing Approach for Thoracic Disc Removal: Cadaveric Morphometric Analysis and Preliminary Clinical Experience

Stillerman CB, Chen TC, Day JD, et al (Univ of Southern California, Los Angeles)

J Neurosurg 83:971–976, 1995   21–2

Background.—When herniated thoracic disks are removed, the transthoracic and lateral extracavitary approaches both reliably relieve myelopathy and radicular pain, but they require more extensive removal of bone than does the transpedicular approach and usually are combined with interbody fusion.

Objective.—A transfacet pedicle-sparing approach was designed to safely perform a microdiscectomy through a limited partial facetectomy without having to remove the pedicle. Morphometric studies were carried out on 15 cadaveric thoracic spine segments to evaluate the pedicle-sparing approach and develop the instruments needed for microdiscectomy. This approach was then used on 6 patients.

Technique.—After the involved disk space was confirmed by anteroposterior fluoroscopy in the prone patient, a 4-cm incision was centered over the appropriate disk space. The posterior elements were exposed and the facet complex partly removed using a high-speed drill. The foraminal soft tissue is coagulated before the lateral annulus was exposed, which was incised with a microknife to remove the disk. Disk tissue was removed using special microangled stomping curettes. No fusion was performed.

Results.—Eight thoracic disks from thoracic levels 7 through 11 were successfully removed from 6 patients. A majority of the disks were located centrolaterally, and half of them were calcified. Both axial pain and myelopathy were consistently improved or totally relieved postoperatively. Radiculopathy resolved in all 3 patients affected. There were no complications, and no patient had recurrent disk-related symptoms.

Discussion.—The transpedicular approach provides a posterolateral path to a herniated thoracic disk and may be used to remove both soft central disks and calcified centrolateral disks at all levels. Minimizing the amount of bone removed and the need for muscle dissection limits perioperative pain and may lessen the risk of chronic back pain developing. Operating time and blood loss both are minimized using this approach. Surgery may be difficult in larger patients, however, and it may be problematic to remove a centrally located disk without having specially designed instruments available.

▶ For years neurosurgeons have used transthoracic or lateral extracavitary approaches to thoracic disk herniation because of the significant risk of paraparesis or paraplegia after a posterior (laminectomy) approach. In this paper, Stillerman et al. provided information about a posterolateral approach that involves less surgery than the former approaches without the same degree of risk of neurologic injury as the latter. I am certain that the simpler transfacet pedicle-sparing approach outlined here will be tried by many neurosurgeons and could conceivably replace the transthoracic and lateral extracavitary operations for many thoracic disk herniations.

R.H. Wilkins, M.D.

Thoracic Vertebrectomy and Reconstruction Using a Microsurgical Thoracoscopic Approach

Dickman CA, Rosenthal D, Karahalios DG, et al (St Joseph's Hosp, Phoenix, Ariz; Johan Wolfgang Goethe Univ, Frankfurt am Main, Germany)
Neurosurgery 38:279–293, 1996   21–3

Background.—Video-assisted thoracoscopic surgery is used widely by cardiothoracic surgeons to treat thoracic cavity abnormalities. This minimally incisional approach has been associated with substantial clinical benefits, including decreases in postoperative pain, ICU and hospital stay, and complication rates. This surgical technique can be applied to anterior thoracic spine abnormalities. Recently investigators have reported using a microsurgical thoracoscopic approach to thoracic discectomy. The development and use of specific surgical techniques for thoracic vertebrectomy, decompression of the thoracic spinal cord, and spinal reconstruction using a microsurgical thoracoscopic approach were described.

Methods.—Seventeen patients with vertebral osteomyelitis, tumors, or compression fractures were treated. Microsurgical thoracoscopic methods were performed using several narrow, flexible, working portals placed in small incisions in the intercostal spaces. Thoracic spine access was obtained through the pleural cavity after temporary deflation of 1 lung using a double-lumen endotracheal tube. The region of interest was exposed by dissecting the parietal pleura, segmental vessels, and rib heads off the surfaces of the involved vertebrae. Spinal decompression and reconstruction were performed using long narrow spine dissection tools. The same amount of spinal dissection was achieved with this technique as with conventional open procedures.

Outcome.—One patient died of a massive myocardial infarction 2 days after surgery. The remainder were followed for 8 months. A second patient died of cancer 6 months after surgery, with no evidence of complications at the surgical site. The 15 survivors had stable clinical and radiographic follow-up assessments. None of the patients had nonunions, loss of fixation, progression of spinal deformity, hardware loosening, displacement of the reconstructive grafts, or persistent pain from spinal instability, spinal cord compression, or nerve root compression. Neurologic outcomes depended mainly on the patient's initial neurologic status.

Conclusion.—Thoracoscopic vertebrectomy is a safe, minimally incisional approach that allows extensive spinal dissection while minimizing muscular incisions and retraction of the chest wall and back. This technique has several advantages over open thoracotomy and posterolateral approaches to anterior spinal abnormalities.

▶ Spinal surgeons such as Dr. Dickman and his colleagues are expanding the indications, techniques, and usefulness of endoscopic spinal surgery in the thoracic and lumbosacral areas. This is an exciting area of development that is altering the field of spinal surgery.

R.H. Wilkins, M.D.

Evaluation of Endoscopy in the Treatment of Rare Meningoceles: Preliminary Results

Raftopoulos C, Balériaux D, Hancq S, et al (Univ Libre de Bruxelles, Belgium)
Surg Neurol 44:308–318, 1995   21–4

Objective.—The use of endoscopic exploration and treatment was evaluated in a review of 5 cases of a rare type of meningocele. Most meningoceles herniate through a defect in either the cranium or the spine, and the location and size of the lesions can make surgery lengthy and complex.

Patients and Methods.—A 1-month-old boy had a large, life-threatening left subtemporal meningocele extending from the anterior foramen lacerum to the buccopharyngeal cavity. All of the other 4 patients had sacral meningoceles. One, a 33-year-old woman, had a huge sacral bilobular meningocele with the largest part located presacrally. A 17-year-old woman had a posterior sacral meningocele consisting of a 75 by 90 mm mass at the superior part of the intergluteal fold. A sacroanal meningocele occurred in another 33-year-old woman, and intrasacral extradural arachnoidoceles occurred in a 30-year-old man. Presenting symptoms varied according to the type of meningocele, ranging from severe respiratory dysfunction in the infant to pain in the lumbosacral area and urinary dysfunction.

Treatment and Outcome.—Two sacral meningoceles were cured through a keyhole opening under endoscopic control. This approach was also used successfully in the infant with the oral cephalocele. Exploration of the posterior sacral meningocele found no communication with normal subarachnoid spaces; a simple suture of the posterior to the anterior walls eliminated the cavity. The case of the arachnoidoceles was particularly complex, involving 1 occult intrasacral meningocele and 2 extradural arachnoidoceles; surgical exploration was carried out using a directable, 2.3-mm endoscope. The extradural space was occluded by injection of a biological adhesive. This patient reported continued slight incontinence.

Discussion.—In these rare cases of meningoceles, endoscopic exploration was able to confirm connections thought to be small and to close such connections by a single stitch or the injection of a biological adhesive. Both length of the procedure and postoperative stay are shortened by the use of endoscopic techniques, which allow extensive exploration through a small aperture.

▶ Raftopoulos et al. added to the variety of indications for endoscopic surgery in the treatment of conditions affecting the CNS.

R.H. Wilkins, M.D.

22 Operative Complications

Orbital Infarction Syndrome After Surgery for Intracranial Aneurysms
Zimmerman CF, Van Patten PD, Golnik KC, et al (Univ of Texas, Dallas; Southern Illinois Univ, Springfield; Med Univ of South Carolina, Charleston)
Ophthalmology 102:594–598, 1995
22–1

Background.—When the ophthalmic artery and its branches become occluded, global orbital infarction can occur as a consequence of ischemia of all intraocular and intraorbital structures. A rare disorder, global orbital infarction, can occur with common carotid occlusion, orbital mucormycosis, giant cell arteritis, and myelofibrosis. It is not usually believed to follow surgery, but the cases of 6 patients who experienced acute unilateral visual loss after surgery for cerebral aneurysm were discussed.

Patients.—Patients underwent frontotemporal craniotomy to clip their aneurysms and had proptosis, ophthalmoplegia, and blindness immediately after surgery.

Case Report.—Woman, 29, had a sudden headache, vomiting, and neck pain. A subarachnoid hemorrhage was diagnosed based on lumbar puncture and CT findings. This was shown to be the result of the rupture of a left anterior communicating artery aneurysm, which was clipped via a left frontotemporal craniotomy. Four hours later, the patient's left pupil was nonreactive to light, and 3 days after surgery, the left eye could not perceive light. Visual acuity was 20/20 in the right eye. The left pupil was 1 mm larger than the right pupil and did have a minimal consensual reaction. Moderate left periorbital edema, chemosis, proptosis, and ptosis were present, and adduction, depression, and elevation were moderately reduced. Left upper facial and corneal sensations were absent. Retinal examination showed left retinal edema and a cherry-red spot, with normal-appearing vessels. Magnetic resonance imaging did not reveal orbital hemorrhage. Three months later, the patient remained blind in the left eye, with a persistent left afferent pupillary defect but a normal consensual pupillary response. The facial anesthesia, ptosis, proptosis, and ophthalmoplegia had resolved.

Results.—Four patients had anterior communicating aneurysms, and the remaining 2 had either a basilar or middle cerebral aneurysm. Five of these were symptomatic, whereas the remaining patient had elective surgery for an asymptomatic aneurysm. All patients developed unilateral proptosis, ophthalmoplegia, and blindness immediately after surgery, which was uncomplicated in 5 cases. In 3 cases, transient numbness developed in the cutaneous distribution of the ophthalmic nerve, with ipsilateral corneal anesthesia. The abnormalities of the fundus included retinal edema, retinal arteriolar narrowing, pigmentary retinopathy, and optic disk pallor. All patients remained blind in the affected eye, although some regained ocular motility. The results of examination were consistent with retinal and choroidal infarction in all cases.

Discussion.—It is possible that the myocutaneous flap that is retracted anteriorly and inferiorly near the orbit in a frontotemporal craniotomy could exert pressure on the globe. This could be of particular significance in people with shallow orbits or orbital congestion. Because visual loss after ophthalmic artery occlusion is irreversible, every precaution must be taken to reduce the risk. This includes controlling increased intracranial pressure, gradually lowering systemic blood pressure, avoiding hypotension and hypovolemia, careful positioning of the patient, and using an aluminum eyeshield in certain cases.

▶ The authors reported a rare but serious complication of aneurysm surgery—orbital infarction, believed to be the result of ophthalmic artery occlusion. Interestingly, none of their patients had an aneurysm in the vicinity of the ophthalmic artery. No mention was made in the 6 case reports about the intraoperative use of temporary vascular clips. In 2 of the case reports, postoperative angiography was commented on, but in neither was there a specific statement about the arteriographic patency of the ophthalmic artery. Thus, the exact reason these 6 patients sustained a presumed ophthalmic artery occlusion is not clear to me.

R.H. Wilkins, M.D.

Correlation of Fornix Damage With Memory Impairment in Six Cases of Colloid Cyst Removal
McMackin D, Cockburn J, Anslow P, et al (Beaumont Hosp, Dublin, Ireland; Oxford Univ, England)
Acta Neurochir (Wien) 135:12–18, 1995   22–2

Background.—Removing a colloid cyst from the third ventricle may result in incapacitating amnesia. High-resolution scanning has suggested that this result can be related to the extent of damage to the fornix. Such damage may be of vascular origin.

Series.—Memory function was evaluated and MRI carried out in 6 unselected patients having a colloid cyst operatively removed from the third ventricle without intentionally sectioning the fornix. Forniceal damage was assessed without knowledge of the psychometric test results.

Clinical Outcome.—One patient described no memory disorder postoperatively and resumed a normal life. Four of the 6 patients described disordered memory, and 1 patient required constant supervision because of severe amnesia.

Imaging Findings.—The right fornix had been destroyed in all 6 patients. All patients had evidence of moderately or severely impaired nonverbal memory function. Only 1 patient who resumed a normal life had an intact left fornix. In 1 other patient the left fornix was partially damaged, whereas in 4 patients the fornix was totally destroyed in both hemispheres. The degree of impaired verbal memory correlated with the severity of damage to the left fornix.

Conclusion.—These findings strongly indicate that bilateral forniceal damage, incurred inadvertently during removal of a colloid cyst from the third ventricle, results in amnesia.

▶ In comparison with the article by D'Esposito et al. (Abstract 30–3), this report focused on the type of fornix injury more likely to be encountered by a neurosurgeon. Among the 6 patients reported, 4 had transcallosal operations and 2 had right frontal transcortical operations. The fornix injury documented by MRI was more extensive than simple division of the column on 1 side to enlarge the foramen of Monro.

R.H. Wilkins, M.D.

The Pathophysiology of Oral Pharyngeal Apraxia and Mutism Following Posterior Fossa Tumor Resection in Children

Dailey AT, McKhann GM II, Berger MS (Univ of Washington, Seattle; Children's Hosp Med Ctr, Seattle)
J Neurosurg 83:467–475, 1995   22–3

Background.—Mutism after posterior fossa tumor resection in children has been previously documented. However, its pathophysiologic mechanisms remain unclear. One series was reviewed to better define the anatomical basis of postoperative mutism.

Patients and Findings.—During 7 years, 110 children underwent posterior fossa tumor resection. Nine of these patients (8.2%) were found to have mutism after surgery. These patients ranged in age from 2.5 to 20 years (mean 8.1 years). Mutism occurred 12 to 48 hours after surgery and lasted from 1.5 to 12 weeks. All the patients had problems coordinating their oral pharyngeal musculature, as evidenced by postoperative drooling and an inability to swallow. Postoperative MR studies confirmed that all of these children had splitting of the entire inferior vermis at surgery. All patients had intact lower cranial nerve function.

Conclusion.—This syndrome of oral pharyngeal motor apraxia with postoperative difficulty in speech and swallowing may result from radical splitting of the inferior vermis. The inferior vermis seems to play a critical role in this postoperative syndrome. The split in the inferior vermis can be limited to less than 1 cm. Should higher access to the fourth ventricle be required, a split above the prepyramidal fissure can be used. Postoperative MRI is useful for excluding noncerebellar causes of mutism and confirming the extent of the inferior vermis split.

Cerebellar Mutism: Report of Seven Cases and Review of the Literature
Erşahin Y, Mutluer S, Çağli S, et al (Ege Univ, Izmir, Turkey)
Neurosurgery 38:60–66, 1995   22–4

Background.—Pathologic conditions of the cerebellum can lead to mutism. Mutism has been described after posterior cranial fossa surgery. Seven cases of cerebellar mutism were described, and 39 cases from an English language literature search were reviewed.

Findings.—A total of 46 cases, 39 from the review, were analyzed. The age of the patients ranged from 2 to 61. Only 4 of the patients in this series were adults. In most cases, the vermis was the site of the lesion, which tended to be large. There were 33 medulloblastomas, 7 astrocytomas, 4 ependymomas, 1 metastatic tumor, and 1 arteriovenous malformation. The latent period for the development of mutism extended up to 6 days. Mutism lasted from 4 days to 4 months. In most cases, dysarthric speech followed the resolution of mutism. Mutism was transient in all patients in this series.

Conclusion.—Cerebellar mutism is a common transient pediatric complication of posterior fossa surgery to resect large midline mass lesions. It is possible that surgical trauma to the dentate nuclei or superior peduncles, followed by edema or ischemia, could cause the development of transient cerebellar mutism, especially after a latency period.

▶ In recent years, several articles (in addition to the 2 abstracted here) have been published about postoperative mutism in neurosurgery, especially after operations for large midline tumors in children.[1–8] Various mechanisms have been proposed to explain this phenomenon.

Based on a review of 25 cases of transient mutism after a posterior fossa approach to cerebellar tumors in children, Aguiar et al.[1] concluded that the mechanism of such transient mutism seems to be a complex of 2 or more factors (e.g., vascular disturbances caused by manipulation or retraction of the cerebellar region around the fourth ventricle and emotional factors), with extensive injury to the vermian and paravermian cerebellar area involving the hemispheric cortex, cerebellar peduncles, fibers of the dentatothalamocortical pathways, and dentate and interpositum nuclei. Van Calenbergh et al.[8] proposed that cerebellar mutism is an extreme form of dysarthria rather than a cognitive deficit or a psychological disturbance. Pollack et al.[7] reviewed 142 patients who underwent resection of infratentorial tumors at the Children's Hospital of Pittsburgh between 1985 and 1994 and found that 12

(8.5%) of them manifested temporary mutism and pseudobulbar symptoms. The authors postulated that this syndrome results from transient impairment of the afferent or efferent pathways of the dentate nuclei that are involved in initiating complex volitional movements.[7] Of interest, in their patients the only factor that was significantly associated with the mutism syndrome was bilateral edema within the brachium pontis. The length of the vermian incision was not a significant factor.

Crutchfield et al.[5] included the case of a 46-year-old man who exhibited mutism after a bifrontal craniotomy for a parasagittal meningioma to support the idea that injury to elements of the dentatothalamocortical pathway, especially bilateral injury, is responsible for the development of postoperative mutism. Frim and Ogilvy[6] used a case in which a cavernous malformation of the right pons (at the level of the middle cerebellar peduncle) was resected via a subtemporal approach to implicate the superior cerebellar hemispheres, the deep cerebellar nuclei, and the nuclear outflow through the superior cerebellar peduncles as the anatomical bases for cerebellar participation in the production of human speech.

Therefore, at this point, the syndrome is well recognized, but its exact mechanism or mechanisms remain a matter of conjecture.

R.H. Wilkins, M.D.

References

1. Aguiar PH, Plese JPP, Ciquini O, et al: Transient mutism following a posterior fossa approach to cerebellar tumors in children: A critical review of the literature. *Childs Nerv Syst* 11:306–310, 1995.
2. Al-Jarallah A, Cook JD, Gascon G, et al: Transient mutism following posterior fossa surgery in children. *J Surg Oncol* 55:126–131, 1994.
3. Asamoto M, Ito H, Suzuki N, et al: Transient mutism after posterior fossa surgery. *Childs Nerv Syst* 10:275–278, 1994.
4. Çakir Y, Karakişi D, Koçanaoğullari O: Cerebellar mutism in an adult: Case report. *Surg Neurol* 41:342–344, 1994.
5. Crutchfield JS, Sawaya R, Meyers CA, et al: Postoperative mutism in neurosurgery. Report of two cases. *J Neurosurg* 81:115–121, 1994.
6. Frim DM, Ogilvy CS: Mutism and cerebellar dysarthria after brain stem surgery: Case report. *Neurosurgery* 26:854–857, 1995.
7. Pollack IF, Polinko P, Albright AL, et al: Mutism and pseudobulbar symptoms after resection of posterior fossa tumors in children: Incidence and pathophysiology. *Neurosurgery* 37:885–893, 1995.
8. Van Calenbergh F, Van De Laar A, Plets C, et al: Transient cerebellar mutism after posterior fossa surgery in children. *Neurosurgery* 37:894–898, 1995.

Vocal Fold Paralysis Following the Anterior Approach to the Cervical Spine

Netterville JL, Koriwchak MJ, Winkle M, et al (Vanderbilt Univ, Nashville, Tenn; Atlanta, Ga)
Ann Otol Rhinol Laryngol 105:85–91, 1996   22–5

Background.—Surgical access to the cervical spine is commonly achieved with the anterior cervical approach. Vocal fold paralysis (VFP) can occur as a complication of this surgery, with a substantial preponderance of right-sided paralysis (94%) over left-sided paralysis (6%). Patients with unilateral VFP after surgery with an anterior cervical approach were studied in an effort to identify the causes of this preponderance.

Methods.—The charts of 16 patients with VFP after disk removal and fusion with an anterior cervical approach were reviewed. In addition, the anatomy of the recurrent laryngeal nerves (RLNs) and the adjacent structures was examined on both sides in anatomical texts, in cadaver dissec-

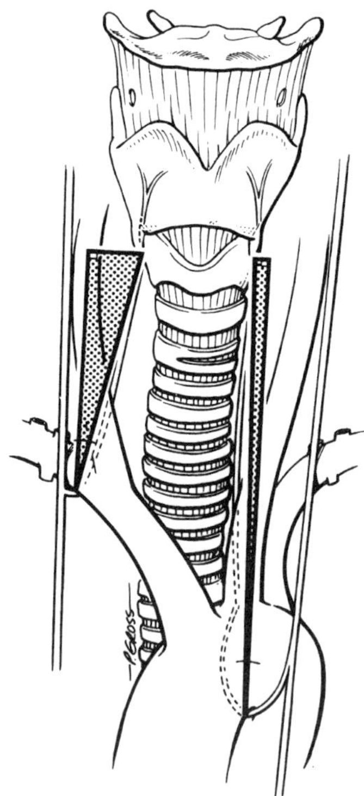

FIGURE 1.—Anatomical drawing of each recurrent laryngeal nerve. Superimposed right triangles resolve course of each recurrent laryngeal nerve into the vertical and horizontal components. The right recurrent laryngeal nerve has a shorter, more oblique course than the left recurrent laryngeal nerve. (Courtesy of Netterville JL, Koriwchak MJ, Winkle M, et al: Vocal fold paralysis following the anterior approach to the cervical spine. *Ann Otol Rhinol Laryngol* 105:85–91, 1996.)

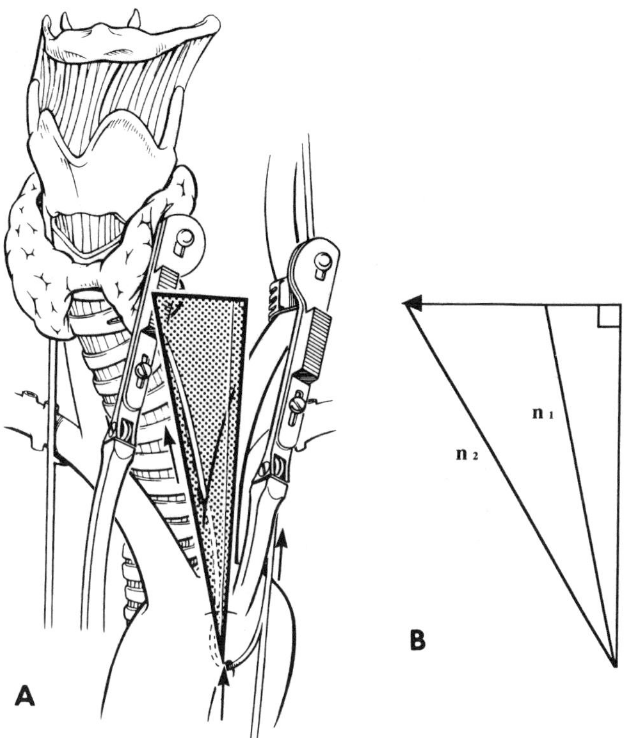

FIGURE 2.—Anatomy (A) and geometry (B) of the left recurrent laryngeal nerve during anterior cervical exposure. Because of the longer, more vertical course of the left recurrent laryngeal nerve, horizontal displacement of the larynx to the right by the Cloward retractor stretches the left recurrent laryngeal nerve only slightly. (Courtesy of Netterville JL, Koriwchak MJ, Winkle M, et al: Vocal fold paralysis following the anterior approach to the cervical spine. *Ann Otol Rhinol Laryngol* 105:85–91, 1996.)

tions, and during observed cervical oncologic procedures requiring the retraction of cervical structures.

Results.—Of the 16 patients with unilateral VFP, 15 had right-sided and 1 had left-sided paralysis. Compared with patients undergoing thyroidectomy or carotid endarterectomy, the patients undergoing disk removal and fusion experienced a greater incidence of dysphagia and aspiration, suggesting trauma to the superior laryngeal, pharyngeal, or recurrent laryngeal branches (or combination thereof) of the vagus nerve. Of the 16 patients, 4 had partial or complete resolution of vocal fold paralysis within 10 months after injury, 8 underwent vocal fold medialization resulting in symptomatic improvement, 2 were awaiting vocal fold medialization 6 and 7 months after injury, and 2 were considering vocal fold medialization at 27 and 45 months after injury. Anatomical examinations revealed that the left RLN is nearly twice as long as the right RLN (9.2 vs. 4.3 cm). In addition, the right RLN has a more oblique course than the left RLN, which describes a more vertical path (Fig 1). During anterior cervical

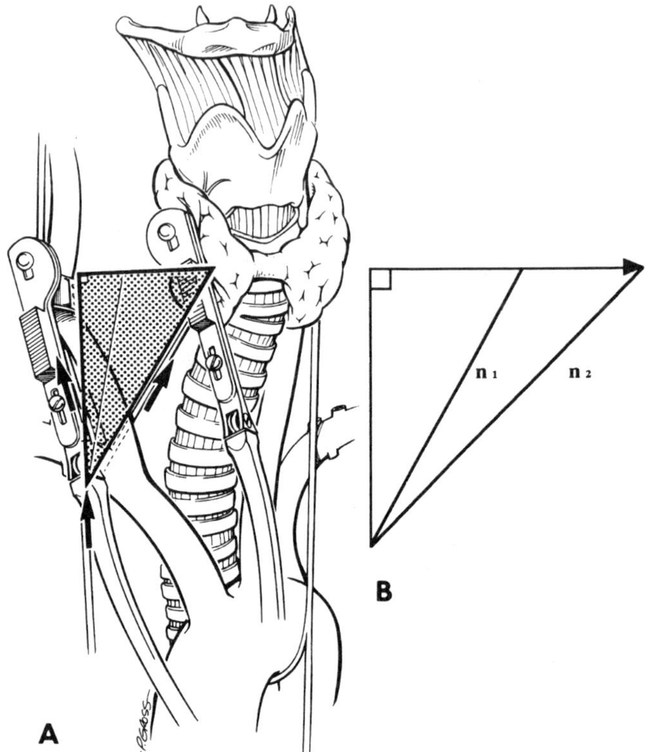

FIGURE 3.—Anatomy (**A**) and geometry (**B**) of the right recurrent laryngeal nerve during anterior cervical exposure. Because of the shorter, more oblique course of the right recurrent laryngeal nerve, horizontal displacement of the larynx to the left by the Cloward retractor stretches the right recurrent laryngeal nerve significantly. (Courtesy of Netterville JL, Koriwchak MJ, Winkle M, et al: Vocal fold paralysis following the anterior approach to the cervical spine. *Ann Otol Rhinol Laryngol* 105:85–91, 1996.)

exposure, horizontal displacement of the larynx with the Cloward retractor stretches the left RLN slightly with displacement to the right (Fig 2) but stretches the right RLN significantly with displacement (Fig 3).

▶ Dr. Netterville and his colleagues provided a thoughtful assessment of the likely mechanisms of vocal fold paralysis related to anterior operations on the cervical spine.

R.H. Wilkins, M.D.

Swallowing Performance Following Anterior Cervical Spine Surgery
Stewart M, Johnston RA, Stewart I, et al (Southern Gen Hosp, Glasgow, Scotland)
Br J Neurosurg 9:605–609, 1995   22–6

Introduction.—Apart from producing a feeling of a lump in the throat, large osteophytes of the anterior cervical spine may produce dysphagia. As many as one fourth of patients with diffuse idiopathic skeletal hyperostosis may be affected. Removing the osteophyte via an anterior cervical approach often cures the dysphagia. The possible effects of cervical spine surgery on swallowing are not well understood.

Objective.—The occurrence of dysphagia was studied in 100 patients seen in a 22-month period who had anterior surgery on the cervical spine for spondylosis producing myelopathy or radiculopathy. A few patients had rheumatic arthritic involvement of the upper cervical spine.

Surgery.—A right-sided oblique approach was taken to the anterior cervical spine in patients with spondylosis. The longus colli muscles were retracted for 1 hour on average. In patients having transoral surgery, the constrictor muscles were partially divided and retracted for about 2 hours.

Findings.—Of the 73 patients contacted 33 (45%) had experienced some dysphagia postoperatively. Most often it began within 1 week of surgery, but in 6 cases it was delayed for longer than 1 month. Nine patients, about one fourth of those affected, were symptomatic for longer than 6 months. The most common problem was difficulty swallowing solid foods, but a few patients had trouble swallowing saliva. Eight patients had painful dysphagia, and 7 coughed. Manometric studies of 5 patients with prolonged dysphagia suggested a hyperactive pharyngoesophageal segment but normally coordinated movements. Results of barium swallow studies were negative.

Conclusion.—Transient dysphagia is not uncommon after surgery on the anterior cervical spine, and there is a risk of persistent difficulty swallowing. A few patients may require balloon dilation or cricopharyngeal myotomy.

▶ Stewart et al. documented the frequency and duration of dysphagia after anterior surgery of the cervical spine. They note that manometric studies of pharyngoesophageal motility may be abnormal despite a normal otolaryngologic examination and normal results of a barium swallow examination.

R.H. Wilkins, M.D.

The Incidence of Complications in Endoscopic Anterior Thoracolumbar Spinal Reconstructive Surgery: A Prospective Multicenter Study Comprising the First 100 Consecutive Cases

McAfee PC, Regan JR, Zdeblick T, et al (Scoliosis and Spine Ctr, Baltimore, Md; Texas Back Inst, Dallas; Univ of Wisconsin Hosp, Madison; et al)
Spine 20:1624–1632, 1995

22–7

Background.—Early perioperative complications in 100 consecutive spinal procedures, 78 of which were video-assisted thoracic surgical (VATS) procedures and 22 were laparoscopic lumbar instrumentation and fusion procedures, were evaluated in a multicenter study. This was the first large series investigating the safety and potential complications of endoscopic surgery for anterior decompression or fusion of the thoracolumbar spine.

Methods.—Video-assisted thoracic surgical procedures included multilevel anterior thoracic releases for deformity in 27 patients, anterior thoracic diskectomies with spinal canal decompression in 41, pyogenic vertebral osteomyelitis decompression in 2, and vertebral corpectomy for neurologic decompression in 8. The mean operative time was 2 hours 34 minutes, and the mean length of stay was 4.97 days.

Anterior laparoscopic interbody stabilization and fusion at L4–L5 or L5–S1 were performed in 22 patients. These are the first cases in the laparoscopic Bagby and Kuslich (BAK) protocol for the Investigational Device Exemption Study for the BAK device. The mean operative time was 4 hours 17 minutes, and the mean length of stay was 5.6 days.

Results.—The most common complications with VATS were transient intercostal neuralgia (6 patients) and atelectasis (5 patients). The most common laparoscopic complication was bone graft donor site infection (2 patients). Two endoscopic cases were converted to open procedures, 1 for extensive pleural adhesions and 1 for a common iliac vein laceration. There were no permanent iatrogenic neurologic injuries, no deep spinal infections, and no long-term sequelae.

Conclusion.—The endoscopic spinal approaches proved to be safe in 100 consecutive cases.

▶ It is amazing what can now be done endoscopically. In regard to spinal surgery, endoscopic approaches through the chest or abdomen are being developed for various anterior operations that until now have been done through an open thoracotomy or open retroperitoneal route. In this paper the authors documented the relative safety of such endoscopic procedures. Innovations such as these are changing the face of spinal surgery. It will be interesting to follow these developments over the next 5 to 10 years.

R.H. Wilkins, M.D.

23 Pituitary Disorders

Recent Advances in Pathogenesis, Diagnosis, and Management of Acromegaly
Melmed S, Ho K, Klibanski A, et al (Univ of California, Los Angeles; St Vincent's Hosp, Sydney, Australia; Harvard Med School, Boston; et al)
J Clin Endocrinol Metab 80:3395–3402, 1995   23–1

Introduction.—Patients with advanced acromegaly are disfigured and disabled, and their life expectancy is shortened by metabolic, respiratory, and cardiovascular complications, as well as neoplastic disease. Prompt diagnosis and effective management can prevent much morbidity and prevent deaths. Pathogenesis, diagnosis, and management were discussed.

Pathogenesis.—Nearly all cases of acromegaly result from hypersecretion of GH by a pituitary adenoma. The basic somatotroph defect may either activate a factor stimulating cell growth or inactivate one that inhibits cell proliferation. A minority of GH-producing tumors have somatic mutations that mimic abnormal signaling by GH-releasing hormone. A number of factors might promote development of a pituitary adenoma. They include disruption of hypothalamic peptides or peptide receptors, peripheral hormonal imbalance, impaired regulation of paracrine angiogenesis, loss of suppressor gene function, and abnormal transduction of pituitary cell signals.

Diagnosis.—Coarse facial features, exaggerated growth of the hands and feet, and soft-tissue hypertrophy are key features of acromegaly. Other clinical sequelae include hyperhidrosis, peripheral neuropathies, visual abnormalities, and sleep apnea. Sleep apnea increases the risks of myocardial infarction, hypertension, and stroke, as well as car accidents. An oral glucose tolerance test can confirm abnormal GH secretion. It also may help to estimate the serum level of insulin-like growth factor–binding protein-3. An anterior pituitary tumor can be confirmed by MRI.

Management.—The chief goals of treating acromegaly are to counter excessive GH secretion and decompress structures impinged on by the adenoma. Small, well-localized microadenomas may be removed by the transsphenoidal approach. Radiotherapy is considered when surgery fails or is not feasible. The next step is administration of the somatostatin analogue octreotide, which may be effective when it is urgently necessary to suppress GH secretion. It may take months or even years to determine precisely how effective treatment has been.

▶ The authors put together a helpful review of recent advances concerning acromegaly.

R.H. Wilkins, M.D.

Conservative Management of Pituitary Apoplexy: A Prospective Study

Maccagnan P, Macedo CLD, Kayath MJ, et al (Escola Paulista de Medicina, São Paulo, Brazil)
J Clin Endocrinol Metab 80:2190–2197, 1995   23–2

Background.—The management of pituitary apoplexy, which appears to be more common than previously thought, is controversial. The wide range of clinical manifestations would suggest that treatment should be based on severity and course. However, surgery has been routinely recommended regardless of the clinical findings, with conservative treatment recommended only for patients with contraindications to surgery. The value and limitations of conservative treatment for pituitary apoplexy were studied.

Methods.—This prospective, nonrandomized study included 12 consecutive patients with pituitary apoplexy. The condition was diagnosed by the clinical findings of sudden headache, visual impairment, or ophthalmoplegia and by CT scanning. Patients consisted of 7 males and 5 females with a median age of 43. The study protocol called for treatment with 2.0 to 16.0 mg of dexamethasone daily; this was given to all patients but 1, who had chronic renal failure and severe hypertension. Surgery was performed if 1 week of dexamethasone therapy failed to improve the patient's visual loss or impaired consciousness or if the neurologic signs and symptoms returned soon after dexamethasone therapy was discontinued.

Results.—Fifty-eight percent of the patients did not require surgery and thus continued to receive dexamethasone treatment. Of these 7 patients, ophthalmoplegia resolved completely in 6 and improved in 1. Follow-up CT showed complete resolution of the tumor in 4 patients and residual masses in 3. All of the surgically treated patients showed residual masses on follow-up CT scans. One patient in each group had a recurrence. Pituitary deficiencies were no more prevalent in the conservatively treated group than in the surgical group. However, conservatively treated patients whose pituitary masses were resolved by the apoplexy had a greater prevalence of pituitary deficiencies. On retrospective analysis of the results, dexamethasone treatment did not appear to improve visual impairment. Complete tumor resolution was predicted by the presence of a large hypodense area within the tumor.

Conclusion.—With appropriate clinical and CT selection, conservative management can often be successful in patients with pituitary apoplexy. This form of treatment is best suited for patients without visual loss or impaired consciousness. Tumor resolution is most likely for patients with a large hypodense area on CT scan.

▶ The authors provided data concerning the nonoperative management of pituitary apoplexy. Although this was a prospective study, there was no initial randomization to nonoperative and operative management, so the 2 forms of management cannot be compared. Even though some of these patients were well managed nonoperatively, it surprised me that the authors would delay surgical treatment of patients with significant visual loss. I therefore agree with their statement, "It is obvious from the present study that patients presenting with major visual disturbances do not benefit from dexamethasone alone and should therefore be operated on promptly."

R.H. Wilkins, M.D.

Endoscopic Management of Lesions of the Sella Turcica

Sethi DS, Pillay PK (Singapore Gen Hosp, Republic of Singapore)
J Laryngol Otol 109:956–962, 1995   23–3

Background.—Endoscopic sinus surgery provides excellent visualization and minimal invasiveness. This approach may be useful in the treatment of lesions of the sella turcica. The transnasal endoscopic technique to manage pituitary adenomas and craniopharyngiomas was described.

Patients and Findings.—The study included 40 patients with sellar lesions. The patients were 22 women and 18 men, ranging in age from 27 to 76. Thirty-eight patients had 2 pituitary adenomas, and 2 had a craniopharyngioma. An otolaryngologic surgeon performed the endoscopic approach to the sphenoid sinus and sella, and a neurosurgeon performed the ablative surgery. In 4 patients, the surgical approach was transethmoid. The transnasal-transsphenoidal endoscopic method provided excellent visualization of the structures in the sphenoid sinus, including the optic nerves, optic chiasm, internal carotid arteries, and sella turcica.

Conclusion.—Endoscopic management of sellar lesions has several distinct advantages over management with the operating microscope. Endoscopes provide better visualization, an angled view, and a wider panoramic perspective of the important anatomical relationships of the sphenoid and sella turcica. Endoscopic management should be included in the armamentarium for pituitary surgery.

▶ The authors demonstrated yet another use for endoscopy—the transsphenoidal resection of pituitary adenomas and craniopharyngiomas. They believed the endoscope provided better illumination, magnification, and visualization during these procedures than the operating microscope. Furthermore, the endoscope has the advantage of angled vision and panoramic perspective. I believe that these techniques will be applied to pituitary surgery with increasing frequency in the next few years.

R.H. Wilkins, M.D.

Delayed Onset of Hyponatremia After Transsphenoidal Surgery for Pituitary Adenomas

Taylor SL, Tyrrell JB, Wilson CB (Univ of California, San Francisco)
Neurosurgery 37:649–654, 1995   23–4

Background.—Hyponatremia has been observed in patients with a variety of intracranial disorders but has been reported only rarely after transsphenoidal resection of pituitary adenomas. However, the symptoms are nonspecific and can appear after hospital discharge. The characteristics of delayed hyponatremia in these patients and its cause have not been established. The frequency, manifestation, and outcome of delayed hyponatremia were clarified in a review of patients treated for hyponatremia after transsphenoidal resection of pituitary adenomas over a 23-year period.

Methods.—A review of the records of 2,297 patients who underwent transsphenoidal resection of pituitary adenomas between 1971 and 1993 revealed 53 patients demonstrating delayed hyponatremia. Eleven patients with conditions known to cause hyponatremia were excluded. The records of the remaining 42 patients were examined for evidence of contributory factors, as well as manifestation, treatment, and outcome.

Results.—Of the 42 patients, 11 were men and 31 were women, who ranged in age from 21 to 79. The symptoms developed 4 to 13 days after surgery and most commonly included nausea and vomiting, headache, and lethargy. Dizziness, confusion, anorexia, and seizures were less common. Hyponatremia was diagnosed after hospital discharge in the majority. In 38 of the 42 patients, serum sodium levels were normal within the 24 hours before the onset of symptoms, suggesting a rapid development of hyponatremia. There were no significant differences in the proportions of men and women. The proportion of adenomas and tumor types were similar to the proportions in the total patient population. No factors that lower serum sodium levels were seen consistently, including glucocorticoid use, diabetes insipidus, or positive or negative fluid balance. The hyponatremia was treated with supplemental sodium and mild fluid restriction (37 patients) or mild fluid restriction alone (4 patients).

Conclusion.—The incidence of delayed hyponatremia after transsphenoidal resection of pituitary adenoma is higher than previously reported, at least 1.8%. Hyponatremia is not related to sex, age, type of adenoma, tumor size, or glucocorticoid tapering. Symptoms are nonspecific. Because untreated delayed hyponatremia may be life threatening, patients should be informed about its symptoms and advised to seek medical attention if they occur.

▶ Taylor et al. called attention to an uncommon but potentially serious sequela of the transsphenoidal resection of a pituitary adenoma—delayed hyponatremia of rapid onset that usually occurs after the patient has left the hospital. This phenomenon was also encountered by Kelly et al.[1] in 9 of 99 consecutive patients.

R.H. Wilkins, M.D.

Reference

1. Kelly DF, Laws ER Jr, Fossett D: Delayed hyponatremia after transsphenoidal surgery for pituitary adenoma: Report of nine cases. *J Neurosurg* 83:363–367, 1995.

24 Acoustic Tumors

Acoustic Neuroma (Vestibular Schwannoma): Growth and Surgical and Nonsurgical Consequences of the Wait-and-See Policy
Charabi S, Thomsen J, Mantoni M, et al (Gentofte Univ Hosp, Hellerup, Denmark; Aarhus Univ, Denmark; Copenhagen Univ)
Otolaryngol Head Neck Surg 113:5–14, 1995   24–1

Objective.—With improvements in surgical and monitoring techniques, the complication rates and mortality associated with removal of vestibular schwannomas (VSs) have become quite low. This has prompted some authors to recommend removal of most tumors after diagnosis, whereas others advocate a more expectant attitude. For a variety of reasons, this "wait-and-see" approach has been offered to elderly patients in particular. The surgical and nonsurgical consequences of the wait-and-see policy were evaluated in a prospective study.

Methods.—The analysis included 123 patients with neuroradiologic evidence of VS evaluated at various centers across Denmark from 1973 to 1993. The patients were 66 females and 57 males with a mean age of 59. The patients had a total of 127 tumors. Neuroradiologic studies were analyzed to estimate the mediolateral and anteroposterior diameters of the tumors and to thus evaluate growth and different growth patterns. The mean patient follow-up was 3.4 years.

Findings.—The tumor grew at a mean annual rate of 3.2 mm/yr, with a mean annual growth rate of 0.72 mL/yr and a mean annual relative growth rate of 41%. Seventy-four percent of the patients had tumor growth, 18% had no growth, and 8% had tumor shrinkage. Twenty-eight percent of patients underwent surgery because of tumor growth, and another 6% received γ-radiation, shunt insertion, or both. Six percent of the patients died of brain-stem herniation caused by tumor compression and 7% died of non–tumor-related causes. Of 28 patients initially regarded as candidates for hearing preservation surgery, 75% lost their candidacy as a result of tumor growth, deterioration of hearing, or both.

Conclusion.—A wait-and-see approach to the management of VSs has some important surgical and nonsurgical implications. Tumor growth can be predicted by the duration of symptoms and by certain tumor neuroradiologic features. High growth rates are related to hearing loss in patients who are candidates for hearing preservation surgery, to tumor growth in treated patients, and to tumor growth in patients who die of tumor-related causes but not to patient age. An observation strategy should not be followed in patients who are candidates for hearing preservation surgery.

▶ Among this series of 127 VSs, a variety of tumor growth patterns were observed. Continuous growth was noted in 51 (40%) tumors, no measurable growth in 23 (18%) tumors, no measurable growth followed by continuous growth in 23 (18%) tumors, negative growth in 10 (8%) tumors, and a variety of positive growth patterns in 20 (16%) tumors. Thus there is some rationale in an initial wait-and-see policy for small tumors because some may grow very slowly, remain dormant, or shrink. However, during such an observation period there is a risk of further hearing loss in patients with some retained hearing. The authors concluded that with few exceptions, such as a patient with a VS of the only hearing ear, patients who are candidates for hearing preservation surgery should be treated rather than observed.

R.H. Wilkins, M.D.

The Limitations of Hearing Preservation in Acoustic Neuroma Surgery: Histological Study of the Interface Between the Eighth Cranial Nerve and the Tumor

Matsunaga T, Kanzaki J, Igarashi M (Keio Univ, Tokyo; Nihon Univ, Tokyo)
Acta Otolaryngol 115:269–272, 1995   24–2

Background.—Most patients who undergo surgical removal of an acoustic neuroma (AN) experience hearing loss because of direct injury to the cochlear nerve and the effects of vascular damage. Tumor size, biological features of the tumor, and individual anatomy may further influence the postoperative hearing loss. The histologic relationships between the eighth cranial nerve and AN were examined in a study of nerve-tumor specimens.

Methods.—Light microscopy and immunohistochemistry were used to examine specimens of the eighth cranial nerve and attached tumor. For light microscopy and immunohistochemistry, specimens from 13 patients were embedded in paraffin and sectioned at 6 µm. They were stained with hematoxylin-eosin; a combination of Luxol fast blue (LFB), Periodic acid–Schiff (PAS) and hematoxylin; and Bodian-LFB-hematoxylin. Rabbit anticow glial fibrillary acidic protein (GFAP) and rabbit antibovine neurofilament 150-kd primary antibodies were used for immunohistochemistry. Another group of specimens from 19 patients were fixed in glutaraldehyde and embedded in Epon, then sectioned at 1.0 µm and stained with methylene blue for light microscopy. Schwannoma cells, normal peripheral nerve fibers, central myelinated nerve fibers, axons within or adjacent to the tumor, and central glial tissue were visualized using these stains. The relationship between myelin and axons could be seen, and the myelin sheaths could be evaluated.

Results.—In 2 of 6 cochlear nerve specimens and 5 of 25 vestibular nerve specimens, the tumor was clearly distinct from the nerve without signs of invasion. No connective tissue separated nerve and tumor, although capillaries were often present in the area between the 2. Moderate invasion by tumor cells was seen in 2 of 6 cochlear nerve specimens and 11 of 25 vestibular nerve specimens. Invasion occurred through the perineurium and endoneurium, and tumor cells pushed through the nerve fibers. Myelinated fibers preserved their arrangement, but the myelin sheaths thinned at the site of invasion. Severe nerve invasion was seen in 2 of 6 cochlear specimens and 9 of 25 vestibular specimens. The eighth cranial nerves in these cases seemed retracted into the tumor tissue at the site of active growth, with nerves and tumor cells intermingled at the point of attachment. The arrangement of myelinated nerve fibers was disrupted, with degenerated myelin sheaths seen near the tumor. The density of myelinated nerve fibers was often low in the cochlear and vestibular sites adjacent to the tumor, and gliosis was present. Finally, hemangioma-like tissue was sometimes detected attached to the surface of cochlear or vestibular nerve, consisting mainly of small arteries and arterioles.

Discussion.—Three types of tumor-nerve interface were seen: sharp demarcation without tumor invasion into adjacent nerve; moderate invasion by tumor cells, with preservation of the arrangement of adjacent myelinated nerve fibers; and severe tumor invasion with disruption and degeneration of myelinated nerve fibers. Even when the boundary between the eighth cranial nerve and the tumor was well demarcated, suggesting greater preservation of hearing after tumor removal, compression by the tumor had led to thinning of the nerve, suggesting that the trauma of surgery and reduced blood flow to the nerve could still cause conduction block. With moderate invasion of the nerve, part of the cochlear nerve may require removal, leading to a range of hearing losses. Severe invasion means that severe damage to the cochlear nerve is unavoidable, and the presence of hemangioma-like tissue means that bleeding is a likely complication of surgery. Finally, the presence of gliosis suggests a reduced likelihood of recovery from surgical injury to the cochlear nerve.

▶ One of the goals of the surgeon treating a small acoustic neuroma in a patient with useful hearing in the same ear is preservation of hearing. Matsunaga et al. showed in this study that the growth pattern of the tumor in relation to the cochlear nerve may destine the attempt to failure no matter how skilled the surgeon and how careful the operation.

R.H. Wilkins, M.D.

Nervus Intermedius Function After Vestibular Schwannoma Removal: Clinical Features and Pathophysiological Mechanisms
Irving RM, Viani L, Hardy DG, et al (Addenbrooke's Hosp, Cambridge, England; Royal Ear Hosp, London)
Laryngoscope 105:809–813, 1995

24–3

Objective.—Few previous reports of facial nerve outcomes after vestibular schwannoma removal have addressed the sensory-autonomic component of this nerve. This situation arises partly because the distress associated with such functions is less apparent to the surgeon and because currently used facial nerve grading systems do not include the functions of the nervus intermedius. The frequency and nature of abnormalities of nervus intermedius function after vestibular schwannoma removal were estimated in a questionnaire study.

Methods.—The study questionnaire was mailed to 257 patients who had undergone vestibular schwannoma surgery. This instrument asked in detail about any abnormalities of lacrimation, including crocodile tears, and of taste. Two hundred twenty-four questionnaires were returned, for a response rate of 87%. The mean follow-up was 4 years.

Results.—Two percent of the patients reported having crocodile tears before surgery, 4% reported dryness of the eye, and 6% had taste abnormalities. After surgery, 44% of the patients had crocodile tears and 72% had an absence of tears or a significant reduction in the production of tears. Forty-eight percent of the patients reported a taste abnormality— either a significant reduction or an alteration in the character of taste. About one third of cases of crocodile tears began within 1 month after surgery, with a second peak onset at about 6 months. Twenty-seven percent of affected patients reported recovery of normal tearing and 42% reported the return of normal taste sensation, whereas crocodile tears resolved in only 6% of cases.

Conclusion.—Patients undergoing vestibular schwannoma surgery are commonly left with nervus intermedius abnormalities. Patients should receive adequate counseling about these symptoms before undergoing surgery. Facial nerve sensory-autonomic dysfunction should be assessed in surgical reports of facial nerve results in cerebellopontine angle surgery.

▶ The authors documented that functions subserved by the nervus intermedius are often altered by the surgical removal of a vestibular schwannoma. Surgeons who remove such tumors should inform their patients preoperatively about possible changes in lacrimation and taste just as they ordinarily inform their patients about possible changes in facial motor function.

R.H. Wilkins, M.D.

Vestibular Adaptation Exercises and Recovery: Acute Stage After Acoustic Neuroma Resection
Herdman SJ, Clendaniel RA, Mattox DE, et al (Univ of Miami, Fla; Duke Univ, Durham, NC; Univ of Maryland, Baltimore; et al)
Otolaryngol Head Neck Surg 113:77–87, 1995

24–4

Introduction.—Animal studies have demonstrated that a lack of visuomotor experience during the acute stage after unilateral vestibular loss can delay the onset of recovery and prolong the recovery period. Patients often avoid movement during this stage because it causes dysequilibrium and nausea. Controlled, prescribed exercises performed during the acute stage were studied to determine whether they would facilitate recovery onset and hasten the rate of recovery.

Subjects.—There were 11 subjects in the experimental and 8 in the control group; all had resection of an acoustic neuroma. Subjective reports and clinical examinations were done before and daily after surgery. Exercises in the experimental group consisted of an X1 viewing paradigm in which patients performed horizontal or vertical head movements while maintaining visual fixation on a target placed within arm's length or across the room. Control group exercises consisted of ambulation plus smooth-pursuit eye movements. All exercises were performed with subjects standing and sitting for 1 minute each, 5 times daily, for a total of 20 minutes.

Results.—Patients in the experimental group reported less dysequilibrium on days 5 and 6 postoperatively. On day 3, 25% of the control subjects and 64% of the experimental group could perform the Romberg test with eyes closed. On day 6, 80% of the experimental and 57% of the control group could maintain the Romberg position with eyes closed for 30 seconds. On day 6, 73% of the subjects in the experimental group had a normal vestibulo-ocular reflex compared with 29% in the control group. All of the control subjects had gait problems on day 6, whereas these were seen in only 40% to 50% of the experimental subjects. Performance on the timed Romberg test on day 3 may help determine which patients will benefit from brief periods of vestibular adaptation exercises.

▶ Herdman et al. showed that the use of simple vestibular adaptation exercises after acoustic neuroma removal results in improved postural stability both in stance and during ambulation. Such brief periods of vestibular adaptation exercises also result in a diminished perception of dysequilibrium during the early stage of recovery.

R.H. Wilkins, M.D.

Impact of Cranioplasty on Headache After Acoustic Neuroma Removal
Harner SG, Beatty CW, Ebersold MJ (Mayo Clinic, Rochester, Minn)
Neurosurgery 36:1097–1100, 1995   24–5

Background.—In a previous review of patients undergoing retrosigmoid removal of an acoustic neuroma, the authors found that the incidence of headache was 23% at 3 months after the procedure and 9% at 2 years. A change in the surgical procedure, including a cranioplasty with methyl methacrylate, was studied to reduce the severity and incidence of these headaches.

Methods.—Beginning in March 1993, all patients undergoing the retrosigmoid removal of an acoustic neuroma had a cranioplasty with methyl methacrylate. This was performed before closure. The 24 patients undergoing the procedure were matched with other patients who had undergone operations by the same surgeons using the retrosigmoid approach without filling the craniectomy defect. The 2 groups were comparable in tumor size, sex, and age. All patients were followed for 3 or more months after surgery.

Findings.—The incidence of postoperative headaches was 4% in the cranioplasty group and 17% in the control group. The 1 patient who had headache after cranioplasty had the largest tumor among the 550 patients in the total series. In all patients with postoperative headache, the headaches were grade 1 or 2. None of the patients died during or after surgery. The use of methyl methacrylate material and the cranioplasty appeared to cause no side effects. Hearing outcomes were similar between groups, with hearing preserved in 3 patients in the control group and in 7 in the cranioplasty group. Mean postoperative facial nerve function was also comparable.

Conclusion.—The cause of postoperative headache in patients undergoing retrosigmoid removal of an acoustic neuroma is not certain. Possibly cervical muscle scars the dura, resulting in traction on the dura from neck motion. Methyl methacrylate inserted as a rigid barrier between these 2 layers is a safe, well-tolerated procedure that appears to reduce the incidence of postoperative headache.

▶ In recent years it has become apparent that a significant percentage of patients who have an acoustic neuroma surgically removed will be bothered by postoperative headaches. The exact cause of this phenomenon is not known. In this paper, Harner et al. showed that a cranioplasty will reduce the incidence of such postoperative headaches; based on this, the authors postulated that scar-related dural traction is the process that causes these headaches and that is prevented by the cranioplasty.

The so-called syndrome of the trephined consists of a constellation of symptoms, including headache, that may accompany a calvarial defect.[1] The effect of atmospheric pressure on the meninges and brain, derangements of CSF hydrodynamics, and regionally impaired blood flow have been thought to be factors in the causation of that syndrome, which can be relieved by a cranioplasty. Perhaps such factors also play a role in causing the headaches that follow acoustic neuroma removal.

R.H. Wilkins, M.D.

Reference

1. Fodstad H, Love JA, Ekstedt J, et al: Effect of cranioplasty on cerebrospinal fluid hydrodynamics in patients with the syndrome of the trephined. *Acta Neurochir (Wien)* 70:21–30, 1984.

25 Other Intracranial Tumors

General

The Applicability of Collins' Law to Childhood Brain Tumors and Its Usefulness as a Predictor of Survival

Brown WD, Tavaré CJ, Sobel EL, et al (Univ of Southern California, Los Angeles)
Neurosurgery 36:1093–1096, 1995   25–1

Background.—In 1955, Collins correlated the recurrence of Wilms' tumor in children with the patient's age plus 9 months. Subsequently the so-called Collins' law (CL) was applied to tumors of "embryonal" origin in the CNS and also to tumors outside the CNS. It has successfully predicted survival in some children with neural tumors, but CL has failed in other cases.

Objective.—The validity of CL was examined in 2,917 patients who were younger than 21 at the time they had initial surgery for 1 of 14 childhood neural tumors. The children were seen at 10 medical centers during a period of nearly 50 years and were entered in the Childhood Brain Tumor Consortium database. Collins' law was considered a good predictor of survival if less than 10% of patients who eventually died remained alive after the period of risk.

Findings.—Anaplastic astrocytomas followed CL, but pilocytic astrocytomas did not. In addition, CL applied to glioblastoma, pineoblastoma, medulloblastoma or "primitive neuroectodermal tumor," teratoma, germinoma, ependymoma, papilloma, and unclassifiable tumors. Collins' law had no predictive value for craniopharyngioma, oligodendroglioma, or astrocytomas of the plain, fibrillary, or protoplasmic type. In cases where CL was predictive of survival, it held when the child was younger than 8 years at the time of diagnosis, but insufficient data were available on older children.

▶ As indicated by the authors, Collins reasoned that a tumor present at birth had to have developed during a period of 9 months or less and that the period of risk for recurrence of such a tumor after treatment (based on the rate of growth unique to that tumor) must be equal to the patient's age plus 9 months. Thus, slowly growing tumors will recur slowly, and quickly growing tumors will recur quickly. Extensions of that concept are that a tumor discovered after birth would have developed during a maximum period of the patient's age plus 9 months and that, after treatment (assuming a constant tumor growth rate), the period of risk of recurrence can be estimated in similar fashion.

In Dorland's medical dictionary, a law is defined as "a uniform or constant fact or principle."[1] Collins' law is not included among the 152 that are listed in that book, which may reflect that CL does not have universal applicability to all tumors, as demonstrated in this study.

R.H. Wilkins, M.D.

Reference

1. *Dorland's Illustrated Medical Dictionary,* ed 28. s.v. "law." Philadelphia, WB Saunders 1994, pp 904–906.

Medulloblastoma and Collins' Law: A Critical Review of the Concept of a Period of Risk for Tumor Recurrence and Patient Survival
Brown WD, Tavaré CJ, Sobel EL, et al (Univ of Southern California, Los Angeles)
Neurosurgery 36:691–697, 1995

25–2

Background.—Collins' law (CL) states that the period of risk for tumor recurrence in Wilms' tumor is the child's age at diganosis plus 9 months. This law has been applied to other tumors of embryonal origin as well, including medulloblastoma (MB). The validity of CL was tested in a large population of children with MB.

Methods and Findings.—Data on 602 children with MB in the Childhood Brain Tumor Consortium (CBTC) were analyzed. Four hundred twenty-one of these children had died. Overall, 16 patients proved to be exceptions to CL. A review of the literature revealed another 22 exceptions to CL. In the CBTC group, all the exceptions were younger than 6 years at initial diagnosis and were followed for a mean of 7.5 years. All the children who were CL exceptions died. However, as age at initial diagnosis increased, the period of observation needed to determine the validity of CL became impractically long.

Conclusion.—In this series, only 3.8% of the patients were exceptions to CL. The application of CL to children younger than 8 years appears to be useful for predicting survival in childhood MB.

▶ Collins' law was originally defined in relation to Wilms' tumor. Among tumors of the CNS, those that most often abide by this law include medulloblastomas, ependymomas, and primitive neuroectodermal tumors. As part of a larger study reviewed in the previous abstract (Abstract 25–1), the authors tested the validity of Collins' law in relation to MB.

R.H. Wilkins, M.D.

Gliomas

Placebo-Controlled Trial of Safety and Efficacy of Intraoperative Controlled Delivery by Biodegradable Polymers of Chemotherapy for Recurrent Gliomas
Brem H, for the Polymer-Brain Tumor Treatment Group (Johns Hopkins Univ, Baltimore, Md; Natl Inst of Neurological Diseases and Stroke, Bethesda, Md; Western Pennsylvania Hosp, Pittsburgh, Pa; et al)
Lancet 345:1008–1012, 1995   25–3

Background.—Effective chemotherapy for brain tumors has proved to be limited because of problems in providing adequate exposure without unacceptable systemic toxicity. One approach is to incorporate drugs into biodegradable polymers that are implanted at the tumor site, allowing prolonged exposure to the tumor with minimal systemic exposure. It is possible to incorporate carmustine, the most effective agent against brain tumors, into the hydrophobic matrix of a poly(carboxyphenoxy-propane/sebacic acid) anhydride polymer.

Trial Design.—A randomized study of carmustine-impregnated polymer was carried out in 222 patients seen at 27 centers with recurrent malignancies of the brain who required reoperation. Biodegradable polymer disks containing 3.85% carmustine were implanted in 110 patients and placebo polymer disks in 112. After the maximum amount of tumor was removed, as many as 8 disks were applied to the surface of the resection cavity. In some cases oxidized regenerated cellulose in sheet form was used to secure the implants.

Results.—Approximately 12% of patients in each group were reoperated on within 6 months of polymer implantation. One fourth of the actively treated patients and 19% of placebo patients received systemic chemotherapy during this period. Median survival was 31 weeks in the carmustine group and 23 weeks in placebo recipients. Nearly two thirds of placebo patients with glioblastoma and 44% of those actively treated had died by 6 months. In these patients, the estimated hazard ratio associated with active treatment was 0.81. On multiple regression analysis, active treatment was significantly beneficial to patients with glioblastoma. Four patients given carmustine and 1 placebo patient developed serious intracranial infection.

Conclusion.—Interstitial chemotherapy using polymer implants appears to be an effective and safe approach to treating recurrent malignant gliomas, particularly glioblastoma.

▶ Brem et al. reported their experience with the treatment of recurrent malignant glioma of the brain using locally applied carmustine that had been impregnated into biodegradable polymer disks from which it was released over a 2- to 3-week period after disk implantation.

R.H. Wilkins, M.D.

Long-Term Outcome of Hypothalamic/Chiasmatic Astrocytomas in Children Treated With Conservative Surgery

Sutton LN, Molloy PT, Sernyak H, et al (Univ of Pennsylvania, Philadelphia; George Washington Univ, Washington, DC)

J Neurosurg 83:583–589, 1995

25–4

Objective.—There is controversy regarding the treatment of astrocytomas of the optic chiasm and hypothalamus, which are histologically benign tumors that occur in childhood. Radical surgery is feasible but carries the risk of damage to the pituitary gland, optic apparatus, hypothalamus, and carotid arteries. Its benefits and risks must therefore be compared with those of standard therapy. The long-term results of patients treated with conservative therapy for hypothalamic/chiasmatic astrocytomas were reported.

Methods.—The retrospective analysis included 33 patients treated for hypothalamic/chiasmatic astrocytomas from 1976 to 1991. Their mean age was 4 years; 13 were 2 years old or younger at diagnosis. All patients met criteria that would have made them candidates for radical surgery if treated today; they had a globular enhancing mass that measured at least 2 cm in the hypothalamic/chiasmatic region. None had CT or MRI evidence of optic nerve or optic radiation involvement, and all were followed for at least 3 years. Treatment varied with age. The patients received either no surgery, less than 50% resection, or biopsy only. This was followed by adjuvant local radiation therapy in 29 patients and by chemotherapy with actinomycin-D and vincristine in 18 patients.

Findings.—Low-grade or pilocytic astrocytoma was confirmed in 32 of the 33 patients. Three patients died of progressive tumor growth, 1 of actual shunt malfunction, and 1 of intercurrent infection. This left 28 patients alive at a mean follow-up of 11 years after diagnosis. Though 5 patients were blind, the other 23 had functional vision in at least 1 eye. Nine patients required thyroid replacement therapy and 8 required growth hormone, but 12 required no endocrine replacement therapy. Sixteen patients were in regular classrooms or had completed regular school; 8 of 9 adult survivors were functioning independently.

Conclusion.—The long-term results of conservative surgery and adjuvant radiation, chemotherapy or both for hypothalamic/chiasmatic astrocytomas were reported. The findings provide a baseline with which to compare the results of radical surgery. Most likely, no single treatment will be best for every patient with hypothalamic/chiasmatic astrocytoma.

▶ The authors documented the relatively indolent nature of hypothalamic/chiasmatic astrocytomas of childhood and argued convincingly that the outcome of any treatment such as radical surgical resection must be compared against the natural history of these lesions.

R.H. Wilkins, M.D.

Meningiomas

Evidence for Clonal Spread in the Development of Multiple Meningiomas

Larson JJ, Tew JM Jr, Simon M, et al (Univ of Cincinnati, Ohio; Mayfield Neurological Inst, Cincinnati, Ohio)
J Neurosurg 83:705–709, 1995
25–5

Introduction.—Two hypotheses have been proposed for the pathogenesis of multiple meningiomas: independent origin or clonal spread. The clonal origin of multiple meningiomas was examined using 2 polymerase chain reaction (PCR) assays for X chromosome inactivation.

Methods.—Tumor specimens were obtained from each meningioma in 4 women with multiple meningiomas, and DNA was isolated from these specimens and from peripheral blood leukocytes (PBLs). The DNA of the active X chromosome was digested with the methylation-sensitive restriction enzyme *Hpa*II. Then 2 polymorphic portions of X chromosome-linked genes, *PGK* and *AR*, were amplified with PCR. The distribution of X chromosome inactivation patterns was calculated.

Results.—In all 4 patients, the DNA samples from the PBLs were heterozygous for either the *PGK* polymorphism (2 patients) or the *AR* polymorphism (2 patients) and demonstrated the normal, polyclonal pattern. However, the DNA samples from the tumor tissue in all 4 patients demonstrated monoclonal PCR amplification patterns. All PCR fragments from the same patient were the same size, indicating identical parental X chromosome inactivation. The probability that each tumor in a patient with multiple meningiomas is a clonal proliferation of the same progenitor cell was 99%.

Conclusion.—Amplification by PCR demonstrated the clonal origin of multiple meningiomas, which share the same parental origin of X chromosome inactivation, regardless of the histologic and karyotypic variations.

▶ This study supported the interesting idea that multiple meningiomas in the same patient, despite being in different anatomical locations, arise from the same clone of cells. The 4 patients reported here had 15 intracranial meningiomas removed. In 1 patient, 6 tumors were located as follows: left frontal convexity, left anterior falx, right posterior falx, right frontal convexity, and right parietal convexity. The authors proposed that such tumors arise from a single transforming event, with the original clone of cells spreading throughout the meninges to the sites of subsequent tumor growth.

R.H. Wilkins, M.D.

Development of Intracranial Meningiomas at the Site of Cranial Fractures Remarks on 15 Cases

Artico M, Cervoni L, Carloia S, et al ("La Sapienza" Univ of Rome)
Acta Neurochir (Wien) 136:132–134, 1995

25–6

Background.—Trauma as a cause of tumor, especially meningioma and glioma, is controversial. The possible correlation between trauma and tumor onset was addressed in a review of 15 patients with posttraumatic intracranial meningioma.

Patients and Findings.—The patients, 9 males and 6 females aged 13 to 69, were selected for review using previously published criteria. All patients had had head trauma characterized by a loss of consciousness and bone fracture on plain films and CT scans. The causes of trauma included motor vehicle accidents, domestic accidents, and blows to the head from a hammer, pickaxe, stick, and falling roof tile. The interval between trauma and the onset of tumor ranged from 4 to 45 years, with a mean of 4 years. Meningioma occurred most frequently in the cerebral convexity. Complete tumor removal was possible in all patients. Eleven tumors were World Health Organization histologic grade I, 3 were grade II, and 1 was grade III. Mean follow-up was 15 years, with a range of 5 to 40 years. Four patients died of unrelated causes. The 11 survivors remained in good neurologic condition.

Conclusion.—Head trauma may contribute to the development of meningioma in some patients. Both neuroradiologic and macroscopic findings indicated that the meningioma occurred at the same site as the trauma in the patients reviewed. Moreover, the trauma produced a bone fracture near a suture in all of these patients.

▶ Although the etiologic relationship between head trauma and intracranial meningioma development is discussed in comprehensive publications dealing with such tumors, most authors conclude that despite occasional interesting anecdotes, there is no conclusive proof that head trauma (a relatively common occurrence) can cause a meningioma to form. Artico et al. presented 15 cases to support the idea that, in fact, a head injury in some patients can result in a meningioma.

R.H. Wilkins, M.D.

Evidence of Meningioma Infiltration Into Cranial Nerves: Clinical Implications for Cavernous Sinus Meningiomas

Larson JJ, van Loveren HR, Balko MG, et al (Univ of Cincinnati, Ohio)
J Neurosurg 83:596–599, 1995

25–7

Objective.—Although good short-term recurrence-free results have been obtained after microsurgical resection of meningiomas of the cavernous sinuses, long-term recurrence and regrowth rates have not been studied. The findings of tumor infiltration into a cranial nerve in 2 patients were documented.

Methods.—Between 1989 and 1993, 36 patients (11 men and 25 women) aged 24 to 75 underwent resection of holocavernous meningiomas. It was the second operation for 8 patients. In 2 patients, a cranial nerve was resected during the cavernous sinus dissection.

> *Case 1.*—Woman, 62, with left-eye blindness was found on MRI to have a 2-cm meningioma of the right cavernous sinus and Meckel's cave 2 years after undergoing resection of a benign meningioma of the left sphenoid wing. Surgical resection and subsequent staining revealed infiltration by a benign meningioma of the third division of the trigeminal nerve.
>
> *Case 2.*—Man, 32, with grand mal seizures and right-eye blindness, was found on MRI to have a large, right holocavernous meningioma. The trochlear nerve was resected when surgery revealed that it was encased by the tumor. The tumor was partially resected; some of it adhered to the right cavernous internal carotid artery. Postoperatively tissue sections showed the benign tumor had infiltrated the trochlear nerve.

Results.—The World Health Organization grading system does not include a category for meningioma infiltration into cranial nerves. Whether cavernous sinus meningiomas should be treated by surgery, radiation, or a combination is a subject of debate, although it is known that recurrence is generally the result of incomplete resection.

Conclusion.—Complete resection of meningiomas infiltrating cranial nerves may not be possible. Procedures with lower morbidity should be considered in these cases.

▶ The authors pointed out that when a meningioma invades a cranial nerve in the cavernous sinus, complete tumor resection is not possible without resection of the involved nerve, and they rightly concluded that "in these circumstances, cavernous sinus dissection in an attempt at complete resection of the tumor, in the long term, may provide no advantage over treatment options with lower morbidity."

R.H. Wilkins, M.D.

Meningiomas of the Tentorial Notch: Surgical Anatomy and Management

Samii M, Carvalho GA, Tatagiba M, et al (Norstadt Hosp, Hannover, Germany)
J Neurosurg 84:375–381, 1996   25–8

Introduction.—The anatomical location of the tentorial notch within the surrounding neurovascular structures makes excision of a tentorial meningioma a complex surgical procedure. The clear preoperative delineation of the location and extension of such a meningioma is crucial. The surgical management and outcomes of 25 tentorial notch meningiomas were reported.

Methods.—Twenty-five patients underwent the surgical resection of tentorial notch meningiomas between 1978 and 1993. Patients underwent preoperative neuroradiologic studies, including CT scanning in all patients, MRI in 13 patients, and angiography in 6 patients. These studies and review of the operative records allowed the establishment of the origin of the tumors. The location of the tumor attachment at the tentorial incisura defined 2 groups: 19 patients with lateral tumors (group 1) and 6 patients with posteromedial tumors (group 2). Surgical technique was chosen based on clinical signs and symptoms, patient age, and the preoperative neuroradiologic studies, with careful attention to the anatomical relationships between the tumor and the surrounding structures.

Results.—The patients included 18 women and 7 men, aged 28 to 72. The most frequent symptom was trigeminal pain, followed by headache, gait disturbance, hearing loss, dizziness, and diplopia. The neurologic signs most frequently indicated impairment of the fifth cranial nerve, followed by impairment of the eighth and seventh cranial nerves. The tumor diameters were as large as 60 by 60 mm, with most greater than 30 by 30 mm. The tumors extended suprainfratentorially in 44% of the patients. Three tumors extended to the foramen magnum, 2 into the internal auditory canal, and 1 into the third and lateral ventricles. There was evidence of brain-stem compression in 88% of the patients. Among the patients in group 1, the lateral suboccipital-retrosigmoid surgical approach was used in 16 patients, and the combined subtemporal-presigmoidal approach in 3 patients. Among the patients in group 2, the infratentorial-supracerebellar approach was used in 4 patients and the occipital-transtentorial approach in 2. Surgical removal was total in 22 patients (88%), subtotal in 2 (8%), and achieved surgical decompression in 1 (4%). Strong tumor adherence to vascular structures, cranial nerves, or the brain stem prevented complete tumor resection in the 3 patients. Postoperative surgical complications included trochlear nerve palsy, partial facial paresis, and transient lower cranial nerve dysfunction. At the time of discharge, 14 patients (56%) returned to their normal activities, 6 (24%) maintained their independence, and 5 (20%) required nursing assistance. Of 21 patients followed for a mean of 5.6 years, 17 resumed their normal activities, 3 needed nursing assistance, and 1 died of unrelated causes.

Conclusion.—Tentorial notch meningiomas can be completely resected with minimal morbidity with a thorough understanding of the neurosurgical anatomy and with the development of microneurosurgical techniques.

▶ Dr. Samii and his colleagues analyzed their experience with meningiomas of the tentorial notch and make useful management recommendations based on that experience, as well as on the publications of others.

R.H. Wilkins, M.D.

Miscellaneous Tumors

Staging, Scoring and Grading of Medulloblastoma: A Postoperative Prognosis Predicting System Based on the Cases of a Single Institute

Sure U, Berghorn WJ, Bertalanffy H, et al (Neurochirurgische Univ Freiburg, Federal Republic of Germany; Nagoya Univ, Japan; Neurochirurgische Univ Aachen, Federal Republic of Germany)
Acta Neurochir (Wien) 132:59–65, 1995

25–9

Purpose.—Overall survival for patients with medulloblastoma has improved, but the condition is serious and outcome is quite variable. Hence, an easily applicable system is needed to predict prognosis. The records of 66 patients undergoing microsurgery and radiotherapy for treatment of medulloblastoma were retrospectively analyzed to establish such an early postoperative prognosis predicting system.

Findings.—Outcomes were compared with respect to patient age, tumor location, histologic diagnosis, degree of resection, and presence of metastases. Prognosis was better in patients older than as opposed to younger than 10 years. Lateral tumors were associated with a better prognosis than were midline tumors with brain-stem infiltration. Prognosis was more favorable for patients undergoing complete rather than subtotal or partial resection; prognosis was also improved if metastases were not present at the time of diagnosis. Histologic designation of the desmoplastic tumor variant carried a better prognosis than did confirmation of classic medulloblastoma characteristics.

Scoring System.—Scoring points were distributed correlating with the degree of inter-subgroup significance according to the individual subgroup prognoses. Each patient received a total score ranging from 0 to 14, and 3 distinct prognostic groups were defined. Of the patients, 44% showed a "good" prognosis (total score 9–14) with a Kaplan-Meier survival rate of 62%. A "moderate" prognosis (total score 5–8) was assigned to 39% of patients, who showed a survival rate of 22%. Seventeen percent of patients showed a total score of 0 to 4 and were considered to have a "poor" prognosis, with a survival rate of 0%. The survival rates between these groups differed significantly; overall median survival time was 55 months.

Discussion.—This newly designed 14-point scoring system allows simple staging and accurate prognostic grading for any single patient. Evaluation of the 5 proposed parameters does not require sophisticated diagnostic equipment. This study did not exclude any patient because of poor postoperative course or incomplete postoperative radiotherapy protocol. The system thus can be applied to any patient with medulloblastoma who undergoes surgery to be followed with standard radiotherapy.

▶ The authors provided a common sense system to predict the prognosis for medulloblastoma treated with surgery and radiotherapy.

R.H. Wilkins, M.D.

26 Pseudotumor Cerebri

Surgical Management of Pseudotumor Cerebri in Pregnancy: Case Report

Shapiro S, Yee R, Brown H (Indiana Univ, Indianapolis)
Neurosurgery 37:829–831, 1995

26–1

Introduction.—Pseudotumor cerebri (PTC) occurs most commonly in obese women and has been associated with pregnancy. Visual loss is common in pregnant women with active pseudotumor. Various treatment options have been used for these patients. The treatment experience with 4 pregnant patients with PTC and refractory progressive severe visual loss was described.

Case 1.—Woman, 24, who was morbidly obese, developed severe headaches and mild vision blurring with bilateral papilledema at 26 weeks' gestation. Visual fields were severely restricted. Results of the CT head scan were normal, but an opening pressure of 50 cm H_2O was found on lumbar puncture. She was treated with acetazolamide and repeat lumbar punctures with drainage, but her visual deterioration progressed. A lumboperitoneal shunt was performed, resulting in immediate and substantial improvement in her vision. She delivered a normal infant vaginally at 34 weeks after induction of labor. She had stable, improved vision thereafter, with no medication.

Case 2.—Woman, 22, who was morbidly obese and had visual loss and an opening pressure of 44 cm H_2O at lumbar puncture was treated with acetazolamide, frequent lumbar punctures, corticosteroid and furosemide, which did not resolve the visual deterioration. A lumboperitoneal shunt with a horizontal-vertical valve was placed. She had improved vision within 1 week and a normal vaginal delivery at 37 weeks.

Case 3.—Woman, 22, who was normal sized, developed visual loss because of PTC at 27 weeks' gestation. Her vision loss progressed despite treatment with lumbar punctures, acetazolamide, prednisone, and furosemide. At 29 weeks' gestation, a lumboperitoneal shunt with a horizontal-vertical valve was placed, resulting in near-normal vision by 4 weeks. A normal infant was delivered vaginally at 36 weeks.

Case 4.—Woman, 36, who was normal sized and had PTC, had a large visual field loss in her right eye at 25 weeks' gestation. Although she was treated with lumbar punctures, acetazolamide, furosemide, and prednisone, her visual fields deteriorated. She was treated with a lumboperitoneal shunt with a horizontal-vertical valve. After initial improvement in vision in the right eye, her vision deteriorated in the left eye, and she required bilateral optic nerve sheath decompression. Premature contractions that developed after surgery required IV therapy and resolved in 1 day. Both visual acuity and visual fields improved to near normal. She delivered a normal infant at 36 weeks.

Discussion.—Treatment for pregnant patients with PTC is nearly the same as for nonpregnant patients with PTC and can include frequent lumbar punctures, acetazolamide, furosemide, corticosteroids, and lumboperitoneal shunting. Lumboperitoneal shunting brought immediate vision improvement in 75% of patients. These patients should be treated by a team including an obstetrician, a neurosurgeon, and an ophthalmologist.

▶ Shapiro et al. showed that pseudotumor cerebri can be managed safely in pregnant patients using the same approaches as in nonpregnant patients, including lumboperitoneal shunting. Interestingly, the intraperitoneal pressure measured during lumboperitoneal shunting in 3 pregnant patients (7, 6, and 6 cm H_2O) was significantly lower than the concurrent CSF pressure (54, 41, and 29 cm H_2O).

R.H. Wilkins, M.D.

27 Intracranial Aneurysms and Intracranial Hemorrhage

Intracranial Aneurysms: MR Angiographic Screening in 400 Asymptomatic Individuals With Increased Familial Risk
Ronkainen A, Puranen MI, Hernesniemi JA, et al (Univ Hosp of Kuopio, Finland)
Radiology 195:35–40, 1995

27–1

Background.—Magnetic resonance angiographic screening in patients with symptomatic intracranial aneurysms (IAs) appears promising. The accuracy and limitations of MR angiographic screening for healthy individuals with a family history of IA were prospectively studied.

Patients and Methods.—Magnetic resonance angiography that used a multislab, 3-dimensional, time-of-flight sequence was performed in 400 healthy individuals from 68 families with histories of aneurysmal subarachnoid hemorrhage. Histories of polycystic kidney disease also were documented in 6 of the 68 families. Intraobserver consistency and interobserver variability were assessed. Positive findings were verified on conventional angiography.

Results.—Thirty-seven individuals had evidence of IAs on MR angiography. Conventional angiography was performed in 32 of these individuals. No significant differences between MR and conventional angiography in the assessment of aneurysm size, location, and orientation, and visibility of the aneurysm neck were observed. Excellent intraobserver consistency and good to excellent interobserver reproducibility were achieved.

Conclusion.—Magnetic resonance angiographic screening is safe and reliable for asymptomatic individuals at increased risk for IA. Screening is advised for those individuals who have 2 or more relatives with IA in their immediate family, even though benefits of such a strategy have not been quantified. When IAs are identified, conventional angiography is still required before surgical intervention.

▶ This is 1 of several studies reported in recent years that have established the value of MR angiography in screening for IAs. Such studies, including this study, have focused on individuals with an increased likelihood of having an IA. Considering the present availability of MR angiography and the expense of the procedure, I doubt that this method would be cost effective in screening an unselected population for IAs, an ultimate goal in attempting to identify IAs before they rupture and while they can be treated with the smallest risk to the patient. Much remains to be done in this regard.

R.H. Wilkins, M.D.

MR Diagnosis of Subacute and Chronic Subarachnoid Hemorrhage: Comparison With CT

Ogawa T, Inugami A, Fujita H, et al (Research Inst of Brain and Blood Vessels, Akita, Japan)
AJR 165:1257–1262, 1995
27–2

Rationale.—Although CT has largely replaced lumbar puncture for diagnosing acute subarachnoid hemorrhage (SAH), scans may appear normal for several days or even weeks after hemorrhage. If MRI were a reliable means of detecting SAH at this stage, many fewer delayed lumbar punctures might be necessary.

Objective.—The reliability of MRI was studied in 37 patients with aneurysmal subarachnoid bleeding. A total of 42 MR studies were done 4 to 75 days after the initial bleeding episode.

Methods.—All patients had CSF examination at the time of MRI. A range of studies, including T1- and T2-weighted images and proton density–weighted images, were carried out using a 0.5-tesla unit. All patients had noncontrast CT scanning within 24 hours of the MR study.

Findings.—Only 46% of CT studies in patients with evidence of SAH from lumbar puncture were positive. In contrast, SAH was demonstrated as a high–signal intensity region by 63% of T1-weighted MR studies. These images were 52% accurate in the subacute stage (first 3 days) and 90% accurate in detecting chronic SAH. Seven patients, however, had positive CT scans but negative T1-weighted MR images. Proton-density–weighted images showed an area of high signal in 9 of 10 patients who had SAH by lumbar puncture. Moderately T2-weighted images were positive in 92% of instances, but conventional T2-weighted images often were falsely negative.

Conclusion.—Magnetic resonance imaging is preferable to CT scanning for documenting subacute and, in particular, chronic SAH.

▶ The authors provided basic comparison data between MRI and CT in regard to the detection of intracranial SAH in the subacute (days 4–14) and chronic (> 14 days) stages.

R.H. Wilkins, M.D.

Familial Aneurysmal Subarachnoid Hemorrhage: A Community-Based Study

Schievink WI, Schaid DJ, Michels VV, et al (Mayo Clinic, Rochester, Minn)
J Neurosurg 83:426–429, 1995
27–3

Background.—Although the familial aggregation associated with intracranial aneurysms has been documented, it may be fortuitous. Intracranial aneurysms are not rare, and most reported familial occurrences involve only 2 members. The familial occurrence of aneurysmal subarachnoid hemorrhage (SAH) was studied in 1 community to determine whether the family members of patients with a ruptured aneurysm are at increased risk of developing an SAH.

Methods.—All 81 patients in Rochester, Minnesota, with an SAH from a proved aneurysmal rupture between 1970 and 1989 were included in the study. These individuals or their families were contacted for information about their family history. The number of SAHs expected among first-degree relatives was determined based on previously established Rochester incidence rates matched for age and sex.

Findings.—Of the index patients, 76 provided complete family histories. Twenty percent had a first- or second-degree relative who had an aneurysmal SAH. Eleven first-degree relatives had aneurysmal SAHs compared with an expected 2.7. Thus first-degree relatives of individuals with SAH had a relative risk of 4.14.

Conclusion.—The familial aggregation of ruptured intracranial aneurysms is not fortuitous. First-degree relatives of patients with a ruptured intracranial aneurysm have a fourfold increase in the risk of aneurysmal SAH.

▶ From time to time, information about familial intracranial aneurysms is published in the medical literature. One of the strengths of the present report is that it is based on the medical record linkage system used for epidemiologic studies in Rochester, Minnesota. As the authors stated, the medical services in that community are provided almost entirely by the Mayo Clinic and its affiliated hospitals and by a smaller group practice, the Olmsted Medical Group, and its affiliated hospital. Medical data concerning all local residents receiving care at those facilities are stored in a common computer database, a fact that ensures virtually complete ascertainment of all diagnosed cases in the population, including diagnoses made at autopsy. Thus, although only 76 patients were included in the present study, the statistical conclusions are valid.

R.H. Wilkins, M.D.

Special Features of Familial Intracranial Aneurysms: Report of 215 Familial Aneurysms

Ronkainen A, Hernesniemi J, Tromp G (Univ Hosp of Kuopio, Finland; Thomas Jefferson Univ, Philadelphia, Pa)
Neurosurgery 37:43–47, 1995   27–4

Background.—There have been no comparisons of familial intracranial aneurysms (FIAs) from a specific population with sporadic aneurysms in the same population. One large series of patients with FIA was reviewed.

Methods.—One hundred sixty-seven family members from 85 families with FIAs in east Finland were studied. Each family had included 2 or more first-degree members with proved instances of subarachnoid hemorrhage (SAH).

Findings.—Two hundred fifteen subjects were found to have FIAs. A slight female preponderance was noted in the patients with FIA. Male patients tended to have SAHs at a significantly younger age than females. Mean age of these patients was lower than in patients with nonfamilial aneurysms. In addition, the FIA patients had smaller aneurysms. Half the FIAs were on the middle cerebral artery, primarily on the right side. Almost one third of the ruptured FIAs were less than 6 mm. Aneurysm frequency at mirror sites in FIA and non-FIA groups did not differ significantly. Compared with randomly selected pairs of patients in the non-FIA group, the frequency of sibling pairs with age at onset within 10 years of each other was more than twice as high.

Conclusion.—There was a slight female preponderance among patients with FIAs, and the most common type of aneurysm was the small right-sided middle cerebral artery aneurysm. Among siblings, FIAs tended to rupture more often within an age interval than would be expected by chance.

▶ Ronkainen et al. studied a large group of patients with familial intracranial aneurysms; 167 patients with FIAs (215 saccular aneurysms) were compared with 983 patients with non-FIAs (1,296 saccular aneurysms). The patients with FIAs were younger and their aneurysms were smaller. Interestingly, half of the FIAs were on the middle cerebral artery, preferentially on the right side.

R.H. Wilkins, M.D.

Aneurysmal and Microaneurysmal "Angiogram-Negative" Subarachnoid Hemorrhage

Tatter SB, Crowell RM, Ogilvy CS (Massachusetts Gen Hosp, Boston)
Neurosurgery 37:48–55, 1995   27–5

Background.—The prognosis of subarachnoid hemorrhage (SAH) in patients with an initially negative cerebral angiogram is more benign than that of untreated aneurysmal SAH. However, hemorrhage recurs in some of these patients, resulting in additional morbidity or mortality. Little is known about the source of hemorrhage in such patients.

Methods and Findings.—Forty patients with angiogram-negative SAH admitted to 1 center from 1989 to 1993 were reviewed. Nine underwent surgical exploration. An arterial bleeding source was discovered in 7 of these explorations: 3 anterior communicating artery complex lesions, 2 middle cerebral artery lesions, 1 internal carotid artery aneurysm arising from the origin of the posterior communicating artery, and 1 vertebral/posterior inferior cerebellar artery aneurysm. Three of the 7 lesions consisted of small aneurysmal sacs. The remaining 4 were microaneurysms too small for a surgical clip. The patient in whom no source of bleeding was found during surgery had a perimesencephalic pattern of blood. Two SAH episodes occurred in 2 of the 4 patients with a microaneurysmal source of bleeding.

Conclusion.—Microaneurysms appear to be the source of a significant percentage of nonperimesencephalic angiogram-negative SAH. These lesions may represent a forme fruste of saccular aneurysms. A protocol for angiogram-negative SAH management was proposed based on the distribution of blood as seen on the patient's first CT.

▶ Ordinarily if a patient has had a spontaneous SAH, especially in a perimesencephalic location, and has had 2 technically adequate 4-vessel angiograms (at least 1 of which is free of vasospasm) that have not shown an aneurysm, arteriovenous malformation, or other obvious source of bleeding, no further investigations are undertaken to look for a source. The authors took the approach of considering surgical exploration in any such patient with a focal hemorrhage in a location suggestive of an aneurysm and for any patient with diffuse SAH and angiographic results suggesting a small abnormality. Among 9 patients who had such surgical exploration, an arterial bleeding source was discovered in 7.

R.H. Wilkins, M.D.

Medical Complications of Aneurysmal Subarachnoid Hemorrhage: A Report of the Multicenter, Cooperative Aneurysm Study
Solenski NJ, Haley EC Jr, Kassell NF, et al (Univ of Virginia Health Sciences Ctr, Charlottesville)
Crit Care Med 23:1007–1017, 1995   27–6

Objective.—Medical (nonneurologic) complications can add to the morbidity and mortality after aneurysmal subarachnoid hemorrhage and can rival the frequency of mortality from neurologic complications. The frequency, severity, and prognostic factors of medical complications of aneurysmal subarachnoid hemorrhage were studied in a large series of patients seen at 51 hospitals in 41 neurosurgical centers in the United States and Canada. In addition, the effects of modern management strategies on the overall frequency of medical complications were evaluated.

Patients.—The study included 457 patients aged 18 and older (mean age 50) with subarachnoid hemorrhage who were randomly assigned to the placebo limb of a large, double-blind, prospective trial of the calcium channel blocker nicarpidine hydrochloride. The majority (59%) arrived within 24 hours (mean 1.0 day) of rupture of an angiographically documented saccular aneurysm. The majority (60%) had good neurologic grades on admission, and 40% had hypertension.

Management.—Nearly two thirds had early surgery, and the majority had prophylactic or therapeutic treatment for vasospasm such as intentional hypervolemia and induced hypertension. Average daily fluid intake during the first 14 days was 4.1 L. Only half of the patients had hemodynamic monitoring. Nearly 80% received anticonvulsant therapy and 70% received corticosteroids.

Outcome.—Virtually all patients had at least 1 medical complication, and 40% had at least 1 severe (life-threatening) complication. The mortality rate from medical complications was 23%, comparable with the mortality rates attributed to the direct effects of the initial hemorrhage (19%), rebleeding (22%), and vasospasm (23%) after aneurysmal rupture. Pulmonary complications accounted for 50% of all deaths from medical complications; the most frequent causes were pneumonia, adult respiratory distress syndrome, and pulmonary emboli.

The most frequent medical complications were anemia, hypertension, cardiac arrhythmia, fever, and electrolyte disturbances. Cardiac rhythm disturbances were frequent, particularly on the day of or day after surgery, but only 5% were life threatening. Pulmonary edema occurred in 23% of the patients, and the majority occurred between days 3 and 7. The frequency of pulmonary edema increased in patients older than 30, in those with poor clinical grade on admission, and on the day of surgery or the day after surgery. Pulmonary edema was not significantly associated with the use of hypertensive hypervolemic therapy. A high (24%) proportion of patients had some degree of hepatic dysfunction, but only 4% had severe hepatic dysfunction. Renal dysfunction occurred in 7% of patients, but 15% of these patients had severe dysfunction. The use of antibiotics and presence of sepsis were independently associated with a higher frequency of renal dysfunction.

Conclusion.—Potentially preventable medical complications after the rupture of an intracranial aneurysm significantly contribute to the overall mortality rate of these patients and equal or exceed deaths from the direct effect of the initial hemorrhage, delayed brain ischemia from vasospasm, or rebleeding. Pulmonary complications are the most common nonneurologic cause of death. These findings underscore the need to recognize, prevent, and correct potential medical complications, particularly during the perioperative period.

▶ The authors showed without question that among patients who have sustained the rupture of an intracranial aneurysm, medical complications are common and have an important influence on management outcome.

R.H. Wilkins, M.D.

Is Transcranial Doppler Sonography Useful in Detecting Late Cerebral Ischaemia After Aneurysmal Subarachnoid Haemorrhage?
Ekelund A, Säveland H, Romner B, et al (Univ Hosp, Lund, Sweden)
Br J Neurosurg 10:19–25, 1996   27–7

Purpose.—Despite efforts to avoid it, vasospasm and delayed ischemic deficit (DID) can occur after aneurysmal subarachnoid hemorrhage (SAH). Imaging techniques to detect vasospasm include angiography and transcranial Doppler sonography (TCD). The clinical value of TCD imaging in patients with aneurysmal SAH was studied.

Methods.—One hundred nine patients with aneurysmal SAH were studied with TCD. The patients underwent TCD an average of 7 days during the first 18 days after SAH. Hunt and Hess grade was I in 13 patients, II in 37 patients, III in 17 patients, IV in 22 patients, and V in 20 patients. Transcranial investigations were performed transtemporally with a 2-MHz transducer and neck examinations with a 4-MHz probe. All patients received the calcium antagonist nimodipine as prophylaxis against cerebral vasospasm. Thirty-four patients who had TCD values of greater than 120 cm/sec but did not have DID participated in a controlled study wherein half received a combination of colloids and crystalloids in addition to dopamine and half received no additional treatment.

Results.—Fifty-seven patients had flow velocities of greater than 120 cm/sec in the middle cerebral artery and 23 of this group had DID. Mean flow velocity in the patients with DID was 170 cm/sec, compared with 155 cm/sec in 34 patients without late evidence of cerebral ischemia. In the controlled study, patients who did and did not receive anti-ischemic therapy had similar mean TCD values and neurologic outcomes. Seven of 12 patients with a rapid increase in flow velocity of 50 cm/sec or more over a 24-hour period had symptomatic vasospasm, and 5 of these patients were left with permanent neurologic deficits.

Conclusion.—In patients with aneurysmal SAH, increasing flow velocity measurements on TCD are correlated with the development of DID. However, there is no strict correlation on an individual basis, which complicates the interpretation of TCD values. Clinical decisions must be based on a combination of factors, possibly including angiography, blood flow measurements, or both. A rapid increase in flow velocity may be a strong predictor of symptomatic vasospasm.

▶ For many years it has been recognized that after the rupture of an intracranial aneurysm, there is a general correlation between the subsequent development of severe angiographic vasospasm and the development of delayed neurologic deficits. It has also been recognized that there are many exceptions to this general rule, probably based on the facts that only the proximal arterial circulation is being visualized and that there are reasons for delayed neurologic deficits in this circumstance other than circulatory insufficiency. In this paper, Ekelund et al. showed that the same sort of relationship, a lack of a strict correlation, exists between the development of increased flow velocity in the middle cerebral artery and the development of delayed neurologic deficits.

R.H. Wilkins, M.D.

CT Angiography in the Examination of Patients With Aneurysm Clips
Vieco PT, Morin EE III, Gross CE (Univ of Vermont, Burlington)
AJNR 17:455–457, 1996   27–8

Introduction.—After intracranial aneurysms are surgically treated, clinical signs may warrant investigation of the clip placement. Complications can include partial clipping of the aneurysm's neck that allows continued filling, improper clip placement that occludes vessels, and clip migration. Currently clip placement is examined postoperatively with catheter angiography. However, CT angiography has shown promise in evaluating intracranial aneurysms. A new CT angiography technique that allows evaluation of both the intracranial aneurysm and the clip was described.

Imaging Technique.—Images were obtained beginning 30 sec after the administration of IV contrast material and were transferred to a GE Advantage Windows Workstation. The data sets were reconstructed with both shaded surface–display (SSD) algorithms, tinted blue, and maximum intensity–projection (MIP) algorithms, tinted red. The MIP images were adjusted to remove bone and vascular detail but retain detail of the clip. The MIP and SSD models were then superimposed.

Methods.—Three patients underwent CT angiography to investigate clip placement after the surgical repair of intracranial aneurysms.

Findings.—In 1 patient, who had 1 clipped aneurysm and 1 aneurysm that was coated with cotton fibers but not clipped, CT angiography showed both the clip and the unclipped aneurysm. In the second patient, who had cortical signs and symptoms suggesting improper clip placement, the CT angiogram revealed appropriate vascular function and clip placement, and the patient's signs resolved. In the third patient, a routine postoperative CT scan suggested clip migration. This finding was confirmed with CT angiography, and the patient underwent repeat surgery.

Discussion.—By superimposing the SSD images, which provide good detail of vasculature, and the MIP images, which give good detail of the clip, the status of a repaired intracranial aneurysm can be reliably evaluated. However, because CT angiography does not totally eliminate beam-hardening artifacts in proximity to the clip, catheter angiography remains the gold standard for postoperative evaluation of clip placement.

▶ The authors presented their experience with CT angiography in patients who have had aneurysms clipped. Computed tomographic angiography[1, 2] has the potential of replacing catheter angiography for postoperative assessment of aneurysm clip placement.

R.H. Wilkins, M.D.

References

1. Hope JKA, Wilson JL, Thomson FJ: Three-dimensional CT angiography in the detection and characterization of intracranial berry aneurysms. *AJNR* 17:439–445, 1996.
2. Ogawa T, et al: Cerebral aneurysms: Evaluation with three-dimensional CT angiography. *AJNR* 17:447–454, 1996.

Recurrent Subarachnoid Hemorrhage From Untreated Ruptured Vertebrobasilar Dissecting Aneurysms
Mizutani T, Aruga T, Kirino T, et al (Showa Gen Hosp, Tokyo; Tokyo Univ Hosp)
Neurosurgery 36:905–913, 1995   27–9

Objective.—Because dissecting aneurysms of the vertebrobasilar artery often bleed, the course of these aneurysms was examined in a series of 42 patients confirmed as having subarachnoid hemorrhage (SAH) arising from such an aneurysm. They represented about 3% of all patients seen from 1985 to 1993 with aneurysmal SAH.

Clinical Aspects.—The average age of the 23 men and 19 women was 53. Thirty-four aneurysms involved 1 vertebral artery, most frequently between the origin of the posterior inferior cerebellar artery and the vertebral artery junction. Eight patients had aneurysms involving both vertebral arteries or both the vertebral artery and another vessel, usually the basilar artery. Most lesions had an irregular fusiform appearance on angiography. About one fourth of the patients initially were transiently comatose. Nearly three fourths of patients remained in good or fair neurologic condition after their initial attack, but this was the case for only 7 of 30 patients having a second rupture.

Management and Outcome.—Twenty-nine patients had 31 operations. Ten patients were not operated on because of their poor clinical state, and 3 others did not have surgery for anatomical reasons. A majority of operations were proximal obliterations of the vertebral artery. Ultimately 9 surgical patients recovered without a deficit, 5 were moderately and 7 were severely disabled, 4 were vegetative, and 4 died. Eleven of the 13 unoperated patients died, 10 of subsequent rupture. In all, 30 patients (71%) subsequently had aneurysmal rupture, 1 of them postoperatively; 14 of these patients died. The second rupture occurred within 24 hours of admission in 40% of all patients and within 1 week of initial SAH in 57%.

Implication.—Patients admitted with SAH from a unilateral dissecting aneurysm of the vertebral artery should have the parent vessel obliterated promptly.

▶ The authors pointed out the risks of recurrent hemorrhage from an untreated ruptured dissecting aneurysm of the vertebrobasilar arterial system and recommended urgent treatment after the initial hemorrhage in an attempt to prevent the occurrence and serious consequences of a second hemorrhage.

R.H. Wilkins, M.D.

28 Vascular Malformations and Fistulas

Genesis of a Dural Arteriovenous Malformation in a Rat Model
Herman JM, Spetzler RF, Bederson JB, et al (Barrow Neurological Inst, Phoenix, Ariz)
J Neurosurg 83:539–545, 1995   28–1

Background.—The development of dural arteriovenous malformations (AVMs) remains incompletely understood. Suggestions that sinus occlusion is a key factor are based mainly on serial angiographic data from patients and limited pathologic information. No model of dural AVM has been available with which to evaluate the putative roles of sinus thrombosis and venous hypertension.

Objective.—A rat model was contrived to determine whether a dural AVM forms in the presence of sinus thrombosis only or if thrombosis is combined with elevated sinus pressure.

Methods.—Two control conditions and 3 experimental situations were contrasted. An arteriovenous fistula (AVF) was formed by joining the right common carotid artery to the external jugular vein, leading to retrograde blood flow through the transverse sinus. The AVF was combined with thrombosis of the sagittal sinus alone and with both sinus thrombosis and occlusion of the vein draining the transverse sinus on the left side. Arterial and sagittal sinus pressures were monitored, and cerebral angiography was repeated after 3 months.

Results.—Creation of an AVF increased the sagittal sinus pressure threefold, and a further increase in pressure was noted when the vein draining the transverse sinus was occluded. Sinus pressure remained significantly elevated after 3 months, declining when the anastomosis was transiently occluded. Some animals in the AVF 2 group exhibited new dural malformations at the 90-day check. All AVF 3 animals had a patent anastomosis at this time.

Pathologic Findings.—Histologic study revealed diffuse sinus dilation and arterialization in the AVF 1 animals. Sagittal sinus occlusion was confirmed in the AVF 2 and AVF 3 groups. All the dural malformations were adjacent to the sagittal sinus and exhibited multiple anomalous arterial and venous channels in the sinus wall or in the adjacent dura. Most animals in these groups had evidence of diffuse cortical ischemia.

Conclusion.—Formation of a dural AVM entails thrombosis of an intracranial venous sinus and increased sinus pressure.

▶ Herman et al. developed a clever method of producing dural AVMs in rats, which will permit the study of this condition in an animal model. In their initial investigation, the authors showed the importance of sinus thrombosis and increased sinus pressure in the genesis of a dural AVM.

R.H. Wilkins, M.D.

Natural History of Intracranial Cavernous Malformations
Aiba T, Tanaka R, Koike T, et al (Niigata Univ, Japan)
J Neurosurg 83:56–59, 1995   28–2

Background.—Since the advent of MRI, the number of intracranial cavernous malformations (ICMs) diagnosed has increased. The natural course of these lesions was investigated in 1 series.

Methods.—The clinical records of 110 patients with ICMs diagnosed histologically or by MRI were reviewed. The mean follow-up was 4.7 years. Sixty-two patients initially had hemorrhages and 25 had seizures. In 23 patients, the diagnosis was incidental. The relationship of the rate of subsequent symptomatic bleeding and age at onset, sex, and location of the initial lesion was determined.

Findings.—The patients with hemorrhage had a high rate of subsequent symptomatic bleeding episodes. This was especially notable in younger female patients. The incidence of bleeding was very low in the other 2 patient groups. In general, outcomes were good in all but those with lesions in the basal ganglia and brain stem. The only death in the hemorrhage group was caused by repeated brain-stem bleeding. Outcomes were excellent in all patients in whom ICM was diagnosed on the basis of seizure or incidental findings.

Conclusion.—The incidence of subsequent symptomatic bleeding, especially in younger females, was high in this series, whereas bleeding episodes were rare in patients whose initial symptoms were nonhemorrhagic. Thus, female hormonal factors are implicated in the pathogenesis of symptomatic bleeding from an ICM. Recurrent hemorrhage in eloquent regions can result in serious neurologic deficits, even when bleeding episodes are mild.

▶ Much is known about the natural history of ICMs. In contrast, until the development of MRI, relatively little was known about the natural history of ICMs. These lesions are easily imaged by MRI, which now permits the detection of asymptomatic, multiple, and familial cavernous malformations to an extent not previously possible. They can then be followed with serial scans, as can symptomatic lesions for which surgical excision is not appropriate. In the present investigation the 62 patients who experienced hemorrhage had the highest incidence of rebleeding; among the 31 who were less than 40 years old, there was a 29% incidence of rebleeding over a mean follow-up time of 3.33 years, and among the 31 older patients the incidence was 14.1% over a 2.9-year period. None of the lesions bled massively, probably because the blood pressure is low in cavernous malformations.

R.H. Wilkins, M.D.

The Natural History of Cerebral Cavernous Malformations
Kondziolka D, Lunsford LD, Kestle JRW (Univ of Pittsburgh, Pa; Univ of British Columbia, Vancouver, Canada)
J Neurosurg 83:820–824, 1995   28–3

Background.—The natural history of unoperated cavernous malformations must be known to determine the value of their surgical removal. The natural history of cavernous malformations and their subsequent need for treatment was studied.

Methods.—Follow-up data about 122 patients enrolled in a prospective study between 1987 and 1993 were analyzed. At entry, mean patient age was 37, with a range of 4 to 82. Malformations were located in the brain-stem in 35% of the patients, the basal ganglia or thalamus in 17%, and a hemispheric region in 48%. Of the patients, 50% had never had a symptomatic hemorrhage; 41% had 1 hemorrhage, 7%, had 2, and 2% had 3. Twenty-three percent of the patients had seizures, and 15% had headaches. Eighty percent of the patients had solitary lesions, and 20% had multiple lesions. Retrospectively, the annual hemorrhage rate was 1.3%. Mean follow-up was 34 months.

Findings.—Nine hemorrhages occurred during follow-up. Six were associated with new neurologic deficits. The prospective annual rate of hemorrhage was 0.6% in patients with no previous bleeding. In patients with previous hemorrhage, this rate was 4.5% (Table 1). Subsequent hemorrhage was not predicted by patient sex, seizures, headache, or solitary vs. multiple lesions. The rate of bleeding episodes did not differ significantly among brain locations. Four patients who had had seizures

TABLE 1.—Annual Hemorrhage Rates for Cavernous Malformations

Clinical Factors	Prospective Annual Hemorrhage Rate
No prior hemorrhage	0.6%
Prior hemorrhage	4.5%
Brain stem location	2.4%
Basal ganglia or thalamus location	2.9%
Hemisphere location	2.7%
Brain stem location with prior hemorrhage	5.0%

(Courtesy of Kondziolka D, Lunsford LD, Kestle JRW: The natural history of cerebral cavernous malformations. *J Neurosurg* 83:820–824, 1995.)

became free of seizure, and 4 who had not had seizures subsequently developed them. Intractable seizures developed in 1 patient. Surgery was performed in 14 patients and radiosurgery in 5. None of the patients died during follow-up.

Conclusion.—The occurrence of previous hemorrhage defines a patient subgroup at increased risk of subsequent hemorrhage. Surgical removal may be considered for patients initially seen with 1 hemorrhage, regardless of the location of the malformation. Current research is defining the role of stereotactic radiosurgery in the treatment of hemorrhagic, intraparenchymal, critically located malformations.

▶ Now that cavernous malformations occurring within the brain can be diagnosed with reasonable certainty by MRI, several authors, including Kondziolka and his colleagues, have attempted to assess the natural history of these lesions[1-6]. Maraire and Awad[4] point out that the behavior of intracranial cavernous malformations is somewhat unpredictable. Some lesions behave aggressively with repetitive hemorrhages, whereas others remain quiescent for many years.[4] Various factors seem to influence lesion behavior, such as lesion location, patient age and gender, state of reproductive cycle, and previous hemorrhage.[4] As the result of their review of this topic, Maraire and Awad[4] recommend that prospective, stratified, hypothesis-driven studies using rigorous epidemiologic methods be undertaken to delineate exactly the patient and lesion factors that influence the clinical aggressiveness of intracranial cavernous malformations.

R.H. Wilkins, M.D.

References

1. Aiba T, Tanaka R, Koike T, et al: Natural history of intracranial cavernous malformations. *J Neurosurg* 83:56–59, 1995.
2. Curling OD Jr, Kelly DL Jr, Elster AD, et al: An analysis of the natural history of cavernous angiomas. *J Neurosurg* 75:702–708, 1991.
3. Fritschi JA, Reulen HJ, Spetzler RF, et al: Cavernous malformations of the brain stem: A review of 139 cases. *Acta Neurochir (Wien)* 130:35–46, 1994.
4. Maraire JN, Awad IA: Intracranial cavernous malformations: Lesion behavior and management strategies. *Neurosurgery* 37:591–605, 1995.
5. Robinson JR, Awad IA, Little JR: Natural history of the cavernous angioma. *J Neurosurg* 75:709–714, 1991.
6. Zabramski JM, Wascher TM, Spetzler RF, et al: The natural history of familial cavernous malformations: Results of an ongoing study. *J Neurosurg* 80:422–432, 1994.

Reduction of Hemorrhage Risk After Stereotactic Radiosurgery for Cavernous Malformations

Kondziolka D, Lunsford LD, Flickinger JC, et al (Univ of Pittsburgh, Pa; Univ of British Columbia, Vancouver, Canada)
J Neurosurg 83:825–831, 1995

28–4

Background.—The benefit of radiosurgery for cavernous malformations is difficult to determine. The natural history of these malformations is unclear, malformation vessels cannot be imaged, and there is no imaging technique that defines cure. However, clinical benefit may be confirmed by a decreased hemorrhage rate over time and a low risk of complications.

Methods.—Forty-seven patients with a hemorrhagic malformation in a critical intraparenchymal location remote from a pial or ependymal surface were chosen for radiosurgery. Of these patients, 44 had had at least 2 hemorrhages before radiosurgery. Mean patient age was 39. Previous attempts at surgical removal had been made in 6 patients. Malformations were found in the pons or midbrain in 24 patients, the medulla in 3, the thalamus in 9, the basal ganglia in 3, deep in a parietal lobe in 4, and deep in a temporal lobe in 4. Hemorrhages had occurred a mean of 4.1 years before radiosurgery. Unlike most other patients with cavernous malformations, these patients had 109 hemorrhages before radiosurgery in 193 observation-years before surgery, for an annual hemorrhage rate of 56.5% including the first hemorrhage, or an annual rate of 32% after the first hemorrhage. Mean follow-up after radiosurgery was 3.6 years.

Findings.—The proportion of patients with hemorrhage after radiosurgery and the mean number of hemorrhages per patient were significantly reduced after radiosurgery. Seven episodes of bleeding occurred in the first 2 years after radiosurgery, for an annual rate of 8.8%. Two to 6 years after radiosurgery, the annual rate declined to 1.1%. The neurologic condition of 26% of the patients worsened and imaging changes were evident after radiosurgery. These deficits were temporary in 8 patients. Another 2 died after surgical resection, and the remaining 2 had new permanent deficits. There was also a significant decrease in the hemorrhage rate after radiosurgery in patients with deep hemorrhagic cavernous malformations, especially after a 2-year latency period.

Conclusion.—Radiosurgery with the γ-unit apparently reduced the rate of hemorrhage in these patients with hemorrhagic cavernous malformations in critical brain regions believed to pose an excessive risk for microsurgical resection. This was especially so after a 2-year latency period. Although the morbidity associated with this treatment was serious, in most patients these delayed effects were temporary. Radiosurgery is not recommended for patients with minimally symptomatic lesions or for patients better treated by open surgical resection.

▶ It is well established that radiosurgery is an effective treatment for certain intracranial arteriovenous malformations. These lesions can be visualized well by angiography, and therefore their obliteration can be documented angiographically. Furthermore, the natural history of intracranial arteriovenous malformations has been established reasonably well, and this provides control data against which the effects of radiosurgery can be compared.

In contrast, the natural history of intracranial cavernous malformations has not yet been determined with the same degree of certainty, and these lesions typically cannot be visualized angiographically. Despite these limitations, Kondziolka and his associates have made a solid step forward with the work summarized here.

R.H. Wilkins, M.D.

29 Cerebrovascular Occlusive Disease

Long-Term Prognosis and Effect of Endarterectomy in Patients With Symptomatic Severe Carotid Stenosis and Contralateral Carotid Stenosis or Occlusion: Results From NASCET

Gasecki AP, for the North American Symptomatic Carotid Endarterectomy Trial (NASCET) Group (Univ of Western Ontario, London, Canada)

J Neurosurg 83:778–782, 1995   29–1

Background.—Results from the North American Symptomatic Carotid Endarterectomy Trial (NASCET) clearly show that endarterectomy benefits patients having severe (≥70%) carotid stenosis and either transient ischemia or a nondisabling stroke. The apparent benefit declines with the

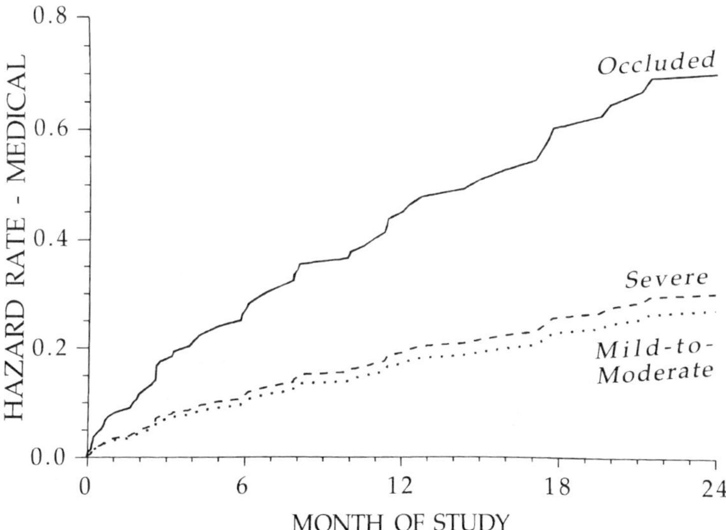

FIGURE 1.—Cumulative hazard curves showing risk (hazard rate) of ipsilateral stroke for medically treated patients at 3 degrees of contralateral carotid artery disease. (Courtesy of Gasecki AP, for the North American Symptomatic Carotid Endarterectomy Trial [NASCET] Group: Long-term prognosis and effect of endarterectomy in patients with symptomatic severe carotid stenosis and contralateral carotid stenosis or occlusion: Results from NASCET. *J Neurosurg* 83:778–782, 1995.)

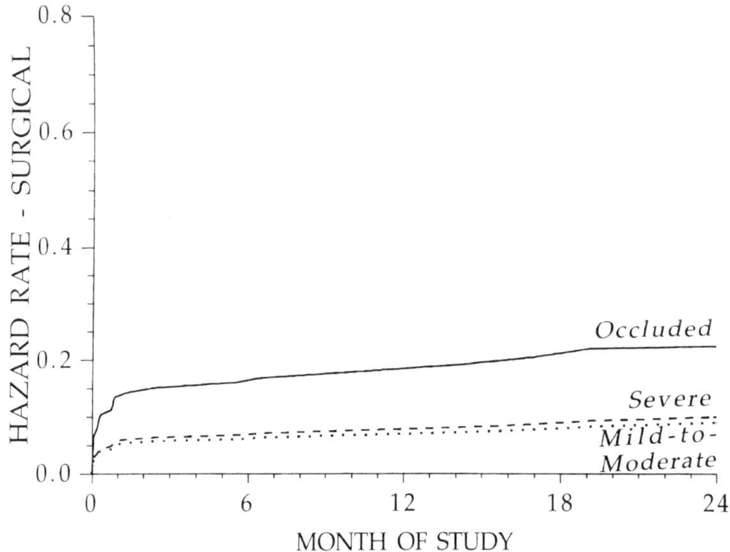

FIGURE 2.—Cumulative hazard curves showing risk (hazard rate) of ipsilateral stroke for surgically treated patients at 3 degrees of contralateral carotid artery disease. (Courtesy of Gasecki AP, for the North American Symptomatic Carotid Endarterectomy Trail [NASCET] Group: Long-term prognosis and effect of endarterectomy in patients with symptomatic severe carotid stenosis and contralateral carotid stenosis or occlusion: Results from NASCET. *J Neurosurg* 83:778–782, 1995.)

degree of carotid stenosis, however, as does the risk of stroke in patients receiving medical treatment. Possibly the presence of disease in the contralateral carotid artery modifies these effects.

Study Population.—The prognostic effects of contralateral carotid disease were examined in 659 patients with 70% to 99% stenosis of a carotid vessel and a recent ischemic event referable to this artery. The risk of ipsilateral stroke—arising from the carotid artery associated with the index symptoms—was compared in 559 patients with less than 70% stenosis of the contralateral carotid artery; 57 patients with 70% to 99% contralateral stenosis; and 43 patients in whom the contralateral carotid artery was occluded. Endarterectomy was planned in 328 patients, whereas 328 were assigned to medical treatment. The average follow-up interval was 18 months.

Findings.—An occluded contralateral carotid artery significantly increased the risk of stroke associated with a severely stenosed index artery. No strokes occurred in the region of the occluded contralateral vessel. The effect of an occluded contralateral carotid artery was much more evident for medically treated patients than for those undergoing endarterectomy (Figs 1–2). The risk of ipsilateral stroke in the first 30 days after surgery was 14% if the contralateral carotid was occluded; 4% if it was severely stenosed but patent; and 5% if it was mildly to moderately narrowed.

Conclusion.—Although an occluded contralateral carotid artery significantly increases the risk of stroke in patients with severe ipsilateral stenosis, endarterectomy of the recently symptomatic vessel remains beneficial.

▶ The authors provided additional conclusions from NASCET. These relate to the effects of contralateral carotid stenosis or occlusion on the results of medical or surgical management of symptomatic significant ipsilateral carotid stenosis.

R.H. Wilkins, M.D.

Endarterectomy for Asymptomatic Carotid Artery Stenosis
Executive Committee for the Asymptomatic Carotid Atherosclerosis Study
(Wake Forest Univ, Winston-Salem, NC)
JAMA 273:1421–1428, 1995   29–2

Background.—In 1987, the Asymptomatic Carotid Atherosclerosis Study (ACAS) was initiated to determine whether the addition of carotid endarterectomy (CEA) to aggressive reduction of modifiable risk factors and treatment with aspirin would decrease the incidence of cerebral infarction in patients with asymptomatic carotid artery stenosis.

Patients and Methods.—Thirty-nine clinical sites in the United States and Canada participated in a 6-year, prospective, randomized trial. A total of 1,662 patients (mean age 67) with asymptomatic carotid artery stenosis of 60% or greater reduction in diameter were enrolled. Of these, 1,659 were available for follow-up. All patients received treatment with daily aspirin and medical risk factor management, and 825 also were randomly assigned to CEA. Transient ischemic attack or cerebral infarction in the distribution of the study artery and any transient ischemic attack, stroke, or mortality observed perioperatively comprised the initial main outcome measures. During the last 9 months of the study, these were changed to cerebral infarction in the distribution of the study artery or any stroke or death perioperatively occurring. The median follow-up was 2.7 years.

Results.—Baseline risk factors for stroke were comparable between the medical and surgical treatment groups. During the perioperative period, 2.3% of the CEA patients had a stroke or died compared with 0.4% of the patients receiving only medical treatment. At median follow-up, the aggregate risk over 5 years for ipsilateral stroke and any stroke or death perioperatively occurring was approximately 5.1% for patients assigned to CEA and 11.0% for those receiving medical treatment only, a statistically significant difference. Similar trends were observed for all subgroups considered, including deciles of stenosis, and for various secondary cerebrovascular end points. When restricted to patients receiving the assigned treatment, results essentially were the same and were nearly identical for patients without previous contralateral symptoms or endarterectomy.

Conclusion.—Carotid endarterectomy performed with less than 3% perioperative morbidity and mortality, combined with aggressive management of modifiable risk factors, can help reduce 5-year risk of ipsilateral stroke in patients with asymptomatic carotid artery stenosis of 60% or greater reduction in diameter. A patient's overall health status also should be considered when candidates are selected for CEA.

▶ This article represents another in a series of studies reported in recent years that defines the value of CEA. This operation was introduced 4 decades ago, and until relatively recently, it was recommended to patients on the intuitive basis that it should help prevent cerebral ischemia and infarction in the distribution of that artery. Subsequent well-designed scientific studies have shown that CEA does have value in certain patient groups. The main caveat in all of these studies is that the surgeons must be able to perform CEA safely, with low morbidity and mortality; otherwise, there is no advantage over medical management.

R.H. Wilkins, M.D.

Cost-Effective Carotid Endarterectomy
Luna G, Adye B (Univ of Washington, Spokane)
Am J Surg 169:516–518, 1995   29–3

Background.—Balancing cost containment with safe surgical practice is a constant challenge to surgeons. Carotid endarterectomy is the most frequently performed vascular procedure in the United States, with annual costs totaling $1.2 billion. Various means to improve the cost-to-reimbursement ratios for this procedure have been proposed and include limiting the extent of preoperative radiographic assessment, eliminating routine admissions to the ICU, and encouraging early postoperative discharge. Surgical results and costs associated with carotid endarterectomy were retrospectively reviewed at the authors' facility and compared with those at other local facilities.

Patients and Findings.—The medical records of all patients undergoing carotid endarterectomies during an 18-month period were reviewed. Sixty-five patients (mean age 70) were identified. All patients underwent preoperative duplex ultrasound scanning, and 62 had cerebral angiography before surgery. Computed tomography was reserved for those patients whose cerebral vascular accident led to a sustained neurologic deficit. After surgery, 56 patients were admitted to the surgical floor, none of whom had postoperative complications or required transfer to the ICU. Eight patients had postoperative cardiac monitoring in the acute care unit. Only 1 patient was admitted to the ICU. This patient had had a perioperative stroke in the recovery room, necessitating further surgical exploration. Only 1 patient died, which occurred as a result of postoperative myocardial infarction. The median length of postoperative hospitalization was 1 day, which was 1.7 days less than at other facilities. The average per-patient hospital cost was $8,060 compared with $11,570 at other facilities. Postoperative ICU admission or overnight stay in the recovery room were routine at other facilities. Factors found to affect charges included ICU admission, length of stay, and complications.

Conclusion.—Limited use of the ICU and short postoperative stays led to a reduction in overall hospital costs. The 1.5% mortality and stroke rates show that these cost-saving practices can be instated without adverse effects to patient outcome.

Short-Stay Carotid Endarterectomy Is Safe and Cost-Effective

Kraiss LW, Kilberg L, Critch S, et al (Univ of Washington, Seattle)
Am J Surg 169:512–515, 1995   29–4

Introduction.—The common protocol for performing carotid endarterectomy (CEA) includes preoperative contrast arteriography, performed using general anesthesia with cerebral perfusion monitoring, and followed by routine admission to the ICU. It would be expected that performing CEA with alternative protocols could be less expensive, provided safety and effectiveness are maintained. A more streamlined protocol, eliminating routine preoperative arteriography, using regional anesthesia, and restricting ICU admission to only high-risk patients, was studied.

Methods.—During a 2-year period, 2 groups of patients underwent CEA performed with either the alternative protocol (group 1, 18 patients) or the conventional protocol (group 2, 178 patients). Group 1 patients routinely underwent preoperative duplex scans and carotid angiography only when occlusion or an atypical disease pattern was indicated. Regional anesthesia was used without cerebral perfusion monitoring. Patients were admitted to the ICU only when clinically indicated. Data on operative risk, perioperative complications, use of vasoactive medication, ICU admission, hospital length of stay, and charges were compared for the 2 groups.

TABLE.—Comparison of Groups Undergoing Carotid Endarterectomy According to the Alternative (Group I) or Conventional (Group II) Protocol

	Group I	Group II	*P* Value
Operations (n)	18	178	
ASA score	2.8 ± 0.1	3.1 ± 0.0	0.12*
Mortality	0 (0%)	1 (1%)	>0.99†
Postoperative stroke	0 (0%)	6 (3%)	>0.99†
Preoperative arteriography	1 (6%)	114 (64%)	<0.0001†
Regional anesthesia	18 (100%)	3 (2%)	<0.0001†
ICU admission	4 (22%)	175 (98%)	<0.0001†
Vasoactive medication	3 (17%)	36 (20%)	>0.99†
Length of stay (d)	1.3 ± 0.1	3.1 ± 0.3	0.03*
Total hospital charges ($)	5,861 ± 229	11,140 ± 729	0.02*

* Two-tailed student's *t* test.
† Fisher's exact test.
Abbreviation: ASA, American society of Anesthesiology.
(Reprinted by permission of the publisher from short-stay carotid endarterectomy is safe and cost-effective by Kraiss LW, Kilberg L, Critch S, et al; *American Journal of Surgery*; 169:512–515; Copyright 1995 by Excerpta Medica Inc.)

Results.—The groups had comparable operative risks. There were no perioperative complications in group 1, whereas there was 1 death and postoperative strokes in 3% of patients in group 2. Preoperative carotid angiography was obtained in 6% of group 1 and 64% of group 2 patients. In group 1, 22% of patients were admitted to the ICU compared with 98% in group 2, even though only 20% of the patients in group 2 received vasoactive medication compared with 17% in group 1. The average length of stay was 1.3 days for group 1 and 3.1 days for group 2 patients. Average hospital charges were $5,861 for patients in group 1 and $11,140 for those in group 2 (Table).

Conclusion.—The results suggest a more favorable complication rate for CEA performed with the alternative protocol, but these findings require confirmation with a larger group. Both the length of stay and hospital charges were significantly reduced with the alternative protocol.

▶ In keeping with the recent emphasis on reducing the costs of medical care by reducing the duration of inpatient hospitalization and by restricting the use of expensive diagnostic procedures and intensive care, the authors of these 2 clinical investigations (Abstracts 29–3 and 29–4) show that CEA can be performed in a less expensive way without an associated increase in morbidity and mortality. In other words, it is possible to improve the cost-effectiveness of this procedure.

R.H. Wilkins, M.D.

Early Discharge After Carotid Endarterectomy

Harbaugh KS, Harbaugh RE (Dartmouth-Hitchcock Med Ctr, Lebanon, NH)
Neurosurgery 37:219–225, 1995   29–5

Rationale.—It is expected that carotid endarterectomy will be done increasingly often in patients with atherosclerotic disease of the carotid vessels, which raises concern over the financial consequences. Complications were reviewed in a series of 233 consecutive procedures done in 195 patients in 1990 to 1994 under the direction of a single neurosurgeon. The goal was to learn whether early discharge and less intensive postoperative monitoring will compromise the outcome.

Patients.—Men constituted nearly two thirds of the series. The average age was 69. Risk factors for atherosclerotic carotid stenosis were present in more than 90% of the patients; the most common were coronary artery disease and hypertension. All but 15 patients were symptomatic and had a transient or fixed hemispheric or retinal ischemic deficit. Four patients had previously had carotid endarterectomy. All operations were done with the patient under general anesthesia.

Outcome.—No patient died perioperatively. Stroke occurred at an overall rate of 2.6%, but the procedural rate of ipsilateral ischemic stroke was 1.3%. Major stroke occurred in 0.9% of the cases. None of the 3 myocardial infarctions were disabling. Patients were discharged after 2.5 days on average, and the interval declined over the course of the study. In the final year of the study the postoperative hospital time averaged 1.6 days. Cervical block anesthesia was used only in the latter half of the review period; it appeared to reduce the mean time to discharge but not to a significant degree.

Conclusion.—Patients who are neurologically and hemodynamically stable immediately after carotid endarterectomy may safely be discharged early. Nearly all patients can be adequately monitored outside of intensive care facilities.

▶ There is a concerted effort, primarily by third-party payers, to reduce medical expenses by reducing the length of hospitalization of patients with various conditions. In this and the following 2 articles (Abstracts 29–6 and 29–7), the authors showed that less intensive monitoring and early discharge after carotid endarterectomy are feasible.

R.H. Wilkins, M.D.

Are One-Day Admissions for Carotid Endarterectomy Feasible?

Collier PE (Sewickley Valley Hosp, Pa)
Am J Surg 170:140–143, 1995   29–6

Objective.—A clinical protocol was developed to care for patients scheduled for elective carotid endarterectomy in a more efficient and standardized manner. The plan was evaluated in 186 patients operated on in a 3½-year period in 1991 to 1994.

Protocol.—The patient and family are educated in the surgeon's office about the procedure and what they can expect. Next they are evaluated by color-flow Doppler imaging and cranial CT scanning rather than cerebral angiography, unless questionable scan findings or symptoms are present. The patient is admitted the same day, is instructed in regional block anesthesia, and undergoes surgery. The arteriotomy is patched if extensive or if the distal internal carotid artery is small in caliber. The patient is monitored in the postanesthesia care unit for at least 3 hours. Discharge is set for the next morning provided that the patient is afebrile and neurologically and hemodynamically stable.

Patients.—The 125 men and 61 women operated on were aged 44 to 84. About half the patients were taking antihypertensive medication, and 15% had evidence of coronary artery disease. One fifth of the patients had had a stroke, whereas about one fourth had asymptomatic stenosis exceeding 80%. Twenty-four patients required general anesthesia.

Results.—The rate of neurologic events was 1.6% and included 1 intracerebral hemorrhage. Only 1.1% of the patients had a permanent deficit. The average savings per patient, when compared with drug-related group reimbursement, was $3,103. About half the patients required intraoperative measures to control blood pressure. The operating time averaged 48 minutes. Only 10% of the patients required intensive care postoperatively. The overall length of stay averaged 1.3 days, and 84% of the patients were discharged after 1 day in the hospital. No patient had to be readmitted. One patient died of myocardial infarction 28 days postoperatively.

Conclusion.—A dedicated team is able to safely and efficiently care for patients needing carotid endarterectomy while conserving substantial resources.

Reduced Length of Stay Following Carotid Endarterectomy Under General Anesthesia

Friedman SG, Tortolani AJ (North Shore Univ Hosp, Manhasset, NY)
Am J Surg 170:235–236, 1995   29–7

Objective.—Traditionally, patients are admitted at least 1 day before carotid endarterectomy (CEA) for angiography and remain in the hospital for 2 to 7 days after the procedure. This prospective study of 72 patients was aimed at determining whether discharge on the first postoperative day is feasible.

Patients.—Sixty-two men and 10 women with an average age of 68 underwent CEA. Eleven patients had sustained a stroke preoperatively. One fifth of the operations were done for high-grade stenosis in asymptomatic patients. About half the patients had coronary artery disease, and more than 40% were hypertensive.

Management.—Whenever possible, cerebral angiography was replaced by MR angiography and duplex scanning, which were performed on an outpatient basis. Conventional cerebral angiography was done in 47% of the patients, mainly early in the study period. All operations employed general anesthesia.

Outcome.—There were no complications from imaging studies, and no patient died or had a stroke after CEA. Two patients described transient ischemic attacks the morning after surgery. Ten patients received nitroprusside intravenously in the recovery room, but only 3 patients required blood pressure control until the next day. In all, 88% of the patients were discharged on the first day after CEA, 11% on the second day, and 1 patient on the third day. The overall average length of stay was 1.1 days. No patient was readmitted on an emergency basis. Five of the 9 later discharges were warranted. No further transient ischemic attacks occurred during an average follow-up of 1 year, but 1 patient had a stroke 9 months postoperatively and was found to have thrombosis at the site of the endarterectomy.

Conclusion.—It is both safe and cost effective to discharge patients the first day after CEA is performed with general anesthesia.

30 Head Trauma

**Motorcycle Helmet Use and Injury Outcome and Hospitalization Costs
From Crashes in Washington State**
Rowland J, Rivara F, Salzberg P, et al (Washington State Dept of Health,
Seattle; Harborview Injury Prevention and Research Ctr, Seattle; Univ of
Washington, Seattle; et al)
Am J Public Health 86:41–45, 1996   30–1

Introduction.—Motorcycle helmets have been shown to significantly
reduce the risk of death from head injury. The effects of helmet use on
motorcycle-related trauma after serious crashes were studied retrospectively using statewide, computer-linked data.

Methods.—The data from statewide crash, hospital, and death records
were linked for 409 motorcycle crash victims and 59 motorcycle fatalities
in Washington State during 1989. The relative risks of various injuries
were calculated for helmeted and unhelmeted riders. The length and cost
of hospitalization were also compared in helmeted and unhelmeted riders.

Results.—The risk of fatal motorcycle crash was significantly higher in
unhelmeted than in helmeted motorcyclists (1.63 relative risk). There was
a slightly elevated risk of hospitalization after a crash for unhelmeted
motorcyclists. However, the relative risk of hospitalization with head
injury was 2.9, of severe or critical head injury was 3.7, and of overall
serious injury was 2.0 among unhelmeted riders. The average length of
hospital stay was 10 days for helmeted riders and 12.6 days for unhelmeted riders, a nonsignificant difference. The average hospitalization cost
did not differ significantly, although the total costs were $3.5 million for
unhelmeted riders and $2.2 million for helmeted riders. Unhelmeted riders
were more likely to be discharged to another care facility and were approximately twice as likely to be readmitted compared with helmeted
riders. The increased risks associated with a lack of helmet use remained
significant after adjustment for other variables associated with head injury.

Conclusion.—Helmet use strongly and independently predicts reductions in head injury, overall injury severity, hospitalization, and fatality
caused by head injury. The cost of medical care would also be reduced with
increased motorcycle helmet use.

▶ Rowland et al. provided data that support the view that helmet use by
motorcyclists is beneficial.

R.H. Wilkins, M.D.

Cerebral Perfusion Pressure: Management Protocol and Clinical Results
Rosner MJ, Rosner SD, Johnson AH (Univ of Alabama, Birmingham)
J Neurosurg 83:949–962, 1995   30–2

Background.—Encouraging results have been achieved with brain-injured patients by basing treatment on the cerebral perfusion pressure (CPP). It has proved possible to increase the CPP by inducing systemic hypertension without risking death from vasogenic edema or uncontrolled intracranial hypertension.

Objective.—The value of CPP management compared with conventional management based on the intracranial pressure (ICP) was studied in 158 patients aged 15 years and older who incurred traumatic brain injury and had a postresuscitation Glasgow Coma Scale (GCS) score of 7 or less. Patients with hypoxemia, traumatic asphyxia, hypotension, or multiple systemic injuries were not included in the study.

Management.—Intravascular volume expansion, CSF drainage, the systemic vasopressors phenylephrine and norepinephrine, and mannitol were used as needed to maintain the CPP at a minimum of 70 mm Hg. In most cases phenylephrine was the primary vasopressor used. Cerebrospinal fluid was drained by ventriculostomy when necessary. The ICP was monitored by a frontal ventriculostomy catheter, and CPP was calculated as the difference between average ICP and mean arterial pressure.

Results.—The average CPP during treatment was 83 mm Hg. The average amount of CSF drained was 100 mL daily. About 40% of patients, especially those with lower GCS scores, required vasopressors. The patients who required vasopressor support had a relatively high ICP, and they also required larger amounts of mannitol. Overall mortality was 29%. Mortality was higher in patients who required vasopressor therapy, but those who survived had as good a neurologic outcome as patients who were treated less intensively. Mortality declined with the initial GCS score; 75% of patients with a score of 7 survived. Most deaths were of patients with GCS scores of 3 to 5 and were a direct result of brain injury. Only 2 surviving patients remained in a vegetative state. Survivors had approximately an 80% chance of recovering well.

Conclusion.—The primary goal of maintaining a CPP of at least 70 mm Hg is an effective approach to treating patients with traumatic brain injury.

▶ Rosner et al. focused attention on the importance of maintaining the cerebral circulation in patients with traumatic brain injury and especially on the value of using the cerebral perfusion pressure as the key parameter to guide therapy. In this paper they showed what can be accomplished in terms of outcome by using this approach in a large group of patients with low initial GCS scores.

R.H. Wilkins, M.D.

Amnesia Following Traumatic Bilateral Fornix Transection

D'Esposito M, Verfaellie M, Alexander MP, et al (Univ of Pennsylvania, Philadelphia; Memory Disorders Research Ctr, Boston; Boston Univ, Mass; et al)
Neurology 45:1546–1550, 1995   30–3

Objective.—Several case reports suggest that the likelihood of severe and persistent memory dysfunction increases with complete disruption of all 3 hippocampal pathways—the proximal fornix, the supracallosal longitudinal striae, and the cingulate bundle. This report shows that isolated damage to the fornix affects on human memory.

> *Case Report.*—Woman, 32, sustained a traumatic penetrating head injury that resulted in a significant and persistent anterograde memory deficit. Language and perception impairments were also evident, but her amnesia was clearly disproportionate. The anterograde amnesia was out of proportion to the limited retrograde amnesia. She had substantial impairments in learning information on several different tasks involving the verbal and visual modalities and the working memory. She retained her ability for procedural learning. Computed tomography revealed a lesion in the region of the proximal, posterior portion of both fornices and hippocampal commissure without evidence of damage to other hippocampal pathways or other critical memory structures such as the hippocampus, thalamus, or basal forebrain.

Implication.—Isolated damage to the proximal fornix, although extremely uncommon, is sufficient to cause amnesia. Isolated anterior fornix damage causing amnesia also has been clearly documented after surgical transection of the fornix during colloid cyst removal. This case report strongly supports the growing body of evidence about the role of fornix lesions on human memory.

▶ The patient described in this report had attended 1 year of college and was a homemaker at the time of her injury. She had no cognitive impairments and no history of drug or alcohol abuse. She sustained a gunshot wound, with the bullet entry in the left parietal area. A left parietal craniotomy was performed for débridement, and she was conscious shortly after surgery. Two months later a ventriculoperitoneal shunt was inserted for hydrocephalus, and further bullet fragments were removed through the previous craniotomy site. The initial neuropsychological evaluation was 4 months after injury. At that time she was taking no medications but had a dense right hemiparesis, left homonymous hemianopsia, and severe proprioceptive loss on her left side.

D'Esposito et al. used this case to support previously published information about the primary importance of the fornix to memory. However, this patient had more than isolated fornix damage and her injury was complicated by hydrocephalus with dilatation of the temporal horns despite the shunt. The authors provided a current review of the subject, which is especially important to the neurosurgeon operating on an anterior third ventricular tumor.

R.H. Wilkins, M.D.

Endoscopic Removal of Organized Chronic Subdural Hematoma
Rodziewicz GS, Chuang WC (SUNY-HSC College of Medicine, Syracuse, NY)
Surg Neurol 43:569–573, 1995   30–4

Introduction.—In the generally elderly and frail patients with chronic subdural hematoma (CSDH), definitive removal of the hematoma often involves unacceptably high anesthetic and surgical risk. An approach that uses surgical endoscopes and allows removal with minimized anesthetic and surgical risk was developed.

Surgical Technique.—With patients under local anesthesia with anesthesia standby to provide sedation and monitoring, the craniectomy was placed eccentrically over the lesion to maximize the view of the hematoma cavity. A 3 by 4 cm dural opening was placed over only the hematoma cavity. The chronic subdural membranes were removed under direct vision and the endoscope was advanced, only under direct vision into the hematoma cavity. When the membranes were encountered, they were removed with graspers, with 1 jaw remaining aligned with the long axis of the grasper, always under direct vision to avoid damaging the brain. The process was continued until the white dura was reached and the majority of the mass of membranes was removed. Jackson-Pratt drains (7 mm) were left in the cavity for 2 to 4 days. After their removal, patients were progressively ambulated. Perioperative phenytoin was administered for seizure prophylaxis.

> *Case 1.*—Right-handed man, 75, with a 2-day history of worsening gait 2 months after a fall underwent CT scanning, which revealed bilateral subdural hematomas. Bilateral twist-drill craniostomies failed to resolve the hematomas. Six days later, the hematomas were removed with the surgical endoscopic approach. Continued resolution of the subdural hematomas was documented by CT scans at 1 week and 1 month and was accompanied by improved gait.
>
> *Case 2.*—Right-handed man, 78, had a 3-day history of unstable gait and left-sided weakness. Computed tomographic scanning detected a right CSDH. The organized hematoma was removed endoscopically under local-standby anesthesia, which resulted in continued resolution of the subdural hematoma, as shown on repeat CT scans and by improvement in the patient's condition.

Conclusion.—Endoscopic removal of organized CSDHs allows access to nearly the entire hematoma cavity with minimal invasion and with local-standby anesthesia. If necessary, the surgeon can safely and rapidly convert to a larger craniotomy.

▶ Endoscopy has been applied successfully to several areas of neurosurgery in recent years, permitting a less invasive approach to achieve the same or better results. In general, endoscopy requires a cavity such as the ventricular system, a unilateral thoracic cavity created by lung deflation, or a peritoneal cavity enlarged by carbon dioxide insufflation. The space created by the accumulation of a CSDH provides another cavity for endoscopy. Rodziewicz and Chuang took advantage of this fact and reported another method of treating these lesions.

R.H. Wilkins, M.D.

Localization of Inactive Cerebrospinal Fluid Fistulas

Eljamel MS, Pidgeon CN (Beaumont Hosp, Dublin, Republic of Ireland)
J Neurosurg 83:795–798, 1995   30–5

Introduction.—Cessation of leakage from a (CSF) fistula is no assurance that the underlying dural tear has healed. Patients may later have recurrent leakage or intracranial infection. In the absence of an active fluid leak, contrast CT cisternography and isotopic cisternography will fail to demonstrate a fistula in more than 40% of patients.

Objective.—The value of MRI for localizing an inactive CSF fistula was studied in 21 patients suspected of having a fistula. Ten patients had posttraumatic meningitis and 11 had intermittent CSF rhinorrhea.

Methods.—Patients first were examined by fine-slice CT, obtaining axial and coronal 1- to 2-mm contiguous slices. An MR study followed, recording heavily T2-weighted images in the axial, coronal, and sagittal planes with a head coil. The studies were interpreted independently by 2 neuroradiologists.

Results.—Computed tomographic scanning demonstrated a bony defect in 7 patients, a fracture in 2, and pneumocephalus in 1. Magnetic resonance imaging revealed a defect containing herniated arachnoid or brain tissue in 11 patients. A CSF signal continuous with that in the basal cisterns was recorded in 5 patients, and a discontinuous signal was recorded in 3 others. Only 2 patients had totally normal MR findings. Exploration confirmed a dural fistula in all 16 patients with positive MR findings and showed no fistula in the 2 patients whose CT study results were positive but who had negative MR findings. In all 3 patients with MR changes suggesting a fistula but with negative findings on CT studies, a dural fistual was confirmed.

Conclusion.—Magnetic resonance imaging is indicated in the examination of a patient with currently inactive CSF leakage before assuming that the dural tear has healed spontaneously.

▶ The authors showed the value of MRI in the identification of inactive CSF fistulas.

R.H. Wilkins, M.D.

Delayed Complications of Ethmoid Fractures: A "Growing Fracture" Phenomenon
Talamonti G, Fontana RA, Versari PP, et al (Niguarda Ca'Granda Hosp, Milan, Italy)
Acta Neurochir (Wien) 137:164–173, 1995   30–6

Background.—Ethmoid fractures are often associated with injuries of arachnoid and olfactory filaments, typically resulting in CSF rhinorrhea. Traumatic CSF rhinorrhea generally occurs soon after the injury and resolves spontaneously or with conservative treatment within a few days. However, delayed complications may occur, though rarely. Ten patients treated for delayed complications of ethmoid bone injuries were described.

Patients.—Ten patients with delayed complications of ethmoid bone lesions were seen over an 11-year period. Of these 10 patients, 6 had meningitis, 3 had recurrences of previously resolved CSF rhinorrhea, and 1 had delayed-onset CSF rhinorrhea. The original injuries were classified as minor in 3 patients, moderate in 4 patients, and severe in 3 patients. All had been discharged neurologically intact except for a permanently impaired sense of smell. None had been treated surgically. The 6 patients with bacterial meningitis were admitted 1 to 31 years after the initial injury. Four patients had a history of multiple meningitis episodes beginning between 2 months and 9 years after the trauma. Of the 3 patients with recurrent CSF rhinorrhea, 2 were admitted 2 months after the trauma, whereas the recurrence in the third patient occurred 25 years after the injury. The patient with delayed CSF rhinorrhea had a sudden episode after sneezing 1 year after a minor head injury. In all patients, ethmoid bone lesions were seen on CT scans. All were treated surgically with intradural repair with a median subfrontal approach using an autologous graft of pericranium or fascia lata.

Results.—All patients had an uneventful postoperative course, with no surgical mortality or morbidity. Aside from the persistent impairment in the sense of smell, all were neurologically intact. There were no episodes of intracranial infection, recurrent CSF leaks, or other neurologic complications during the follow-up of 1 to 12 years.

Discussion.—Patients with ethmoid bone injuries may experience delayed complications, including recurrent or delayed-onset CSF rhinorrhea and meningitis, which can occur even after minor head trauma and at widely varying intervals from the initial trauma. These delayed complications may be explained by mechanisms similar to that occurring in growing skull fractures in children. Normal brain pulsations, transmitted to the herniated encephalocele, may gradually erode the thin ethmoid bone, thus enlarging the bone defect. Surgical repair of the defects with a graft is recommended for the management of patients with delayed complications.

▶ It is well known that some calvarial fractures in young children may enlarge with time. The authors presented evidence that ethmoid fractures in older patients may also enlarge, giving rise to delayed complications such as meningitis and CSF rhinorrhea.

R.H. Wilkins, M.D.

31 Epilepsy

Extent of Medial Temporal Resection on Outcome From Anterior Temporal Lobectomy: A Randomized Prospective Study
Wyler AR, Hermann BP, Somes G (Swedish Med Ctr, Seattle; Baptist Mem Hosp, Memphis, Tenn; Univ of Tennessee, Memphis)
Neurosurgery 37:982–991, 1995
31–1

Introduction.—Anterior temporal lobectomy (ATL) is the most common operative approach to controlling complex partial seizures. Success rates have varied substantially at different centers, in part because of a lack of consensus on how much temporal lobe tissue to remove. Agreement is growing that seizures are best controlled by removing most or all of the hippocampus.

Objective.—A blinded, randomized study was planned in a prospective series of 70 patients aged 18 to 40, with medically refractory seizures originating from the mesial region of 1 temporal lobe, who underwent ATL. In 34 patients the hippocampus was resected posteriorly to the anterior edge of the cerebral peduncle, whereas in 36 patients it was totally resected up to the level of the superior colliculus. Lateral cortical resection was equally extensive in the 2 groups.

Results.—After 1 year, 69% of patients having total hippocampectomy and 38% of those having partial hippocampectomy were free of seizures. The extent of resection was the only significant predictor of outcome on logistic regression analysis, although younger patients tended to do better. The advantage of total hippocampectomy persisted after 4 years of follow-up. Total hippocampal resection did not impair verbal memory function. In patients having left ATL, the degree of hippocampal sclerosis predicted future verbal memory function. Complications developed in 7% of patients and were similarly frequent in the 2 surgical groups.

Conclusion.—In patients undergoing ATL for medically refractory seizures, aggressive hippocampectomy promotes seizure control without compromising memory function.

▶ Wyler et al. made a case for extensive hippocampectomy as part of ATL for the control of complex partial seizures.

R.H. Wilkins, M.D.

32 Infections

Pott's Puffy Tumor: The Forgotten Entity: Case Report
Babu RP, Todor R, Kasoff SS (New York Med College, Valhalla)
J Neurosurg 84:110–112, 1996   32–1

Introduction.—Pott's puffy tumor was originally described as a subperiosteal abscess and osteomyelitis of the frontal bone after frontal sinus infection. Just 11 cases of this lesion have been reported in the antibiotic era. A case of Pott's puffy tumor occurring after frontal sinusitis was reported.

Case Report.—Man, 20, developed a gradually enlarging mass on his forehead after an episode of frontal sinusitis, for which he received antibiotics. Examination showed a soft, fluctuant, nontender swelling of the forehead, and laboratory studies revealed a white blood cell count of 7,800/mm^3 and an erythrocyte sedimentation rate of 30 mm/hour. Computed tomography and MRI scans revealed a subgaleal mass with destruction of the frontal bone. An epidural collection was present, but the brain parenchyma was normal. The preoperative diagnosis of Pott's puffy tumor was confirmed at bifrontal craniotomy. A massive amount of granulation tissue was removed from the subgaleal plane, and a moderate amount of granulation tissue was carefully scraped away from the dura. All abnormal bone was removed before the craniotomy flap was replaced. The patient recovered without incident. Tissue cultures grew *Streptococcus viridans*, and the patient received a 6-week course of IV penicillin.

Discussion.—Because of the availability of antibiotic treatment, Pott's puffy tumor has become a rare complication of frontal sinusitis. However, this potentially dangerous lesion can still occur in patients with partially treated frontal sinusitis. Treatment is surgical, including drainage of the abscess and removal of the osteomyelitic bone.

▶ Disease processes can have diverse manifestations; these variations from typical patterns provide a diagnostic challenge for both the novice and

the experienced physician. It is therefore refreshing to occasionally encounter a well-documented "text-book case" such as that presented here.

R.H. Wilkins, M.D.

Medical and Surgical Treatment in Neurocysticercosis—a Magnetic Resonance Study of 161 Cases
Martinez HR, Rangel-Guerra R, Arredondo-Estrada JH, et al (Hosp Univ UANL, Monterrey, Mexico; Univ de Monterrey, Mexico)
J Neurol Sci 130:25–34, 1995   32–2

Introduction.—The most common neuroparasitosis, neurocysticercosis (NCC), is caused by CNS infestation with the larvae of *Taenia solium*. The use of MRI has aided in the diagnosis of active NCC. Introduction of the cysticidal agents praziquantel (PZQ) and albendazole (ABZ) has improved the outcome and resulted in the revision of indications for surgical management in patients with NCC. Experience with 161 patients with active NCC was reported.

Methods.—Between 1986 and 1994, 161 patients with active NCC were treated. All were diagnosed with MRI. There were 4 groups of patients, classified by the predominant cyst localization: brain parenchymal cysts, ventricular cysts, subarachnoidal cysts, and cysticercus racemose. Albendazole, 15 mg/kg daily, was given to 126 patients for 10 days. Ten patients were treated with PZQ, 50 mg/kg/daily, for 15 days. All patients had follow-up MRI 1 month after treatment to document the persistence or disappearance of cysts or morphologic changes in the lesions.

Results.—Of the 85 patients with brain parenchymal cysts, 79 were treated with ABZ, with an effectiveness rate of 89.8%; 6 were treated with PZQ, with 50% effectiveness; and 5 were treated with surgery. Of the surgical patients, 3 had MR images of an irregular cystic structure suggesting a neoplastic lesion, and the other 2 had persistent cysts after medical treatment. Of the 24 patients with ventricular cysts, 20 were treated surgically, whereas ABZ treatment resulted in the disappearance of cysts in the lateral ventricle in 2 patients and, in conjunction with ventricular shunt placement, clinical improvement in 2 patients with fourth ventricular cysts. Forty-six patients had subarachnoidal NCC. The cysts disappeared in 75% of the patients treated with PZQ and in 100% of those treated with ABZ. One cyst in the spinal subarachnoidal space was removed surgically. Of the 6 patients with cysticercus racemose, 4 were treated surgically, with 1 death, and 2 were successfully treated with multiple courses of ABZ.

Conclusion.—Antiparasitic drugs, particularly ABZ, can be used effectively to treat parenchymal and subarachnoid NCC, as well as racemose cysts without intracranial hypertension. Surgical treatment is indicated in patients with refractory parenchymal cysts or those that produce intractable seizures, and in patients with ventricular cysts. However, ventricular cysts may also be managed with ABZ and ventricular shunt.

▶ The authors document the value of MRI in diagnosing NCC and in monitoring the results of treatment of the various types of NCC. In addition, they show that most of these patients can be effectively treated with medication, without the need for a surgical procedure.

R.H. Wilkins, M.D.

An Endoscopic Approach to Cysticercosis Cysts of the Posterior Third Ventricle
Neal JH (Marshfield Clinic, Wis)
Neurosurgery 36:1040–1043, 1995   32–3

Introduction.—Patients with intraventricular cysticercosis often have solitary cysticercosis cysts of the third ventricle. These cysts can cause acute hydrocephalus and sudden death. A transcortical transforaminal approach with a flexible endoscope was attempted in 2 patients to remove third ventricular cysts with a less invasive method.

> *Case 1.*—Woman, 20, had a headache and progressive lethargy during 1 day. Hydrocephalus involving the lateral and third ventricles was detected with CT. Cysticercosis antibodies were identified in the CSF. Magnetic resonance imaging revealed a cystic lesion in the posterior third ventricle. Endoscopic surgery with a transforaminal approach was planned. A preoperative ventriculogram showed that the cyst had migrated to the fourth ventricle, and it was uneventfully removed with a suboccipital craniotomy.
>
> *Case 2.*—Woman, 21, had a 2-day history of headaches, nausea, vomiting, and lethargy. Hydrocephalus involving the lateral and third ventricles was revealed on a CT scan of the brain. She did not have detectable cysticercosis titers in the CSF or serum. Magnetic resonance imaging revealed a cyst in the posterior third ventricle. With stereotactic guidance, a rigid endoscope was inserted into the lateral ventricle until the foramen of Monro was visualized. A ureteroscope was then introduced through the endoscope's outer cannula. The flexible endoscope navigated the foramen of Monro to visualize the anterior and then the posterior third ventricle. The cyst was removed with aspiration while the endoscope was removed. The cyst was removed intact, and the patient did not need ventricular shunting.

Discussion.—Because these cysts can migrate, preoperative imaging should be performed immediately before any planned resection of a third ventricular cyst. It is feasible to remove a third ventricular cysticercosis cyst using a minimally invasive endoscopic technique, which obviates ventricular shunting or open craniotomy. However, endoscopic experience is crucial to minimize the risks of injury to neurovascular or ventricular structures. The procedure may be inappropriate for patients with evidence of ependymitis.

▶ The authors showed that it is feasible to remove a cysticercosis cyst from the third ventricle with the use of a minimally invasive endoscopic technique.

R.H. Wilkins, M.D.

33 Hydrocephalus and Developmental Defects

Hydrocephalus Associated With Intramedullary Low-Grade Glioma: Illustrative Cases and Review of the Literature
Cinalli G, Sainte-Rose C, Lellouch-Tubiana A, et al (Univ René Descartes, Paris; Hôpital Necker-Enfants Malades, Paris)
J Neurosurg 83:480–485, 1995   33–1

Background.—More than 200 cases of hydrocephalus associated with intraspinal tumors have been reported; before the advent of CT and MRI, this association was considered rare. The causative link between hydrocephalus and intraspinal tumors is easily understood in the case of malignancies but less so for benign lesions, especially intramedullary spinal cord low-grade gliomas. Eight cases of hydrocephalus associated with intramedullary low-grade glioma in children were reported, along with a review of 38 cases from the literature.

Patients.—The children were treated at 1 hospital over a 15-year period. There were 4 girls and 4 boys ranging in age from 3 to 8 years. All had benign intramedullary spinal cord glial tumors. The first sign of disease in all 8 children was intracranial hypertension related to hydrocephalus, with or without other neurologic disturbances. All patients had a shunt placed before the tumor was diagnosed or operated on. Neuroradiologic studies showed contrast enhancement of the intracranial subarachnoid spaces. This was a progressive finding in 6 patients, suggesting that the tumor was spreading in the subarachnoid space. Subarachnoid tumor spread was histologically confirmed in 2 patients. Seven patients had signs of cerebral dysfunction other than those associated with hydrocephalus during follow-up, including seizures, sudden onset of slowly regressing symptoms, and insidious neurologic deterioration.

Literature Review.—Of 125 cases of intramedullary tumors associated with hydrocephalus identified from the literature, 38 were intramedullary low-grade gliomas. Intracranial leptomeningeal seeding was present in 15 of these cases. The hydrocephalus was diagnosed before the tumor in 18 cases and afterward in 18; spontaneous resolution of ventricular dilation occurred in 3 of the former cases and in 1 of the latter.

Discussion.—The problem of hydrocephalus associated with intramedullary low-grade glioma was reviewed. Several possible causes of this unusual association have been advanced, including increased CSF viscosity resulting from elevated fluid protein content, obliteration of the cisterna magna caused by rostral extension of the tumor, and blockage of the subarachnoid pathways of CSF resorption. One theory holds that CSF hydrodynamics could be altered by the presence of fibrinogen in the CSF and its transformation into fibrin at the level of the basal cisterns and Pacchioni's granulations. This could lead to communicating-type hydrocephalus. Leptomeningeal fibrosis would result and predispose to secondary implantation of tumor elements in the subarachnoid spaces of the intracranial compartment.

▶ Cinalli et al. reviewed the unusual association of intramedullary low-grade glioma and hydrocephalus and discussed the possible mechanisms that might explain a cause and effect relationship between the 2 conditions.

R.H. Wilkins, M.D.

Clinical Experience With a New Pressure-Adjustable Shunt Valve

Reinprecht A, Czech T, Dietrich W (Univ of Vienna)
Acta Neurochir (Wien) 134:119–124, 1995   33–2

Introduction.—A new programmable valve shunt system, the Codman Medos, provides 18 possible pressure selections between 30 and 200 mm H_2O, thereby allowing the patients' specific pressure demands to be met. Researchers report the results of their first 2 years of clinical use of the system in 90 patients who underwent shunt surgery.

Methods.—The Codman Medos system uses a noninvasively adjustable pressure setting of a flat spring in the inlet valve unit. An external programmer activates a stepper motor within the valve housing to change the pressure setting of the spring. Pressure can be adjusted after implantation of the valve by positioning the external programmer above the inlet valve. A pressure selector button is used to choose the desired pressure. The patient group included 15 children younger than 16 years: 9 with hydrocephalus, 3 with congenital cysts, 2 with shunt overdrainage, and 1 with spina bifida. The most common diagnoses in adult patients were idiopathic normal-pressure hydrocephalus in 32, neoplastic hydrocephalus in 14, and posthemorrhagic hydrocephalus in 12. Valve pressure was programmed to 200 mm H_2O before insertion in all adults; in children, pressure was programmed according to age and ventricular size. Pressure settings were subsequently adjusted in response to the clinical course.

Results.—Of the 11 complications, 4 were infections, 5 were subdural effusions, and 2 were catheter obstructions. The 4 patients with infection underwent removal of the infected shunt system, external ventricular drainage, and antibiotic therapy, followed by insertion of a new programmable shunt system. Five patients had overdrainage phenomenon with subdural fluid collections. At a median follow-up of 13 months, 64 of the 90 patients had excellent results with resolution of signs and symptoms, 19 patients had a good outcome but residual symptoms remained, and 7—all adults—showed no clinical improvement. The valve operating pressure was adjusted during the shunting procedure in all children and in all but 20 adult patients.

Conclusion.—The pressure-adjustable valve system used in these patients yielded good clinical results. In addition to the advantage of meeting specific patient pressure demands, the design of the valve allows insertion even in small infants without technical difficulties or cutaneous complications.

▶ If a shunt system with a pressure valve is used to treat hydrocephalus or drain an intracranial fluid collection, the choice of the valve is usually based on an educated guess about the level of resistance that will be necessary to permit adequate drainage but also avoid the problems caused by overdrainage. The advantage of a programmable valve such as the valve used in this study is that the valve pressure can be adjusted postoperatively to tailor its function to the needs of the individual patient. Whether this attractive feature will actually improve the neurologic outcome and reduce the complications related to overdrainage will need to be proved in a prospective randomized study.

R.H. Wilkins, M.D.

Shunt Failure in Adult Hydrocephalus: Flow-Controlled Shunt Versus Differential Pressure Shunts: A Cooperative Study in 289 Patients
Decq P, Barat J-L, Duplessis E, et al (Hôpital Henri Mondor, Creteil, France; Hôpital Bretonneau, Tours, France)
Surg Neurol 43:333–339, 1995   33–3

Background.—Although the use of ventricular shunts has dramatically improved the outcomes of patients with hydrocephalus, many complications are still associated with them. Because of the large number of shunt designs in current use and the different techniques of insertion, the problem of shunt malfunction is very complex. The efficiency of flow-controlled shunts in decreasing shunt failure in adults with hydrocephalus was investigated.

Methods.—Two hundred eighty-nine patients in 3 neurosurgical departments were included in the retrospective, comparative study. One hundred forty-two patients underwent surgery with a conventional differential pressure (DP) shunt, and 147 patients underwent surgery with the flow-controlled (FC) system. The analysis included the first complication that required surgical revision within 2 years of implantation.

Findings.—The 1-year actuarial risk of shunt infection was 8.3% in the DP group and 10.9% in the FC group. This difference was nonsignificant.

The 1-year actual risk of mechanical complications was 38% for the DP group and 10% for the FC group. This difference resulted primarily from a reduction in complications associated with the overdrainage phenomenon.

Conclusion.—The use of an FC system reduced the risk of mechanical complications associated with the hydrodynamic properties of shunts used in adults with hydrocephalus. Complications related to overdrainage were especially decreased.

▶ In this retrospective study the authors found that there were fewer complications caused by overdrainage when they used an FC shunt (Orbis-Sigma valve) to treat adult hydrocephalus than when they used a DP shunt.

R.H. Wilkins, M.D.

The Natural History of Arachnoid Cysts: Endoscopic and Cine-Mode MRI Evidence of a Slit-Valve Mechanism

Santamarta D, Aguas J, Ferrer E (Hosp Clínic i Provincial, Barcelona)
Minim Invasive Neurosurg 38:133–137, 1995   33–4

Background.—Arachnoid cysts, considered a developmental abnormality of the arachnoid, are space-occupying lesions filled with CSF-like content and surrounded by a membrane resembling arachnoid mater. These cysts are thought to originate from a splitting or duplication of this membrane. The exact causes and natural history of these cysts are debated. The different hypotheses proposed include agenesis of brain structures, arachnoiditis, active fluid secretion, and a pulsatile pump mechanism. A patient with a suprasellar arachnoid cyst in which a slit-valve mechanism was seen by cine-mode MRI before surgery and confirmed during endoscopy was presented.

> *Case Report.*—Boy, 9, had endocrine disorders consisting of precocious puberty and diabetes insipidus. A large suprasellar cyst, isointense with CSF, was seen on MRI. The lateral ventricles were dilated asymmetrically, and the third ventricle was completely collapsed. The pituitary stalk and the optic chiasm were compressed. The CSF flow dynamics were studied by cone-phase contrast MRI. Images were acquired using a technique with cardiac gating and velocity encoding. The images were arranged in a cine loop, obtained according to the direction and velocity of flow. Axial cine-phase contrast MRI was acquired with anteroposterior codification of flow. Determination of flow velocity was allowed. Egress of CSF from the cyst was hardly detected by axial cine-phase contrast MRI. The jet velocity was 20 cm/sec. At surgery, the suprasellar cyst was fenestrated endoscopically; during the procedure the small communication between the subarachnoid space and the cyst was

seen and photographed and the slit-valve mechanism was confirmed. One year later, MRI showed a partially collapsed cyst filling the suprasellar region.

Conclusion.—The mechanism by which arachnoid cysts enlarge may be explained by the presence of a slit in the wall, acting as a functional one-way valve between the subarachnoid space and cyst. The result would be an increase in pressure inside the cyst and microvilli development in the luminal surface to compensate for the CSF intake. A pressure gradient would exist between the subarachnoid space and cyst responsible for the one-way valve. The images obtained in the patient described suggest that arterial inflow is the mechanism responsible for an increase in pressure in the subarachnoid space, creating a pressure gradient from the subarachnoid space to the cyst.

▶ The question of how arachnoid cysts fill has been a matter of conjecture. Endoscopic and cine-mode MRI techniques offer a way of answering the question, and the present case is a step in that direction.

R.H. Wilkins, M.D.

Disappearance of Arachnoid Cysts After Head Injury

Mori T, Fujimoto M, Sakae K, et al (Saiseikai Shigaken Hosp, Shiga, Japan; Kyoto Prefectural Univ, Japan)
Neurosurgery 36:938–942, 1995

33–5

Introduction.—Arachnoid cysts are often incidentally found by CT and are usually believed to be congenital anomalies. Because the natural history of arachnoid cysts is unknown, their management is controversial. There have been rare reports of the spontaneous disappearance of arachnoid cysts. The disappearance of these cysts after head injury suggests the possibility of a natural cure, obviating surgery.

Methods.—Five male patients aged 9 months to 29 years who had sustained head injuries were studied. Each had acute or chronic subdural hematomas or effusion and arachnoid cysts. Only 2 were surgically treated. The patients were followed with CT scans to assess the cyst size and the associated lesions.

Results.—In the 2 patients with acute subdural hematoma, the hematoma transformed into a subdural effusion, which was gradually absorbed within 5 and 10 months. The cyst completely disappeared in 1 patient at 5 months, when the effusion was absorbed (Fig 1); however, the cyst size was unchanged 2 years after injury in the other patient. In the patient with subdural effusion at admission, the size of the arachnoid cyst gradually decreased but did not disappear. The 2 patients with chronic subdural hematoma were managed with surgical irrigation and subdural drainage. Postoperative CT scans showed the shrinking and disappearance

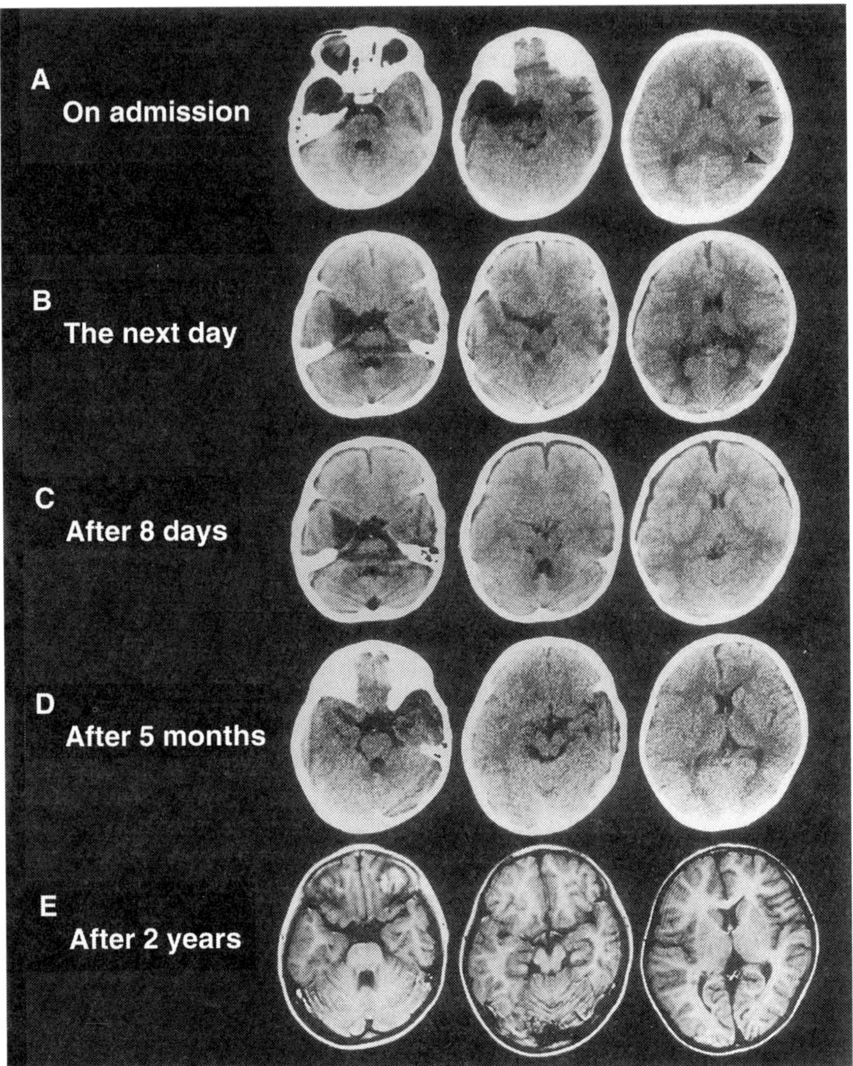

FIGURE 1.—B, CT scan performed at admission shows a low-density area in the anterior portion of the right middle fossa and a thin acute subdural hematoma (*arrows*). C, CT scan performed on the day after admission shows a thin subdural effusion instead of a hematoma. D, follow-up CT scan performed after the head injury shows bilateral subdural effusion. E, follow-up scan performed 5 months after the first examination. The arachnoid cyst and subdural effusion have disappeared. F, MR images. (Courtesy of Mori T, Fujimoto M, Sakae K, et al: Disappearance of arachnoid cysts after head injury. *Neurosurgery* 36:938–942, 1995.)

of the cysts within 2.5 months in 1 patient and within 9 months in the other patient.

Discussion.—A head injury may result in a tear of the outer wall of the cyst, resulting in an osmotic gradient between the subdural space and the cystic space, causing the outflow of cyst fluid and reducing the size of the cyst. The cyst fluid leakage into the subdural space is then absorbed, although the effusion may become a chronic subdural hematoma, requiring irrigation. The cyst wall may be ruptured by minor head injuries and may silently disappear. Therefore, asymptomatic patients should be followed without surgery, and patients with chronic subdural hematoma should be managed with irrigation only and imaging follow-up.

▶ The authors documented that a presumed arachnoid cyst may resolve after a head injury, probably by rupture of the cyst wall and either gradual absorption of the resulting subdural effusion or surgical drainage of the resulting chronic subdural hematoma.

R.H. Wilkins, M.D.

Posterior Fossa Volume and Response to Suboccipital Decompression in Patients With Chiari I Malformation

Badie B, Mendoza D, Batzdorf U (Univ of California, Los Angeles)
Neurosurgery 37:214–218, 1995   33–6

Background.—A smaller posterior fossa (PF) volume may be 1 mechanism responsible for tonsillar herniation through the foramen magnum in

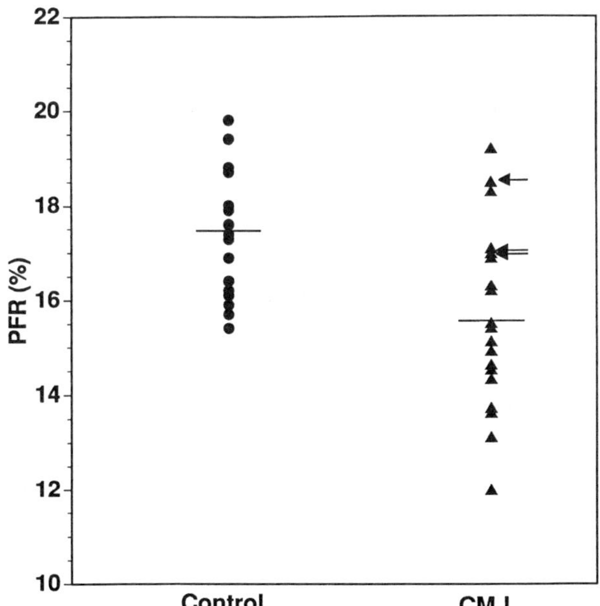

FIGURE 2.—Posterior fossa ratios in control patients (*circles*) and patients with Chiari I malformation (*triangles*). *Horizontal bars* mark the mean value for each group (17.5 for control patients vs. 15.6 for CMI patients; *P* = 0.0008). *Arrows* point to the results for 3 patients with CMI who did not respond to suboccipital decompression. *Abbreviations: PFR,* posterior fossa ratio; *CMI,* Chiari I malformation. (Courtesy of Badie B, Mendoza D, Batzdorf U: Posterior fossa volume and response to suboccipital decompression in patients with Chiari I malformation. *Neurosurgery* 37:214–218, 1995.)

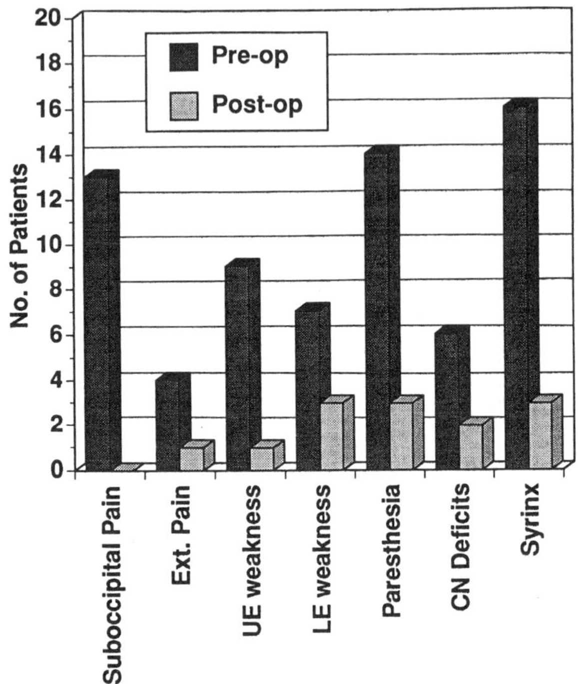

FIGURE 5.—Symptoms, neurologic findings, and presence of syringomyelia in patients with Chiari I malformation before and after posterior fossa decompression. Postoperative evaluation represents partial or complete resolution of symptoms and signs. *Abbreviations: Ext.*, extremity; *UE*, upper extremity; *LE*, lower extremity; *CN*, cranial nerve; *Pre-op*, preoperative; *Post-op*, postoperative. (Courtesy of Badie B, Mendoza D, Batzdorf U: Posterior fossa volume and response to suboccipital decompression in patients with Chiari I malformation. *Neurosurgery* 37:214–218, 1995.)

patients with a Chiari I malformation (CMI). Although previous radiologic analyses of cranial anatomy have suggested that patients with CMI have smaller PF volumes, an association of PF volume with decompressive surgery has not been documented. The ratio of PF volume to supratentorial volume (PF ratio; PFR) was calculated from the MR images of patients with and without CMI, and the relationship of this value to the responses of patients to suboccipital decompression was determined.

Methods and Findings.—The MR images of 20 patients with CMI and 20 control subjects were studied retrospectively with a computerized image analyzer. The mean PFR in patients with CMI was 15.6, significantly smaller than in the control group, which had a mean PFR of 17.5. Although the PFR did not correlate with the extent of tonsillar herniation in patients with CMI, it was directly associated with patient age. Younger patients with CMI but not control patients had smaller PFRs. Decompressive surgery elicited clinical and radiographic responses in all but 3 patients. In patients not benefiting from such surgery, PFRs were normal (Figs 2 and 5).

Conclusion.—Most patients with CMI have smaller PFRs. A smaller PF volume may be the main cause of tonsillar herniation. Patients with CMI and smaller PFRs tend to experience symptoms earlier than do patients with normal PFRs. Suboccipital decompression tends to be more beneficial in patients with smaller PFRs.

▶ The authors confirmed the fact that patients with the CMI tend to have a small PF. As one might expect, the tighter the space, the earlier the symptoms and the better the response to surgical decompression. Whether the small PF is a primary cause of the tonsillar herniation remains a matter of conjecture.

R.H. Wilkins, M.D.

Surgical Indication and Results of Foramen Magnum Decompression Versus Syringosubarachnoid Shunting for Syringomyelia Associated With Chiari I Malformation
Hida K, Iwasaki Y, Koyanagi I, et al (Univ of Hokkaido, Sapporo, Japan)
Neurosurgery 37:673–679, 1995   33–7

Objective.—The results of surgery for syringomyelia were compared in 33 symptomatic patients with Chiari I malformations whose initial operation was foramen magnum decompression (FMD) and 37 similar patients who underwent syringosubarachnoid (SS) shunt surgery. The patients were operated on between 1982 and 1993.

Patients.—The patients' ages ranged from 3 to 59 years (average age 29). None had spinal dysraphism or syringobulbia. Nearly two thirds of patients had motor weakness, and all but 4% had disordered sensation. Pain was present in 39% of patients. One fourth had a lower cranial nerve palsy or nystagmus. Autonomic dysfunction was identified in 16% of patients. Nearly 60% of patients, mainly those who were younger, had scoliosis.

Surgery.—The SS shunt is preferred in patients who have a large syrinx in a widened spinal cord. The laminectomy is done at the level where the syrinx is largest. The dura is incised microsurgically and joined to the stump of the arachnoid membranes. The myelotomy is done by making a 2-mm surgical section posteriorly in the midline or posterolaterally along the dorsal root entry zone. The Sapporo shunt tube, a soft catheter, is used. The FMD consists of removing the occipital bone around the foramen magnum and the C1 arch.

Results.—No patients died or had major complications. The neurologic conditions of 82% of the patients improved after FMD during an average follow-up of 38 months. Simple FMD, with only partial dural resection, was as effective as FMD with dural plasty. The neurologic conditions of all but 3% of patients improved after SS shunting, during an average follow-up of 75 months. Pain was more effectively relieved by the SS shunt procedure. Magnetic resonance imaging confirmed a reduction in size of the syrinx in all patients in both groups, but this occurred more rapidly after SS shunting (2 vs. 6 weeks on average). Further surgery was done in 9% of the patients undergoing FMD and 19% of those in the SS shunt group. In the latter patients, technical problems were chiefly responsible. Two patients in the FMD group had meningitis postoperatively and kyphosis developed in 1.

Conclusion.—The SS shunt seems to be a more effective initial operation than FMD for patients having syringomyelia with Chiari I malformation, especially those with larger syringes.

▶ As anyone who treats syringomyelia knows, no single treatment is perfect, and patients may require several operations during their lifetime. The present retrospective study was not ideal because the patients were not randomized to specific operations. Yet it did shed light on what can be accomplished by the 2 main surgical techniques used currently to treat syringomyelia associated with the Chiari I malformation.

R.H. Wilkins, M.D.

Human Tails and Associated Spinal Anomalies
James HE, Canty TG (Univ of California, San Diego)
Clin Pediatr 34:286–288, 1995   33–8

Introduction.—In the literature, human tails have been classified as either true tail (a persistent vestigial tail with no associated disorders or involvement of neural elements) or pseudotail (with spinal cord involvement). Neuroimaging is recommended with both types before surgery is performed. The neuroimaging and operative findings in 3 patients with tail-like appendages were described.

Case 1.—Boy, newborn, had a 15-cm tail-like appendage attached to an elevated, skin-covered soft-tissue mass in the midlumbar region, with a small cutaneous hemangioma. Spinal MRI revealed high-signal intensity from the base of the tail through the subcutaneous tissue and into the lumbosacral canal, penetrating the subarachnoid space. The conus was low in the lumbar region. The tethered cord was released with microsurgery using a carbon dioxide laser, with good results.

Case 2.—Girl, newborn, had an appendage 5-cm long and 1-cm wide attached to the right paraspinal midlumbar region by a depressible, skin-covered soft-tissue mass with a small hemangioma. Computed tomography revealed a hypodense image suggestive of a lipoma that migrated from the subcutaneous tissues into the spinal canal and laterally displaced the nerve roots in the conus. The lipoma was microsurgically resected with the use of intraoperative monitoring of nerve root function. During 12 years of follow-up, there was no recurrence of the lipoma or neurologic sequelae.

Case 3.—Boy, neonate, had a midforearm amputation defect and a 5-cm tail-like appendage attached to a large, skin-covered soft-tissue mass with a small hemangioma. Spinal MRI revealed a normal conus and a dorsal lumbosacral junction defect. Surgery revealed a discontinuous tract from the base of the tail that did not penetrate the dura. The mass and appendage were resected. During 5 years of follow-up the child had normal neurologic development.

Discussion.—Two of the 3 patients had neural structure involvement in their tail-like appendages. It is suggested that all patients with midline or near-midline appendages undergo neuroimaging with MRI or high-resolution spinal ultrasonography to characterize the surgical anatomy and guide surgical intervention.

▶ It is well known that certain skin lesions may be associated with spinal dysraphism, including hemangioma, hypertrichosis, dermal sinus, and subcutaneous lipoma. In this context, a tail or pseudotail may be present in a newborn infant—a phenomenon that can induce fright or embarrassment in the parents and curiosity in medical personnel. The authors stressed that neural structures are often involved in patients with a tail or pseudotail, and they recommended that appropriate neuroimaging be performed before surgical removal of the appendage to permit the simultaneous correction of coexisting abnormalities, such as tethering of the spinal cord.

R.H. Wilkins, M.D.

34 Spinal Disorders

Degenerative Diseases

Determinants of Lumbar Disc Degeneraton: A Study Relating Lifetime Exposures and Magnetic Resonance Imaging Findings in Identical Twins

Battié MC, Videman T, Gibbons LE, et al (Univ of Alberta, Edmonton, Canada; Univ of Helsinki; Univ of Jyväskylä, Finland; et al)
Spine 20:2601–2612, 1995   34–1

Introduction.—The causes of most back symptoms are unknown. However, structural and biochemical changes associated with disk degeneration are strongly suspected to be the cause of back pain, particularly when associated with radicular pain. Several factors have been suggested as accelerators of degenerative disk changes. The effects of lifetime exposures to these commonly suspected risk factors on disk degeneration were studied in twins examined with MRI.

Methods.—Identical twin pairs were selected from the Finnish Twin Cohort. Data collected previously indicated discordance in the selected twin pairs in 1 of the following 5 risk factors: occupational materials handling, sedentary work, exercise participation, vehicular vibration, and cigarette smoking. A detailed, structured interview was conducted with each subject to review the lifetime work history and to collect data on sport and leisure time activities. Each job was then categorized by the type and degree of physical loading, and leisure time physical loading was evaluated. The participants were asked about their histories of back pain. All were examined with MRI to evaluate disk degeneration. The influence of the risk factors and the effects of twinship on the MRI findings were analyzed.

Results.—The identified risk factors were stronger determinants of upper than of lower lumbar disk degeneration. The only statistically significant associations were between disk height narrowing and occupational physical loading and between decreased signal intensity and greater leisure time physical loading. In multivariate analyses, occupational physical loading was the only significant predictor of twin differences in upper lumbar disk degeneration, and there were no significant predictors of twin differences in the lower lumbar region. Twinship, reflecting the influences of genetics and early shared environment, accounted for the majority of variability in disk degeneration in both the upper and lower lumbar regions.

Conclusion.—The widely suspected environmental and behavioral factors have little effect on the process of disk degeneration. Disk degeneration is likely to be most dependent on genetic and early environmental influences, as well as unidentified factors.

▶ This work, which won the 1995 Volvo Award in Clinical Sciences, provided epidemiologic evidence that factors previously thought to accelerate lumbar disk degeneration, such as long-term vocations and avocations that heavily load the lumbar spine, actually play a small role. The results of their investigation suggest that disk degeneration is more likely related to genetic and early environmental influences, as well as to other, as yet unidentified, factors.

R.H. Wilkins, M.D.

Magnetic Resonance Neurography for Cervical Radiculopathy: A Preliminary Report
Dailey AT, Tsuruda JS, Goodkin R, et al (Univ of Washington, Seattle; Univ of Utah, Salt Lake City; Univ of California, Los Angeles)
Neurosurgery 38:488–492, 1996   34–2

Introduction.—Clinical history, physical examination, electrodiagnostic studies, and radiologic images must be carefully correlated to determine diagnosis and treatment of cervical radiculopathy. Magnetic resonance neurography (MRN) techniques were used to directly image symptomatic spinal nerve roots in 3 patients with cervical radiculopathy and 1 normal volunteer to determine whether MRN could detect signal changes in cervical spinal nerves subjected to compression from either a disk or an osteophyte.

Methods.—Three patients with radiographic evidence of herniated cervical disks on MRI and symptoms of cervical radiculopathy underwent MRN studies. For comparison, 1 asymptomatic volunteer was evaluated by MRN. A 1.5-tesla MR scanner was used. Imaging sequences used to view the cervical spine and spinal nerves were coronal T1-weighted conventional spin-echo sequences, T2-weighted fast spin-echo sequences in the coronal and axial planes, and axial and coronal fast spin-echo multiplanar short tau inversion recovery (FMPIR) sequences.

 Patient 1.—Man, 50, had a 2-year history of neck pain and shooting pain radiating in a C6 distribution down the right arm. He had trace weakness in the right biceps and normal reflexes. All electrical studies were normal. A large disk bulge at C5-6 that was more prominent on the right side was seen on conventional MRI. A MRN examination of the cervical spinal nerves showed increased signal exclusively located in the right C6 spinal nerve (Fig 2A). Quantitative analysis of the axial FMPIR sequence confirmed this finding.

Patient 2.—Man, 45, had a 1-year history of shooting pains in the neck and in the right upper extremity and tingling and numb-

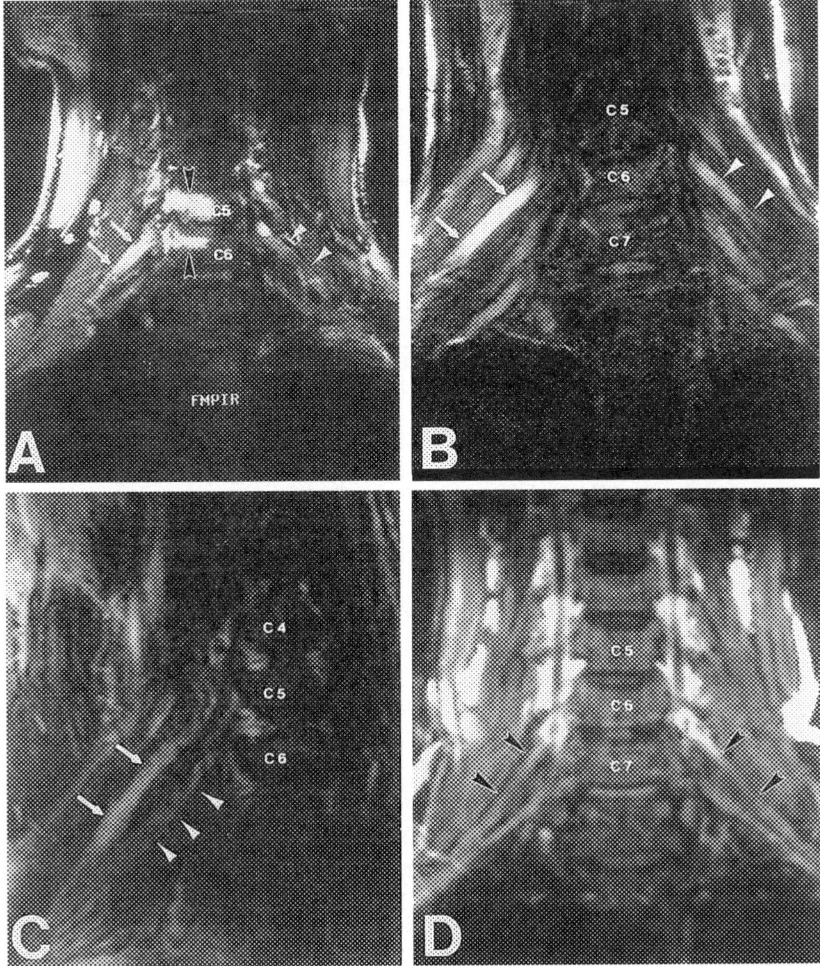

FIGURE 2.—**A**, coronal FMPIR from patient 1. Note the markedly higher signal in the right C6 spinal nerve (*arrows*) compared with the left (*white arrowheads*). Also note the degenerative reactive marrow changes in the C5 and C6 vertebral bodies (*black arrowheads*). **B**, coronal FMPIR image from patient 2. Again note the higher signal in the right C6 nerve (*arrows*) compared with the asymptomatic left C6 spinal nerve (*arrowheads*). **C**, coronal T2-weighted fast spin-echo image from patient 3. The right spinal nerves are visible in this image, which shows higher signal in the C5 nerve (*arrows*), corresponding to the electromyographic results, than in the adjacent C6 nerve (*arrowheads*). **D**, coronal FMPIR from an asymptomatic volunteer (patient 4). No differences in signal intensity are identified when the right and left C6 spinal nerves (*arrowheads*) are compared. *Abbreviation: FMPIR*, fast spin-echo multiplanar short tau recovery. (Courtesy of Daily AT, Tsuruda JS, Goodkin R, et al: Magnetic resonance neurography of cervical radiculopathy: A preliminary report. *Neurosurgery* 38:488–492, 1996.)

ness in the right C6 dermatome. There was grade 4+/5 weakness in the right biceps and brachioradialis and a diminished right biceps reflex. Sensory examination was normal. The electromyogram was normal, but increased latencies consistent with a neurapraxic injury of the right C6 spinal nerve were detected on nerve conduction studies. A disk bulge and osteophyte were observed on conventional MRI at the C5-6 level. Cervical spinal nerve MRN showed increased signal in the right C6 spinal nerve (Fig 2B). This finding was confirmed by quantitative analysis.

Patient 3.—Man 54, had a 4-week history of paraspinal muscle spasm in the neck and sharp pain radiating down the right arm and into the dorsum of the right hand. He experienced grade 4/5 weakness in the right deltoid, biceps, and triceps muscles. Sensation to light touch and pinprick was diminished in the right C5 and C6 dermatomes. Results of electrical studies were consistent with an axonotmetic injury of the right C5 spinal nerve. Multiple ventral compressions throughout the spinal canal were seen on CT and were most prominent at C4-5 and C5-6. Osteophytes and bulging disks at C4-5 and C5-6 were seen on conventional MRI. The MRN of the cervical spinal nerves indicated the right C5 spinal nerve had higher signal intensity than the adjacent C6 and C7 nerves (Fig 2C). The patient was not able to tolerate the axial FMPIR study, so quantitative analysis could not be performed.

Patient 4.—Woman, 38, was a volunteer with no history of neck pain or radiculopathic upper extremity pain or weakness. There was no evidence of cervical disk degeneration or spondylosis on conventional MRI. All cervical spinal nerves from C5 to C8 had similar signal intensities on axial and coronal FMPIR sequences (Fig 2D).

Conclusion.—There is a potential for MRN to directly image changes in compressed spinal nerves in patients with cervical radiculopathy. Sensitivity and specificity are yet to be determined using a much larger series of symptomatic and asymptomatic research subjects.

▶ This is an intriguing report of an MRI technique[1,2] that may prove to be of value in identifying the nerve root involved in a radiculopathy when it cannot be identified precisely by history, neurologic examination, electrodiagnostic testing, or radiologic imaging.

R.H. Wilkins, M.D.

References

1. Filler AG, Howe FA, Hayes CE, et al: Magnetic resonance neurography. *Lancet* 341:659–661, 1993.
2. Howe FA, Filler AG, Bell BA, et al: Magnetic resonance neurography. *Magn Reson Med* 28:328–338, 1992.

Contrast-Enhanced MR Imaging in Acute Lumbar Radiculopathy: A Pilot Study of the Natural History
Modic MT, Ross JS, Obuchowski NA, et al (Cleveland Clinic Found, Ohio)
Radiology 195:429–435, 1995   34–3

Background.—In current medical practice, imaging studies are used in assessing sciatica when true radicular symptoms are present, when nerve root irritation is evident at physical examination, and when, in the presence of motor weakness, 4 to 6 weeks of conservative management has been unsuccessful. Although sound empirical data support a conservative imaging approach, it has never been tested specifically with gadolinium-enhanced MRI. Clinical findings and contrast material–enhanced MR images were prospectively studied in patients with acute lumbar radiculopathy.

Methods.—Twenty-five patients were included. Physical examination and MRI were done at the initial assessment, at 6 weeks, and at 6 months. Magnetic resonance studies consisted of T1-weighted sagittal and axial images, T2-weighted sagittal spin-echo or fast spin-echo images, and T1-weighted sagittal and axial images obtained after IV administration of gadopentetate dimeglumine.

Findings.—Eighteen patients had a herniated nucleus pulposus (HNP) at 1 or more levels. Two patients had synovial cysts and stenosis. Findings were normal in 5 patients. Neurologic symptoms were marginally more severe in patients with an HNP than in those without an HNP at initial assessment. Twenty-two patients completed the 6-week examinations, and 14, the 6-month examinations. Three patients were excluded from the study after undergoing surgery. At 6 weeks, 36% of HNPs larger than 6 mm were substantially reduced. At 6 months, more than 60% of these HNPs were markedly reduced.

Conclusion.—For level and side of HNP and radicular symptoms, agreement between clinical and MR findings was excellent. Pain and disability were uncorrelated with disk size, behavior, and type.

▶ When a patient is seen with the symptoms of lower lumbar or first sacral radiculopathy and has the appropriate abnormalities on physical examination, an MRI study of the lumbosacral spine ordinarily will demonstrate the cause, which most frequently is a lumbar disk herniation. Presently the standard therapeutic approach in the United States is to initially treat the patient with rest and medication and then with a hemilaminectomy and diskectomy if there has been no significant improvement. The assumption has been that the disk herniation will remain as a compressive force, like a stone in a shoe. However, it has become apparent, through studies such as this, that the disk herniation frequently will become smaller during the ensuing weeks and months. Therefore, if the patient's symptoms and findings are resolving or are at a tolerable level, nonoperative treatment may be the best approach.

R.H. Wilkins, M.D.

Randomised Comparison of Chiropractic and Hospital Outpatient Management for Low Back Pain: Results From Extended Follow Up
Meade TW, Dyer S, Browne W, et al (St Bartholomew's Hosp, London; Northwick Park Hosp, Harrow, England)
BMJ 311:349–351, 1995

34–4

Background.—In a previous study the authors demonstrated greater improvement in patients with low back pain treated by chiropractic than in those receiving hospital outpatient management. The trial was "pragmatic" in that the therapists were permitted to treat the patients as they would in everyday practice. The results after up to 3 years' follow-up are reported.

Methods.—The randomized trial included 741 adult patients with low back pain for which manipulation was not contraindicated. The patients were assigned to receive care either at a chiropractic clinic or in a hospital outpatient department. The groups were compared on an intention-to-treat basis for change in total Oswestry questionnaire score and pain score, as well for patient satisfaction.

Results.—At 3 years, the improvement in total Oswestry score was about 29% greater for the patients treated by chiropractic. The benefits of chiropractic on pain were particularly apparent. Patients assigned to the chiropractic group received further treatments for back pain after the end of the study. Chiropractic care was rated as more helpful than hospital management regardless of whether the patients were initially referred to the study from a chiropractor or a hospital.

Conclusion.—Three years' follow-up confirmed the advantages of chiropractic care over hospital outpatient management for patients with low back pain. Patients receiving chiropractic care derived more benefit and reported greater long-term satisfaction. The advantages of chiropractic may result from the greater number of treatments administered over longer periods. More research is needed to identify the effective components of chiropractic care.

▶ This study demonstrated the beneficial effect of chiropractic on low back pain. I find that patients are almost always complimentary of their chiropractor, even if they do not get adequate relief, and I suspect that few malpractice suits are directed against chiropractors. Patients generally feel that the chiropractor is trying to help them. I think that the time spent with the patient and the hands-on approach of the chiropractor are largely responsible for that feeling. This should serve as a reminder to modern neurosurgeons, whose focus may tend toward technology, that personal interactions with patients are important to patient satisfaction and healing no matter how good the measurable outcome of a neurosurgical procedure.

R.H. Wilkins, M.D.

Efficacy of Epidural Steroid Injections for Low-Back Pain and Sciatica: A Systematic Review of Randomized Clinical Trials
Koes BW, Scholten RJPM, Mens JMA, et al (Vrije Univ, Amsterdam; Erasmus Univ, Rotterdam, The Netherlands)
Pain 63:279–288, 1995
34–5

Introduction.—There are many therapeutic interventions for low back pain and sciatica. The efficacy of epidural steroid injections was assessed with a meta-analysis of published randomized clinical trials, with specific attention to the methodological quality of the studies.

Methods.—A literature search was performed to identify published randomized clinical trials of epidural steroid injections for the treatment of back pain, sciatica, or both. The 12 identified published trials were scored for methodological quality based on assessment of 4 categories: study population, interventions, effect measurement, and data presentation and analysis.

Results.—The 12 studies had widely varying methodological scores ranging from 17 to 72. Four of the studies had scores higher than 60 points. The most common methodological problems were noncomparable baseline characteristics, small sample size, a lack of comparison with a relevant treatment modality, noncomparable cointerventions, unclear patient blinding, and lack of long-term follow-up. Overall, half of the trials reported better results with epidural steroid injection than with the reference treatment, whereas the other half reported either no difference in efficacy or better outcomes with the reference treatment. Of the 4 studies with the highest methodological scores, 2 reported the superiority of epidural steroid treatment and the other 2 reported equal effects of steroid injection and reference treatment. Outcome and methodological quality were not clearly related.

Conclusion.—Most studies of the efficacy of epidural steroid injections for the treatment of low back pain and sciatica have been methodologically flawed, which has prevented the establishment of the treatment's efficacy. Therefore, future research should use careful methodology. There is no current evidence of efficacy of epidural steroid injections in patients with back pain without sciatica. More study is needed to determine which population of patients would be most likely to benefit from this treatment.

▶ The authors provided a worthwhile review of the subject of epidural steroid injections for the treatment of low back pain and sciatica. They concluded that the efficacy of this form of treatment has not yet been established.

R.H. Wilkins, M.D.

A Meta-Analysis on the Efficacy of Epidural Corticosteroids in the Treatment of Sciatica

Watts RW, Silagy CA (Flinders Univ, Bedford Park, South Australia)
Anaesth Intensive Care 23:564–569, 1995

34–6

Background.—Low back pain and sciatica are frequently treated with epidural corticosteroid agents. However, studies of its efficacy have generally been too small to report statistically significant effects. A meta-analysis of all randomized trials of epidural steroids was performed to evaluate efficacy in the treatment of sciatica.

Methods.—Eleven randomized trials of epidural treatment for sciatica were identified from a MEDLINE search and were assessed for methodological quality. Included were data on diagnosis, duration of symptoms, randomization process, epidural technique, corticosteroid use, additional treatments, control, and the number of patients involved. Relief of pain was the main measure of efficacy.

Results.—The 11 placebo-controlled trials involved 907 patients and had generally good quality. The pooled odds ratio for at least 75% pain relief was 2.61 and for near complete relief was 2.79. The efficacy appears to be independent of injection route, with odds ratios of 3.80 for caudal epidural steroids and 2.43 for lumbar epidural steroids. The odds ratio was 3.59 for short-term relief and 1.87 for long-term relief. There was significant variation among studies in short-term but not long-term pain relief, suggesting that selection of patients and assessment of response influenced short-term efficacy. Adverse events were rare and included dural taps, transient headache, transient increase in pain, and irregular periods.

Conclusion.—Pooled data from randomized trials provide evidence of the efficacy of caudal or lumbar epidural steroid treatment of lumbosacral radicular pain.

▶ The epidural administration of a corticosteroid preparation is a commonly used form of nonoperative therapy for back and leg pain caused by intervertebral disk disease or spondylosis. By means of their meta-analysis, Watts and Silagy provided support for this form of treatment.

R.H. Wilkins, M.D.

Fragment Excision Versus Conventional Disc Removal in the Microsurgical Treatment of Herniated Lumbar Disc

Faulhauer K, Manicke C (Brüderkrankenhaus Trier, Federal Republic of Germany)
Acta Neurochir (Wien) 133:107–111, 1995

34–7

Introduction.—In their experience with microsurgery for herniated lumbar disks, the authors found it difficult to inspect the dorsal aspect of the disk during medial or lateral foraminotomy. They therefore decided to remove only the herniated disk fragment. Despite fears that such patients would be prone to recurrence, the patients actually had fewer recurrences and reported feeling better because of the less marked sequelae of instability. Follow-up studies were reviewed to determine whether these initially good results were maintained over time.

Methods.—The analysis included 2 groups of patients who underwent lumbar disk surgery: 100 who had conventional microdiskectomy and 100 who had removal of only the herniated disk fragment. The latter group included 43 patients with classic mediolateral herniation, 29 with a fragment located in the proximal foraminal part of the upper nerve root, and 28 with a fragment in the distal foramen or extraforaminally. The mean follow-up was 43 months. The 2 groups were compared for true recurrences and for postoperative instability problems.

Results.—The recurrence rate was 2% in the fragment excision group and 7% in the conventional microdiskectomy group. The instability rate was 16% after fragment excision and 30% after conventional diskectomy. The average duration of clinical instability was 10 weeks in the former group and 15 weeks in the latter. Two patients in the fragment excision group and 4 in the conventional microdiskectomy group had severe postoperative instability.

Conclusion.—In selected lumbar disk surgery patients, simple fragment excision may lower the rate of repeat herniation and the severity of instability compared with conventional microdiskectomy. The routine performance of interspace evacuation in all cases does not appear to be justified.

▶ Since the beginning of surgery for lumbar disk disease, opinion has differed regarding how to deal with a free-fragment disk herniation. Should only the free fragment be removed, or should, in addition, as much of the nucleus pulposus as possible be removed through the rent in the annulus fibrosus to reduce the likelihood of recurrent disk herniation? The present study extended this discussion to free-fragment disk herniation treated microsurgically. In their paper the authors spoke of postoperative instability, namely, persisting mechanical low back pain with associated lumbar stiffness and an alteration in posture.

This was not a prospective randomized trial. Although all of the operations were performed by 1 surgeon, the comparisons between the 2 groups are not entirely valid. Free-fragment removal as the sole maneuver was done only if the annular opening was small, and the combined procedure was done only if the herniation was in continuity with the disk and not dislocated away from it. Even so, it does appear that simple free-fragment disk removal is the procedure of choice if the annular opening is small, especially if the extruded fragment or fragments are displaced above or below the disk from which they originated.

R.H. Wilkins, M.D.

Measurement of Exercise Tolerance on the Treadmill in Patients With Symptomatic Lumbar Spinal Stenosis: A Useful Indicator of Functional Status and Surgical Outcome
Deen HG Jr, Zimmerman RS, Lyons MK, et al (Mayo Clin Scottsdale, Ariz)
J Neurosurg 83:27–30, 1995
34–8

Background.—Treadmill testing may be useful in the assessment of patients with lumbar spinal stenosis. The value of determining exercise tolerance on a treadmill in evaluating preoperative functional status and postoperative progress in patients undergoing decompressive laminectomy for lumbar spinal stenosis was investigated.

Methods.—Twenty patients with intractable neurogenic claudication and radiographically confirmed severe lumbar spinal stenosis were included. Mean age was 73. All patients underwent lumbar decompressive laminectomy. Before and 2 months after surgery, ambulation was assessed quantitatively on a treadmill at a 0-degree ramp incline at 1.2 mph and the patient's preferred walking speed. Assessments were terminated after 15 minutes or at the onset of severe symptoms.

Findings.—The mean time to initial symptoms in the preoperative 1.2-mph trial was 2.7 minutes. The mean time to severe symptoms was 5.5 minutes. At the same speed after surgery, 65% of the patients were able to walk without symptoms for 15 minutes. The mean time to first symptoms was 11.1 minutes, and the mean time to severe symptoms was 11.8 minutes. Findings in the preferred walking speed trials were similar. The treadmill test was associated with no complications.

Conclusion.—Exercise stress testing on a treadmill is a safe, easy, quantifiable method for evaluating baseline function status in patients with lumbar spinal stenosis and neurogenic claudication. The results of testing are also useful in assessing outcomes after laminectomy and in guiding the subsequent management of patients with residual symptoms.

▶ The syndrome of neurogenic claudication caused by lumbar spinal stenosis has been well recognized for many years. Typically the severity of the syndrome has been assessed only by the history: How far can you walk before you have to rest? How severe are your symptoms? Given the widespread availability of treadmill testing and its use in assessing the cardiovascular system, it is surprising that such testing to quantify neurogenic claudication has not been used until now.

R.H. Wilkins, M.D.

Changes in Epidural Pressure During Walking in Patients With Lumbar Spinal Stenosis
Takahashi K, Kagechika K, Takino T, et al (Ishikawa Prefectural Central Hosp, Japan; Kanazawa Univ, Japan)
Spine 20:2746–2749, 1995   34–9

Background.—The most common symptom of lumbar spinal stenosis is neurogenic intermittent claudication. The pathogenesis of neurogenic intermittent claudication is unclear. However, investigators have speculated that it may be caused by either compression of the nerve roots or nerve root ischemia. The pathogenesis of neurogenic intermittent claudication was investigated by analyzing epidural pressure changes during walking in patients with and without lumbar spinal stenosis.

Methods.—Twelve patients with lumbar spinal stenosis who had cauda equina, radicular symptoms, or both at the L4-5 level, and neurogenic intermittent claudication and 7 control subjects with normal spinal canals were studied. A catheter transducer was inserted into the epidural space at the L4-5 level. Epidural pressure was measured continuously in 7 patients and the 7 controls during both simple walking and walking with lumbar flexion on a treadmill set at a velocity of 2 km/hour. Epidural pressure changes were correlated with gait phases, using foot switches to record gait patterns in 5 patients.

Results.—Both patients and controls demonstrated a pattern of increase and decrease in epidural pressure during walking. The peak values of pressure increase were significantly greater during both simple walking and walking with lumbar flexion in patients with spinal stenosis than in the controls. Among the patients, the peak values of pressure increase were significantly lower during walking with lumbar flexion than during simple walking and were not significantly different from the values recorded among controls during simple walking. The pressure increase was recorded during the double-supporting phase of each gait cycle.

Conclusion.—Repeated intermittent increases of epidural pressure at the level of spinal stenosis may cause intermittent compression of the nerve roots, which may induce physiologic changes, including nerve root ischemia, thus causing intermittent claudication.

▶ The exact mechanisms that result in neurogenic intermittent claudication have been debated. With this study, the authors provided evidence that the appropriate nerve roots are compressed as the patient walks.

R.H. Wilkins, M.D.

Surgical Treatment for Ossification of the Posterior Longitudinal Ligament of the Cervical Spine

Kawano H, Handa Y, Ishii H, et al (Miyazaki Med College, Japan; Fukui Med School, Matsuoka Yoshida-gun, Japan)
J Spinal Disord 8:145–150, 1995

34–10

Background.—Ossification of the posterior longitudinal ligament (OPLL) is an uncommon condition with an unknown cause. As OPLL grows, the spinal cord and nerve roots become compressed, causing neurologic deterioration. OPLL is treated by posterior surgical decompression or by the use of an anterior approach with removal of the ossified portion of the ligament. Results obtained with these 2 methods in 75 patients were described.

Methods.—Patients aged 39 to 74 had symptomatic OPLL. They were followed for an average of 65 months. The extent of lower and upper extremity motor function, sensory function, and performance were rated using the neurosurgical cervical spine scale (NCSS). The type and shape of OPLL were estimated, and the contraction rate (CR) of the vertebral column was calculated. Thirty-seven patients had continuous OPLL (COPLL), 29 had segmental OPLL (SOPLL), 5 had mixed COPLL and SOPLL (MOPLL), and the remaining 4 had circumscribed disk OPLL (DOPLL). The goal of anterior surgery was to remove the OPLL to reduce or eliminate compression of the nerve root, spinal cord, and vascular system. Anterior decompression (AD) was used in 48 patients and posterior decompression (PD) in the rest. Anterior decompression was used for 14 patients with COPLL, 27 with SOPLL, 3 with MOPLL and all patients with DOPLL. Posterior decompression was performed for OPLL extending over 4 or more vertebral bodies that was localized in the high cervical area and extended to the thoracic spine or that was accompanied by acute spinal cord injury.

Results.—The average CR was 57.5% in patients in the AD group and 43.2% in patients in the PD group. The length of the affected area ranged from 2 to 7 vertebral bodies in COPLL, from 1 to 5 vertebral bodies in SOPLL, and from 3 to 8 vertebral bodies in MOPLL. The mean improvement postoperatively in the NCSS score was 78% for patients in the AD group and 46.1% for patients in the PD group, with complete cure in 24 patients in the AD group and 1 patient in the PD group. On follow-up of 70 patients, the NCSS score decreased in patients in the PD group from 10.4 to 9.7 points, whereas it increased for patients in the AD group from 12.9 to 13.0.

Discussion.—Surgery was performed to attempt to remove the OPLL as much as possible except when drilling this ossified structure would put patients with extremely narrow thecoperiosteal diameters at risk. It is likely that the NCSS score decreased among patients in the PD group because of progression of residual OPLL. Anterior decompression seemed superior to PD, although the latter method was required in some cases.

▶ The authors provided a careful analysis of the outcomes of anterior and posterior decompressive surgery in the treatment of ossification of the OPLL in a relatively large group of patients. They use a parameter that I was unfamiliar with—the CR of the vertebral column. This is defined by the formula CR = (APD−TPD)/APD × 100(%), where APD is anteroposterior diameter and TPD is thecoperiosteal diameter. It reflects the degree of narrowing of the spinal canal.

R.H. Wilkins, M.D.

Trauma

Validity of the Three-Column Theory of Thoracolumbar Fractures: A Biomechanic Investigation

Panjabi MM, Oxland TR, Kifune M, et al (Yale Univ, New Haven, Conn; Spine-Tech, Inc, Minneapolis)
Spine 20:1122–1127, 1995   34–11

Introduction.—The stability of the injured spine must be evaluated when treatment is considered. The 3-column theory of spinal fractures has been introduced, which evaluates the status of the anterior column (the anterior vertebral body, anterior anulus fibrosis, and anterior longitudinal ligament), the middle column (the middle osteoligamentous complex), and the posterior column (the posterior osseous arch and posterior ligamentous complex). This theory of the spine was related to spinal instability using CT and biomechanical experiments to evaluate the significance to stability of injuries in each of the columns.

Methods.—A high-speed trauma model was used to produce burst fractures in 16 cadaveric thoracolumbar human spine specimens in either of 2 ways: simple axial compression or flexion-compression. Multidirectional flexibility tests, with 6 physiologic loads, were performed before and after the trauma, and instability was quantified with stereophotographs. Injury severity was graded in 14 sectors of the 3 columns on CT scans, with grade 0 reflecting intact status, grade 1 reflecting partial fracture, and grade 2 reflecting complete fracture.

Results.—The fracture patterns varied with each type of trauma load. The flexion moment and injury scores were significantly greater with the flexion-compression trauma load than with the simple axial compression trauma load. In both groups, the injury score of the middle column had the highest correlation with 8 of the 9 flexibility parameters.

Discussion.—These biomechanical findings provide the first objective evidence of the validity of the 3-column theory of thoracolumbar spinal fractures and suggest that the middle column is the primary determinant of spinal stability.

▶ The standard approach to scientific advancement is the development of a hypothesis to explain an observed phenomenon, followed by adequate testing to prove or disprove the hypothesis. In 1983, Denis[1] advanced the idea of the 3-column spine and its significance in the classification of acute thoracolumbar spinal injuries. Panjabi and associates are well qualified to test this hypothesis and did so in the manner described. Their results support Denis' concept.

R.H. Wilkins, M.D.

Reference

1. Denis F: The three column spine and its significance in the classification of acute thoracolumbar spinal injuries. *Spine* 8:817–831, 1983.

Vertebral Column Injuries and Lap-Shoulder Belts
Huelke DF, Mackay GM, Morris A (Univ of Michigan, Ann Arbor; Univ of Birmingham, England)
J Trauma 38:547–556, 1995 34–12

Introduction.—Vertebral or spinal cord injuries have been rarely reported in car occupants wearing lap-shoulder belts. Reports of cervical, thoracic, and lumbar spine injuries were reviewed from experimental, medical, and engineering sources.

Methods.—Cases of vertebral column fractures or fracture dislocations were reviewed from the data banks from university field crash investigators and from the National Accident Severity Study. Only cases involving front seat occupants who were wearing 3-point lap-shoulder belts during survivable frontal crashes with no evidence of head impact or forehead/ face injury were included.

Results.—Most cervical spine injuries involved the forward subluxation of C5–C7 or fracture-dislocation injuries in the higher cervical vertebrae. These were caused by neck flexion over the shoulder restraint. Transverse process fractures, vertebral fractures, compression fractures, wedge fractures, and fracture/dislocations were seen in the thoracolumbar spine. Any of these injuries could occur with low-speed impact.

Discussion.—Inertial forces of the mass of the head acting on the neck are enough to injure the cervical spine as a result of forward flexion. Specific injuries may vary depending on the type of flexion and the presence or absence of some rotation. Thoracolumbar fractures can occur with relatively low impact accidents and are unrelated to age, height, weight, or seat location. These findings underscore the importance of testing and monitoring the performance and limitations of restraints.

▶ The development and use of belt restraints for occupants of motor vehicles have been of benefit to people involved in motor vehicle accidents. These restraints reduce the likelihood of the occupant striking the interior of the vehicle or being ejected from it. However, there are limits to the protection afforded by belt restraints, and they may themselves cause injury. For example, lap belts may cause acute flexion injuries of the thoracolumbar spine. Although these injuries are largely prevented by the use of lap-shoulder belts, such 3-point restraints do not restrain the head and neck. Thus, the cervical spine may be injured from the inertial forces of the mass of the head acting on the neck.

The authors concluded that when all crash types are considered, at all impact speeds, belt restraints are effective in reducing the frequency of injuries and deaths. Yet, in some specific crashes, the belt restraint systems are associated with injury to specific body areas. It is probable that the incidence of cervical and thoracolumbar spinal injuries can be further reduced in frontal crashes if an air bag system is also used.

R.H. Wilkins, M.D.

Utility of MR Imaging in Pediatric Spinal Cord Injury

Felsberg GJ, Tien RD, Osumi AK, et al (Duke Univ, Durham, NC)
Pediatr Radiol 25:131–135, 1995   34–13

Background.—Children reportedly sustain 1% to 10% of the nearly 10,000 traumatic spinal cord injuries occurring each year in the United States. The ability of MRI to detect acute and subacute spinal cord injuries in children was retrospectively reviewed.

Patients and Methods.—The MR images of 22 children with suspected traumatic spinal cord injuries occurring during a 6-year period were evaluated. Patient age ranged from 8 months to 18 years. The mean time between injury and MR examination was 60 hours. Findings on MRI were compared with physical examination results and with those obtained on radiographic and CT assessment.

Results.—The MR images showed abnormalities in 12 patients. Spinal cord contusions, 5 of which were hemorrhagic, were observed in 7 patients. All 5 children with MR evidence of spinal cord hemorrhagic contusions remained severely disabled with residual paralysis/paresis on follow-up. Abnormal radiographic and CT findings were seen in only 2 of the 7 patients with cord contusion. The MR images also showed traumatic changes occurring outside the cord in 5 patients. These included ligamentous injury, disk herniation, and epidural hematomas. Vertebral fractures in 4 of the 5 children with neck or back pain were observed on both MR and CT images; however, ligamentous injury and epidural hemorrhage were shown only on the MR images.

Conclusion.—In children with acute and subacute spinal cord injuries, MRI is able to provide information not obtained by radiographs and CT scans, and it is useful in predicting future neurologic function.

▶ It has become apparent in recent years that MRI can provide diagnostic information about patients with spinal cord injury that cannot be obtained by any other method. The identification of ligamentous disruption, epidural hematoma formation, and acute disk herniation is important in treatment decisions, but of greater importance is the identification of changes within the spinal cord that are critical to prognosis. All of this is especially true in children, who are more likely than adults to have spinal cord injury without radiographic abnormality (i.e., by radiologic diagnostic methods other than MRI).

R.H. Wilkins, M.D.

Open Reduction of Traumatic Atlanto-Axial Rotatory Dislocation With Use of the Extreme Lateral Approach: A Report of Two Cases
Crockard HA, Rogers MA (Natl Hosp for Neurology and Neurosurgery, London)
J Bone Joint Surg (Am) 78A:431–436, 1996   34–14

Introduction.—Early closed reduction of atlantoaxial rotatory dislocation is ideal, with distraction and derotation, held by external bracing. However, when this strategy fails, the joint may fuse in its malaligned position (Fig 1), which can result in torticollis and facial asymmetry. An operative approach to irreducible atlantoaxial rotatory dislocation was described.

Surgical Technique.—Patients were placed in the true lateral position. After palpation of the tip of the transverse process of the atlas, the approach to the cephalad 3 cervical vertebrae was accomplished with an incision from the mastoid process along the posterior margin of the posterior triangle using the fat planes under the sternocleidomastoid that extend caudally to the vertebral artery (Fig 3). The dissection continued through the prevertebral fascia, the fat plane posteromedial to the levator scapulae and splenius cervicis muscles to the vertebral artery between the axis and atlas and the second cervical nerve root (Fig 4). If the vertebral artery had to be mobilized, attachments of the inferior oblique, splenius cervicis, and levator scapulae muscles to the tip of the transverse foramen of the first cervical vertebra were detached.

> *Case 1.*—Girl, 10 years, experienced severe neck pain, dysesthesia, and torticollis after undergoing biopsy of a cervical lymph node under general anesthesia. An atlantoaxial rotatory dislocation and partial occipitoatlantal dislocation were confirmed by radiographic studies (see Fig 1). After 3 months, she was treated ineffectively with a manipulation of the cervical spine and traction. Subsequent laminectomy at the first and second cervical levels was also ineffective. The patient then underwent open reduction. It was necessary to remove a substantial amount of fibrous tissue and articular cartilage from between the joints and to use an osteotome to divide the odontoid, using a bilateral approach. Two years postoperatively she had full neck flexion and extension, lateral rotation of 60 degrees to the right or left, and no neurologic sequelae.

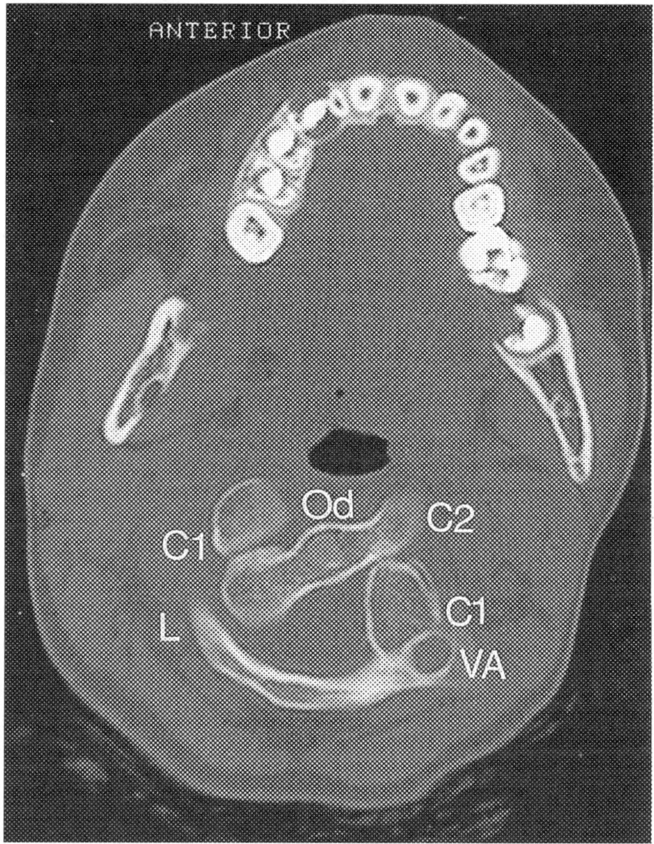

FIGURE 1.—Computed tomography scan of girl in case 1 showing complete bilateral atlantoaxial rotatory dislocation. *Abbreviations: C1*, the articular surface of the lateral mass of the atlas; *Od*, the base of the odontoid process; *C2*, the axis; *VA*, the vertebral artery in the transverse foramen; *L*, the lamina of the atlas. (Courtesy of Crockard HA, Rogers MA: Open reduction of traumatic atlanto-axial rotatory dislocation with use of the extreme lateral approach: A report of two cases. *J Bone Joint Surg [Am]* 78A:431–436, 1996.)

Case 2.—Girl, 4 years, had severe neck pain and torticollis after a motor vehicle accident. An atlantoaxial rotatory injury, revealed by radiographs, was treated initially with analgesics and a collar, followed by several weeks of continuous traction, which failed to correct the dislocation. She underwent open reduction, which required mobilization of the vertebral artery and removal of fibrous tissue and articular cartilage from the joint surfaces to relocate the joint. Two years postoperatively she had no torticollis, 90 degrees of lateral rotation to the right, 70 degrees of lateral rotation to the left, and no neurologic sequelae.

Discussion.—Successful closed reduction must be performed immediately after the injury. If this is not possible, traction will not be useful. In

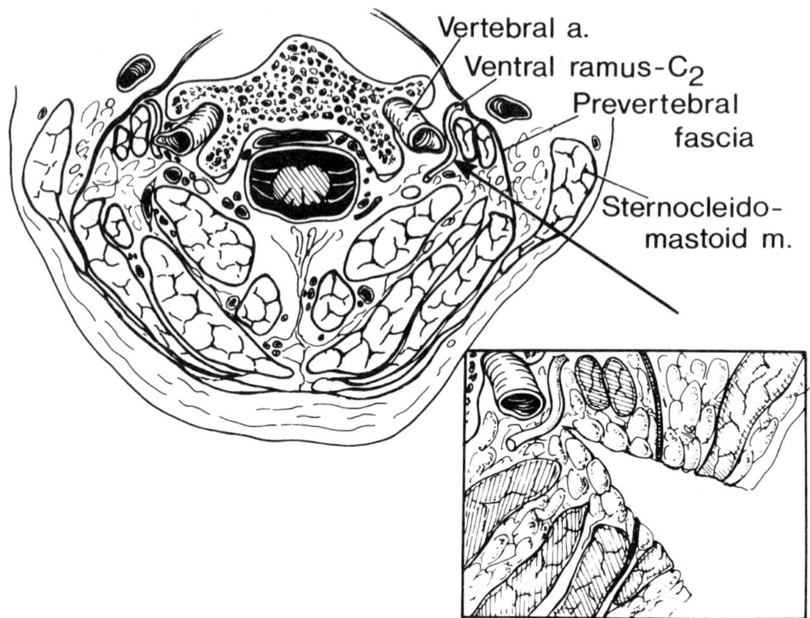

FIGURE 3.—With the extreme lateral approach, a vertical incision is made in the sternocleidomastoid muscle to gain access to the fibrofatty layer leading caudad to the lateral masses of the first and second cervical vertebrae. (Courtesy of Crockard HA, Rogers MA: Open reduction of traumatic atlanto-axial rotatory dislocation with use of the extreme lateral approach: A report of two cases. *J Bone Joint Surg [Am]* 78A:431–436, 1996.)

patients with irreducible atlantoaxial rotatory injuries, open reduction will be necessary. However, because of the potential for complications, the procedure should be performed only by surgeons who regularly operate on the cephalad part of the cervical spine.

▶ Traumatic atlantoaxial rotatory dislocation presents a problem in management if the abnormal alignment cannot be reduced by distraction and derotation. In this paper Crockard and Rogers described a surgical technique that permits the restoration of normal anatomical relationships.

R.H. Wilkins, M.D.

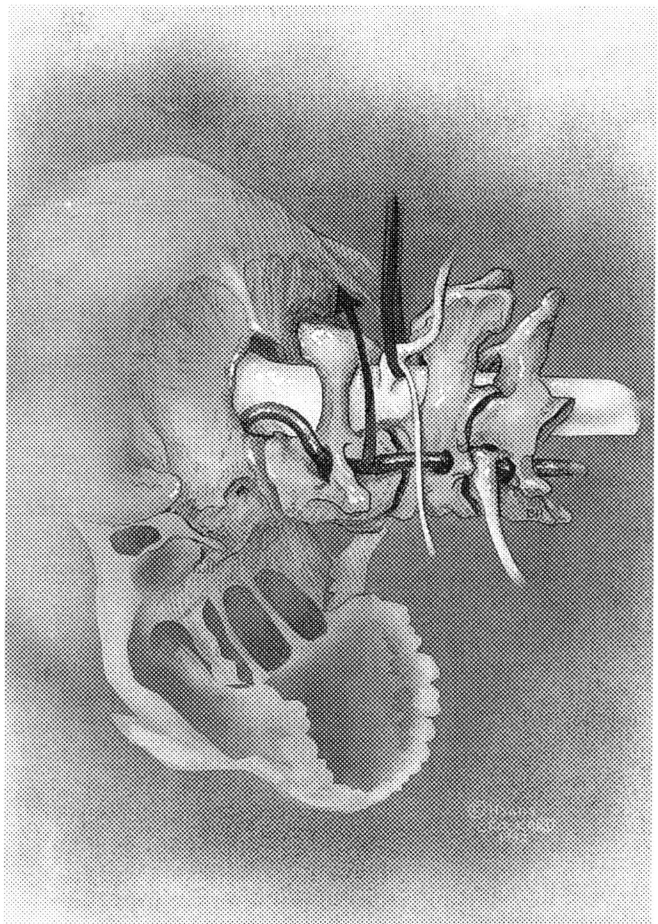

FIGURE 4.—Elevation of the second cervical nerve root exposes the vertebral artery and, deep to it, the joint between the first and second cervical vertebrae. Mobilization of the vertebral artery from the transverse foramen (*arrow*) exposes all of the joint. (Courtesy of Crockard HA, Rogers MA: Open reduction of traumatic atlanto-axial rotatory dislocation with use of the extreme lateral approach: A report of two cases. *J Bone Joint Surg [Am]* 78A:431–436, 1996.)

Injuries Involving the Transverse Atlantal Ligament: Classification and Treatment Guidelines Based Upon Experience With 39 Injuries

Dickman CA, Greene KA, Sonntag VKH (St Joseph's Hosp and Med Ctr, Phoenix, Ariz)
Neurosurgery 38:44–50, 1996

34–15

Background.—No comprehensive studies of acute traumatic disruptions of the transverse atlantal ligament have been published. The in vivo pathoanatomy of injuries involving the transverse atlantal ligament was documented for the first time.

Methods and Findings.—Thirty-nine patients underwent comprehensive anatomical and clinical assessment. Upper cervical spinal injuries were examined on plain radiographs, thin-section CT, and MRI. Sixteen injuries were classified as type I (disruptions of the substance of the ligament) and 23 were classified as type II (fractures and avulsions involving the tubercle for insertion of the transverse ligament on the C1 lateral mass; Fig 1). The clinical characteristics of these 2 injury types could be used to determine treatment. Type I injuries were unable to heal satisfactorily without internal fixation. Early surgery was most effective for such injuries. Initial treatment with rigid cervical orthosis was most effective for type II injuries, which resulted in an incompetent transverse ligament physiologically even though the ligament substance was not torn. These injuries had a 74% success rate when managed nonoperatively. Surgery was appropriate for patients with type II injuries showing nonunion with persistent instability after 3 to 4 months of immobilization. The rate of immobilization failure was 26% among patients with type II injuries, indicating the need for close monitoring to identify patients subsequently needing surgery.

Conclusion.—Treatment of upper cervical spinal injury must be based on the extent of injury to the ligaments and bone structures involved. Early surgery for internal fixation is indicated for type I injuries, which are unable to heal otherwise. Nonoperative treatment using external immobilization is sufficient for three fourths of the patients with type II injuries.

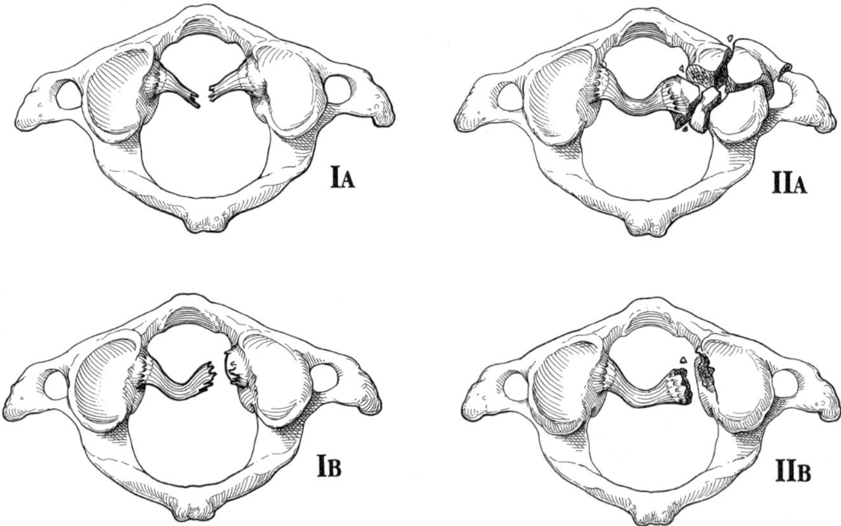

FIGURE 1.—Classification of injuries to the transverse atlantal ligament. Type I injuries disrupt the ligament substance in its midportion (**IA**) or at its periosteal insertion (**IB**). Type II injuries disconnect the tubercle for insertion of the transverse ligament from the C1 lateral mass involving a comminuted C1 lateral mass (**IIA**) or avulsing the tubercle from an intact lateral mass (**IIB**). (Courtesy of Dickman CA, Greene KA, Sonntag VKH: Injuries involving the transverse atlantal ligament: Classification and treatment guidelines based upon experience with 39 injuries. *Neurosurgery* 38:44–50, 1996. From Barrow Neurological Institute.)

▶ It is well recognized in the area of spinal trauma that reunited bone fragments have a high likelihood of healing, whereas ligamentous disruption may not result in firm healing and thus may cause continuing spinal instability at the level of the injury. Dickman et al. assessed a series of patients with injuries involving the transverse atlantal ligament and both classified these injuries and developed sound treatment guidelines based on their experience.

R.H. Wilkins, M.D.

Nonoperative Management of Types II and III Odontoid Fractures: The Philadelphia Collar Versus the Halo Vest
Polin RS, Szabo T, Bogaev CA, et al (Univ of Virginia, Charlottesville)
Neurosurgery 38:450–457, 1996   34–16

Introduction.—There have been many attempts to find options to the halo apparatus for the nonsurgical management of odontoid fractures. The nonsurgical management of odontoid fractures was compared in patients managed in cervical orthoses and halo vests.

Methods.—Of the 54 patients, 36 had type II fractures and 18 had type III fractures. Average patient age was 50.7. Patients were nonrandomly assigned by their attending physician into halo vest and rigid orthosis groups.

Results.—Twenty patients in the type II fracture group were treated in the halo vest and 16 were treated in a neck orthosis. Five patients in the type II group showed a persistent, unhealed fracture line, but were stable to flexion/extension, 7 remained unstable to flexion/extension, and 4 eventually required late surgical intervention for persistent instability (Table 3). One patient died of aspiration pneumonia after receiving a closed head injury in the hospital when attempting to walk while in the halo vest. Significantly more patients younger than 40 (9/82%) in the type II group achieved fracture union, compared with patients older than 60 (7/50%).

Five of 18 patients in the type III fracture group were managed in the halo vest. The remaining 5 wore a rigid orthosis. All patients with type III odontoid fractures showed fracture healing and stability to flexion/extension on postimmobilization radiographs.

A comparison of 16 patients managed in the rigid cervical orthosis and 20 patients placed in the halo vest for type II fractures showed similar rates of late surgical intervention. The overall rate of instability was 27% (4 of 15) in the cervical orthosis group and 16% (3 of 19) in the halo vest group. Treatment failures were observed in 7 of 15 patients managed in a rigid collar and in 5 of 19 patients with halo vests (see Table 3). This difference in healing between groups was not significant. The mean age of type II patients managed in a rigid collar was 69 and was 48.5 for those in halo vest. The age difference was significant.

Conclusion.—There was an overall 23% incidence of late instability to flexion/extension in patients with type II odontoid fractures. In patients

TABLE 3.—Comparison of Treatment of Type II Fractures With Cervical Orthoses and Halo Vests

Patient Group (No.)	Average Displacement (mm)	Average Age (yr)	No. of Patients Healed/Stable*	No. of Patients Not Healed/Stable†	No. of Patients Healed/Stable‡	No. of Patients Not Healed§
All (35)	4.0	53	22	5	1	7
Cervical orthosis (16)	3.5	68	8	3	1	4
Halo vest (19)	4.5	44	14	2	0	3

Note: No statistical difference between nonsurgical treatment groups was demonstrated. One early death in the halo group was excluded.
* No evidence of instability to flexion/extension and solid bone fusion across fracture line.
† No evidence of instability to flexion/exstension but no solid bone fusion across fracture line.
‡ Instability to flexion/extension but solid bone fusion across fracture line.
§ Neither stability to flexion/extension nor solid bone fusion across fracture line.
(Courtesy of Polin RS, Szabo T, Bogaev CA, et al: Nonoperative management of types II and III odontoid fractures: The Philadelphia collar versus the halo vest. *Neurosurgery* 38:450–457, 1996.)

with type III fractures, there was a 34% rate of fracture line persistence with no late instability. Four patients with type II fracture required late fusion. No patients with type III fracture required surgery. There was no significant between-group difference in the rate of instability and the need for late fusion in patients managed with a rigid collar or halo vest. Because the halo vest is associated with morbidity and discomfort, all patients with type III fractures should be managed in a rigid collar. It is also recommended that in the nonoperative management of type II fractures that the rigid collar orthosis be used instead of the halo vest because there was no difference in patient outcome in this series.

▶ The authors supplied data to support their contention that a rigid cervical orthosis is as effective as halo immobilization in the treatment of type II and III odontoid fractures, with better patient comfort and less risk.

R.H. Wilkins, M.D.

Clinical Syndromes Associated With Disproportionate Weakness of the Upper Versus the Lower Extremities After Cervical Spinal Cord Injury
Levi ADO, Tator CH, Bunge RP (Univ of Toronto; Univ of Miami, Fla)
Neurosurgery 38:179–185, 1996   34–17

Background.—Patients with cervical spinal cord injuries initially seen with hand and arm weakness or paralysis and relatively preserved lower extremity strength are usually considered to have cruciate paralysis or acute central cervical spinal cord injury. The presence of a localized injury in a somatotopically organized corticospinal tract has been assumed, which would explain the pathophysiologic findings of dissociated strength in the upper vs. lower extremities. However, evidence suggests that there is no somatotopic organization in the corticospinal tract in the medulla or cervical spinal cord in primates. An alternative hypothesis for these 2 syndromes was presented.

Alternative Hypothesis.—Greater hand and arm weakness relative to leg weakness can occur when injury affects the corticospinal tract (CST) anywhere from the medulla to the cervical enlargement. Because the main function of the CST is to subserve fine motor movements to the distal musculature, especially of the upper limbs, CST injury tends to result in relatively greater dysfunction in the hand and arms than in the legs. Relative leg movement and locomotor activity is retained because other fiber tracts in the spinal cord can mediate these motor activities.

Conclusion.—The alternative mechanism proposed is consistent with the evidence of no somatotopic organization to the CST in monkey or human cervical spinal cords. This mechanism also unifies a spectrum of cervical spinal cord injuries, resulting in similar clinical syndromes, such as cruciate paralysis and acute central cervical spinal cord injury.

▶ The authors provided a unifying explanation for disproportionate limb weakness in patients with cervicomedullary or cervical spinal cord injury.

R.H. Wilkins, M.D.

Post-Traumatic Syringomyelia (Cystic Myelopathy): A Prospective Study of 449 Patients With Spinal Cord Injury

Schurch B, Wichmann W, Rossier AB (Zurich Univ, Switzerland; Univ Hosp, Zurich, Switzerland; Tufts Univ, Boston)
J Neurol Neurosurg Psychiatry 60:61–67, 1996   34–18

Background.—Posttraumatic syringomyelia (PTS) is being reported with increasing frequency, perhaps because of the greater use of MRI for early diagnosis. A group of 449 traumatic paraplegic and tetraplegic patients was studied prospectively to determine the incidence of PTS and to correlate its presence with common symptoms and signs.

Methods.—The study group included all patients with posttraumatic spinal injury admitted to the Swiss Paraplegic Centre from 1987 through 1993. Patients were followed until July 1, 1994, and most were seen clinically at least once yearly. In most cases MRI was performed on the day of injury, then annually after diagnosis of PTS. Each scan was read by 2 radiologists.

Results.—A diagnosis of PTS was confirmed by MRI in 20 (4.45%) patients. The diagnosis was made at a mean of 9.4 years after the spinal injury; the first symptoms of PTS occurred at a mean of 7.2 years after the trauma. Thus, diagnosis was delayed for a mean of 2.3 years after symptom onset. The most common symptom was a dull aching or burning pain that was made worse by coughing or straining. In 10 of 12 patients, pain was located at or above the site of the original injury. Two patients had numbness but no pain. Sensory disturbances and decreased deep tendon reflexes in the upper or lower limbs were the most common clinical signs of PTS.

Seven patients were managed surgically and 13 were treated conservatively, including 3 who refused surgery. Pain disappeared in 6 patients treated surgically and motor improvement was noted in 5. All patients treated conservatively remained stable clinically except for those who had refused surgery. Findings at MRI indicated that cord compression, tense syrinx, and kyphosis at the fracture site were related to enlargement of the syrinx and further neurologic deterioration.

Conclusion.—Regular evaluation of patients with spinal cord injury is necessary to diagnose PTS, because symptoms may be delayed for many years after the injury. Progressive muscle weakness, severe pain, or both are indications for surgery. In operated patients, neurologic improvement or stabilization correlated with collapse of the cyst.

▶ Schurch et al. provided a current account of PTS.

R.H. Wilkins, M.D.

Low-Velocity Gunshot Wounds to the Spine With an Associated Transperitoneal Injury
Lin SS, Vaccaro AR, Reisch S, et al (Thomas Jefferson Univ Hosp, Philadelphia)
J Spinal Disord 8:136–144, 1995   34–19

Background.—Civilian gunshot wounds to the spine, usually caused by low-velocity missiles, are treated differently from high-velocity combat injuries in several ways, 1 of which is the use of débridement. This procedure, with operative decompression, seems to increase morbidity without improving neurologic status, and nonoperative treatment is often favored for patients with incomplete neurologic deficits and without neural compression. When the gunshot wound is accompanied by a transperitoneal injury, the role of débridement is particularly controversial because of the risk of meningitis and other infections secondary to viscus perforation and bacterial contamination. Outcomes for 29 patients treated at 1 spinal cord injury center where routine débridement of the spinal wound is not practiced were reviewed.

Methods.—The patients (25 males and 4 females) were admitted to the Regional Spinal Cord Injury Center of Delaware Valley of Thomas Jefferson University between 1979 and 1992 with low-velocity gunshot wounds to the spine associated with a transperitoneal injury. Their charts and radiographs were reviewed to determine initial neurologic status and neurologic status at follow-up (average 44.9 months), as well as the presence of postinjury infectious complications. All patients underwent emergency exploratory laparotomy soon after arrival at the hospital, without débridement of the missile tract or removal of the bullet unless it was easily accessible. Colon injuries were treated by colostomy and Hartmann's pouch or colectomy and primary anastomosis. Parenchymal injuries were treated as needed.

Results.—Fourteen of the patients had multiple gunshot wounds, resulting in a total of 32 spinal injuries and 53 intra-abdominal injuries in 29 patients. Sixteen patients had viscus injuries, and 17 had parenchymal injuries. In 9 cases, entrance and exit wounds were present without retained bullet fragments, whereas 20 patients had retained fragments in or around the spine. Seventeen of the 21 patients with a parenchymal or noncolonic viscous injury (or both) received IV antibiotics for at least 5 days, and the remaining 4 received antibiotics for 48 hours or less. One (4.7%) of these 21 patients subsequently developed an infectious complication (subdiaphragmatic abscess). All 8 patients with a colonic injury received antibiotics for at least 5 days. Psoas abscesses developed in 2 (25%) of these 8 patients. Spinal infections did not develop in any patient.

Discussion.—Patients with low-velocity gunshot wounds and transperitoneal injuries do not require spinal débridement and may be treated with parenteral antibiotics to reduce the risk of infectious complications. The low morbidity among patients with noncolonic viscus or parenchymal injuries is similar to that in other published studies, and the lower infection rate in these patients with colonic injuries may result from the longer use of antibiotics (≥5 days).

▶ The neurosurgeon is occasionally asked to treat a patient with a low-velocity gunshot wound of the spine in whom the bullet has also passed through the peritoneal cavity. Lin et al. showed that antibiotic treatment seems to be sufficient to prevent spinal infection, without the need for spinal débridement.

R.H. Wilkins, M.D.

Neoplasms

Magnetic Resonance Imaging Differentiation of Compression Spine Fractures or Vertebral Lesions Caused by Osteoporosis or Tumor
Rupp RE, Ebraheim NA, Coombs RJ (Med College of Ohio, Toledo)
Spine 20:2499–2504, 1995
34–20

Background.—It often is difficult to accurately assess compression fractures of the spine radiographically if malignancy is a possibility, especially in elderly patients who are at risk of osteoporotic fracture. Characteristic MR findings have been described, but most studies have included a limited number of biopsy-confirmed cases.

Objective.—The MR findings of 34 patients with either an atraumatic compression fracture of the spine or a vertebral lesion of unknown origin who underwent MRI before biopsy were reviewed. Twenty patients had lumbar spinal lesions, 13 had thoracic spinal lesions, and 1 had a cervical spinal lesion.

Methods.—Sagittal and axial T1- and T2-weighted images were recorded in all patients. Twenty-one patients, 12 with tumor and 9 with osteoporosis, had contrast studies. The definitive diagnosis was made by CT-guided percutaneous biopsy in 32 cases and open biopsy in 2.

Findings.—A primary spinal tumor or metastatic disease was detected in 18 patients, whereas 16 had biopsy findings of osteoporosis. The findings of decreased signal activity on T1-weighted images and increased T2-weighted signal were sensitive signs of tumor involvement but were not specific. Normal marrow findings in a compressed vertebral body on T1-weighted images were consistent with osteoporosis. Contrast enhancement, posterior vertebral expansion, and involvement of multiple levels all failed to distinguish between osteoporotic and neoplastic involvement. Involvement of a pedicle and an adjacent soft-tissue mass were specific findings of neoplastic disease.

Conclusion.—Magnetic resonance imaging may permit a distinction between osteoporotic and neoplastic disease in patients with a compression fracture of the spine or an unknown vertebral lesion.

▶ The radiologic differentiation of vertebral lesions due to osteoporosis from those caused by neoplastic growth can be difficult. The authors provided helpful guidelines for making this differentiation with MRI.

R.H. Wilkins, M.D.

Spinal Tumors in Patients With Neurofibromatosis Type 2: MR Imaging Study of Frequency, Multiplicity, and Variety

Mautner V-F, Tatagiba M, Lindenau M, et al (Allgemeines Krankenhaus Hamburg Ochsenzoll, Hamburg, Germany; Nordstadtkrankenhaus Hannover, Germany; Hamburg-Othmarschen MRI Inst, Hamburg, Germany; et al)

AJR 165:951–955, 1995

34–21

Background.—Neurofibromatosis type 2 (NF2), a rare autosomal dominant disorder, results in various CNS tumors. Bilateral vestibular schwannomas are the hallmark of the disease. Patients with a single symptomatic spinal tumor sometimes have multiple asymptomatic spinal lesions. The frequency, multiplicity, and variety of spinal tumors in patients with NF2 were reported.

Methods.—Seventy-three patients with NF2 underwent MRI of the whole spinal canal. Patient age ranged from 4 to 69.

Findings.—Of the patients, 89% showed evidence of spinal tumors on MR images. Multiplicity of tumors was found in 41 patients (56%). Intramedullary tumors were seen on MR in 24 patients, including 3 pathologically proved ependymomas. Two patients had a syrinx associated with the tumor. Intradural extramedullary and extradural tumors were seen on the cervical spine images of 36 patients, on thoracic spine images of 40, and on lumbar spine images of 49. Ten schwannomas, 7 meningiomas, and 2 neurofibromas were proved pathologically. Tumor type was confirmed by histologic assessment of 22 tumors in 19 patients.

Conclusion.—Spinal tumors are common in patients with NF2. These tumors are often multiple and of a variety of histologic types. The presence of multiple spinal tumors of different pathologic types strongly suggests NF2. Detecting spinal tumors in patients who do not meet the diagnostic criteria for NF2 may enable the diagnosis in at-risk family members, thus permitting appropriate genetic counseling.

▶ These authors documented that patients with NF2 frequently have intraspinal tumors and often have multiple intraspinal tumors.

R.H. Wilkins, M.D.

Long-Term Outcome After Removal of Spinal Schwannoma: A Clinico-pathological Study of 187 Cases

Seppälä MT, Haltia MJJ, Sankila RJ, et al (Helsinki Univ; Finnish Cancer Registry, Helsinki)
J Neurosurg 83:621–626, 1995

34–22

Introduction.—Nearly one third of all primary spinal tumors are schwannomas. Ordinarily these neoplasms are benign and can be totally removed. Patients who are not too disabled at the time of resection have an encouraging short-term outcome, but late complications such as spinal deformity and arachnoiditis are possible.

Series.—The long-term outcome was assessed in 187 patients operated on for spinal schwannoma at a single neurosurgery department from 1953 to 1985. The median follow-up interval was just short of 13 years.

Early Surgical Results.—All the schwannomas were removed by partial or total laminectomy. Fourteen patients had an emergency operation. Two thirds of the tumors were completely intradural. There were 2 primary operative deaths, and a third patient died after a second reoperation. Ten percent of patients had postoperative complications. Of 142 patients examined a few months postoperatively, 78% were improved and 7% were worse. All but 10 of 53 patients who were unable to walk before surgery regained ambulatory function.

Long-Term Outcome.—Local or radiating pain was the most common problem at follow-up, reported by more than half the patients, but pain usually was mild or intermittent. Of 127 assessable patients, 43% had returned to their previous work and another 3% to less demanding work. Twenty-eight patients (22%) were unable to work. Cystic myelopathy developed in 2 patients during follow-up, and 8 (6%) had spinal arachnoiditis or medullary atrophy. Spinal deformity developed in 6% of those followed up. Eleven of 20 incompletely removed tumors recurred, but reoperation was performed on only 2.

Conclusion.—Spinal schwannomas are, in general, benign tumors associated with long-term survival. The results of resection correlate closely with the patient's preoperative status.

▶ Seppälä et al. analyzed patient outcome after the resection of a spinal schwannoma in a relatively large series. The unique feature of their report is the information they collected about long-term results. Of note is the fact that among 127 patients followed up for a median time of 12.9 years, only 27 (21%) were asymptomatic.

R.H. Wilkins, M.D.

Miscellaneous Disorders

MRI of 'Idiopathic' Juvenile Scoliosis: A Prospective Study

Evans SC, Edgar MA, Hall-Craggs MA, et al (Middlesex Hosp, London)
J Bone Joint Surg (Br) 78B:314–317, 1996   34–23

Objective.—Juvenile idiopathic scoliosis is relatively uncommon. With the availability of MRI, studies have found a preponderance of syringomyelia, often associated with Chiari I malformation, in the juvenile age group. Recent reviews have identified a possible association between syringomyelia and some cases of idiopathic scoliosis. Patients with juvenile scoliosis were prospectively studied by MRI.

Methods.—The study included 31 consecutive patients with idiopathic scoliosis detected between the ages of 4 and 12 years. Twenty-four were girls (mean age 9 years), and 7 were boys (mean age 7 years). All underwent MRI scanning of the hind brain and spinal cord to seek evidence of syrinx formation, spinal dysraphism, and cord neoplasms.

Results.—Twenty-six percent of patients had a significant neuroanatomic abnormality detected on MRI. Six of these 8 patients had Chiari I malformation associated with a syrinx, 1 had isolated Chiari I malformation, and 1 had astrocytoma of the cervical spinal cord. Four of these patients had a left-sided thoracic curve compared with only 3 of 23 patients with normal neuroanatomical findings. None of the clinical features examined could distinguish between patients with and without MRI abnormalities. Unilateral absence of abdominal reflexes was found in 12% of patients with neuroanatomic abnormalities and 9% of those without.

Conclusion.—Magnetic resonance imaging of the hind brain and spinal cord detects Chiari I malformation and other neuroanatomic abnormalities in many patients with apparent "idiopathic" juvenile scoliosis. It is potentially dangerous to undertake surgical treatment of scoliosis in a patient with undecompressed syringomyelia, and significant improvement may follow decompression of the foramen magnum. Thus, MRI scanning should be mandatory for all patients with juvenile-onset scoliosis.

▶ Evans et al. reminded us that juvenile scoliosis is not always idiopathic and that preoperative assessment by MRI may reveal the cause and lead to safer surgical treatment.

R.H. Wilkins, M.D.

Pathological Basis of Spinal Cord Cavitation in Syringomyelia: Analysis of 105 Autopsy Cases

Milhorat TH, Capocelli AL Jr, Anzil AP, et al (State Univ of New York Health Science Ctr, Brooklyn; Kings County Hosp Ctr, Brooklyn, NY)
J Neurosurg 82:802–812, 1995

34–24

Background.—The pathogenesis of cavitary formation in syringomyelia may have clinical importance and therapeutic implications for patients. Three distinct cavitary patterns in brain and spinal cord autopsy specimens taken from 105 patients with non-neoplastic syringomyelia were identified.

Methods.—Clinical data and general autopsy data on 105 patients who underwent a standard complete autopsy were collected. Material from the brain and spinal cord was fixed and stained for histologic examination.

Results.—A communicating syrinx is defined as a tubular dilatation of the central canal that is continuous with the fourth ventricle; it is associated with hydrocephalus. A noncommunicating or isolated syrinx consists of a focal dilatation of the central canal that is separated at variable distances from the fourth ventricle; it is associated with Chiari I malformation, basilar impression, and arachnoiditis. The third pattern found is associated with spinal cord injury, such as trauma and hemorrhage; it does not communicate with the central canal and is therefore identified as an extracanalicular syrinx.

Conclusion.—Syringomyelia has at least 3 cavitary patterns that likely have prognostic and therapeutic implications. Prognosis correlates with histologic findings.

▶ Dr. Milhorat has studied the pathology and pathophysiology of syringomyelia for a number of years. This paper is representative of his important contributions to what is known about this perplexing condition.

R.H. Wilkins, M.D.

Synovial Cysts of the Lumbar Spine: Diagnosis, Surgical Management, and Pathogenesis Report of Eight Cases

Yarde WL, Arnold PM, Kepes JJ, et al (Univ of Kansas, Kansas City)
Surg Neurol 43:459–465, 1995

34–25

Background.—Intraspinal extradural synovial cysts, which usually arise from the zygoapophyseal joint capsule, are filled with clear or xanthochromic fluid and have a synovial-like lining with communication to a synovial sheath or joint capsule. These cysts—most commonly occurring at the L4–5 level, sometimes at the L5–S1 and L3–4 levels—are an unusual cause of lower back pain and radiculopathy. Eight patients with lumbar synovial cysts were reviewed.

Patients.—The patients were evaluated by a neurosurgery service over a 5½-year period. The symptoms included lower extremity radiculopathy in all patients and dysesthesia in some. Symptoms had been present for 2 to 16 months and were progressive in all patients. Plain radiographs of the lumbar spine showed moderate to severe degenerative changes. Magnetic resonance imaging was performed in all patients and helped in making the correct diagnosis in 4. Computed tomographic myelography was done in 4 patients but was not helpful. Laminectomy or hemilaminectomy and cyst excision were performed in all patients, who were followed for at least 1 year.

Outcomes.—Histopathologic examination confirmed the presence of a synovial cyst. Seven of the 8 patients had dramatic pain relief after surgery, including complete resolution of pain in 5. One patient had persistent pain, which resolved after removal of scar tissue 6 months after the initial operation. Lower extremity weakness resolved in 5 of 5 cases, and dysesthesia was lessened or the same in all patients. Lumbar fusion was done at the same time as cyst excision in 2 patients with spondylolisthesis.

Discussion.—Synovial cysts of the lumbar spine are an uncommon cause of pain and radiculopathy. Magnetic resonance imaging appears to be the most reliable diagnostic study. Surgery is a safe and effective treatment that often yields dramatic improvement.

▶ Just a decade ago, synovial and ganglion cysts of the spinal canal were considered a rarity. With the widespread use of postmyelographic CT scanning and MRI it has become apparent that these lesions are not rare. In the lumbar region, where they are most often found, they must be included in the differential diagnosis of disk herniation.

R.H. Wilkins, M.D.

Pigmented Villonodular Synovitis of the Spine: A Clinical, Radiological, and Morphological Study of 12 Cases

Giannini C, Scheithauer BW, Wenger DE, et al (Mayo Clinic, Rochester, Minn)
J Neurosurg 84:592–597, 1996

34–26

Objective.—Pigmented villonodular synovitis (PVNS) is a lesion involving the synovial membrane of joints or tendon sheaths that usually affects the appendicular skeleton in young patients. Pigmented villonodular synovitis involving the axial skeleton is rare, so little information regarding its natural history, treatment, or prognosis is available. The clinical and pathologic findings of 22 cases of PVNS of the spine were reviewed.

Methods.—Thirteen cases of PVNS involving the spine were identified, of which 10 had pathologic and radiographic material available for review; 2 of these 13 cases were excluded. The study also included 11 previously reported cases from the literature, including additional follow-up in 6 patients.

Findings.—Patients consisted of 12 women and 10 men (age range 21–81). The posterior elements of vertebrae were involved at all spinal

TABLE 3.—Treatment and Follow-Up of 22 Patients With Pigmented Villonodular Synovitis of the Spine

Treatment	No. of Cases	Recurrence of Lesion	Follow-Up Information	Duration of Follow Up (mos)*
gross-total removal	17	3 (18%)	11 cases free of disease after 1st operation	56.8 (6–132)
			3 cases of recurrence within 1 yr; patients underwent reresection; all free of disease	43 (10–96)
			3 cases in which data are not available	NA
subtotal removal/ biopsy only	3/1	none	all cases stable	37.5 (8–84)
unknown	1	NA	NA	NA

* Values represent mean. Range is provided within parentheses.
Abbreviation: NA, not available.
(Courtesy of Giannini C, Scheithauer BW, Wenger DE, et al: Pigmented villonodular synovitis of the spine: A clinical, radiological, and morphological study of 12 cases. *J Neurosurg* 84:592–597, 1996.)

levels, though the cervical and lumbar regions were most frequently affected. Eighty-nine percent of patients had facet joint involvement, and 70% had extension into the epidural space. Of 17 patients treated by gross total tumor removal, 11 were disease free at a mean follow-up of 57 months. Four patients treated with subtotal tumor removal or biopsy only were in stable condition without disease progression at a mean follow-up of 38 months (Table 3). Local recurrence rate was 18%, but repeat surgical excision was apparently curative.

Conclusion.—Pigmented villonodular synovitis of the axial skeleton is rare. The present review strengthens the theory that the condition originates in the synovial membrane lining the diarthrodial joints of the vertebral arches. The differential diagnosis may be difficult because of the unusual location of the disease and its ability to cause bone destruction. Treatment should consist of gross total removal; subtotal resection may also control the disease.

▶ The authors reviewed their experience with an unusual condition, PVNS of the spine and also summarized the limited information about it in the medical literature. Although the associated destruction of bone may suggest a malignant lesion, the overall outlook with surgical treatment is good, as shown in Table 3.

R.H. Wilkins, M.D.

Spontaneous Spinal Cerebrospinal Fluid Leaks and Intracranial Hypotension

Schievink WI, Meyer FB, Atkinson JLD, et al (Mayo Clinic, Rochester, Minn)
J Neurosurg 84:598–605, 1996
34–27

Introduction.—Some cases of spontaneous intracranial hypotension are attributed to spinal CSF leaks. However, few studies have provided radiographic or surgical documentation of such leaks. Eleven patients with spontaneous intracranial hypotension associated with radiographically confirmed spinal CSF leaks were reported.

Patients.—The patients, seen over a 10-year period, were 6 women and 5 men (mean age 38). The most prominent and debilitating symptom was postural headache, with other symptoms including nausea, vomiting, sixth cranial nerve paresis, and local back pain.

Findings.—In all 11 patients, a spinal CSF leak was documented by indium-111 radionuclide cisternography or CT myelography. The leak was found in the cervical spine in 2 patients, the cervicothoracic junction in 2, the thoracic spine in 5, and the lumbar spine in 1. False negative results were obtained in 30% of radionuclide cisternography studies. Cranial imaging findings included subdural fluid collections, meningeal enhancement, and downward cerebellar displacement resembling a Chiari I malformation.

Outcomes.—Most patients responded to supportive therapy or an epidural blood patch. Surgery was performed in 4 patients whose CSF leak resulted from leaking meningeal diverticula. The diverticula were successfully ligated in 3 of these patients, but the fourth had an extensive and inoperable complex of diverticula. Other findings included an unusual body habitus and joint hypermobility in 2 patients and spontaneous retinal detachment at a young age in 2.

Conclusion.—Though unusual, spontaneous spinal CSF leaks can cause spontaneous intracranial hypotension. The most frequent location of these leaks is the cervicothoracic junction or thoracic spine; associated meningeal diverticula may be present as well. The best study to demonstrate CSF leaks is CT myelography. Although the condition is self-limiting in most cases, surgery may be useful in some patients with leaking meningeal diverticula. Some patients may have an underlying connective tissue disorder.

▶ As the authors stated, and documented with their own series, spontaneous spinal CSF leaks are uncommon, but they are increasingly recognized as a cause of spontaneous intracranial hypotension.

R.H. Wilkins, M.D.

Surgical Management of Spinal Epidural Hematoma: Relationship Between Surgical Timing and Neurological Outcome

Lawton MT, Porter RW, Heiserman JE, et al (St Joseph's Hosp and Med Ctr, Phoenix, Ariz; Arizona State Univ, Tempe)
J Neurosurg 83:1–7, 1995

34–28

Background.—Spinal epidural hematoma (SEH) is uncommon, and authorities disagree on how urgently surgery should be done. One series was reviewed to determine the relationship between surgical timing and neurologic outcomes.

Methods.—Thirty patients with SEH were included in the review. The cause was spinal surgery in 12 SEHs, epidural catheters in 7, vascular lesions in 4, anticoagulation medications in 3, trauma in 2, and spontaneous in 2. Most patients' initial symptom was pain. Neurologic deficits developed in all patients. Eight patients had complete motor and sensory loss, 6 had complete motor loss with some sensation, and 16 had incomplete loss of motor function. The mean interval from onset of the initial symptoms to the maximum neurologic deficit was 13 hours. The mean interval from symptom onset to surgery was 23 hours. Treatment for all patients consisted of surgical evacuation of the hematoma.

Outcomes.—At a mean follow-up of 11 months, symptoms improved after surgery in 26 patients and remained unchanged in 4. Forty-three percent of the patients recovered completely, and 44% recovered functionally. Surgical mortality was 3%. This 1 death resulted from a pulmonary embolus. Preoperative neurologic status was associated with outcome, as was promptness of surgery, with neurologic recovery increasing as the interval from symptom onset to surgery decreased. Patients undergoing surgery within 12 hours had better neurologic outcomes than did patients with identical Frankel grades preoperatively whose treatment was delayed past that time.

Conclusion.—Neurologic recovery among patients with SEHs is maximized by rapid diagnosis and emergency surgery. Complete neurologic lesions or long-standing compression can also be substantially improved with surgical treatment.

▶ This study underscored the need for prompt recognition and evacuation of an epidural hematoma. The average postoperative Frankel grade (in numerical equivalents) decreased from 4.7/5 in patients operated on within 6 hours of symptom onset to 3.7/5 in those operated on after more than 24 hours, and there was a corresponding decrease in complete recovery rates from 67% to 12%. Of incidental interest, the cause of the hematoma was iatrogenic in 22 of 30 patients in this study.

R.H. Wilkins, M.D.

Microvascular Anatomy of Dural Arteriovenous Abnormalities of the Spine: A Microangiographic Study

McCutcheon IE, Doppman JL, Oldfield EH (Natl Inst of Neurological Disorders and Stroke, Bethesda, Md; Natl Insts of Health, Bethesda, Md)
J Neurosurg 84:215–220, 1996   34–29

Background.—Most cases of vascular abnormalities of the spinal cord are believed to result from an abnormal communication between a dural artery and medullary vein on the dura in the area of a sensory nerve root. The inability of spinal arteriography to depict these small lesions leaves the question of etiology unsettled. If an arteriovenous malformation (AVM) is present at the site of dural AV shunting, the lesion would have a congenital origin; if a direct AV fistula (AVF) is present, the lesion would be acquired. The vascular structure of dural AV abnormalities was detailed in an ex vivo study using microangiographic techniques.

Methods.—The study included 6 patients with myelopathy and confirmed spinal dural vascular malformations. All underwent en bloc resection of the involved dural root sleeve, proximal nerve root, and adjacent spinal dura. All of the lesions were between T6 and T12, at which levels resection of the dorsal nerve root causes little clinical deficit. In the microangiographic study, the vessel associated with the abnormality was cannulated for slow injection of a dilute solution of barium sulfate, during which sequential fine-grain radiography was performed.

Results.—All specimens showed a direct communication between the arterial and venous components of the lesion, and none showed the capillary glomus of a true AVM. The involved arteries split into daughter vessels, which rejoined within the outer dural layer. The serpentine loops then crossed to the inner dural surface to empty into the medullary vein, with no intervening capillary plexus. The dura also showed numerous medium to small collateral vessels arising from adjacent intercostal or lumbar arteries and converging at the fistula site to join the single medullary vein.

Conclusion.—Dural AV abnormalities of the spine were demonstrated to be direct AVFs that connect the dural branch of the radiculo-medullary-dural artery with the intradural medullary vein. The findings explain why spinal dural AVFs have a multiple segmental arterial supply and a single draining medullary vein, as well as the tendency for flow to return to the arteriovenous shunt after embolic occlusion. If embolization is selected as the treatment approach, all feeding vessels must be permanently occluded. In some patients, simply dividing the engorged medullary vein that drains the lesion may provide lasting occlusion of the AVF.

▶ The authors demonstrated the specific vascular connections of 6 dural AVFs of the spine. These observations have clinical relevance, as discussed in the paper.

R.H. Wilkins, M.D.

Preoperative Percutaneous Injection of Methyl Methacrylate and *N*-Butyl Cyanoacrylate in Vertebral Hemangiomas

Cotten A, Deramond H, Cortet B, et al (B Hosp, Lille, France; Hosp Nord, Amiens, France)
AJNR 17:137–142, 1996

34–30

Background.—Vertebral hemangioma, a common benign lesion of the spine, is often discovered incidentally. In those rare cases of a painful or aggressive lesion, surgical decompression is performed. Potential complications of surgery include profuse intraoperative bleeding, postoperative

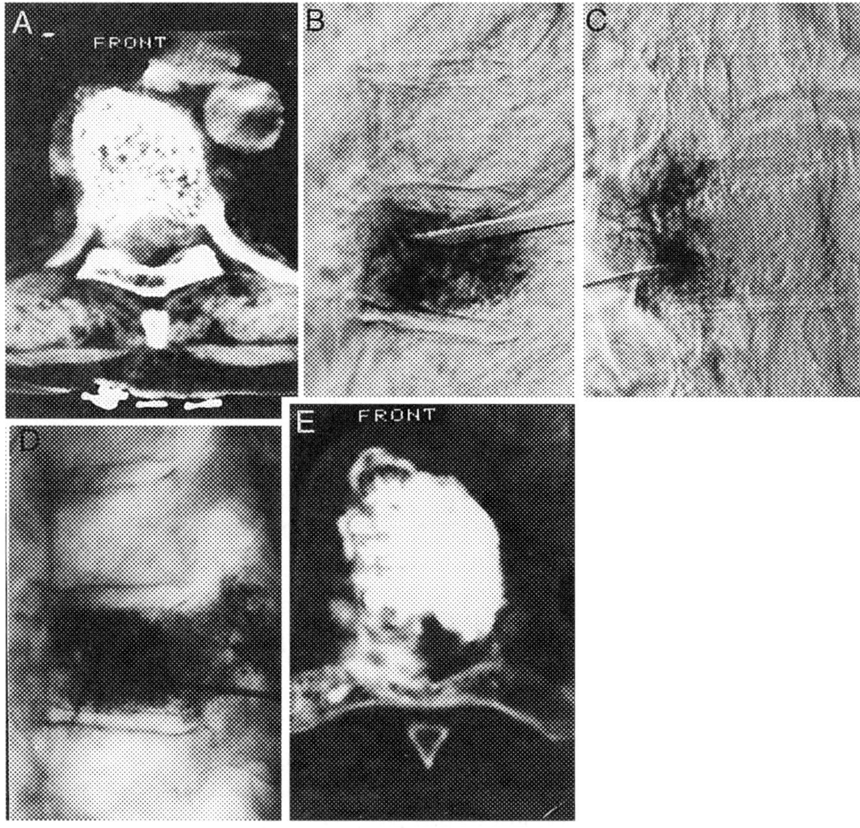

FIGURE 1.—**A,** unenhanced CT scan showing hemangioma of the body and right posterior arch of T8, with epidural component. **B,** lateral subtraction screening view showing percutaneous injection of cement into the T8 vertebral body to strengthen it. **C,** frontal subtraction screening view showing injection of N-butyl cyanoacrylate that diffuses into the epidural component of the hemangioma to optimize the blood loss during surgery. **D,** lateral subtraction screening view showing injection of N-butyl cyanoacrylate that diffuses into the epidural component of the hemangioma. **E,** unenchanced CT scan showing filling of the body of T8 by cement and diffusion of N-butyl cyanoacrylate into the right posterior arch and epidural component of the hemangioma. (Courtesy of Cotten A, Deramond H, Cortet B, et al: Preoperative percutaneous injection of methyl methacrylate and N-butyl cyanoacrylate in vertebral hemangiomas. *AJNR* 17;137–142, 1996; Copyright by American Society of Neuroradiology.)

epidural hematoma formation, and vertebral collapse. The 4 patients reported were treated preoperatively with percutaneous injections of methyl methacrylate into the vertebral body to prevent vertebral collapse and *N*-butyl cyanoacrylate into the posterior arch to minimize blood loss (Fig 1).

Patients and Methods.—Patients consisted of 2 men (aged 55 and 61 years) and 2 women (aged 63 and 71). One experienced intermittent spinal claudication, and 3 had progressive spinal cord compression. All showed the characteristic honeycombed appearance of a thoracic (3) or lumbar (1) vertebral hemangioma on CT scans. Epidural extension was present in 3 cases. The treatment consisted of 3 parts: arterial embolization was performed initially in 3 cases; 1 day later, the percutaneous injections designed to strengthen the vertebral body and to optimize hemostasis during surgery were administered; on the third day decompressive laminectomy and epidural hemangioma (when present) excision were performed.

Results.—The percutaneous injections were completed without complication and laminectomy was performed with insignificant blood loss. In 3 cases the epidural component was excised without difficulty. The patients were followed for an average of 20 months, and none showed radiographic evidence of vertebral collapse. Each patient experienced improvement in pain and neurologic symptoms in the 15 days after surgery, and the improvement in clinical status was maintained throughout follow-up.

Conclusion.—The combination of percutaneous injections used in these patients with symptomatic vertebral hemangiomas was successful in preventing the potential complications of laminectomy. Intraoperative blood loss was minimal, and strengthening of the vertebral body prevented subsequent collapse.

▶ Cotten et al. made a strong case for the preoperative percutaneous injection of symptomatic vertebral hemangiomas using methyl methacrylate and *N*-butyl cyanoacrylate.

R.H. Wilkins, M.D.

35 Peripheral Nerve Disorders

Outcome Following Conservative Management of Thoracic Outlet Syndrome
Novak CB, Collins ED, Mackinnon SE (Washington Univ, St Louis)
J Hand Surg (Am) 20:542–548, 1995   35–1

Introduction.—There have been several outcome studies of surgical treatment for thoracic outlet syndrome (TOS). Although conservative management is recommended as the initial treatment for TOS, few studies of its outcomes have been published. The subjective outcomes of patients receiving conservative management for TOS were reported.

Methods.—The study included 37 women and 5 men (mean age 38) with a clinical diagnosis of TOS who had completed a program of conservative management at least 6 months previously. Their symptoms had been present for a mean of 38 months before treatment, and their mean follow-up since the end of treatment was 1 year. Treatment consisted of posture modification and a specific physical therapy program emphasizing patient independence with effective home exercise. Data on the subjective outcomes of treatment were collected in a telephone interview.

Results.—Symptoms improved in 25 patients, were unchanged in 10, and worsened in 7. Seventeen patients reported full ability to participate in work and recreational activities, whereas 7 reported limitations in both areas. Factors associated with a poor overall outcome included obesity, workers' compensation, and associated carpal or cubital tunnel syndrome. Thirty-eight patients reported improvement in neck and shoulder symptoms. Patients without concomitant distal nerve compression reported significantly greater improvement in hand and arm pain.

Conclusion.—Conservative management yields good outcomes for many patients with TOS. The physical therapy program used in this study predictably relieves proximal neck and shoulder symptoms and hand symptoms for patients who do not have carpal or cubital tunnel syndromes. When these associated syndromes are present, patients are less likely to gain relief from symptoms of hand paresthesia and numbness.

▶ In this study the clinical diagnosis of thoracic outlet syndrome was based on patient complaints and physical findings and on the exclusion of other pathologic processes. The symptoms included pain in the cervical, scapular, and suprascapular regions that radiated to the upper extremity, as well as paresthesia or numbness extending to the hand; the symptoms were exacerbated by upper extremity work, particularly in positions above 90 degrees of shoulder flexion. Physical findings included scalene tenderness and positive provocative maneuvers, including arm elevation for 60 sec. There was no evidence of vascular insufficiency as determined by the Allen test. The treatment program, which consisted of 7 components, was comprehensive and effective. Patients with bona fide thoracic outlet syndrome should be managed in this fashion initially, and surgical treatment should be reserved for those who do not obtain sufficient relief.

R.H. Wilkins, M.D.

Anterior Interosseous Nerve Lesions: Clinical and Electrophysiological Features

Seror P (Electromyographic Lab, Paris)
J Bone Joint Surg (Br) 78B:238–241, 1996   35–2

Bacgkround.—Lesions of the anterior interosseous nerve (AIN), a motor branch of the median nerve, produce a characteristic pinch deformity between the thumb and index finger (Fig 1). Such lesions are rare and prone to misdiagnosis as tendon injuries. The clinical and electrophysiologic findings in a series of patients with AIN lesions were reviewed.

Patients.—The study included 13 patients with 14 complete or incomplete lesions of the AIN who were referred for electrophysiologic studies. Seven cases had the complete, classical pinch abnormality. The remaining 7 patients had partial motor weakness, involving isolated palsy of the

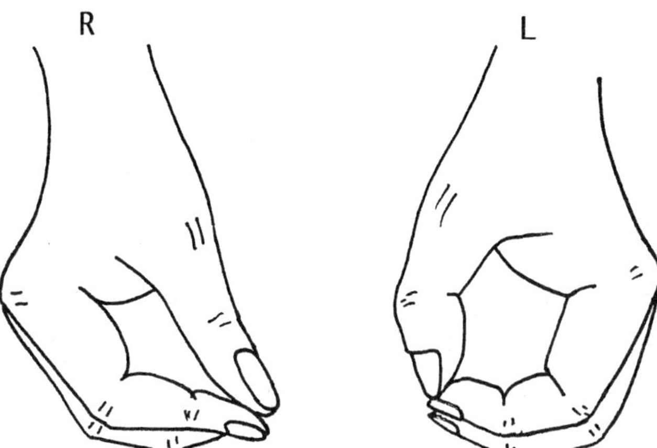

FIGURE 1.—Characteristic involvement of pinch of the right hand due to a complete lesion of the anterior interosseous nerve with palsy of flexor pollicis longus and flexor profundus of the index finger. The pinch of the left hand is normal. (Courtesy of Seror P: Anterior interosseous nerve lesions: Clinical and electrophysiologic features. *J Bone Joint Surg [Br]* 78B:238–241, 1996.)

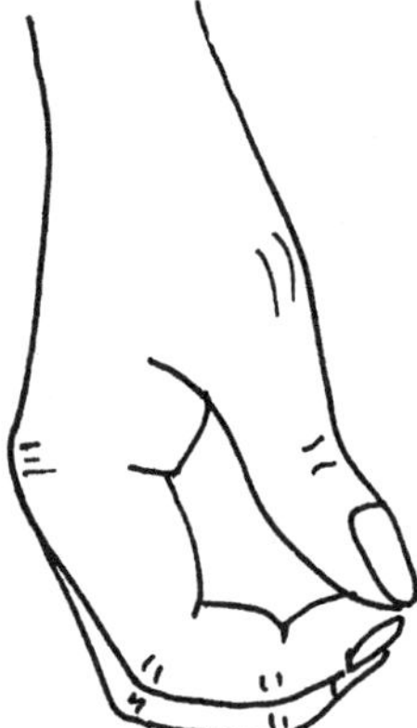

FIGURE 2.—Isolated palsy of flexor pollicis longus. (Courtesy of Seror P: Anterior interosseous nerve lesions: Clinical and electrophysiologic features. *J Bone Joint Surg [Br]* 78B:238–241, 1996.)

flexor pollicis longus in 3 (Fig 2) and isolated palsy of the index finger in 4 (Fig 3). The condition was initially misdiagnosed as tendon rupture in 3 patients. Of the rest, only 3 initially had a correct clinical diagnosis of an AIN lesion.

Findings.—Five of the AIN lesions proved to be of mechanical origin, and 7 were caused by "neuritis." Electrophysiologic abnormalities, mainly of the pronator quadratus, were present in all cases. The mean compound motor action potential of the pronator quadratus was 1.1 mV compared with a normal value of 7 to 24 mV. The main trunk of the median nerve was functioning normally in all cases. At least 7 patients had a spontaneous recovery. Surgical release was performed in 1 patient, producing a partial recovery.

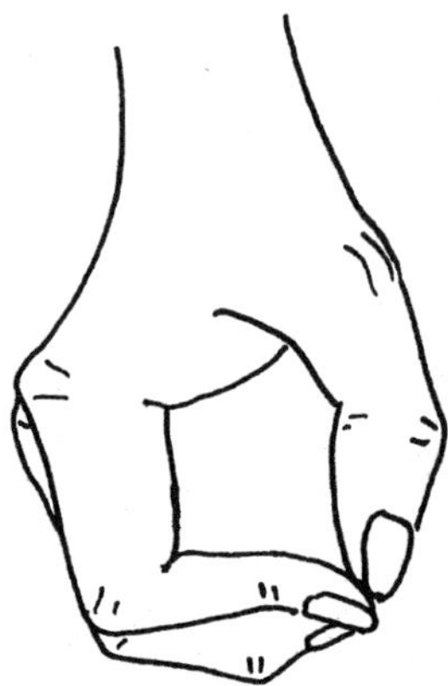

FIGURE 3.—Isolated palsy of flexor profundus of the index finger. (Courtesy of Seror P: Anterior interosseous nerve lesions: Clinical and electrophysiologic features. *J Bone Joint Surg [Br]* 78B:238–241, 1996.)

Conclusion.—Lesions of the AIN are rare but can result from either mechanical or inflammatory conditions. In about half of cases, the clinical findings resemble those of single tendon rupture. Electrodiagnostic testing, especially of the pronator quadratus, is needed to determine the site and severity of the lesion. Spontaneous late recovery is possible, so surgery should be delayed for at least 1 year in patients with nontraumatic AIN injuries.

▶ Seror presented a consecutive series of 13 patients with lesions of the anterior interosseous nerve and used this opportunity to review the subject.

R.H. Wilkins, M.D.

Operative Treatment of Meralgia Paresthetica: Transection Versus Neurolysis
van Eerten PV, Polder TW, Broere CAJ (Univ Hosp Nijmegen, The Netherlands)
Neurosurgery 37:63–65, 1995   35–3

Background.—The best operative technique for the treatment of meralgia paresthetica (MP) has not been definitively established. The outcomes of transection and neurolysis were compared in 1 series.
Methods.—Between 1974 and 1992, 21 patients with MP were treated surgically after conservative therapy failed. Patient ages at the time of surgery ranged from 21 to 71. Ten underwent neurolysis, and 11 underwent transection. The choice of procedure was random. Five neurosurgeons performed all the procedures. Mean follow-up was 74 months.
Outcomes.—Twelve patients achieved complete relief of their initial symptoms. Among those undergoing transection, 9 had complete relief and 2 had partial relief. There were no failures in this group. Among those undergoing neurolysis, 3 had complete relief and 3 had partial relief. Four treatment failures occurred in this group.
Conclusion.—A direct comparison of neurolysis and transection demonstrated that transection is superior in patients with MP. Surgery is indicated for such patients only when pain is severe and persistent despite adequate conservative treatment.

▶ Because meralgia paresthetica is infrequent, it would be difficult to set up a prospective study comparing the results of nerve transection and neurolysis (decompression), especially if the study is restricted to 1 institution and 1 surgeon. The authors did the next best thing: They conducted a retrospective review of cases treated at 1 institution by 5 surgeons, 4 of whom performed both types of operation studied. I would have predicted better results from neurolysis (providing that the nerve was decompressed well), but the opposite was so, probably because of patient preference for loss of sensation rather than alteration of sensation.

R.H. Wilkins, M.D.

Surgical Outcome for Intra- and Extrapelvic Femoral Nerve Lesions
Kim DH, Kline DG (Louisiana State Univ, New Orleans)
J Neurosurg 83:783–790, 1995   35–4

Introduction.—The femoral and sciatic nerve complexes are responsible for major functional innervation of the lower extremity. Because of a lack of data, it is very difficult to predict the surgical outcomes of femoral nerve lesions. The outcomes of 94 patients with such lesions were presented.

Patients.—Ninety-four patients with femoral nerve lesions were treated at 1 university medical center over a 20-year period. Seventy-eight of these patients had traumatic neuropathies, and 54 underwent surgery for the indications of persistent complete functional loss or pain. The femoral nerve was most commonly injured iatrogenically in such operations as inguinal herniorrhaphy, total hip replacement, and intra-abdominal vascular or gynecologic operations. Other, less common operations included appendectomy, lumbar sympathectomy, and laparoscopic surgery. Noniatrogenic causes included gunshot and stab wounds, nerve laceration by glass, and stretch or contusive injuries in patients with pelvic fractures. The remaining 16 patients had tumors involving the femoral nerve: 8 had neurofibromas, 4 had schwannomas, 1 had a neurogenic sarcoma, 2 had ganglion cysts, and 1 had a leiomyosarcoma.

Treatment and Outcomes.—Surgery was successful in most of the patients with tumors. Of the 78 patients with traumatic neuropathies, 45 had no evidence of clinical or electrical recovery. These patients underwent exploration and evaluation by intraoperative nerve stimulation and recording of nerve action potentials (NAPs), as did some patients with partial injuries. Thirteen patients with complete loss of nerve function preoperative had recordable NAPs and underwent neurolysis. All 13 had recovery of function to at least grade 3. Sural graft repairs, with grafts measuring 1.5 to 14.0 cm, were performed in 27 patients. By 2 years postoperatively, most of these patients had some degree of nerve regeneration and had regained grade 3 or 4 function. Of 5 patients with suture repair, 4 recovered grade 3 or better function.

Conclusion.—A large series of patients with femoral nerve lesions is reviewed. Good functional results can be obtained even in severe and proximal injuries that require lengthy graft repairs. Most injuries are iatrogenic. Early assessment of the severity of injury will help in deciding whether to perform surgical exploration. Even in patients with complete clinical deficits, direct intraoperative recording of NAPs is needed to provide objective evidence for or against axonal regeneration.

▶ This is a worthwhile review of 1 aspect of the large experience of Dr. Kline with various disorders of peripheral nerves managed by a neurosurgeon.

R.H. Wilkins, M.D.

Peripheral Nerve Biopsies

Anthony DC, Crain BJ (Harvard Med School, Boston; Children's Hosp, Boston)
Arch Pathol Lab Med 120:26–34, 1996

35–5

Introduction.—Nerve biopsy specimens are often referred to specialized laboratories for evaluation, but the ability of these laboratories to evaluate a specimen may be affected by the initial handling procedures. In response to a needs assessment conducted by the College of American Pathologists, detailed guidelines and procedures for handling peripheral nerve biopsies were offered.

Clinical Classification and Symptoms Categories.—Processing by the reference laboratory is aided by a knowledge of the rationale for the biopsy and the duration and progression of symptoms. Four types of onset have been described: acute, subacute, chronic progressive, and chronic relapsing (Table). Information on the distribution of involvement can help to limit the differential diagnosis, as does a determination of predominant type of involvement: motor, sensory, or autonomic. Processing of the biopsy specimen should take into account 5 broad categories of clinical manifestation: acute ascending neuropathy, subacute sensorimotor neuropathy, chronic peripheral neuropathies, hereditary peripheral neuropathies, and mononeuropathy or multiple mononeuropathies.

Biopsy Process.—Before the biopsy, the clinical differential diagnosis, goal of the biopsy, and planned site for obtaining the specimen should be discussed. The sural nerve is generally the most informative site for quantitative assessment, and the biopsy should secure a straight specimen without creating distortion artifacts. Care must be taken to avoid applying pressure or traction to the nerve. Specimens are transported as soon as possible after biopsy. It is important to retain a length of the nerve as a straight linear segment (Fig 1). Freezing provides the options of performing immunofluorescence, special stains, or biochemical or genetic studies. The

TABLE.—Evaluation of a Peripheral Nerve Biopsy Specimen

Clinical Diagnosis	Paraffin Embedding	Resin Embedding	Frozen Section	Teased Fiber	EM
Normal nerve (eg, vagotomy)	+	−	−	−	−
Nerve tumor	+	±	−	−	±
Acute ascending neuropathy	±	+	±	+	±
Subacute symmetric neuropathy	+	+	±	±	−
Subacute asymmetric neuropathy	+	+	±	±	±
Chronic progressive neuropathy	+	+	±	+	±
Chronic relapsing neuropathy	+	+	±	+	±
Hereditary neuropathy, adult	±	+	±	±	±
Hereditary neuropathy, childhood	±	+	+	±	+
Mononeuropathy or multineuropathy	+	+	±	+	±

Note: Plus sign indicates it is used routinely for diagnostic evaluation; *minus sign* indicates it is not generally necessary for diagnosis; *plus or minus sign* indicates it may be necessary for diagnosis in some cases.

Abbreviation: EM, electron microscopy.

(Courtesy of Anthony DC, Crain BJ: Peripheral nerve biopsies. *Arch Pathol Lab Med* 120:26–34, 1996.)

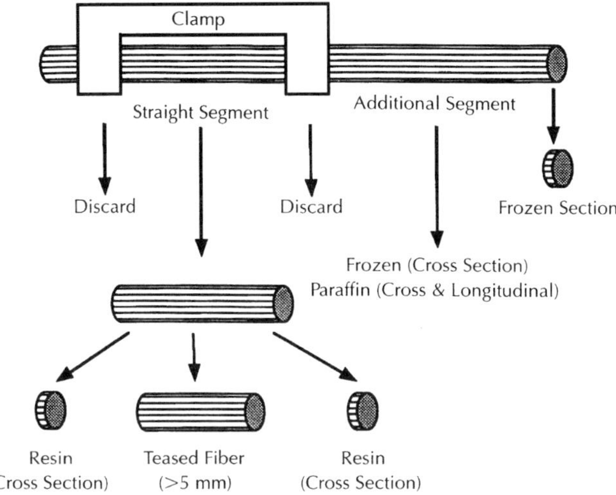

FIGURE 1.—Dividing a nerve biopsy specimen. The portion of the nerve specimen that is fixed as a straight segment is used for resin embedding and teased fiber analysis. Additional segments can be used for intraoperative frozen section, retention of a frozen specimen for possible biochemical analyses, and paraffin embedding. (Courtesy of Anthony DC, Crain BJ: Peripheral nerve biopsies. *Arch Pathol Lab Med* 120:26–34, 1996.)

most difficult procedural issue is handling the glutaraldehyde-fixed tissue once a straight segment has been fixed. Fixed specimens should be sent separately from frozen sections to avoid freezing artifact in the fixed specimen.

Processing a Peripheral Nerve Biopsy Specimen.—Different types of information are provided by the 5 commonly used methods to evaluate the biopsy specimens: resin (plastic) embedding, routine hematoxylin and eosin staining, frozen sections, teased fiber analysis, and electron microscopy. The specific uses of each type are discussed. It is important to recognize the various artifacts of preparation that may appear at magnification.

Interpretation of Peripheral Nerve Biopsy Specimen.—Axonal degeneration and axonal regeneration are the most common pathologic findings, often occurring in combination. The second most common pathologic process is demyelination. Axonal regeneration and remyelination can often be distinguished by the teased fiber preparation; axonal degeneration is identified in resin-embedded sections.

▶ Anthony and Crain prepared an excellent current review of the procedure of peripheral nerve biopsy, with emphasis on the pathologic aspects.

R.H. Wilkins, M.D.

36 Autonomic Dysfunction

Percutaneous Radiofrequency Upper Thoracic Sympathectomy
Wilkinson HA (Univ of Massachusetts, Worcester)
Neurosurgery 38:715–725, 1996   36–1

Purpose.—Since its initial description in 1984, the technique of percutaneous radiofrequency upper thoracic sympathectomy has evolved in some important ways. In the phase I procedure, lesions were made until sympatholysis was achieved. Subsequently phase II focused on efforts to precisely place a smaller number of lesions, based on anatomical findings. Most recently, in phase III, at least 3 lesions are made rostrocaudally in each ganglion in an attempt to destroy the entire fusiform ganglion. Fifteen years of experience with percutaneous radiofrequency upper thoracic sympathectomy was reviewed and analyzed.

Methods.—The experience included 148 unilateral or bilateral sympathectomies in 247 limbs of 110 patients using the phase I to III percutaneous radiofrequency technique. Most of the procedures were performed on an outpatient basis. The patients were 65 females and 45 males ranging in age from 10 to 81. Surgical sympathectomy had failed in 4 patients. The indications for sympathectomy included hyperhidrosis, vascular occlusion, chronic vasculopathies such as Raynaud's disease, painful causalgia or reflex sympathetic dystrophy, or Prinzmetal's angina. All procedural modifications were made on the basis of anatomic, clinical, and radiographic correlations and patient follow-up.

Technique.—The phase III technique uses neuroleptanalgesia with only superficial local anesthesia. General anesthesia, intubation, and lung collapse are not needed. The ganglion lesions are created using 2 18-gauge radiofrequency TIC needle electrodes. C-arm fluoroscopy and electrical stimulation, which produces a sensory awareness threshold of greater than 1.0 V, are used to target the lesion sites. Bilateral finger plethysmography and hand skin temperature monitoring are used to assess the immediate effectiveness of the lesions.

Results.—The rate of treatment failure or major recurrence was 25% overall; however, the phase III procedure decreased the frequency of early and late treatment failures. In patients treated with this procedure, sympathetic activity was completely or largely interrupted in 96% of limbs at 2 years and 91% of limbs at 3 years. Success rates were 83% at 2 years and 72% at 3 years with the phase I procedure and 77% at 2 years and 71% at 3 years with the phase II procedure. There were 6 cases of symptomatic pneumothorax, but this was the only serious complication. Repeat operations were easily and effectively performed, when necessary.

Conclusion.—Percutaneous radiofrequency sympathectomy is a safe, effective, and relatively simple technique. There are few severe recurrences with the most recent modification of the procedure. Percutaneous radiofrequency sympathectomy can be performed using supplemented local anesthesia, permits immediate assessment of the results, and can be easily repeated if needed or desired.

▶ Dr. Wilkinson began performing percutaneous radiofrequency upper thoracic sympathectomy in 1979 and has developed this procedure in 3 phases. With his phase III technique (used since 1988), he documented that the sympathetic activity continues to be completely or largely interrupted in 96% of operated limbs after 2 years and in 91% after 3 years. The risks of this procedure are low, and in Dr. Wilkinson's hands it compares quite favorably with open or endoscopic upper thoracic sympathectomy.

R.H. Wilkins, M.D.

Cardiopulmonary Exercise Testing Following Bilateral Thoracoscopic Sympathicolysis in Patients With Essential Hyperhidrosis
Noppen M, Herregodts P, Dendale P, et al (Univ of Brussels, Belgium)
Thorax 50:1097–1100, 1995　　　　　　　　　　　　　　　　　　　36–2

Background.—Essential hyperhidrosis is ascribed to overactivity of the sympathetic nerve fibers passing through the dorsal sympathetic ganglia D2 and D3. Interrupting the sympathetic chain thoracoscopically has proved to be an effective and safe treatment when lesser measures fail, but the D2 and D3 ganglia are directly in the path of cardiac sympathetic innervation. Many patients are unable to exercise maximally after excision of these ganglia by the supraclavicular approach.

Objective and Methods.—The effect of thoracoscopic sympathicolysis on the cardiopulmonary response to exercise was studied in 22 women and 4 men (average age 27) with severe, treatment-resistant essential hyperhidrosis. Studies were repeated 1 month after bilateral lysis of the D2 and D3 ganglia. Fourteen healthy participants also underwent cycle ergometer exercise testing.

Results.—Palmar hyperhidrosis was relieved in all patients. The patients had higher peak exercise heart rates than control participants before surgery, although the difference was not significant. After sympathicolysis the resting and peak heart rates decreased significantly, and the oxygen pulse increased. There were no significant differences from healthy participants.

Conclusion.—In contrast to open surgical sympathectomy, there is no substantial impairment of exercise capacity after thoracoscopic lysis of the dorsal sympathetic ganglia.

▶ As a result of their study, Noppen et al. concluded that "D2–D3 thorascopic sympathicolysis causes a small and asymptomatic reduction in maximal and resting heart rate and is not associated with a decrease in exercise capacity, in contrast with the detrimental effects on exercise capacity of open surgical sympathectomy." They postulated that this difference relates to the facts that thoracoscopic sympathicolysis is a more precise and accurate way of interrupting the sympathetic chain and that the procedure has less effect on lung volumes and airflow rates than open surgery.

R.H. Wilkins, M.D.

37 Functional Neurosurgery

The Results, Indications, and Physiology of Posteroventral Pallidotomy for Patients With Parkinson's Disease
Iacono RP, Shima F, Lonser RR, et al (Loma Linda Univ, Calif; Kyushu Univ, Fukuoka, Japan)
Neurosurgery 36:1118–1127, 1995   37–1

Background.—Stereotactic surgery for Parkinson's disease was once indicated only in patients with active motor manifestations refractory to drug treatment. The refinement of Leskell's posteroventral pallidotomy has enabled surgical treatment of both akinetic and hyperkinetic symptoms. The outcomes of 126 patients undergoing posteroventral pallidotomy were reviewed.

Methods.—Fifty-eight of the patients had a unilateral procedure and 68, bilateral. Two scales were used to objectively assess symptoms before and after surgery. Postoperative assessments were performed at 1 week and periodically between 1 and 12 months.

Findings.—Individual motor subscores on the Unified Parkinson's Disease Rating Scale were significantly decreased. The most dramatic outcomes, however, were akinetic symptom reversal and the elimination of dyskinesia and profound "off" periods. Complications occurred in 6.3% of the patients and included permanent (2 patients) and transient (1 patient) partial pericentral hemianopsia, and transient hemiparesis unassociated with hemorrhage.

Conclusion.—Pallidotomy substantially improves akinesia, off states, gait freezing, appendicular bradykinesia, dyskinesia, dystonia, tremor, and rigidity. Postural instability is also improved but to a lesser extent. Posteroventral pallidotomy is a valuable addition to treatment methods for Parkinson's disease that is resistant to medical therapy.

Ventroposterior Medial Pallidotomy in Patients With Advanced Parkinson's Disease

Sutton JP, Couldwell W, Lew MF, et al (Univ of Southern California, Los Angeles)
Neurosurgery 36:1112–1117, 1995   37–2

Background.—Ventroposterior medial pallidotomy appears to be beneficial in treating moderately severe Parkinson's disease. The effects of this surgery in patients with advanced, medically refractory Parkinson's disease were investigated in a pilot study.

Methods.—The 5 patients selected for the procedure had advanced Parkinson's disease with disabling symptoms. Mean patient age was 67 and mean duration of disease was 11.6 years. The average Hoehn and Yahr stage when "off" was 3.9. Previous medical treatment had been ineffective in all patients. Motor fluctuations were severe in most patients, with peak-dose dyskinesias or dystonia. Unilateral pallidotomies were done in 3 patients, 2 of whom underwent another pallidotomy after 8 weeks. In the remaining 2 patients, staged bilateral pallidotomies were done.

Findings.—Overall function did not significantly change after the first operation. Contralateral peak-dose dyskinesias and dystonia were markedly reduced in all 3 patients with these symptoms. After unilateral ventroposterior medial pallidotomy, pre-existing depression worsened in 2 patients, new visual field defects were detected in 2, gait freezing was increased in 1, speech worsened in 1, swallowing possibly worsened in 1, and transient facial weakness occurred in 2.

Conclusion.—In selected patients with Parkinson's disease, ventroposterolateral pallidotomy can decrease or eliminate contralateral peak-dose dyskinesia or dystonia. At least 1 patient had a dramatic improvement in the Hoehn and Yahr score. However, outcomes varied among patients, and some were adversely affected. Functional improvement was nonsignificant.

▶ These reports (Abstracts 37–1 and 37–2) added to the growing body of information about the benefits and limitations of pallidotomy for patients with Parkinson's disease.

R.H. Wilkins, M.D.

Stereotactic Ventral Pallidotomy for Parkinson's Disease

Dogali M, Fazzini E, Kolodny E, et al (New York Univ; North Shore Univ Hosp, Manhasset, NY; Cornell Univ, Manhasset, NY)
Neurology 45:753–761, 1995   37–3

Background.—Treatment for Parkinson's disease (PD) using dopaminergic agents is effective for several years but is often followed by deterioration, which can be accompanied by levodopa-induced dyskinesias and unpredictable clinical responses. Several surgical procedures have been advocated to alleviate the symptoms of PD, many of which have focused on destruction of parts of the globus pallidus. However, accurate localization of surgically placed lesions in this structure has been difficult. A state of the art, image-directed stereotactic method was used to destroy the ventral medial globus pallidus in patients with medically intractable PD.

Methods.—The study included 25 patients with PD responsive to levodopa. All had bradykinesia and rigidity-predominant PD with response fluctuations including "off" parkinsonism and "on" chorea-kinetic dystonia. Of these, 18 formed the surgical group, and 7 formed the nonsurgical group, who wanted surgery but preferred to wait until long-term results from other patients were available. All patients underwent neurologic, visual field, and radiologic investigation, including MRI. Neurologic testing was conducted at baseline, within 1 week of surgery, and every 3 months thereafter for 1 year. Nonsurgical patients were examined on a comparable schedule. Patients' movements were recorded on videotape and blindly rated by 2 investigators. Surgery was performed with patients under local anesthesia; and a stereotactic frame centered in the MRI or CT scanner was used; after the first 10 patients, only the MR scanner was used. Multiple overlapping lesions were made at the target site. Comparisons in function were made between surgical subjects and age-, disease-, and antiparkinsonian medication–matched nonsurgical controls.

Results.—No perioperative morbidity or mortality occurred, and all surgical patients had improved rigidity and contralateral finger dexterity and arm-hand movement between 2 points after surgery. A significant decrease (65%) in Unified Parkinson's Disease Rating Scale scores, as well as Activities of Daily Living scores, was seen in the surgical patients when medication was withdrawn for 12 hours 1 week after surgery and during follow-up. The Core Assessment Program for Intracerebral Transplantation scores also improved significantly for the contralateral (38.2%) and ipsilateral (24.2%) limb. Walk scores also improved by 45%. One year after surgery, 8 patients used an increased dosage of levodopa or dopamine agonist, and 8 patients decreased or eliminated such drugs. One patient continued on the same dosage. Tolerance by surgical patients of larger drug doses resulted from reduced dyskinesia.

Discussion.—Signs and symptoms of PD improved significantly after pallidotomy, and patients reported improvements in overall functioning when in their "best on" status. This improvement continued throughout the course of the study.

▶ There has been a resurgence of interest in pallidotomy, especially as a method of treating patients with Parkinson's disease who develop deterioration of function after years of dopaminergic therapy. Dogali et al documented what can be achieved by such an approach.

R.H. Wilkins, M.D.

Neuropathological Evidence of Graft Survival and Striatal Reinnervation After the Transplantation of Fetal Mesencephalic Tissue in a Patient With Parkinson's Disease

Kordower JH, Freeman TB, Snow BJ, et al (Rush-Presbyterian-St Luke's Med Ctr, Chicago; Univ of South Florida, Tampa; Univ of British Columbia, Vancouver; et al)

N Engl J Med 332:1118–1124, 1995   37–4

Background.—Clinical trials are in progress to determine whether grafts of fetal nigral neurons, implanted in patients with Parkinson's disease, will survive, produce dopamine, and improve motor function. Positron emission tomography using fluorodopa have been done to assess graft viability, but it does not distinguish between sprouting host dopaminergic neurons and those that are grafted. There is no direct evidence that these grafts are able to innervate the striatum.

Objective.—It was possible to examine the brain of a parkinsonian patient who had considerable improvement, as well as increased fluorodopa uptake, after receiving bilateral grafts of fetal ventral mesencephalic tissue and who died 18 months later of pulmonary embolism.

Case Report.—Man, 59, had had Parkinson's disease for 8 years. Carbidopa-levodopa therapy initially led to considerable improvement, but later the patient had fluctuating motor function, dyskinesia, and dystonia during "on" periods, as well as a progressively worsening gait and bradykinesia. He had had to stop working and was unresponsive to higher doses of medication, continuous-release treatment, and added selegiline or dopamine agonists.

Nigral tissue from 7 embryos was placed in the postcommissural putamen using a stereotactic needle. Cyclosporine was given starting 3 weeks before initial implantation and was continued for 8 weeks after a second procedure. The patient became able to perform all daily activities independently and to exercise actively. Motor problems during "on" periods were virtually eliminated. Objective disease scores were improved 15 months postoperatively. Fluorodopa uptake in the putamen increased. The patient died of massive pulmonary embolism 18 months after the implant procedure, when recovering from ankle fusion.

Extensive loss of neurons was evident in the midbrain, and there were extracellular deposits of neuromelanin. Large viable transplants were seen bilaterally at all transplant sites within the putamen. Many implants were larger than at the time of transplantation. All graft sites contained clusters of tyrosine hydroxylase-immunoreactive neurons. Dopaminergic neurons were found along the periphery of the transplants, which were well integrated within the host striatum. Dopaminergic processes crossed the graft-host interface to innervate the parkinsonian striatum.

Conclusion.—The clinical improvement in this parkinsonian patient was associated with reinnervation of the putamen by viable dopaminergic neurons of embryonic origin.

▶ This is an important case report. As the authors pointed out, there have been few pathologic studies after the transplantation of fetal nigral tissue, and long-term survival of grafted nigral neurons had not been demonstrated before this case. In the present case, the implants not only survived but also enlarged, and the dopaminergic neurons innervated the patient's striatum.

R.H. Wilkins, M.D.

38 Miscellaneous Topics

A Proposed Model of Cerebrospinal Fluid Circulation: Observations With Radionuclide Cisternography
Greitz D, Hannerz J (Karolinska Hosp, Stockholm)
AJNR 17:431–438, 1996   38–1

Background.—Currently CSF circulation is believed to demonstrate a 2-directional flow in the spinal canal, with active cranially directed circulation in the anterior compartment and downwardly directed bulk flow in the posterior compartment. These concepts were based on radionuclide cisternography (RC) findings. The ability to detect bulk flows in subarachnoid spaces with radionuclide scanning was investigated. A flow phantom representing the subarachnoid spaces was used to clarify the scanning findings.

Methods.—The CSF circulation was investigated with RC in 10 women with venous vasculitis and high intracranial pressure. Radionuclide cisternography scanning was performed 15 and 30 minutes and 1, 1.5, 3, 6, and 24 hours after injection of radionuclide and contrast material. Computed tomography scans were also obtained at 0.5, 3, and 6 hours after injection, and RC tomography was performed 6 hours after injection. A model of CSF circulation was constructed with a flow phantom containing water and blue dye with a higher specific weight. The upward distribution of blue dye after injection into the lower part of the U-shaped tube was evaluated with a pulsatile flow with and without an additional tube representing the spinal cord. Second, water was added to pulsating blue dye to study inflow and outflow into the tube.

Results.—Of the 10 patients, 9 demonstrated normal CSF circulation, with a well-defined convexity maximum and no filling in the lateral ventricles. The tracer was maximally concentrated at the site of injection in the lumbar region without moving toward the convexity. The tracer injected in the conus region quickly reached the foramen magnum, within 15 minutes but took 3 to 6 hours to reach the sacral end of the thecal sac. Cranial distribution appeared normal. Lumbar injection resulted in longer delays, requiring 5 to 7 hours to reach the convexity. All patients demonstrated reduced activity in the basal cistern, cisterna magna, cervical, and thoracic areas after 24 hours, with remaining activity occurring primarily in brain tissue and the spinal cord, not in the subarachnoid spaces. However, activity in the lumbosacral area remained high after 24 hours.

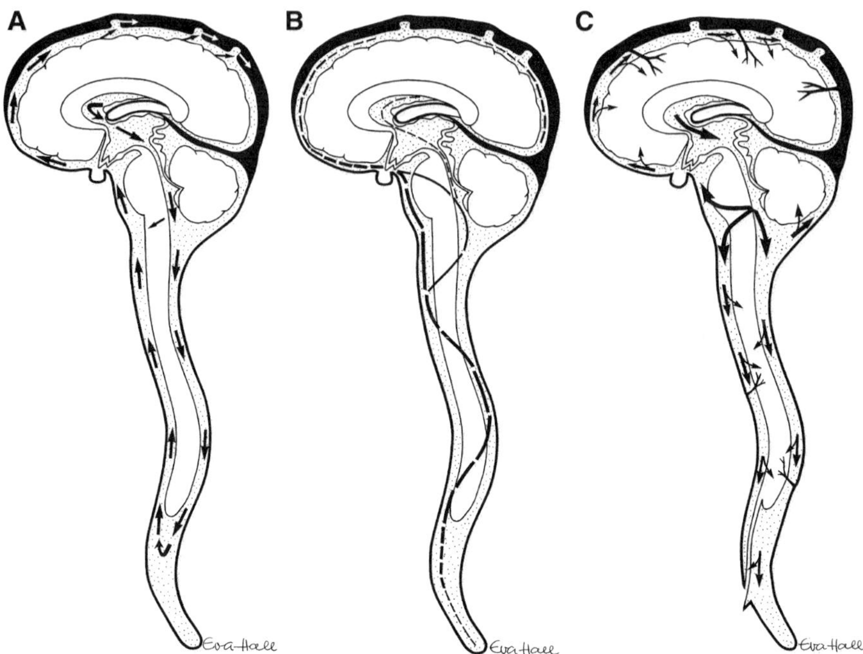

FIGURE 5.—Diagram showing the commonly accepted bulk flow model (**A**) and the 2 types of CSF circulation related to the proposed concept of the circulation (**B** and **C**). The dominant pulsatile flow shown in **B** is responsible for the rapid spread of tracers within the extraventricular CSF spaces, and the comparatively small, almost minute, bulk flow (**C**) explains the appearance of the cisternogram in normal cases causing washout of tracer in the ventricular system and the basal cisterns. **B**, there is a dominant pulsatile flow with a fast-velocity compartment in the brain stem–cord area and slow velocities at the upper and lower ends of the subarachnoid spaces. The amplitude and velocity are indicated by the length of the segments of the *dashed line*. The systolic and diastolic flows in the spinal canal follow 1 main channel, which is located toward the convexities showing a meandering S-shaped route caused by centrifugal forces and lower resistance in wider subarachnoid spaces. **C**, the minute bulk flows are exaggerated for clearer illustration. The thickness of the *arrows* is related to the magnitude of the bulk flow, which decreases in both directions from the foramen magnum. The CSF is resorbed everywhere in the CNS by the circulating blood. The spinal nerves, including the cauda equina, are represented solely by 1 caudal root in this schematic drawing. (Courtesy of Greitz D, Hannerz J: A proposed model of cerebrospinal fluid circulation: Observations with radionuclide cisternography. *AJNR* 17:431–438, 1996; Copyright by American Society of Neuroradiology.)

Upward distribution of the tracer dye in the flow phantom model moved 5 cm in 17 hours with simple diffusion, 50 cm in 17 hours with pulsations, and 80 cm in 30 minutes with pulsations and a cord tube. With inflow at the foramen magnum and outflow at the convexity, washout occurred at the convexity without creating a convexity maximum, although a lumbar maximum did occur after the convexity washout. With both inflow and outflow of water at the foramen magnum, a maximum occurred at both the lumbar region and the convexity.

Conclusion.—The findings of convexity maximum and the lumbosacral area and local dilution of tracer at the foramen magnum conflict with the concept of the pacchionian granulations as the main pathway of CSF outflow. Cerebrospinal fluid may possibly be resorbed into the capillary bloodflow through the extracellular spaces of the brain (Fig 5).

▶ Greitz and Hannerz raised the interesting possibility that the presently accepted concepts of CSF circulation and absorption are erroneous. It will be interesting to see if any additional support for their alternative hypotheses is forthcoming.

R.H. Wilkins, M.D.

Long-Term Results of Peripheral Nerve Stimulation for Reflex Sympathetic Dystrophy
Hassenbusch SJ, Stanton-Hicks M, Schoppa D, et al (MD Anderson Cancer Ctr, Houston; Cleveland Clinic Found, Ohio)
J Neurosurg 84:415–423, 1996   38–2

Background.—Reflex sympathetic dystrophy (RSD) is typically managed successfully with medication, blocks, or infusions. However, peripheral nerve stimulation (PNS) is a treatment strategy that has been used with some success in patients with severe RSD. Its efficacy in patients with severe RSD with symptoms related to the distribution of just 1 major peripheral nerve was assessed prospectively.

Methods.—A 2-day trial of PNS was offered to patients with pain related to PNS entirely or mainly in the distribution of 1 major peripheral nerve that was refractory to other conservative RSD treatments. A permanent implanted generator connected to the electrode was programmed in patients experiencing at least 50% reductions in pain and objective improvements in the physical examination categories of vasomotor tone, trophic changes, and somatic motor changes. The patients were seen for follow-up assessments at intervals of 2 to 6 weeks. Results were considered good if pain was reduced by at least 50% and there were improvements in at least 2 physical categories and fair if pain was reduced by at least 50% and there was improvement in none or 1 physical category or if pain was reduced by 25% to 49% and there was improvement in at least 1 physical category.

Results.—Thirty-two patients underwent the 2-day trial, and the permanent generator was placed in 30 patients. Of these 30 patients, PNS was successful in 19 (63%), with 10 having consistently good results and 9 having fair relief, with a follow-up of more than 2 years. In the patients with successful treatment, the mean pain score was reduced from 8.3 to 3.5. Vasomotor tone was markedly improved, but less significant improvements were seen in motor weakness and trophic changes. Activity levels increased substantially, with improvements in working ability, as well as sleeping, motor strength, and driving. Treatment failures occurred at a mean of 1.3 years after treatment began, with a reversal of pain relief and no significant improvements in the physical categories or activity levels.

Complications included the need for electrode implantation revision in 8 patients (27%), with generators detaching from the anchoring sutures in 2 patients and cosmetic revisions in 2.

Conclusion.—Peripheral nerve stimulation can be effective in the treatment of RSD localized in the distribution of just 1 major peripheral nerve that is refractory to conservative management. A comparative study is needed to determine the relative efficacy of PNS and spinal cord stimulation in these patients.

▶ The authors reported the results of PNS for severe RSD or complex regional pain syndrome in 30 patients, 19 of whom experienced good or fair long-term relief.

R.H. Wilkins, M.D.

Subject Index*

A

Abdominal
   migraine, prevalence and clinical
      features of, 97: 109
Abscess
   brain
      otitis media and, suppurative,
         95: 175
      polymicrobial, hereditary
         hemorrhagic telangiectasia
         presenting with, 96: 342
      spinal epidural, bacterial, review of,
         95: 497
      subperiosteal, and suppurative otitis
         media, 95: 175
Abuse
   child, causing retinal hemorrhage,
      95: 435
   cocaine, long-term, cerebral perfusion
      and neuropsychological
      consequences of, 95: 190
   solvent
      chronic, causing white matter
         changes, 97: 207
      vapor, causing leukoencephalopathy,
         comparison to
         adrenoleukodystrophy, 96: 153
Academic
   performance in children with
      neurofibromatosis type 1, 97: 186
Accessory
   nerve neurotization in infants with
      brachial plexus birth palsy, 96: 426
Accidents
   head injury and retinal hemorrhage due
      to, 95: 435
   motor vehicle, and Alzheimer's disease,
      95: 66
Acetazolamide
   in vestibulopathy, familial, 95: 275
Acetylcholine
   receptor channel openings, prolonged,
      due to mutation in M2 domain of e
      subunit causing congenital
      myasthenic syndrome, 96: 69
Acetylcholinesterase
   staining for sensory/motor-differentiated
      nerve repair in hand, 95: 526
Acetylsalicylic acid (*see* Aspirin)
Acidosis
   lactic
      in MELAS (*see* MELAS)

pyruvate dehydrogenase deficiency
   and, 96: 116
Aciduria
   glutaric, type I, dystonia and dyskinesia
      in, 96: 112
Acoustic
   neurinoma (*see* Neuroma, acoustic)
   neuroma (*see* Neuroma, acoustic)
   schwannoma, cystic, MRI of, 95: 339
Acquired immunodeficiency syndrome (*see*
   AIDS)
Acromegaly
   pituitary adenoma in, GH-secreting
      adenomectomy for, transsphenoidal,
         95: 334
      surgical results, 95: 331
   recent advances in pathogenesis,
      diagnosis, and management of,
         97: 337
   sleep apnea in
      effect of octreotide on, 96: 221
      perioperative management and
         surgical outcome, 96: 281
ACTH (*see* Adrenocorticotropic,
   hormone)
Actinomycin-D
   in astrocytoma,
      hypothalamic/chiasmatic, after
      conservative surgery, long-term
      outcome, in children, 97: 352
Activity
   ordinary, for acute low back pain,
      96: 213
Acupuncture
   needles, sensory and electric stimulation
      through, effect on postural control
      after stroke, 96: 24
   in stroke patients, 95: 255
Acyclovir
   in meningitis, benign recurrent
      lymphocytic, due to herpes simplex
      virus infection, 96: 160
Acyl–coenzyme A
   dehydrogenase deficiency,
      medium-chain, clinical course of,
         96: 113
Adenocarcinoma
   salivary gland, invading skull base,
      charged particle irradiation of,
         96: 276
Adenoma
   pituitary

Author Index